# Smart Nanomaterials Technology



**Series Editors**

Azamal Husen, Department of Biotechnology, Smt. S. S. Patel Nootan Science & Commerce College, Sankalchand Patel University, Gujarat, Ethiopia

Mohammad Jawaid, Chemical and Petroleum Engineering, United Arab Emirates University, Al Ain, United Arab Emirates

Nanotechnology is a rapidly growing scientific field and has attracted a great interest over the last few years because of its abundant applications in different fields like biology, physics and chemistry. This science deals with the production of minute particles called nanomaterials having dimensions between 1 and 100 nm which may serve as building blocks for various physical and biological systems. On the other hand, there is the class of smart materials where the material that can stimuli by external factors and results a new kind of functional properties. The combination of these two classes forms a new class of smart nanomaterials, which produces unique functional material properties and a great opportunity to larger span of application. Smart nanomaterials have been employed by researchers to use it effectively in agricultural production, soil improvement, disease management, energy and environment, medical science, pharmaceuticals, engineering, food, animal husbandry and forestry sectors.

This book series in Smart Nanomaterials Technology aims to comprehensively cover topics in the fabrication, synthesis and application of these materials for applications in the following fields:

- Energy Systems—Renewable energy, energy storage (supercapacitors and electrochemical cells), hydrogen storage, photocatalytic water splitting for hydrogen production
- Biomedical—controlled release of drugs, treatment of various diseases, biosensors,
- Agricultural—agricultural production, soil improvement, disease management, animal feed, egg, milk and meat production/processing,
- Forestry—wood preservation, protection, disease management
- Environment—wastewater treatment, separation of hazardous contaminants from wastewater, indoor air filters.

Dilfuza Jabborova · Deepranjan Sarkar · Rakesh S. ·
Rahul Datta · Sachidanand Singh
Editors

# Nanomaterials in Agroforestry Systems

Springer

*Editors*
Dilfuza Jabborova
Academy of Sciences of the Republic of Uzbekistan
Institute of Genetics and Plant Experimental Biology
Kibray, Uzbekistan

Rakesh S.
Resilient Farm and Food Systems
International Crops Research Institute for the Semi-Arid Tropics
Hyderabad, Telangana, India

Sachidanand Singh
Department of Biotechnology
School of Energy Technology
Pandit Deendayal Energy University
Gandhinagar, Gujarat, India

Deepranjan Sarkar
Department of Food Agriculture and Natural Resources
School of Environment Resources and Development
Asian Institute of Technology
Klong Luang, Pathum Thani
Thailand

Rahul Datta
Department of Geology and Pedology
Mendel University in Brno
Brno, Czech Republic

ISSN 3004-8273 ISSN 3004-8281 (electronic)
Smart Nanomaterials Technology
ISBN 978-981-96-1339-7 ISBN 978-981-96-1337-3 (eBook)
https://doi.org/10.1007/978-981-96-1337-3



This Springer imprint is published by the registered company Springer Nature Singapore Pte Ltd.
The registered company address is: 152 Beach Road, #21-01/04 Gateway East, Singapore 189721, Singapore

# Preface

Agroforestry is a good option to deal with a lot of challenges that we face related to food security, livelihoods, biodiversity, climate change, etc. The socio-ecological impacts of agroforestry packages even under degraded ecosystems are quite impressive. Exploring the nanoscale dimension for managing natural resources is common nowadays. Nanotechnology has a very high potential to improve the resource use efficiency of the agroforestry sector. The recent applications of nanomaterials in crops and trees have been highlighted in this book.

The book focuses on the green synthesis of nanoparticles, nutrient management, stress management, crop and tree production, risk assessment, etc. Land restoration is vital for sustainable food production systems. Agroforestry initiatives leading to carbon sequestration provide a decarbonization framework under changing climate scenarios. Furthermore, the applications of smart nanostructured materials improve the productivity of agroforestry systems in stressful environments like salinity and aridity. It is essential to study nanoparticle-tree interactions to harness benefits like nitrogen fixation and minimize the potential toxicity of nanoparticles. The targeted delivery approach for controlling insects, pathogens, and other pests in comparison to conventional agrochemicals attracts researchers to explore emerging nano-agrochemicals. Chapters on bioenergy production and nanopesticidal effects on honeybees reflect that modern technologies will not sustain in the long term if they do not address energy and biodiversity aspects. Biosafety and bioremediation knowledge help us to avoid indiscriminate use of nano-enabled products and track the released product or pollutant. To obtain reliable conclusions in nanoscience research, we have also included one chapter on statistical techniques.

An attempt was made to cover different nanoproducts and management practices applied in agroforestry systems. We appreciate each and every contributor for their superb work. This book will be useful for students, researchers, stakeholders, farmers, and policymakers working in nanotechnology and agroforestry practices. We welcome positive feedback and constructive criticism from the readers.

Kibray, Uzbekistan Dilfuza Jabborova
Klong Luang, Thailand Deepranjan Sarkar
Hyderabad, India Rakesh S.
Gandhinagar, India Sachidanand Singh
Brno, Czech Republic Rahul Datta

# Contents

# Editors and Contributors

## About the Editors

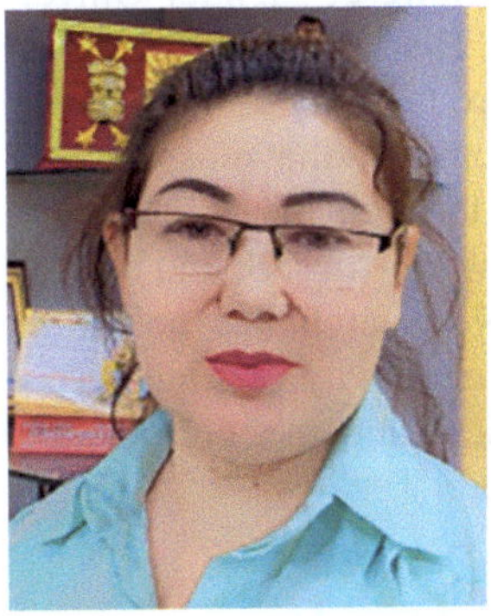

**Dr. Dilfuza Jabborova** is Head of Laboratory Medicinal Plants Genetics and Biotechnology, Institute of Genetics and Plant Experimental Biology, Academy of Sciences of the Republic of Uzbekistan. She is an expert in plant microbe interaction, crop physiology, soil biochemistry, microbial ecology and biological control of plant diseases. She is currently working on the use of microbial inoculants for biological control, plant growth promotion, and sustainable agriculture. She has published her research outputs in reputed international journals having high impact factor. She is listed in, top 2% of scientists of the world in the list released by Stanford University in collaboration with Elsevier.

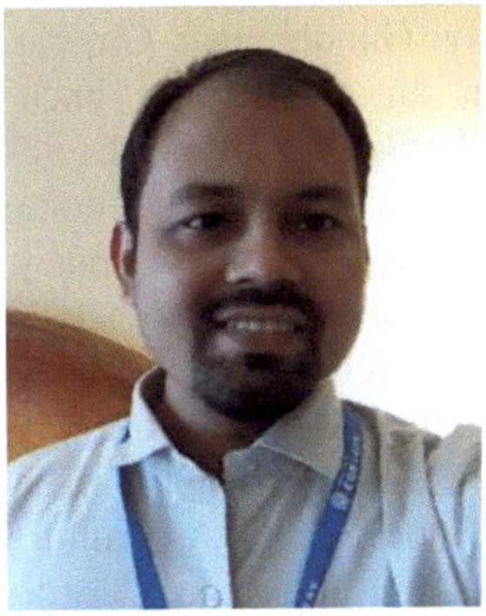

**Deepranjan Sarkar** is working as a Postdoctoral Research Fellow at the Department of Food, Agriculture and Natural Resources, School of Environment, Resources and Development, Asian Institute of Technology (AIT), Thailand. Before joining AIT, he served as an Assistant Professor (Soil Science) at the Integral University, Lucknow, India, and also as a Consultant at the International Rice Research Institute (IRRI), India. His research interests include Soil Fertility, Plant Nutrition, Regenerative Agriculture, Resource Use Efficiency, Rice–Wheat Systems, Microbial Interactions, Carbon Sequestration, Land Restoration, Climate Change, and UN-SDGs.

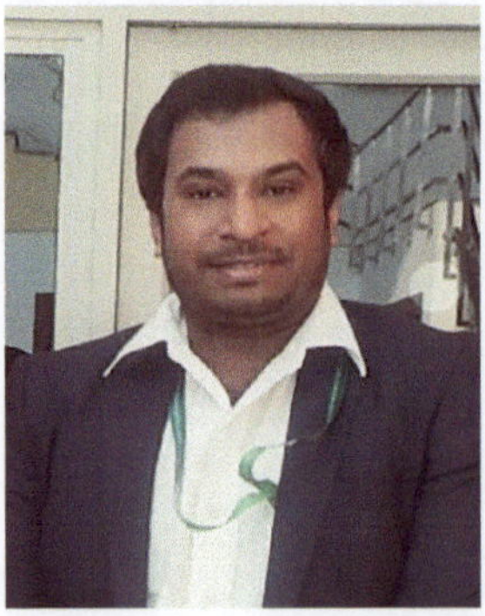

**Rakesh S.** is working as an Associate Scientist at the International Crops Research Institute for the Semi-Arid Tropics (ICRISAT), Hyderabad, India. Before joining ICRISAT, he served as a Research Associate at ICAR-National Academy of Agricultural Research Management (NAARM), Hyderabad, and also as a Senior Research Fellow in the Australian (ACIAR) funding Project "Sustainable and Resilient Farming System Intensification- SRFSI" at UBKV, West Bengal. His research interests include Carbon Sequestration; Carbon Dynamics; Conservation Agriculture; Nutrient Management; Crop Production; Soil Fertility; Environmental Sustainability; Integrated Nutrient Management, Land Restoration, and Climate Change Adaptation.

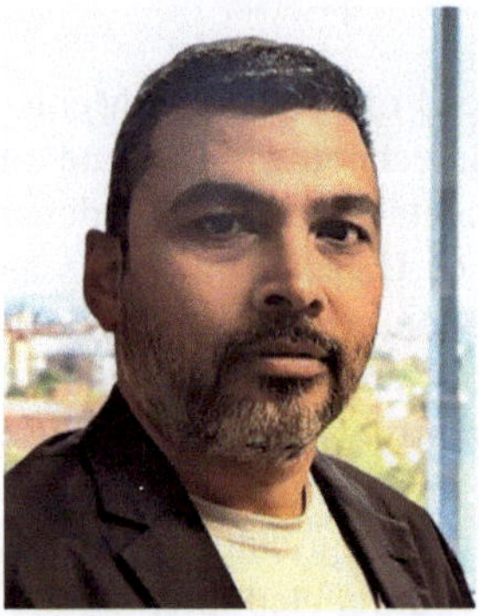

**Rahul Datta** is Assistant Professor in the field of Soil Science currently is working at Mendel University in Brno, Czech Republic. His research has focused largely on increasing crop productivity using "green" and sustainable methods. Some of the most notable problems he has addressed through his research are drought stress, heavy metal toxicity in soil, and climate change greenhouse gas. His research has helped in increasing the quality and productivity of staple crops like wheat maize, barley, rice, and other crops like mangoes, spinach, and cotton.

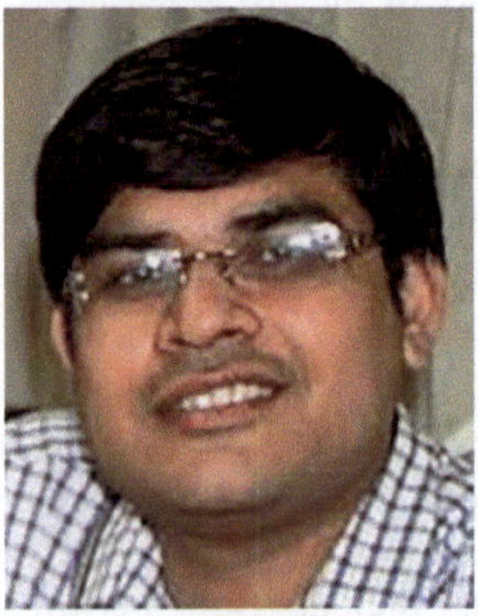

**Dr. Sachidanand Singh** presently working as an Associate Professor and Head in the Department of Biotechnology, School of Energy Technology, Pandit Deendayal Enenrgy University, Gandhinagar Gujarat. His education belongs from an engineering background i.e., B.Tech. in Biotechnology, M.Tech. Bioinformatics, PhD, and Postdoctoral experience come from Ohio State University, College of Pharmacy, USA. He has more than 14 years of experience in teaching, administration, and research. He has served as Professor and Head Internal Quality Assurance Cell and Dean of Allied Sciences at Sankalchand Patel University, Gujarat, Dean of Biotechnology and Agriculture Sciences, NAAC SSR Head, and Research Coordinator at Shri Ramswaroop Memorial University. Work experience includes Karunya University, Shri Ramswaroop Memorial University, Vignan University, and

Sankalchand Patel University. His research area includes Plant Biotechnology, metagenomics, Systems Biology, Network Biology, Micro RNA-based studies, Expression Data Analytics, Next-generation Sequencing, and Statistical Genetics. His present focus also includes understanding the Canonical and non-canonical pathways of miRNA Biogenesis, Dynamics, and mechanisms of miRNA-mediated Gene Regulation. He teaches different subjects, especially Genomics and Proteomics, Microarray and Image Analysis, Drug Design, and Molecular Modeling for graduate and postgraduate students. He has been involved in various assignments given by the University authority from time to time as an Online teaching platform, Research Initiatives, Biogas Plant, NAAC, NBA, and other council approvals. He has published more than 60 research and review articles in peer-reviewed journals, 9 Patents published among which 4 are granted. He has completed one SERB, Govt. of India-funded project, and two University research grant projects. He has received several awards in his area of research and for his teaching strategies. He has organized different conferences and workshops and received Govt. funds for the same. He has shared his area of expertise with different colleges and universities as an invited speaker at different conferences and workshops. He has guided 36 B.Tech. and 10 M.Tech. projects. He has awarded 3 PhD students under him in the field of Herbal products, drug Design, and integration with network biology. Dr. Sachidanand Singh, presently working as an Associate Professor and Head in the Department of Biotechnology, School of Energy Technology, Pandit Deendayal Enenrgy University, Gandhinagar Gujarat. His education belongs from an engineering background i.e., B.Tech. in Biotechnology, M.Tech. Bioinformatics, PhD, and Postdoctoral experience come from Ohio State University, College of Pharmacy, USA. He has more than 14 years of experience in teaching, administration, and research. He has served as Professor and Head Internal Quality Assurance Cell and Dean of Allied Sciences at Sankalchand Patel University, Gujarat, Dean of Biotechnology and Agriculture Sciences, NAAC SSR Head, and Research Coordinator at Shri Ramswaroop Memorial University. Work experience includes Karunya University, Shri Ramswaroop Memorial University, Vignan University, and

Sankalchand Patel University. His research area includes Plant Biotechnology, metagenomics, Systems Biology, Network Biology, Micro RNA-based studies, Expression Data Analytics, Next-generation Sequencing, and Statistical Genetics. His present focus also includes understanding the Canonical and non-canonical pathways of miRNA Biogenesis, Dynamics, and mechanisms of miRNA-mediated Gene Regulation. He teaches different subjects, especially Genomics and Proteomics, Microarray and Image Analysis, Drug Design, and Molecular Modeling for graduate and postgraduate students. He has been involved in various assignments given by the University authority from time to time as an Online teaching platform, Research Initiatives, Biogas Plant, NAAC, NBA, and other council approvals. He has published more than 60 research and review articles in peer-reviewed journals, 9 Patents published among which 4 are granted. He has completed one SERB, Govt. of India-funded project, and two University research grant projects. He has received several awards in his area of research and for his teaching strategies. He has organized different conferences and workshops and received Govt. funds for the same. He has shared his area of expertise with different colleges and universities as an invited speaker at different conferences and workshops. He has guided 36 B.Tech. and 10 M.Tech. projects. He has awarded 3 PhD students under him in the field of Herbal products, drug Design, and integration with network biology. He has already edited three Books under Springer and Taylor and Francis publishing group. He has a collaboration with Mendel University Czech Republic, Europe, Lund University, Sweden and Monash University Australia.

## Contributors

**Faheem Ahmad** Department of Botany, Aligarh Muslim University, Aligarh, India

**Mohammed Gulzar Ahmed** Department of Pharmaceutics, Yenepoya Pharmacy College and Research Centre, Yenepoya (Deemed to Be University), Mangaluru, Karnataka, India

**Ajith S.** International Maize and Wheat Improvement Centre (CIMMYT), Delhi, India;
Department of Agricultural Statistics, Uttar Banga Krishi Viswavidyalaya, Cooch Behar, West Bengal, India

**Laura Aliotta** Department of Civil and Industrial Engineering (DICI), University of Pisa, Pisa, Italy;
Research Unit DICI-UNIPI, National Interuniversity Consortium of Materials Science and Technology (INSTM), Pisa, Italy

**Sumaira Anjum** Department of Biotechnology, Kinnaird College for Women, Lahore, Pakistan

**K. Aravinthraju** Department of Agricultural Entomology, Tamil Nadu Agricultural University, Coimbatore, Tamil Nadu, India

**Iqra Attique** Department of Biotechnology, Kinnaird College for Women, Lahore, Pakistan

**Mohan Ganesh Balaga** Assistant Professor, Department of Entomology, Sri Kinjarapu Yerrannaidu College of Agricultural Sciences (SKYCAS), Etcherla, Srikakulam, Andhra Pradesh, India

**Adalberto Benavides-Mendoza** Departmento de Horticultura, Universidad Autónoma Agraria Antonio Narro, Saltillo, Mexico

**Marcelino Cabrera-De la Fuente** Departmento de Horticultura, Universidad Autónoma Agraria Antonio Narro, Saltillo, Mexico

**Monika Chaudhary** School of Biological Engineering and Life Sciences, Shobhit Institute of Engineering and Technology (NAAC Accredited Grade 'A', Deemed to-Be-University) NH-58, Modipuram, Meerut, India

**Maria-Beatrice Coltelli** Department of Civil and Industrial Engineering (DICI), University of Pisa, Pisa, Italy;
Research Unit DICI-UNIPI, National Interuniversity Consortium of Materials Science and Technology (INSTM), Pisa, Italy

**Jyoti G. Koliyar-Jatinder Das** Department of Environmental Sciences, SIES (Nerul) College of Arts, Science and Commerce (Autonomous), Thane District, Nerul, Navi Mumbai, Maharashtra, India

**Rahul Datta** Department of Geology and Pedology, Faculty of Forestry and Wood Technology, Mendel University in Brno, Brno, Czech Republic

**Manoj Kanti Debnath** Department of Agricultural Statistics, Uttar Banga Krishi Viswavidyalaya, Cooch Behar, West Bengal, India

**Vijay Devra** Janki Devi Bajaj Government Girls College Kota, Kota, Rajasthan, India

**Amarendra Nath Dey** Department of Forestry, Cooch Behar, West Bengal, India

**Dinesha S.** Department of Forestry, North-Eastern Hill University, Tura Campus, Tura, Meghalaya, India

**Vinod Kumar Dubey** Department of Genetics & Plant Breeding, College of Agriculture, Acharya Narendra Deva University of Agriculture and Technology, Ayodhya, Uttar Pradesh, India

**Paola Fincheira** Centro de Excelencia en Investigación Biotecnológica Aplicada Al Medio Ambiente (CIBAMA), Universidad de La Frontera, Temuco, CP, Chile

**Sabuj Ganguly** BSM&TC (BTSSO), Central Silk Board, Baripada, Odisha, India

**Amar P. Garg** Swami Vivekanand Subharti University, Subhartipuram, Meerut, India

**Vito Gigante** Department of Civil and Industrial Engineering (DICI), University of Pisa, Pisa, Italy;
Research Unit DICI-UNIPI, National Interuniversity Consortium of Materials Science and Technology (INSTM), Pisa, Italy

**Yolanda González-García** National Institute of Forestry, Agricultural and Livestock Research, Northwest Regional Research Center, Todos Santos Experimental Field, La Paz, Mexico

**Magín González-Moscoso** Department of Nanotechnology, Polytechnic University of Chiapas, Suchiapa, Mexico

**B. H. Jaswanth Gowda** Department of Pharmaceutics, Yenepoya Pharmacy College and Research Centre, Yenepoya (Deemed to Be University), Mangaluru, Karnataka, India;
School of Pharmacy, Medical Biology Centre, Queen's University Belfast, Belfast, UK

**K. Gurushankar** Department of General Pathology, Saveetha Dental College and Hospitals, Saveetha University, Saveetha Institute of Medical and Technical Sciences (SIMATS), Chennai, Tamil Nadu, India

**Mubashra Inam** Department of Biotechnology, Kinnaird College for Women, Lahore, Pakistan

**Dilfuza Jabborova** Institute of Genetics and Plant Experimental Biology, Kibray, Uzbekistan

**Deepika Jeengar** Department of Entomology, College of Agriculture, Govind Ballabh Pant University of Agriculture and Technology, Pantnagar, Uttarakhand, India

**Run Jing** School of Environmental Science and Engineering, Tianjin University, Tianjin, P.R. China

**Antonio Juárez-Maldonado** Department of Botany, Autonomous Agrarian University Antonio Narro, Saltillo, Mexico

**Pranjal Kr Kaman** Department of Plant Pathology, Assam Agricultural University, Jorhat, Assam, India

**Karthik Kannan** Department of Mechanical Engineering and Advanced Institute of Manufacturing With High-Tech Innovations, National Chung Cheng University, Chiayi County, Taiwan

**Karthik R.** Department of Entomology, Assam Agricultural University, Jorhat, Assam, India

**Alagesan Keerthana** Department of Entomology, Tamil Nadu Agricultural University, Coimbatore, Tamil Nadu, India

**Laxmanarayanan M.** ICAR-National Bureau of Soil Survey and Land Use Planning, Nagpur, Maharashtra, India

**Andrea Lazzeri** Department of Civil and Industrial Engineering (DICI), University of Pisa, Pisa, Italy;
Research Unit DICI-UNIPI, National Interuniversity Consortium of Materials Science and Technology (INSTM), Pisa, Italy

**Anna Lesiak** Institut de Chimie de Nice (ICN) UMR CNRS 7272, Parc Valrose, Université Côte d'Azur, Nice, France

**Xuebin Lu** School of Environmental Science and Engineering, Tianjin University, Tianjin, P.R. China;
School of Ecology and Environment, Tibet University, Lhasa, P.R. China

**Jadeyegowda Madegowda** College of Forestry, KSN UAHS, Shivamogga, Karnataka, India

**Pramod Mall** Department of Entomology, College of Agriculture, G B Pant University of Agriculture and Technology, Pantnagar, Uttarakhand, India

**Chaitanya Metha** Department of Quality Assurance and Pharmaceutical Analysis, SVKM's Dr. Bhanuben Nanavati College of Pharmacy, Mumbai, Maharashtra, India

**Anamika Mishra** School of Bio-Sciences and Technology (SBST), Vellore Institute of Technology (VIT), Vellore, Tamil Nadu, India

**Shatakshi Mishra** School of Bio-Sciences and Technology (SBST), Vellore Institute of Technology (VIT), Vellore, Tamil Nadu, India

**Sourav Mohanto** Department of Pharmaceutics, Yenepoya Pharmacy College and Research Centre, Yenepoya (Deemed to Be University), Mangaluru, Karnataka, India

**A. V. Moorthy** Department of Entomology, College of Agriculture, G B Pant University of Agriculture and Technology, Pantnagar, Uttarakhand, India

**Sagnik Nag** Jeffrey Cheah School of Medicine and Health Sciences (JCSMHS), Monash University Malaysia, Selangor, Malaysia;
School of Bio-Sciences and Technology (SBST), Vellore Institute of Technology (VIT), Vellore, Tamil Nadu, India

**Arati Ningombam** ICAR Research Complex for North Eastern Hill Region, Manipur Centre, Lamphelpat, Manipur, India

**Arindam Pal** Department of Entomology, Post Graduate College of Agriculture, Dr. Rajendra Prasad Central Agricultural University, Samastipur, Pusa, Bihar, India

**Janardhan Pallavi** School of Bio-Sciences and Technology (SBST), Vellore Institute of Technology (VIT), Vellore, Tamil Nadu, India

**Renu Pandey** Department of Entomology, College of Agriculture, G B Pant University of Agriculture and Technology, Pantnagar, Uttarakhand, India

**Ashwani Kumar Patel** Department of Mycology and Plant Pathology, Institute of Agricultural Sciences, Banaras Hindu University, Varanasi, Uttar Pradesh, India

**Shrutee Pawar** Department of Quality Assurance and Pharmaceutical Analysis, SVKM's Dr. Bhanuben Nanavati College of Pharmacy, Mumbai, Maharashtra, India

**Rocío Maricela Peralta-Manjarrez** Departmento de Horticultura, Universidad Autónoma Agraria Antonio Narro, Saltillo, Mexico

**Priya** Department of Entomology, Post Graduate College of Agriculture, Dr. Rajendra Prasad Central Agricultural University, Samastipur, Pusa, Bihar, India

**Hermes Pérez-Hernández** Department of Botany, Autonomous Agrarian University Antonio Narro, Saltillo, Mexico

**Rakesh S.** International Crops Research Institute for the Semi-Arid Tropics, Patancheru, Hyderabad, Telangana, India

**Vandana Sahu** Department of Mycology and Plant Pathology, Institute of Agricultural Sciences, Banaras Hindu University, Varanasi, Uttar Pradesh, India

**K. Sankara Rao** Department of Entomology, Bihar Agricultural University, Bhagalpur, India

**Laishram Santhalembi** ICAR Research Complex for North Eastern Hill Region, Manipur Centre, Lamphelpat, Manipur, India

**Savitha Santosh** Central Research Institute for Dryland Agriculture, Hyderabad, Telangana, India

**Deepranjan Sarkar** Agricultural Systems and Engineering, Department of Food, Agriculture and Natural Resources, School of Environment, Resources and Development, Asian Institute of Technology, Klong Luang, Pathum Thani, Thailand

**Shawon Shriya Sarkar** Department of Forest Biology and Tree Improvement, Forest College and Research Institute, Tamil Nadu Agricultural University, Tamil Nadu, India

**Ajit Kumar Savani** ICAR-National Academy of Agricultural Research Management, Hyderabad, Telangana, India

**Shikha** Department of Soil Science, College of Agriculture, G. B. Pant University of Agriculture and Technology, Pantnagar, Uttarakhand, India

**Vithanala Shiva Sai Swaroop** Department of Plant Pathology, Assam Agricultural University, Jorhat, Assam, India

**Sachidanand Singh** Department of Biotechnology, School of Energy Technology, Pandit Deendayal Energy University, Gandhinagar, Gujarat, India

**H. Soundharya** School of Bio-Sciences and Technology (SBST), Vellore Institute of Technology (VIT), Vellore, Tamil Nadu, India

**B. Stany** School of Bio-Sciences and Technology (SBST), Vellore Institute of Technology (VIT), Vellore, Tamil Nadu, India

**Vetriselvan Subramaniyan** Jeffrey Cheah School of Medicine and Health Sciences (JCSMHS), Monash University Malaysia, Selangor, Malaysia

**Vyshnavi Sunil** Department of Entomology, College of Agriculture, Kerala Agricultural University, Vellayani, Thiruvananthapuram, Kerala, India

**Kottam Sushma** Department of Plant Pathology, CoH, Dr YSRHU, Anantharajupeta, Andhra Pradesh, India

**Vasanti Suvarna** Department of Pharmaceutical Analysis, SVKM's Dr. Bhanuben Nanavati College of Pharmacy, Mumbai, Maharashtra, India

**Vinaya Tari** Department of Biology, Faculty of Science and Technology, Universitas Airlangga, Surabaya, East Java, Indonesia

**Sushmita Thokchom** Department of Entomology, Assam Agricultural University, Jorhat, Assam, India

**Gonzalo Tortella** Centro de Excelencia en Investigación Biotecnológica Aplicada Al Medio Ambiente (CIBAMA), Universidad de La Frontera, Temuco, CP, Chile; Departamento de Ingeniería Química, Facultad de Ingeniería y Ciencias, Universidad de La Frontera, Temuco, Chile

**Toushif P. K.** Department of Forestry, Mizoram University, Aizawl, Mizoram, India

**M. Vani Praveena** Acharya N.G. Ranga Agricultural University, Guntur, Andhra Pradesh, India

**Balraju Wagmare** Govindh Ballabh Pant National Institute of Himalayan Environment and Sustainable Development, Sikkim, India

**Dwi Kusuma Wahyuni** Department of Biology, Faculty of Science and Technology, Universitas Airlangga, Surabaya, East Java, Indonesia

**Jingfei Wang** School of Environmental Science and Engineering, Tianjin University, Tianjin, P.R. China

**Karolina Waszkowska** LPHIA, SFR MATRIX, University of Angers, Angers, France

**Kai Yan** School of Environmental Science and Engineering, Tianjin University, Tianjin, P.R. China

**Zhihao Yu** School of Environmental Science and Engineering, Tianjin University, Tianjin, P.R. China

# An Overview of Nanotechnology in Agroforestry Systems

**Shawon Shriya Sarkar, Ajith S., Shikha, Rakesh S., Deepranjan Sarkar, Rahul Datta, and Sachidanand Singh**

**Abstract** The field of nanotechnology is rapidly developing with diverse applications in medicine, biotechnology, electronics, energy, agriculture, and environmental remediation. Agroforestry is emerging as a viable option for managing the land-use systems. The use of nanomaterials or nanoproducts is undoubtedly increasing to manage the resources of modern agriculture. For the concurrent production of crops and trees, a targeted delivery approach is essential. Nano-based formulations are used in tree-crop systems for meeting nutrient requirements, controlling pests, improving tolerance to environmental stresses, reducing pollution, etc. to attain food security at the global level. However, technological innovation should be assessed for fate and potential risks as a part of sustainable landscape management.

S. S. Sarkar
Department of Forest Biology and Tree Improvement, Forest College and Research Institute, Tamil Nadu Agricultural University, Tamil Nadu, India

Ajith S.
International Maize and Wheat Improvement Centre (CIMMYT), Delhi, India

Shikha
Department of Soil Science, College of Agriculture, G. B. Pant University of Agriculture and Technology, Pantnagar, Uttarakhand, India

Rakesh S. (✉)
International Crops Research Institute for the Semi-Arid Tropics, Hyderabad, India
e-mail: rakisavan.940@gmail.com

D. Sarkar
Agricultural Systems and Engineering, Department of Food, Agriculture and Natural Resources, School of Environment, Resources and Development, Asian Institute of Technology, Klong Luang, Pathum Thani, Thailand

R. Datta
Department of Geology and Pedology, Faculty of Forestry and Wood Technology, Mendel University in Brno, Brno, Czech Republic

S. Singh
Department of Biotechnology, School of Energy Technology, Pandit Deendayal Energy University, Gandhinagar, Gujarat, India



D. Jabborova et al. (eds.), *Nanomaterials in Agroforestry Systems*, Smart Nanomaterials Technology, https://doi.org/10.1007/978-981-96-1337-3_1

Statistical techniques have a vital role in speeding up the research and development cycle of nanoscience. In this chapter, we attempted to provide a brief synopsis regarding the prospects of nanoparticle application in agroforestry systems.

**Keywords** Nanoparticles · Green synthesis · Nutrient management · Stress management · Ecotoxicity testing · Response surface methodology

## 1 Introduction

Nanoparticles are gaining popularity because of their distinct physicochemical properties. Particles that fall between 1 and 100 nm in size, at the minimum in one of the three dimensions, are referred to as nanoparticles [41]. In 1959, Richard Feynman, an American physicist introduced the idea of nanotechnology, and in 1974, the term "nanotechnology" was originally used and defined by Japanese scientist Norio Taniguchi [12]. Several scientists and organizations have defined nanotechnology in terms of design, properties, synthesis, and applications. These definitions provide a range of perspectives on nanotechnology, highlighting its focus on manipulating matter at the atomic and molecular scale to achieve novel properties and functionalities. Thus, nanotechnology operates within the nanoscale dimensions and offers various uses for societal benefits by exploring the unique physical and chemical characteristics of nanomaterials [13].

The rising global population and climate change urgency demand advancements in agriculture. Nanotechnology which got recognition for its potential where traditional methods fall short has seen significant growth in agriculture over the past decade. Nano-based technologies have shown promising results in soil and crop management, offering enhanced yield and protection for sustainable agriculture [22, 68]. Similarly, such strategies are also beneficial in agroforestry systems for soil fertility management, pest management, enhanced farm production, and assuring the agroforestry products' quality and safety [63, 70]. It is thought that nanotechnology will provide the platform to convert forest resources into high-value goods useful for building, biomedical, and coating purposes, as well as smart paper and nano-packaging [28].

Agroforestry systems offer both financial and environmental advantages when they deliberately mix crops with trees and/or shrubs. But obstacles including poor tree germplasm, restricted access to input and output markets, unstable land tenure, and insufficient technical expertise prevent smallholder farmers from widely implementing agroforestry [63]. Nanotechnology developments can aid in removing these obstacles. As mentioned earlier, the technology that manipulates matter at nanoscale scales is finding use in agriculture. New nanotechnology-based instruments are being developed for improved plant protection, real-time field-level monitoring, soil remediation, and tailored seed and agrichemical delivery. Agroforestry applications for many nanomaterials, such as nanofertilizers, nanoherbicides, nanopesticides, and nanosensors have been suggested [20]. Agroforestry systems that maintain soil health and the environment are well-suited for certain materials like carbon nanomaterials, gradual nutrient release, biodegradability, and high reactivity. These materials include nano-clay and metal/metal oxide nanomaterials. This is a transformative opportunity to enhance our understanding of nano-enabled strategies for implementing effective and sustainable farming practices in agroforestry systems.

## 2 Nano-Enabled Agrochemicals

With the help of various nanomaterials, many chemical forms can be given to plants more efficiently for increased yield—a practice known as "nano-enabled agrochemicals". Materials with an exterior diameter between 1 and 100 nm are referred to as nanomaterials, regardless of whether they are accidentally, naturally occurring, or artificially made. Nano-enabled agrochemicals offer a range of benefits for agroforestry systems, for example, ensuring adequate plant nutrition is essential for enhancing system productivity and guaranteeing food security for the world's expanding population. The precision delivery systems ensure precise delivery of agrochemicals, such as pesticides, herbicides, and fertilizers to target plants in agroforestry systems. Nanoformulations enable controlled release mechanisms, ensuring that the active ingredients are delivered at the right time and in the right amounts, thereby minimizing wastage and environmental pollution [43, 66]. These advancements also contribute to reduced environmental and bioaccumulation impacts by lowering the amount of chemicals required and minimizing off-target effects [17, 27, 30]. Improved nutrient management practices are adopted for efficient utilization of fertilizers, nanoscale nutrient carriers can improve nutrient uptake by plant roots, leading to healthier and more resilient agroforestry crops. Recently, the application of nanobiopesticides as eco-friendly alternatives to synthetic pesticides and fungicides and support for natural pest management strategies have generated great attention [2, 47]. These nanoparticles or nanoproducts that are designed to be used as pesticides are synthesized using biological control agents or plants having excellent biocompatibility and biodegradability features. Moreover, carbon-based nanomaterials can act as soil amendments and improve the fertility and productivity of sandy soils [42].

## 3 Synthesis of Nanoparticles

### *3.1 Top-Down Approach*

This method refers to the disintegration of the bulk material into nanosized structures or particles (Fig. 1). The process is attained by using several techniques like electro-explosion, sputtering, mechanical milling, chemical etching, and laser ablation [1, 9].

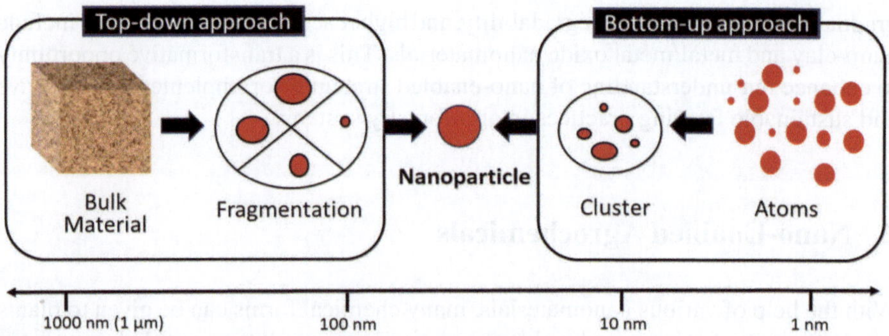


**Fig. 1** Common approaches for the synthesis of nanoparticles

### *3.2 Bottom-Up Approach*

The accumulation of a material from the bottom specifically atom-by-atom or molecule-by-molecule is known as the bottom-up approach. Methods like chemical vapor deposition, sol–gel, soft and hard templating, hydrothermal, solvothermal, and laser pyrolysis are used to produce nanoparticles [9, 10].

### *3.3 Green Synthesis*

Green synthesis utilizes the production of nanomaterials using sustainable methods, and natural resources, typically involving plant extracts, microorganisms, or other biocompatible sources as innovative solutions that offer various fronts in agroforestry systems. There is an increasing trend in the publication of research papers related to the biosynthesis of nanoparticles which indicates that the researchers are attracted toward the exploration of natural resources for the synthesis of nanomaterials [69]. The biosynthesis of nanoparticles has gained growing importance in the face of cost-effective and environmentally sustainable nanoproducts [31].

Plant extract-mediated synthesis facilitates the eco-friendly synthesis of nanoparticles using a variety of phytochemicals, such as polyphenols, flavonoids, and terpenoids, which can act as reducing and stabilizing agents, harnessing these natural compounds for sustainable agriculture [25]. Bioactive nanoparticles synthesized using plant extracts or microbial sources can possess inherent bioactivity and play an essential role in crop management, offering targeted delivery of nutrients and pest control agents. Zinc oxide nanoparticles can be synthesized from fresh leaves of *Azadirachta indica*, leaf extract of *Aloe vera*, flower of *Trifolium pratense*, bacterial strain (*Pseudomonas aeruginosa*), etc. [5]. With increasing heavy metal pollution

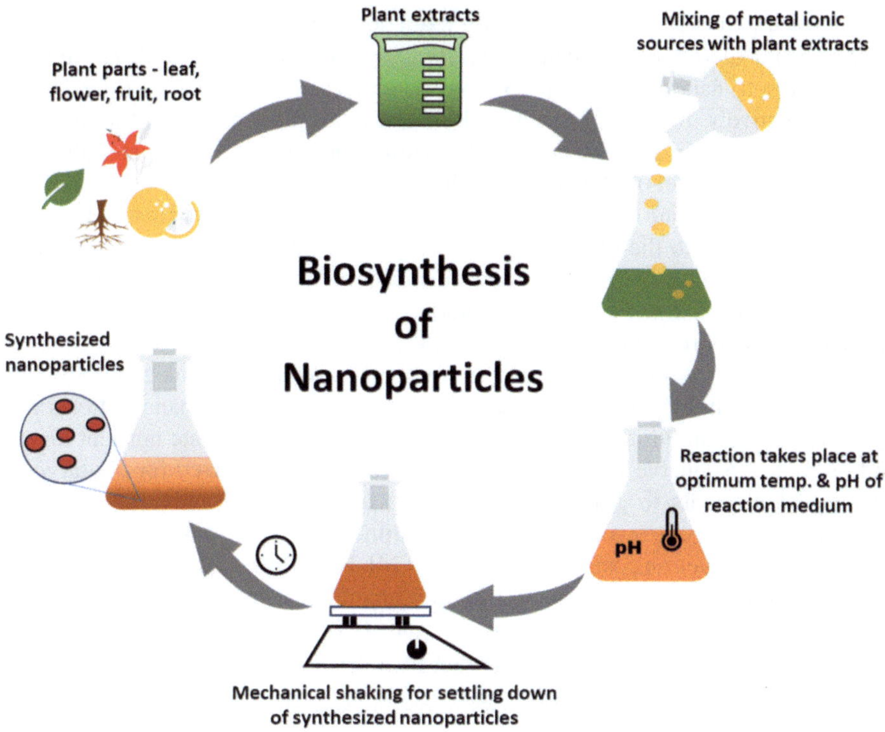


**Fig. 2** Schematic representation of nanoparticle synthesis using biological (or green) method

concerns, phytoremediation using biosynthesized nanoparticles is an emerging clean-up method to aid in soil remediation [49]. A systematic protocol for the biosynthesis of nanoparticles is presented in Fig. 2.

## 4 Applications of Nanomaterials

### *4.1 Soil Fertility and Nutrient Management*

Globally, the production of healthy food is dependent on good soil. Preserving present healthy soils and repairing damaged soils offer pragmatic solutions to global challenges of the twenty-first century [36]. Researchers and enterprises are concentrating on solutions that give the greatest nutrient availability and the least amount of environmental disturbance to achieve the Sustainable Development Goals [55]. According to Shang et al. [59], substituting conventional fertilizers with their nano-enabled equivalents can significantly boost nutrient delivery efficiency, lower pollution levels, and enhance soil health. To study phosphorus (P) phytoavailability, Zahra et al. [76]

grew lettuce plants for 90 days in sandy loam soil amended with titanium dioxide ($TiO_2$) and magnetite ($Fe_3O_4$) nanomaterials at 0–250 mg/kg (six levels). The authors found that both nanomaterials, at 150 mg/kg, increased the uptake of P by 74 and 89%, respectively. In a study conducted by Gui et al. [26], butterhead lettuce was grown for 30 days in soil amended with cerium oxide ($CeO_2$) nanomaterials at 0–1000 mg/kg (four levels). The findings indicated that $CeO_2$ nanoparticles, at 100 mg/kg, increased the nitrate (a major nitrogen source for higher plants) content in leaves by 38.2%, relative to the untreated plants. The foliar spray of nanofertilizers such as silver nanoparticles (15 mL/L) and zinc nanoparticles (12.5 mL/L) improved total chlorophyll, leaf area, shoot diameter, flower percentage, fruit yield, and fruit physicochemical properties of peach trees [40].

With respect to soil fertility and nutrient management, nanotechnology will play a key role in agroforestry systems by employing different nanoparticles and nanocomposites, aiming to improve nutrient use efficiency, mitigate nutrient losses, and promote sustainable food systems. Nanofertilizers are utilized for the targeted delivery of nutrients to plants, optimizing uptake efficiency, reducing waste by protecting them from leaching or volatilization losses, and ensuring controlled release; thus production costs can be reduced [74]. Nanomaterials such as nanoclays and nanocomposites can be explored for soil amendment in agroforestry practices to improve soil structure, water retention, and nutrient availability. Nano-biochar enhances nutrient management by serving as a carrier for essential elements and promoting microbial activity [18].

## 4.2 *Stress Management*

Significant losses in crop output are caused by both biotic and abiotic stresses. Yet, the percentage of worldwide crop output lost to biotic stressors varies depending on the principal crop and the area [57]. Insect infestations reduce primary food and cash crop yields by 15% to 20% [53]. Similarly, abiotic stresses alter plants' morphology, physiology, biochemistry, and molecular makeup, affecting their capacity to grow, develop, and produce [8]. Such stresses include heat, drought, waterlogging, heavy metals, and mineral toxicity [24, 56]. They have the potential to significantly reduce the yield by 50% or more [35]. Nanotechnology offers promising solutions to mitigate different stresses and enhance resilience in agroforestry practices for managing both biotic and abiotic stresses. For example, nanopesticides improve their efficacy by enhancing their delivery, adhesion to plant surfaces, and penetration into plant tissues [66]. Nanoformulations used for weed control are known as nanoherbicides and they can be classified into organic (PCL atrazine, carbon nanotubes_diuron, biochar_2,4-D), inorganic (Zn-layered hydroxide_4CPA, SMSs NPs_2,4-D, clay-imazaquin, nanoclay_2,4-D), or hybrid ($Fe_3O_4$ NPs coated with hollow silica spheres_glyphosate) nanoparticles [23]. Silver nanoparticles exhibit antimicrobial properties, which can be utilized to combat plant pathogens, such as bacteria, fungi, and viruses [11]. They can be incorporated into coatings and films, or used as sprays to protect plants from diseases. Nanosensors can detect early signs of pest infestations or disease outbreaks, enabling prompt intervention and targeted pest management strategies while minimizing environmental impact.

When metal-based nanoparticles (like zinc oxide) are applied, root morphology is altered, and more lateral roots and root biomass are formed. As a result, water intake is enhanced and better water status is maintained under drought stress [52]. Thakur et al. [67] reported that zinc oxide and titanium dioxide nanoparticle pretreatment dramatically increased wheat's resistance to heat stress by increasing enzyme activities (superoxide dismutase and guaiacol peroxidase. Similarly, the salt stress tolerance of tomato plants was observed to increase with the application of copper nanoparticles as foliar spray; enhancing the plant's antioxidant systems under saline conditions [48]. The application of zero-valent iron nanoparticles in contaminated soil reduced the bioavailability of heavy metals (lead and cadmium) and helped in seedling establishment and increasing biomass of Persian maple tree seedlings [65]. Zinc oxide nanoparticles synthesized from *Azadirachta indica* (neem tree) extracts increased maize growth in chromium-contaminated soil [38]. To tackle diverse phyto-stresses, nanobiostimulants are gaining wide interest among researchers for bioactive properties and safety concerns (biodegradability, biocompatibility). Seed nanopriming with nanobiostimulant (nano zinc sulfide) can boost seed germination and antioxidant defense system of rice [34].

## 5 Fate of Nanomaterials

### *5.1 Translocation of Nanomaterials in Soil and Plant*

The pattern of absorption, bioaccumulation, bioavailability, and biotransformation of nanomaterial in the ecosystem is very complex. Such processes are governed by nanoparticle's type, size, morphology, chemical makeup, surface chemistry, solubility, and stability, and also plant species [23, 54, 72]. In soil, the engineered nanoproducts interact with a variety of organic or inorganic ligands which might change the porosity of the soil, consequently affecting soil aggregation and water movement [73]. Nanoparticles undergo a variety of transformations like adsorption–desorption, dissolution, aggregation-sedimentation, degradation, and biotransformation, when they are discharged into the soil [14]. They can accumulate in soil if they have properties, such as less solubility and high resistance to degradation [45, 73].

Plants absorb (uptake) the nanomaterials through roots and leaves using diffusion, infiltration, and endocytosis mechanisms, or with the help of ion channels and transporters [58, 72]. With the entry of nanoparticles through the root epidermis or leaf stomata (or cuticle), they may be translocated to other plant components, including stems, flowers, and fruits. However, sometimes they accumulate in roots and do not move from roots to shoots due to the inhibitory effect of the Casparian strip [16] or rigid cell wall [71]. Several fates of nanoparticles like aggregation, dissolution, transformation, and deposition in plants are reported [64]. Understanding soil transport and plant uptake of nanomaterials is crucial for assessing the environmental impact and efficacy of nanotechnology in enhancing agroforestry practices while ensuring sustainability and safety.

### *5.2 Ecotoxicity Assessment*

Nanoparticles can potentially accumulate in soil and affect soil microorganisms (microbicidal) if applied at higher concentrations; thus hampering microbial diversity and activity, e.g., nutrient mineralization, nitrogen fixation, and plant growth promotion [33]. The toxic effect (13.3% mortality) of silver nanoparticles on soil earthworms was reported at 200 mg/kg after 28 days of exposure [62]. Monitoring the toxicity of nanoparticles to plants and assessing their persistence in the environment is essential. Gui et al. [26] reported the beneficial impact of $CeO_2$ nanoparticles on lettuce growth at 100 mg/kg, however, plant growth was reduced at 1000 mg/kg. Thus, following standard protocols for specific organisms (maintained at specific conditions, age) and exposure (acute or chronic toxicity) to measure endpoints including survivability, growth, behavioral changes, enzymatic activity, fecundity, genotoxicity, bioaccumulation, and ecological interactions within food webs aid in ecotoxicological studies [15, 51]. The use of representative species from various trophic levels or phases in a food chain, such as primary producers, grazers, and predators, may be intriguing since certain toxins will build up in the food chain (a process known as biomagnification) (Fig. 3). The distribution of nanoparticle within the tissues (a process known as bioaccumulation) of organisms also needs to be evaluated.

## 6 Risk Management

Finally, incorporating risk management strategies is imperative when implementing nanotechnology in agroforestry systems. Nanomaterials possess unique properties that may introduce uncertainties regarding their environmental impacts, such as soil and water contamination and potential toxicity to plants and organisms. Effective risk management involves a thorough evaluation of nanomaterial properties, exposure pathways, and ecological interactions. Implementing preventive measures related to manufacturing, processing, packaging, and storage systems can mitigate potential risks. Additionally, regulatory frameworks should be established to ensure the safe use and disposal of nanomaterials in agroforestry systems. Inhalation and skin contact will negatively affect human health. On the positive side, nanotechnology is a potential tool to address the risk of invasive alien species and forest fires arising due to changes in land-use patterns [60]. Collaboration among researchers, policymakers, and stakeholders is essential to develop comprehensive risk management

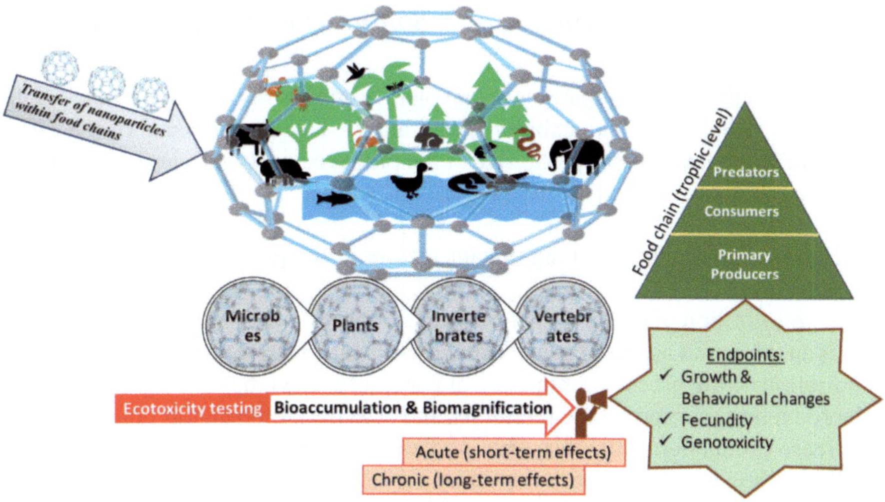


**Fig. 3** Focal points of ecotoxicity testing of nanoparticles at different trophic levels

strategies that promote sustainable and responsible integration of nanotechnology in agroforestry systems and balance innovation with environmental protection.

## 7 Statistical Approaches in Nanotechnology

The proper use of appropriate statistical techniques is highly essential for obtaining scientific and reliable conclusions and it reduces drudgery in research as well [6]. Statistical techniques have made a sizable impact on the nanotechnology field in the past and still play an important role in tackling the challenges that arise in the development of nanotechnology [75]. These techniques and methodologies have highly contributed to the rapid growth and development of nanotechnology in terms of data collection, designing of an experiment, estimation of treatment effects, testing of hypothesis, and quality control of nanomaterial synthesis [37].

Statistically designed experiments play a vital role in speeding up the research and development cycle of nanoscience and also help to create more robust, reliable, and quality nanomaterials [44]. The design of experiments is becoming increasingly important to the advancement of the science of nanotechnology as well as in the field of nanomanufacturing. Sampling distributions and other methods help to evaluate the quality of nanomaterials in quality control experiments [29]. The data-based modeling of properties of nanostructures has attained huge attraction due to the advent of advanced machine learning techniques [21].

### *7.1 Optimization of Nanoparticle Synthesis and Application*

Controlled synthesis of nanoparticles from plant origin results in nanoparticles of the desired size, uniformity, and stability which are the key determinants of the effectiveness of nanomaterials [61]. The size of the produced nanoparticles is determined by various factors involved in the preparation such as reaction conditions, types of materials used, and their concentration [7]. Factorial experiments are useful in the determination of the most significant factors in the process of biosynthesis of nanoparticles [32].

The optimization of profound determinants of properties of synthesized nanoparticles is an important aspect of standardizing the most effective nanomaterial [3]. The optimization of the process parameters in nanoparticle synthesis is essential during bulk production to improve the reliability and stability of the nanoproduct and also to increase production [19]. Response surface methodology (RSM) has become a popular method nowadays for the optimization of processes [50]. It is a systematic approach to find out the ideal process parameters required to obtain nanoparticles of desired properties [4]. The RSM is highly helpful in obtaining high-efficiency nanomaterials through the optimization of various process parameters of the synthesis of nanoparticles [46]. This methodology is also useful in optimizing nanotubes used in the delivery system to enhance the nutrient use efficiency of plants [39].

## 8 Conclusion

The challenges of agroforestry systems are many and various where precise application of management strategies needs a lot of research. Besides, the application of nanotechnology in the field of agroforestry is still relatively new. The synthesis of nanoparticles of desired physicochemical properties is essential for improving the efficiency of nanomaterials. For the transfer of technology to land, there is a requirement for the comprehension of researchers and policymakers, training and workshops, and consistent financing for this emerging area to flourish. Nanosensors can be useful tools to detect changes in moisture content, nutrient levels, and pest infestations. Nanoparticles can improve resource use efficiency in tree-crop systems by reducing leaching losses or having low impacts on non-target organisms. Research on the fate, transport, and ecotoxicological consequences of nanoparticles in food systems is essential for sustainable nanotechnology-related management practices. Green synthesis or production of nanoparticles from organic resources is a promising approach in terms of biocompatibility and biodegradability concerns. The application of artificial intelligence and machine learning models is the need of the hour to study the complex interaction of nanoparticles with different kinds of flora and fauna in agroforestry systems and their short- and long-term impacts. However, the regulatory aspects of nanoformulations cannot be overlooked.

## References


1. Abbas M, Yan K, Li J, Zafar S, Hasnain Z, Aslam N (2022) Agri-nanotechnology and tree nanobionics: Augmentation in crop yield, biosafety, and biomass accumulation. Front Bioeng Biotechnol 10:853045. https://doi.org/10.3389/fbioe.2022.853045
2. Abdollahdokht D, Gao Y, Faramarz S, Poustforoosh A, Abbasi M, Asadikaram G, Nematollahi MH (2022) Conventional agrochemicals towards nano-biopesticides: An overview on recent advances. Chem Biol Technol Agric 9:13. https://doi.org/10.1186/s40538-021-00281-0
3. Acharya NN, Lin DK (2008) Understanding a ZnO nanorods fabrication process: a supersaturated design approach. Int J Nanomanuf 2(4):319–330. https://doi.org/10.1504/IJNM.2008.022559
4. Adibah N, Firdianti BE, Suprapto S (2023) Synthesis of silver nanoparticles using response surface methodology. J Nano- Electron Phys 15(3): 03001. https://doi.org/10.21272/jnep.15(3).03001
5. Agarwal H, Kumar SV, Rajeshkumar S (2017) A review on green synthesis of zinc oxide nanoparticles–An eco-friendly approach. Resour-Effic Technol 3:406–413
6. Ajith S, Ramesh D, Karthik R (2021) Statistics for Scientific Agricultural Research. In: Kaur R, Bakshi B (eds) Recent Advances in Scientific Research. Lap Lambert Academic Publisher, Chişinău, pp 141–165
7. Alnaddaf LM, Almuhammady AK, Salem KF, Alloosh MT, Saleh MM, Al-Khayri JM (2021) Green synthesis of nanoparticles using different plant extracts and their characterizations. In: Al-Khayri JM, Ansari MI, Singh AK (eds) Nanobiotechnology: Mitigation of Abiotic Stress in Plants. Springer, Cham, pp 165–199. https://doi.org/10.1007/978-3-030-73606-4_8
8. Ansari WA, Atri N, Pandey M, Singh AK, Singh B, Pandey S (2019) Influence of drought stress on morphological, physiological and biochemical attributes of plants: A review. Biosci Biotech Res Asia 16. https://doi.org/10.13005/bbra/2785
9. Arora S, Murmu G, Mukherjee K, Saha S, Maity D (2022) A comprehensive overview of nanotechnology in sustainable agriculture. J Biotechnol 355:21–41
10. Baig N, Kammakakam I, Falath W (2021) Nanomaterials: A review of synthesis methods, properties, recent progress, and challenges. Mater Adv 2:1821–1871
11. Bamal D, Singh A, Chaudhary G, Kumar M, Singh M, Rani N, Mundlia P, Sehrawat AR (2021) Silver nanoparticles biosynthesis, characterization, antimicrobial activities, applications, cytotoxicity and safety issues: An updated review. Nanomaterials 11:2086. https://doi.org/10.3390/nano11082086
12. Bayda S, Adeel M, Tuccinardi T, Cordani M, Rizzolio F (2020) The history of nanoscience and nanotechnology: from chemical–physical applications to nanomedicine. Molecules 25(1):112. https://doi.org/10.3390/molecules25010112
13. Bhushan B (2017) Introduction to nanotechnology. In: Bhushan B (ed) Springer handbook of nanotechnology. Springer Handbooks, Springer, Berlin, Heidelberg, pp 1–19
14. Bolan S, Sharma S, Mukherjee S, Zhou P, Mandal J, Srivastava P et al (2024) The distribution, fate, and environmental impacts of food additive nanomaterials in soil and aquatic ecosystems. Sci Total Environ 916:170013. https://doi.org/10.1016/j.scitotenv.2024.170013
15. Boros BV, Ostafe V (2020) Evaluation of ecotoxicology assessment methods of nanomaterials and their effects. Nanomaterials 10:610. https://doi.org/10.3390/nano10040610
16. Cai F, Wu X, Zhang H, Shen X, Zhang M, Chen W et al (2017) Impact of $TiO_2$ nanoparticles on lead uptake and bioaccumulation in rice (*Oryza sativa* L.). NanoImpact 5:101–108
17. Chaud M, Souto EB, Zielinska A, Severino P, Batain F, Oliveira-Junior J, Alves T (2021) Nanopesticides in agriculture: Benefits and challenge in agricultural productivity, toxicological risks to human health and environment. Toxics 9:131. 10.3390%2Ftoxics9060131
18. Chausali N, Saxena J, Prasad R (2021) Nanobiochar and biochar based nanocomposites: Advances and applications. J Agric Food Res 5:100191. https://doi.org/10.1016/j.jafr.2021.100191

19. Chowdhury S, Yusof F, Faruck MO, Sulaiman N (2016) Process optimization of silver nanoparticle synthesis using response surface methodology. Procedia Eng 148:992–999. https://doi.org/10.1016/j.proeng.2016.06.552
20. El-Ramady H, Abdalla N, Sári D, Ferroudj A, Muthu A, Prokisch J, Fawzy ZF, Brevik EC, Solberg SØ (2023) Nanofarming: Promising solutions for the future of the global agricultural industry. Agronomy 13:1600. https://doi.org/10.3390/agronomy13061600
21. Fan Z, Hu X, Gao RX (2022) Indirect measurement methods for quality and process control in nanomanufacturing. Nanomanufacturing Metrol 5:209–229. https://doi.org/10.1007/s41871-022-00148-4
22. Fatima F, Hashim A, Anees S (2021) Efficacy of nanoparticles as nanofertilizer production: a review. Environ Sci Pollut Res 28:1292–1303
23. Forini MM, Pontes MS, Antunes DR, de Lima PH, Santos JS, Santiago EF, Grillo R (2022) Nano-enabled weed management in agriculture: From strategic design to enhanced herbicidal activity. Plant Nano Biol 1:100008. https://doi.org/10.1016/j.plana.2022.100008
24. Franco JA, Bañón S, Vicente MJ, Miralles J, Martínez-Sánchez JJ (2011) Root development in horticultural plants grown under abiotic stress conditions–a review. J Hortic Sci Biotechnol 86:543–556
25. Gauba A, Hari SK, Ramamoorthy V, Vellasamy S, Govindan G, Arasu MV (2023) The versatility of green synthesized zinc oxide nanoparticles in sustainable agriculture: A review on metal-microbe interaction that rewards agriculture. Physiol Mol Plant Pathol 125:102023. https://doi.org/10.1016/j.pmpp.2023.102023
26. Gui X, Zhang Z, Liu S, Ma Y, Zhang P, He X et al (2015) Fate and phytotoxicity of $CeO_2$ nanoparticles on lettuce cultured in the potting soil environment. PLoS ONE 10:e0134261. https://doi.org/10.1371/journal.pone.0134261
27. Hajji-Hedfi L, Chhipa H (2021) Nano-based pesticides: challenges for pest and disease management. Euro-Mediterr J Environ Integr 6:69. https://doi.org/10.1007/s41207-021-00279-y
28. Husen A, Jawaid M (eds) (2020) Nanomaterials for agriculture and forestry applications. Elsevier, Amsterdam, p 532
29. Hussain N, Tahir MH, Jamal F, Ameeq M, Shafiq S, Mendy JT (2024) An acceptance sampling plan for the odd exponential-logarithmic Fréchet distribution: applications to quality control data. Cogent Eng 11(1):2304497. https://doi.org/10.1080/23311916.2024.2304497
30. Iavicoli I, Leso V, Beezhold DH, Shvedova AA (2017) Nanotechnology in agriculture: Opportunities, toxicological implications, and occupational risks. Toxicol Appl Pharmacol 329:96–111
31. Jadoun S, Arif R, Jangid NK, Meena RK (2021) Green synthesis of nanoparticles using plant extracts: A review. Environ Chem Lett 19:355–374
32. Keijok WJ, Pereira RHA, Alvarez LAC, Prado AR, da Silva AR, Ribeiro J, Guimarães MCC (2019) Controlled biosynthesis of gold nanoparticles with *Coffea arabica* using factorial design. Sci Rep 9:16019. https://doi.org/10.1038/s41598-019-52496-9
33. Khan ST, Adil SF, Shaik MR, Alkhathlan HZ, Khan M, Khan M (2022) Engineered nanomaterials in soil: Their impact on soil microbiome and plant health. Plants 11:109. https://doi.org/10.3390/plants11010109
34. Khepar V, Sidhu A, kaur Mankoo R, Manchanda P, Sharma AB, (2024) Nanobiostimulant action of trigolic formulated zinc sulfide nanoparticles (ZnS-T NPs) on rice seeds by triggering antioxidant defense network and plant growth specific transcription factors. Plant Physiol Biochem 210:108605. https://doi.org/10.1016/j.plaphy.2024.108605
35. Kumar S (2020) Abiotic stresses and their effects on plant growth, yield and nutritional quality of agricultural produce. Int J Food Sci Agric 4:367–378
36. Lal R, Bouma J, Brevik E, Dawson L, Field DJ, Glaser B et al (2021) Soils and sustainable development goals of the United Nations: An International Union of Soil Sciences perspective. Geoderma Reg 25:e00398. https://doi.org/10.1016/j.geodrs.2021.e00398
37. Lu JC, Jeng SL, Wang K (2009) A review of statistical methods for quality improvement and control in nanotechnology. J Qual Technol 41(2):148–164. https://doi.org/10.1080/00224065.2009.11917770

38. Mehmood S, Ou W, Ahmed W, Bundschuh J, Rizwan M, Mahmood M et al (2023) ZnO nanoparticles mediated by *Azadirachta indica* as nano fertilizer: Improvement in physiological and biochemical indices of *Zea mays* grown in Cr-contaminated soil. Environ Pollut 339:122755. https://doi.org/10.1016/j.envpol.2023.122755
39. Mohamad Yatim N, Shaaban A, Dimin MF, Yusof F, Abd Razak J (2016) Application of response surface methodology for optimization of urea grafted multiwalled carbon nanotubes in enhancing nitrogen use efficiency and nitrogen uptake by paddy plants. J Nanotechnol:1250739. https://doi.org/10.1155/2016/1250739
40. Mosa WFA, El-Shehawi AM, Mackled MI, Salem MZ, Ghareeb RY, Hafez EE, Behiry SI, Abdelsalam NR (2021) Productivity performance of peach trees, insecticidal and antibacterial bioactivities of leaf extracts as affected by nanofertilizers foliar application. Sci Rep 11:10205. https://doi.org/10.1038/s41598-021-89885-y
41. Nagarajan R (2008) Nanoparticles: building blocks for nanotechnology. In: Nagarajan R, Hatton TA (eds) Nanoparticles: Synthesis, Stabilization, Passivation, and Functionalization. American Chemical Society, Washington, DC, pp 2–14
42. Nepal J, Xin X, Maltais-Landry G, Ahmad W, Pereira J, Santra S et al (2023) Carbon nanomaterials are a superior soil amendment for sandy soils than biochar based on impacts on lettuce growth, physiology and soil biochemical quality. NanoImpact 31:100480. https://doi.org/10.1016/j.impact.2023.100480
43. Nair R, Varghese SH, Nair BG, Maekawa T, Yoshida Y, Kumar DS (2010) Nanoparticulate material delivery to plants. Plant Sci 179(3):154–163
44. Nembhard HB, Acharya N, Aktan M, Kim S (2005) Design issues and analysis of experiments in nanomanufacturing. In: Badiru AB (ed) Handbook of Industrial and Systems Engineering. CRC Press, Boca Raton, pp 367–386
45. Ogunkunle CO, Oyedeji S, Okoro HK, Adimula V (2021) Interaction of nanoparticles with soil. In: Amrane A, Mohan D, Nguyen TA, Assadi AA, Yasin G (eds) Nanomaterials for soil remediation. Elsevier, Amsterdam, pp 101–132
46. Othman AM, Elsayed MA, Elshafei AM, Hassan MM (2017) Application of response surface methodology to optimize the extracellular fungal mediated nanosilver green synthesis. J Genet Eng Biotechnol 15(2):497–504. https://doi.org/10.1016/j.jgeb.2017.08.003
47. Pan X, Guo X, Zhai T, Zhang D, Rao W, Cao F, Guan X (2023) Nanobiopesticides in sustainable agriculture: developments, challenges, and perspectives. Environmental Sci: Nano 10:41–61
48. Pérez-Labrada F, López-Vargas ER, Ortega-Ortiz H, Cadenas-Pliego G, Benavides-Mendoza A, Juárez-Maldonado A (2019) Responses of tomato plants under saline stress to foliar application of copper nanoparticles. Plants 8:151. https://doi.org/10.3390/plants8060151
49. Prakash P, Chandran SS (2023) Nano-phytoremediation of heavy metals from soil: a critical review. Pollutants 3:360–380
50. Rakhmanova A, Kalybekkyzy S, Soltabayev B, Bissenbay A, Kassenova N, Bakenov Z, Mentbayeva A (2022) Application of response surface methodology for optimization of nanosized zinc oxide synthesis conditions by electrospinning technique. Nanomaterials 12(10):1733. https://doi.org/10.3390/nano12101733
51. Rana S, Kalaichelvan P (2013) Ecotoxicity of nanoparticles. Int Sch Res Notices 2013:574648. https://doi.org/10.1155/2013/574648
52. Rasheed A, Li H, Tahir MM, Mahmood A, Nawaz M, Shah AN et al (2022) The role of nanoparticles in plant biochemical, physiological, and molecular responses under drought stress: A review. Front Plant Sci 13:976179. https://doi.org/10.3389/fpls.2022.976179
53. Rathee M, Dalal P (2018) Emerging insect pests in Indian agriculture. Indian J Entomol 80:267–281
54. Rico CM, Majumdar S, Duarte-Gardea M, Peralta-Videa JR, Gardea-Torresdey JL (2011) Interaction of nanoparticles with edible plants and their possible implications in the food chain. J Agric Food Chem 59:3485–3498
55. Sarkar D, Rakshit A (2023) Amalgamation of farmers' bio-priming knowledge in integrated nutrient management for sustainable management of red cabbage soil under Middle Gangetic Plains, India. Environ Manag 72:382–395

56. Sarkar D, Pal S, Mehjabeen M, Singh V, Singh S, Pul S, Garg J, Rakshit A, Singh HB (2018) Addressing stresses in agriculture through bio-priming intervention. In: Rakshit A, Singh HB (eds) Advances in Seed Priming. Springer, Singapore, pp 107–113
57. Savary S, Willocquet L, Pethybridge SJ, Esker P, McRoberts N, Nelson A (2019) The global burden of pathogens and pests on major food crops. Nat Ecol Evol 3:430–439
58. Sembada AA, Lenggoro IW (2024) Transport of nanoparticles into plants and their detection methods. Nanomaterials 14:131. https://doi.org/10.3390/nano14020131
59. Shang Y, Hasan MK, Ahammed GJ, Li M, Yin H, Zhou J (2019) Applications of nanotechnology in plant growth and crop protection: a review. Molecules 24:2558. https://doi.org/10.3390/molecules24142558
60. Singh D, Arya S, Gupta B, Kaushik D, Arya VS, Kumar U, Singh K (2021) Applications of nanotechnology in forest management. J Nanosci Nanotechnol 21:3466–3480
61. Singh H, Desimone MF, Pandya S, Jasani S, George N, Adnan M, Aldarhami A, Bazaid AS, Alderhami SA (2023) Revisiting the green synthesis of nanoparticles: uncovering influences of plant extracts as reducing agents for enhanced synthesis efficiency and its biomedical applications. Int J Nanomedicine 18:4727–4750. https://doi.org/10.2147/IJN.S419369
62. Singh K, Thakur SS, Ahmed N, Alharby HF, Al-Ghamdi AJ, Al-Solami HM, Bahattab O, Yadav S (2022) Ecotoxicity assessment for environmental risk and consideration for assessing the impact of silver nanoparticles on soil earthworms. Heliyon 8:e11167. https://doi.org/10.1016/j.heliyon.2022.e11167
63. Singh M, Upadhyay L, Badekhan A, Shil S, Gautam SK, Anand A (2024) Leveraging remote sensing and nanotechnology to overcome barriers to agroforestry adoption by small holder farmers. J Sci Res Rep 30:113–140
64. Su Y, Ashworth V, Kim C, Adeleye AS, Rolshausen P, Roper C, White J, Jassby D (2019) Delivery, uptake, fate, and transport of engineered nanoparticles in plants: a critical review and data analysis. Environ Sci Nano 6:2311–2331
65. Tafazoli M, Hojjati SM, Biparva P, Kooch Y, Lamersdorf N (2017) Reduction of soil heavy metal bioavailability by nanoparticles and cellulosic wastes improved the biomass of tree seedlings. J Plant Nutr Soil Sci 180:683–693
66. Tang Y, Zhao W, Zhu G, Tan Z, Huang L, Zhang P, Gao L, Rui Y (2024) Nano-pesticides and fertilizers: solutions for global food security. Nanomaterials 14:90. https://doi.org/10.3390/nano14010090
67. Thakur S, Asthir B, Kaur G, Kalia A, Sharma A (2021) Zinc oxide and titanium dioxide nanoparticles influence heat stress tolerance mediated by antioxidant defense system in wheat. Cereal Res Commun 50:385–396
68. Usman M, Farooq M, Wakeel A, Nawaz A, Cheema SA, ur Rehman H, Ashraf I, Sanaullah M, (2020) Nanotechnology in agriculture: Current status, challenges and future opportunities. Sci Total Environ 721:137778. https://doi.org/10.1016/j.scitotenv.2020.137778
69. Vanlalveni C, Lallianrawna S, Biswas A, Selvaraj M, Changmai B, Rokhum SL (2021) Green synthesis of silver nanoparticles using plant extracts and their antimicrobial activities: A review of recent literature. RSC Adv 11:2804–2837. https://doi.org/10.1039/D0RA09941D
70. Wagay OA, Khan S, Rafeeq J, Pala NA, Bhat GM, Dutt V et al (2023) Nanotechnology and its potential application in forest and forest-based industries: a review. SKUAST J Res 25:527–537
71. Wang K, Wang Y, Li K, Wan Y, Wang Q, Zhuang Z, Guo Y, Li H (2020) Uptake, translocation and biotransformation of selenium nanoparticles in rice seedlings (*Oryza sativa* L.). J Nanobiotechnology 18:103. https://doi.org/10.1186/s12951-020-00659-6
72. Wang X, Xie H, Wang P, Yin H (2023) Nanoparticles in plants: Uptake, transport and physiological activity in leaf and root. Materials 16:3097. https://doi.org/10.3390/ma16083097
73. Xu Z, Long X, Jia Y, Zhao D, Pan X (2022) Occurrence, transport, and toxicity of nanomaterials in soil ecosystems: a review. Environ Chem Lett 20:3943–3969
74. Yadav A, Yadav K, Abd-Elsalam KA (2023) Nanofertilizers: Types, delivery and advantages in agricultural sustainability. Agrochemicals 2:296–336

75. Yuangyai C, Nembhard HB (2015) Design of experiments: a key to innovation in nanotechnology. In: Ahmed W, Jackson MJ (eds) Emerging nanotechnologies for manufacturing, 2nd edn. William Andrew Publishing, Waltham, pp 230–254
76. Zahra Z, Arshad M, Rafique R, Mahmood A, Habib A, Qazi IA, Khan SA (2015) Metallic nanoparticle ($TiO_2$ and $Fe_3O_4$) application modifies rhizosphere phosphorus availability and uptake by *Lactuca sativa*. J Agric Food Chem 63:6876–6882

# Synthesis of Nanoparticles

# Role of Agroforestry Plants in the Synthesis of Nanoparticles

**Vijay Devra**

**Abstract** Rising scientifically, the topic of green technology has attracted a lot of attention recently because of its numerous applications. It is a multidisciplinary field that is safe, non-hazardous and ecologically friendly in contrast to the chemical and physical processes used for producing nanoparticles. Variations in the biomaterials employed during the synthesis process will result in differing nanoparticle sizes, forms and biological functions. It is reported that agroforestry plants contain various phytochemicals, viz. carotenoids, vitamins, minerals, amino acids, sterols, glycosides, alkaloids, flavonoids and phenolics, they play roles as reducing as well as stabilizing agents during the synthesis of nanoparticles. This chapter provides an overview of the most recent research on distinct green synthesis techniques that rely on diverse agroforestry plant components, agro-waste & agricultural biomass for the development of nanoparticles. By minimizing the need for dangerous chemicals and promoting "biosynthesis," the use of these materials lowers the cost of synthesis.

**Keywords** Agroforestry plants · Plant components · Agro-wastes · Agricultural biomass

## 1 Introduction

Man has co-evolved with plants and their derived products since antiquity. Plant-based products are being used in modern life to offer living conditions, and health benefits, and to support humans in the treatment of many disorders [36]. Plant discovery for new bioactive phyto compounds and the advancement of current technology is a fast-expanding topic of study [28]. Plants have emerged as a source for nanoparticle fabrication in the last decade. This is a significant scientific discovery since it is viewed as a green methodology contributing to a global effort to protect the planet from future damage caused by man-made contaminants [79]. Developing sustainable technologies, creating and using materials, and replacing

V. Devra (✉)
Janki Devi Bajaj Government Girls College Kota, Kota, Rajasthan, India
e-mail: v_devra1@rediffmail.com

 
D. Jabborova et al. (eds.), *Nanomaterials in Agroforestry Systems*, Smart Nanomaterials Technology, https://doi.org/10.1007/978-981-96-1337-3_2

existing nanotechnology-related products with novel, non-toxic ones are all aspects of "sustainable" nanotechnology [85].

Several researchers have recently become interested in nanotechnology, which is the process of working with material with at least one dimension scaled between one and one hundred nanometres [34, 94]. Numerous novel and practical nanoscale materials have been produced due to research on nanoparticles (NPs). Nanomaterials (NMs) with nanoscale dimensions demonstrated unique features when compared to their bulk counterparts, as documented in several research [76]. In contrast to methods based on either chemical or physical, green synthesized NPs are thought to be environmentally beneficial since they are less hazardous, require suitable equipment to produce and contain fewer harmful compounds [92, 93]. Although nanoparticles production from plant or plant component extract is gaining popularity, biological synthesis still uses bacteria, fungi, algae and various plant parts [94]. According to Husen and Iqbal [33], biological methods or environmentally friendly technology have become important tools for producing NPs with acceptable potential qualities and assistance in getting beyond the limitations and disadvantages of chemical and physical synthesis. Many researchers have recently developed nanoparticles (NPs) using various plant parts, such as leaves [63], stem [86], bark [20], pulp [73], latex [8], seeds [34], flowers [41], fruits [52] and root [89]. Since plant roots include a variety of nutrients and food reserves, they can be regarded as one of the essential components for the manufacturing of NPs [103].

In addition, they contain proteins, enzymes, carbohydrates, phenolics, alkaloids, flavonoids and terpenoids, among other chemical components. These metabolites play a vital function in stabilizing and capping metal ions and converting them into desirable nanoparticles. The following topics are briefly reviewed in this chapter: (1) The most recent methods for generating metal-oxide nanoparticles (NPs) from agro-forestry plants; (2) Agri-food waste; and (3) Agricultural biomass, with applications in several cutting-edge domains [38].

## 2 Nanoparticles Synthesis from Agroforestry Plant Parts

One environmentally benign approach in nanotechnology has been the creation of metal nanoparticles through plant-mediated processes. Plants are highly inclined to synthesize them because they are sustainable, reusable and give the nanoparticles a built-in stabilizing agent straight away. A recent study found that the eco-friendly production of nanoparticles of metallic materials utilizing various plant segments are crucial straightforward, affordable and reliable method [60]. Many plants and herbs include higher antioxidants in the photochemical components of leaves, stems, seeds and fruits. As a result, the benefit of antioxidants derived from plants offers a significant opportunity for biological research and technology to collaborate on the creation of nanoparticles [72]. These synthesis methods can be used with minimal detrimental effects on the environment, establishing new benchmarks for extraordinarily environmentally friendly and sustainable technologies. Various plant parts

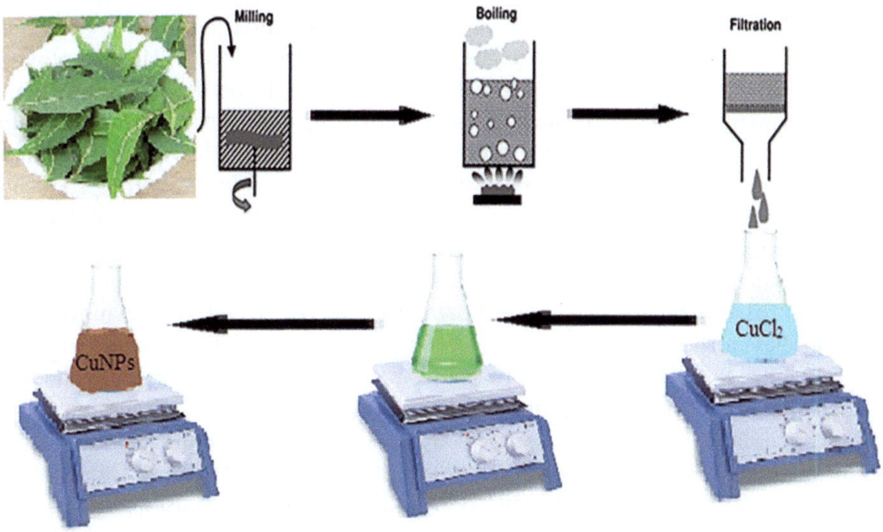


**Fig. 1** Sustainable nanoparticles production with agroforestry plants

are used for the synthesis of metallic nanoparticles [84]. Alkaloids, polysaccharides, terpenoids, bioactive polyphenol proteins and other plant extracts are essential for reducing and eventually stabilizing ionic metallic particles [87]. At room temperature, thoroughly mix the metal solution of salt into the Plant-derived extracts (Fig. 1). A shift in the reaction solution's colour denotes the start of the biological reduction of salt instants and the formation of nanoparticles [82].

To create green nanoparticles with plant assistance, follow these three procedures: activation, growth and termination [64]. During the activation stage, plant metabolites react to remove metal ions from their salt solution. A metal atom is nucleated when metal ions transition from oxidation states of mono- or divalent metals to zero-valent states. Next comes the "development" phase, in which the nanoparticles come together to create different structures, including rectangles, circles, blocks, strings and strands [4]. When plant biomolecules cap the nanoparticle during the later stages of termination, it enters its stable phase.

## *2.1 Leaf Extracts*

Several researchers have confirmed that using different plant leaf extracts to produce metallic nanoparticles is an environmentally benign method. According to Nilavukkarasi et al. [67], extract of C. zeylanica leaves was used for the production of silver nanoparticles and they show good antiproliferative features and remarkable efficacy against harmful bacteria as reported by toxicology research. Machado et al. [57] investigated the feasibility of utilizing a range of leaf samples to produce iron nanoparticles. The extract from the leaf capacity as an antioxidant was also evaluated. The green tea and oak pomegranate extracts were the richest. Water employed as a solvent in the manufacture of leaf extract is known to be the least expensive and environmentally friendly method of synthesizing nanoparticles. Azadirachta indica (Neem) leaf was utilized to synthesize AgNPs using a low-cost reductant, which had the greatest absorption peak in UV light. It was found that the produced AgNPs had visible spectra at 433 nm. The oxidative destruction of harmful dyes by advanced oxidation processes in the presence of water has demonstrated the exceptional catalytic capabilities of synthesized AgNPs [65]. Previous studies employing leaf extract from Pisonia grandis have shown that Zinc Oxide and Magnesium Oxide Nanoparticles can be biosynthesized in an economically and environmentally sustainable way [40]. A GCMS analysis revealed that the plant extract contained fifty phytochemicals [95]. According to FTIR investigations, biological components that contain phenolic compounds in an extract are essential for stabilizing characteristics on zinc and magnesium nanoparticles. Another study [2] that employed Cassia alata leaf broth to demonstrate phyto-assisted ZnO NP synthesis also used zinc acetate (0.01 M). SEM data show an abundance of nanoparticles with spherical shapes in the 60–80 nm size range. It was found that biosynthesized $TiO_2$ nanoparticles ranged in size from 15 to 50 nm and had round forms [101]. Additionally, they examined the role of $TiO_2$, which showed broad-spectrum antibacterial action against a wide variety of infections.

## 2.2 *Fruit Substance*

Scientists have used fruit to create metallic nanoparticles. Terminates chebula fruit extract was used to create iron and palladium nanoparticles [50]. The polyphenol-rich T. chebula extract exhibits a redox potential of 0.63 V vs. saturated calomel electrode, according to cyclic voltammetry measurements, which reduces the concentration of iron chloride to FeNPs. Prosopis farcta fruit extract was used as a reducing agent in the synthesis of silver nanoparticles [81]. The study found that the overall flavonoid and phenolic component level of green-silver nanoparticles was higher than that of the plant extract by themselves. Compared to P. farcta fruit extract alone, green-silver nanoparticles exhibited greater reactive and antimicrobial properties. Nakkala et al. [66] described the generation of gold nanoparticles using fruit extract of Piper longum, along with details on their experimental catalytic and antioxidant activities. According to the researchers' findings, these significantly catalytic AuNPs can be used to remove harmful colours from industrial effluents [102].

## 2.3 Seed Extract

Citrullus colocynthis seed extract in aqueous form was used to create AgNPs as agent for stabilization and reduction [9]. AgNPs that were biosynthesized demonstrated potent antibacterial activities against Pseudomonas aeruginosa, E. coli, Methicillin-resistant S. aureus and bacterium Staphylococcus aureus. A different study created a green way using an aqueous extract of Durio zibethinus seed to produce silver nanoparticles by analysing the antibacterial, catalytic and toxic characteristics. AgNPs showed greater photocatalytic activity against blue methylene and antibacterial activity against brine shrimp [98]. Synthesized AgNPs have potential applications in nanotechnology, biology, water, pharmaceuticals and biosensors in the future [83].

## 2.4 Extract from Bark

The extract from the bark of Mimusops elengi was used to produce AuNPs in a green manner at room temperature. The bark extract's polyphenols functioned as agent that reduces and stabilizes. Synthesized AuNPs have played a catalytic role in the breakdown of nitrophenol into the corresponding aminophenol, as shown by Majumdar et al. [59]. Using a $PdCl_2$ solution, palladium nanoparticles (PdNPs) were created in an easy and eco-friendly manner [46]. Gum ghatti is a non-hazardous renewable organic material made from the Anogeissus latifolia timber, was utilised by researchers as a stabilizing and reducing agent. The produced particles exhibit remarkable catalytic behaviour in environmental remediation. Spruce bark (Picea abies L.) was successfully employed in a study to synthesize AgNPs using it as a biosource of low-cost, non-hazardous reducing and stabilizing compounds [31]. According to Tanase et al. [99], several parameters' influence on the carefully regulated synthesis of AgNPs were examined. These comprised the length of incubation period, the extract/salt silver nitrate ratio and the reactant concentration.

## 2.5 Root Extract

Furthermore, studies with the use of root extract of Lantana camara and Cibotium barometz [78, 104] for the production of silver nanoparticles. Another study describes a straightforward, affordable, eco-friendly and green synthesis method that uses extract from the roots of Asparagus racemosus as a capping agent and synthesis reducer producing crystalline, uniformly spherical nano silver particles with dimensions between 10 and 17 nm when optimized conditions [51]. The generated AgNPs were evaluated in relation to certain microbiological organisms.

## 2.6 *Extract from Flowers*

In another study, Nyctanthes arbor-tristis aqueous floral extract was employed as a natural reducing substance to create ZnO nanoparticles [39]. The study found that the diameter variation of these NPs was 12–32 nm. However, studies are being conducted to determine the NPs' antifungal potential. Another straightforward and environmentally friendly synthesis of PdNPs was described by Shaik et al. [88], using the L. Origanum vulgare extract's aerial component as a biodegrading reagent. The reduction as well as stabilizing factors are brought about by the phytochemicals that are currently present in the Organum vulgare extract. FTIR data confirms that the Organum vulgare extract acts as a reductant and renders the NPs functional. Kar and Ray [43] developed an innovative, eco-friendly method for synthesizing NiNPs. A modification directed towards the magnet in the final product. The production of metallic nanostructures from the resources of plants is shown in Table 1, and information about further recent investigations is provided.

# 3 Synthesis of Nanoparticles Using Agro-Wastes

Many agricultural byproducts are relevant in nanobiotechnology, and growing the use of harvesting residues as substitutes for biological materials for sustainable nanotechnology has attracted a lot of interest [21]. Dry and ground agricultural waste materials can be extracted using hot water in a simple procedure to produce extracts that include active biomolecules that facilitate the development of nanoparticles (Table 2). The environment serves as a "treasure" for waste products, particularly food waste, which is useful for the generation of nanoparticles [90]. In view of the advantages, it offers in terms of technology, economics and the environment, the process of producing nanomaterials utilizing agricultural waste as a substrate is rapidly achieving acceptance [83]. Agro-wastes, which might be from kitchen, horticultural, or aquaculture operations, are rich in polyphenolic compounds, lignin, cellulose and chitin, among other significant bio compounds [24].

A sustainable process for the manufacture of AuNPs from leftover Citrullus lunatus var (watermelon) waste was described by Chamsa-ard et al. [18]. The antimicrobial characteristics of several extracted and synthetic materials. By using the Kirby-Bauer resistivity approach, AuNPs were assumed. According to the study, the resulting AuNPs have antimicrobial properties against the bacterium Staphylococcus epidermidis and Escherichia coli. Dang et al. [19] investigated a room-temperature, ecologically sustainable method for generating gold nanoparticles with excess Macadamia shells. The structural analysis results show that the gold nanoparticles were circular, rectangular and polygonal in shape and that they were crystal-like, with dimensions that varied between 50 and 2 µm. The antimicrobial efficacy of biosynthesized gold nanoparticles against the bacterium Staphylococcus epidermidis and Escherichia coli was demonstrated. One more study reported the production of

**Table 1** Utilizing agroforestry plant parts for biogenic synthesis of nanoparticles

| Biological agent | Nanoparticles | Dimensions (nm) and morphology | The potential uses | Citations |
|---|---|---|---|---|
| Extract of leaves | | | | |
| Capparis zeylanical | Ag nanoparticles | 23 nm, round | Antibacterial and antiproliferative properties | Nilavukkarasi et al. [67] |
| Azadirachta indica | Cu nanoparticles | 48 nm, cubic | Regarding orange G dye degradation | Nagar and Devra [63] |
| C. alata | Zinc oxide nanoparticles | 60 nm, round in shape | Antimicrobial agent that targets E. Coli | Agarwal et al. [2] |
| Azadirachta indica | Ag nanoparticles | 9 nm, round in shape | Catalyst for the deterioration of fabric colours | Nagar and Devra [65] |
| Azadirachta indica | Fe nanoparticles | | Catalyst for the deterioration of textile dyes | Rathore and Devra [79] |
| Folearia vulgaria | CuO nanoparticles | 25 nm | Potentials for dermatological wound healing, antifungal, antibacterial and antioxidant properties without cytotoxicity | Zangeneh et al. [109] |
| Globulus eucalyptus | Cu oxide nanoparticles | 16.7–22.5 nm | Strong antibacterial and biofilm-preventing substance | Ali et al. [5] |
| Achillea millefolium | CuO nanoparticles | 28 nm, semi round in shape | Applications in biomedicine | Rabiee et al. [75] |
| Plukenetia volubilis L | $Cu_2O$ nanoparticles | 6–10 nm, round in shape | Decomposition of organic contaminants in water using nano catalyst | Kumar et al. [49] |
| Extract of fruit | | | | |
| Syzygium cumini | Ag nanoparticles | | Nanomedicine applications | Chakravarty et al. [17] |
| Phyllanthus emblica | Ag nanoparticles | 30 nm, hexagonal | Antibacterial uses | Renuka et al. (2020) |
| Prosopis farcta | Ag nanoparticles | 12.6 nm | Applications in biomedicine | Salari et al. [81] |
| Extract of seed | | | | |

(continued)

**Table 1** (continued)

| Biological agent | Nanoparticles | Dimensions (nm) and morphology | The potential uses | Citations |
|---|---|---|---|---|
| Pimpinella anisum | Ag & Au nanoparticles | 18–22 nm,16-22 nm, round in shape | Antibacterial and antifungal substances | Zayed et al. [110] |
| Pepo cucurbita | Titanium oxide nanoparticles | Three-dimensional, greater than 100 nm | Numerous uses | Abisharani et al. [1] |
| Durio zibenthinus | Ag nanoparticles | 20–75 nm, round, cylindrical form | Applications such as photocatalysis and antibacterial | Sumitha et al. [98] |
| Extract of bark | | | | |
| Terminalia arjuna | Au nanoparticles | 20–50 nm, round shape | Potential for neuroprotection through anti-amyloidogenic, anticholinesterase and antioxidant properties | Suganthy et al. [97] |
| The picea abies | Ag nanoparticles | Compact 226-nm cubs | Antimicrobial substance | Tanase et al. [99] |
| Extract of erythrina caffra | Ag nanoparticles | ~16 nm, round in form | Antimicrobial substance | Shaik et al. [89] |
| Cinnamomum verum | Mn nanoparticles | 50–100 nm, round shape | Antimicrobial agents and photocatalysts | Kamran et al. [42] |
| Extract of root | | | | |
| Cibotium barometz | Au nanoparticles | 6–28 nm, round shape | Antibacterial action against escherichia coli among other pathogens | Wang et al. [104] |
| Lantana camara | Au nanoparticles | 11–32 nm, round shape | Cytotoxic and antioxidant qualities | Ramkumar et al. [78] |
| A. racemosus | Ag nanoparticles | 10–17 nanometer, round | Applications in biomedicine and biopharmaceuticals | Kumar et al. [51] |
| V. Vigenis berberis | Ag nanoparticles | 30–70 round | Antimicrobial substance | Behravan et al. [12] |
| Extract of flower | | | | |
| Wyetanthes arbortristis | ZnO nanoparticles | 12–32 nm crystalline nature | Anti-fungal substance | Jamdagni et al. [39] |
| Hibiscus rosa sinesis | Ni nanoparticles | | | Kar & Ray [43] |
| L. Origanum vulgare | Pd nanoparticles | ~2 nm, round | Utilizing catalysts | Shaik et al. [88] |

(continued)

**Table 1** (continued)

| Biological agent | Nanoparticles | Dimensions (nm) and morphology | The potential uses | Citations |
|---|---|---|---|---|
| Acuminate bauhinia | Ag nanoparticles | 17 nm uniform | On MSCs, osteogenic differentiation and proliferation | Hu et al. [32] |
| Astragalus magnifera | Ag nanoparticles | 10–20 nm, round | Antimicrobial substance | Ameen et al. [6] |

$Cu/Cu_2O/CuO$ NPs for various applications utilizing polyphenols from pomegranate extract. The results showed that when synthesized nanoparticles were aimed toward the electrode surface, they performed well electrochemically [26]. Bibi et al. [13] proposed that cobalt nitrate hexahydrate was used as a precursor and Peel extract from the fruit of Punica granatum was used as a reducer to make the artificial cobalt oxide NPs. For the environmentally friendly formation of silver nanoparticles, the peel of orange pith and citrus debris make excellent substrates and reducing reagents. According to Lopez-Tellez et al. [56], the bio-reduction process produced NPs with a reasonable size distribution that is approximately 5 nm in spherical form. The orange peel aqueous extract was used in the one-pot synthesis of green Ag Nanoparticles with an average particle size of 15–20 nm, as reported by Saratale et al. [84]. The produced AgNPs show anticancer action against C6 cells of rat glial tumours and are very efficient against a variety of microbial infections. In a two-step procedure that involved atom creation and atom compounding, [53] investigated the method for producing palladium nanoparticles (PdNPs) from watermelon peel. Using the WRAE accessible reducing groups, a specific amount of the palladium ions in the solution must be reduced initially. Based on the FTIR data of the particles, the polyhydroxy compounds groups of WRAE have been discovered in the production and restoration of PdNPs. Additionally, the Suzuki coupling reaction made use of the synthesized palladium nanoparticles' catalytic effectiveness. These findings imply that agro-waste and watermelon rind can be used to generate Pd-to-Pd NPs for catalytic purposes. Mango peel extract, a typical agricultural waste, was employed as a reducer and stabilizer to produce small and monodisperse GNPs. Krishnaswamy et al. [48] evaluated the potential for using food waste to create AuNPs that are obtained during grape processing. The high concentration of polyphenolic chemicals found in grape seeds, skin and stem, including epicatechin, catechin, proanthocyanidin and tannins, may be the compound accountable for stabilizing and reducing the concentration of AuNPs [10].

The concept is based on biomass extract's capacity to act as a stabilizing and reducing agent. Bankar and Associates [11] used extract from banana peels to create palladium nanoparticles. The water-based extract was produced by boiling the banana peel in water, and after that, acetone was added to the residue. When palladium chloride was mixed with the resulting precipitate, palladium was reduced and helped to

**Table 2** Biogenic synthesis of nanoparticles using agro-waste & agricultural biomass

| Biological agent | Nanoparticles | Dimensions (nm) and morphology | The potential uses | Citations |
|---|---|---|---|---|
| Agro-waste | | | | |
| Waste watermelon | Au nanoparticles | 100 nm-2.5 um, hexagonal, triangle and sphere | Uses in pharmacies | Chamsa-ard et al. [18] |
| Cane sugar biomass | $Cu_2O$ nanoparticles | 38.1 nm, erratic | Harmful coloured pollutants decomposition using solar energy | Yadav et al. [106] |
| Macaddamia nut shells | Au nanoparticles | 50 nm-2 um, hexagon, triangle and sphere | Uses in pharmacies | Dang et al. [19] |
| Extract from pomegranate peel | Cu oxide nanoparticles | 5–20 nm, almost round in shape | The use as catalysts and capacitors | Fuku et al. [26] |
| Shells of walnuts | Cu nanoparticles | 15–20 nm, 60–80 nm, Agglomerated | Applications in foodstuffs and medicine | Mehdizadeh et al. [62] |
| Peels of oranges | Ag nanoparticles | 15–20 nm, round in shape | Antimicrobial, antitumor and anti-inflammatory effects against disease in humans | Saratale et al. [84] |
| Waste corn-cob | Ag & Au nanoparticles | AgNPs-2–28 nm, spherical, AuNPs-5–50 nm multiple shape | Used in the sewage treatment process | Doan et al. [22] |
| Coffee ground wastes | Ag nanoparticles | 8.2–10.4 nm, spherical | It is environmentally favourable because of plant waste | Zuorro et al. [113] |
| Agricultural biomass | | | | |
| Agri-biomass derived lignin | ZnO nanocomposite | 3–5 nm, spherical | Uses as antibacterial and UV-blocking components for usage in a variety of sectors | Kaur et al. [44] |

(continued)

**Table 2** (continued)

| Biological agent | Nanoparticles | Dimensions (nm) and morphology | The potential uses | Citations |
|---|---|---|---|---|
| Biomass from agricultural waste | Metal oxide nanomaterials | | Applications of nanomaterials generated from agricultural leftovers, particularly in catalysis | Zamani et al. [108] |
| Silica rice husk | AgNPs/$SiO_2$ | 25 nm, spherical | Uses of silica rice husk-derived nanomaterial, especially in catalysis | Andas and Adam [7] |
| Rice husk biomass | Pd (0) ($Fe_3O_4$@$SiO_2$-Pd) | 31–73 nm, spherical | Used as a Suzuki coupling reaction nanocatalyst that is magnetically recoverable | Khazaei et al. [45] |
| Rice husk silica | Nano $Sio_2$ | Very tiny crystalline NPs | Materials made of nano silica have been created for a variety of technical uses | Hussain et al. [35] |
| Rice husk silica | $Mg_2SiO_4$ | 80–85 nm, spherical | A less expensive method of creating nano-crystallite forsterite particles, making it suitable for large-scale manufacturing of the same | Mathur et al. [61] |
| Sugar cane bagasse | $TiO_2$NPs | 5–20 nm | Used as photo-catalyst | Xue et al. [105] |
| Sugar cane bagasse | Magnetic iron oxide nanoparticles | 50–200 nm | Used for the adsorption of $Cr^{6+}$ found in leather industry wastewater | Jabasingh et al. [37] |
| Sugarcane leafy trash | Carbonaceous composite with a sponge-like hybrid MgO structure | MgO flakes with carbon sponge shaped like nanotubes | Utilized as an adsorbent to remove methylene blue (MB), Pb (II) and arsenate (As(V)) | Li et al. [55] |

(continued)

**Table 2** (continued)

| Biological agent | Nanoparticles | Dimensions (nm) and morphology | The potential uses | Citations |
|---|---|---|---|---|
| Bagasse from sugar cane | Nanocomposite of bagasse from sugar cane & $Fe_3O_4$ | | Utilized as absorbents in the treatment of effluents containing hazardous metal ion contamination | Carvalho et al. [16] |
| Wheat straw | Nano $SiO_2$ | 100–200 nm | Apply for pyrano synthesis [2, 3-c] derivatives of pyrazoles | Patel et al. [71] |
| Wheat straw | AgNPs, AuNPs, CuNPs, NiNPs | | Utilized in the fields of food processing, medical, water treatment, textile engineering, sensors, imaging and catalysis | Sharma et al. [91] |
| Wheat straw | Lignocellulosic nanomaterials | | Bioplastics applications | Pascoli et al. [69] |

form nanoparticles. Later, using a mango peel extract produced in water, [107] synthesized AuNPs. The generated nanomaterials have sizes between 6.03 and 18.01 nm. In a different study, Zuorro et al. [113] used phenolic extracts from spent coffee ground wastes and bioactive compounds produced in aqueous ethanol solvent to assess the feasibility of AgNP production. It also conforms with the concepts of the circular economy and is environmentally benign due to the utilization of plant waste and aqueous ethanol as a solvent. A facile thermal decomposition technique was used to synthesize Ferric oxide nanocomposites from the lignocellulosic agricultural waste of papaya leaves [3]. The iron (II) and (III) solutions were mixed with cleaned and dried papaya leaf powder, followed by NaOH solution was added. Following drying at 353 K, the black precipitate ($Fe_3O_4$-NC) was heated to calcine in an air-filled furnace to yield nanoparticles with a size range of 18–46 nm. With a 96% removal effectiveness, $Fe_3O_4$-NC was shown to be the most effective nanocomposite for chlorazol black. The production of supported hydrous aluminium oxide nanoparticles utilizing tea waste was documented by Cai et al. [15]. Supported porous alumina was utilized to defluoridate drinking water by the anion exchange of fluoride with sulphate ions. Another study reported that pine needles might be used to generate nanocomposites of nanocellulose and $NiFe_2O_4$ nanoparticles [30]. Carbon nanofibers (CNF) derived from pine needles were synthesized to produce these nanocomposites. The authors observed that supported $NiFe_2O_4$ functions as a powerful catalytic system for the reduction of nitrophenols and the oxidative decomposition of Remazol Black 5 (RB5). Activated carbon-supported 10 nm titanium oxide nanoparticles with 10 nm size derived from hazelnut shells or olive residues are employed in the photodegradation of methylene blue as the catalyst. [23]. Guo et al. [29] used porous carbon obtained from honey pomelo peel to synthesize $NiCo_2O_4$ nanocomposites. After mixing urea, Co (II), and Ni (II) solution with porous carbon and Carbon-supported $NiCo_2O_4$ nanosheets were obtained by heating it to 120 °C. Recently, several methods for producing biomass fuels, proteins, fertilizers and carbon from the accessible waste biomass have been developed for commercial application [47].

## 4 Nanoparticles Synthesis Employing Crop Biomass

The most plentiful renewable biomass on the planet, agricultural biomass has long helped humans and animals survive (Vani et al. 2023). There have been initiatives in the past several years to investigate novel approaches for reducing waste generation and increasing the value of solid agro-industrial wastes [27]. The main crops that produce a lot of trash, including shells, sorghum, husks and biomass, are rice, corn, wheat and sugarcane [80]. The advancement of nanomaterials has impacted the environment by creating new opportunities for applications in various industries, such as technological devices, the universe, farming, power generation and medicine [58]. Many techniques, including milling, aggregation, precipitation and others, were developed over the preceding period to create nanostructures [100]. Numerous techniques can synthesize a wide range of nanomaterials. Particularly for rice materials and debris (Fig. 2), biomass from agricultural waste has continuously drawn attention as an affordable, environmentally friendly energy resource [77]. Cellulose and lignin make up the majority of the cell walls of agro-waste. The substance Lignin is expected to be a beneficial good and a significant resource with a range of applications, according to Zhu et al. [112] (Table 2). Since natural biomass and biomolecules are being used to create nanomaterials, additional possibilities are now easily available. For example, lignocellulosic and chrysotile fibres can be used to create nanocomposites [68]. Eutrophication and water bloom are the results of agricultural practices that continuously add phosphates to water bodies. It might be difficult to remove phosphate from wastewater economically and efficiently. By using in situ hydrothermal synthesis, wheat straw and UiO-66 nanoparticles, a unique composite of the material nanocomposites (St + @UiO-66) has been developed by [74]. According to research done in [39] by Kaur et al. cellulose had been extracted from inexpensive waste biomass to aid in the synthesis of ZnO nanocomposite. Even at high ionic strength, nanocomposites demonstrated twice the adsorption capability of an individual. Composites showed remarkable antioxidant, UV-blocking and antibacterial activities because of the lignin content, which ZnO further increased [70].

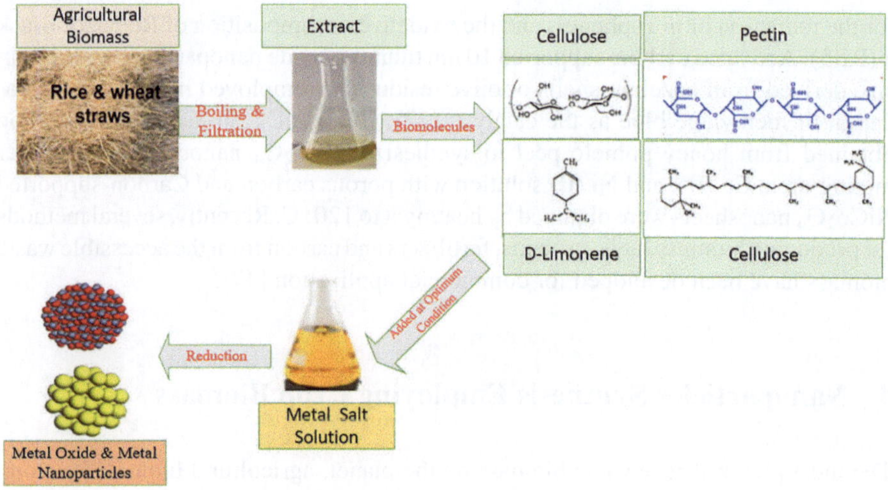


**Fig. 2** Synthesis of nanoparticles using agricultural biomass

## *4.1 Rice Husk*

Using a solid-state technique and silica recovered from rice husks [54, 61] generated nanoparticles of silica by acid-washing rice husk from Vietnam. The environmental conditions, duration and concentration of surfactant were utilized to regulate the nanoparticle morphology. Thus, it was shown that silica-supported imidazole could be produced using these organo-functionalized $SiO_2$NPs [108]. The fusion temperature of the rice husk mostly influences mesopore diameters and pore volumes. Mesoporous silicas have been generated from sodium silicate solution using rice kernel charcoal, NaOH solution, and CTAB as an agent that drives structure [111]. The silica materials' specific surface area, pore size and standard diameter of pores have been demonstrated to have a mesoporous structure [7]. In a different study, 14 nm-sized silica/carbon hybrid nanoparticles were produced by pyrolyzing powdered rice husk in a high pressure and temperature reactor [14]. Using this nanotechnology, a renewable and recyclable polymer called Ecoflex was converted into a nanocomposite, using a 3D printing technique. Palladium ($Fe_3O_4$NP@$SiO_2$-Pd) is supported by silica-coated magnetic nanoparticles ($Fe_3O_4$NP@$SiO_2$), which are made by dispersing $Fe_3O_4$ nanoparticles and silica obtained from rice husks in ammonia solution [45]. Le et al. synthesized silica nanoparticles in [54]. Next, employing this nanomaterial as a catalyst, in the presence of a remained eggshell, which serves as an affordable and sustainable solid base. Investigations were done on the Suzuki linking of aryl iodides and bromides that are electron-rich or electron-poor, preparation for 80–85 nm forsterite ($Mg_2SiO_4$) nanoparticles).

### 4.2 *Sugarcane Biomass*

Sugarcane bagasse is a widely available biological produced by agriculture from the sugarcane and alcohol industries. The quantity of biomass templates significantly affected size control when using SCB to adjust the size of titanium oxide nanoparticles ($TiO_2$NPs) [105]. $TiO_2$NPs supported by SCBs range in size 5–20 nm. Methyl orange was used as an azo dye with the availability of visible light to assess the catalytic activity of $TiO_2$NPs supported by sugar cane bagasse. Jabasingh and associates [37] used ammonia and sugar cane bagasse to coprecipitate Fe(III)/Fe(II) in an inert atmosphere to create 50–200 nm metallic FeO nanoparticles. This magnetic material has the potential to facilitate $Cr^{6+}$ adsorption. Additionally, magnesium oxide hybrid carbon-based nanocomposite that resembles sponges was created by thermal breakdown under N2 flow using sorghum leaves and magnesium acetate as a reactive substrate [55]. This nanomaterial was made of carbon sponge that resembled nanotubes and flakes of magnesium oxide that were the size of nanometres [96].

### 4.3 *Wheat Straw*

Patel and colleagues [71] calcined wheat straw that had been acid-washed, treated the straw with NaOH solution, then neutralized it with HCl to generate 100–200 nm silica nanoparticles. A four-component, one-pot method for synthesizing derivatives of pyrano [2, 3-c] pyrazole was used to study this catalyst. In another study, KOH-containing wheat straw was calcined in an inert atmosphere using salt of ferric nitrate and grain straw are used to produce a spongy carbon-supported $Fe_2O_3$ tiny layer [25].

## 5 Conclusion

To synthesize metal nanoparticles, a variety of techniques are used as physical, chemical-based and physiological methods. The majority of these issues have to do with shape, size distribution, stability, crystalline growth control and nanoparticle aggregation. Agricultural byproducts and plant derived metal particles are more stable than those derived from other creatures. Furthermore, producing uniformly sized metal nanoparticles for industrial and scale-up applications uses a simple, eco-friendly process. Numerous plant and waste material biomolecules, including polysaccharides, alcoholic compounds, alkaloids, proteins and enzymes, might contribute to creating, stabilization and biodegradation of metal NPs. Future studies will concentrate on recombinant organisms and the adjustment of reaction parameters to process an enormous quantity of enzymes, proteins and other macromolecules participating in the creation of nanoparticles. Furthermore, the increasing need for safe and ecologically friendly biomedical technologies is catered to through their sustainable synthesis techniques. Upcoming initiatives to mitigate the negative effects of pollution and improve ecosystem sustainability may benefit from producing innovative green nanomaterials and their use in extensive environmental restoration programmes.

## References


1. Abisharani JM, Devikala S, Kumar RD, Arthanareeswari M, Kamaraj P (2019) Green synthesis of $TiO_2$ nanoparticles using Cucurbita pepo [ka1] seeds extract. Mater Today: Proc 14:302–307
2. Agarwal H, Kumar SV, Rajeshkumar S (2017) A review on green synthesis of zinc oxide nanoparticles–an eco-friendly approach. Resour Effic Technol 3(4):406–13
3. Ahmed MJK, Ahmaruzzaman M (2015) Fabrication and characterization of novel lignocellulosic biomass tailored $Fe_3O_4$ nanocomposites: influence of annealing temperature and chlorazol black E sequestration. RSC Adv 5:107466–107473
4. Akhtar MS, Panwar J, Yun YS (2013) Biogenic synthesis of metallic nanoparticles by plant extracts. ACS Sustain Chem Eng 1(6):591–602
5. Ali K, Ahmed B, Ansari SM, Saquib Q, Al-Khedhairy AA, Dwivedi S, Alshaeri M, Khan MS, Musarrat J (2019) Comparative in situ ROS mediated killing of bacteria with bulk analogue, *Eucalyptus* leaf extract (ELE)-capped and bare surface copper oxide nanoparticles. Mater Sci Eng C 100:747–758
6. Ameen F, Srinivasan P, Selvankumar T, Kamala-Kannan S, Al Nadhari S, Almansob A, Dawoud T, Govarthanan M, (2019) Phytosynthesis of silver nanoparticles using *Mangifera indica* flower extract as bioreductant and their broad-spectrum antibacterial activity. Bioorg Chem 88:102970
7. Andas J, Adam F (2016) One-pot synthesis of nanoscale silver supported biomass-derived silica. Mater Today Proc 3:1345–1350
8. Arsalani S, Guidelli EJ, Silveira MA, Salmon CEG, Araujo JFDF, Bruno AC et al (2019) Magnetic $Fe_3O_4$ nanoparticles coated by natural rubber latex as MRI contrast agent. J Magn Magn Mater 475: 458–464
9. Azizi S, Mohamad R, Rahim RA, Ariff MR, AB, (2017) Hydrogel beads bio-nanocomposite based on kappa-carrageenan and green synthesized silver nanoparticles for biomedical applications. Int J Biol Macromol 104:423–431
10. Bala JM, Vennila JJ, Ganesh S, Sachidanand SSS (2011) Analysis of active components in Acanthus ilicifolius leaves for their potential chemoprotective activity against hepatocellular carcinoma: an in silico approach
11. Bankar A, Joshi B, Kumar AR, Zinjarde S (2010) Banana peel extract mediated novel route for the synthesis of silver nanoparticles. Colloids Surf A 368(1–3):58–63
12. Behravan M, Panahi AH, Naghizadeh A, Ziaee M, Mahdavi R, Mirzapour A (2019) Facile green synthesis of silver nanoparticles using *Berberis vulgaris* leaf and root aqueous extract and its antibacterial activity. Int J Biol Macromol 124:148–154
13. Bibi I, Nazar N, Iqbal M, Kamal S, Nawaz H, Nouren S, Safa Y, Jilani K, Sultan M, Ata S, Rehman F, Abbas M (2017) Green and eco-friendly synthesis of cobalt-oxide nanoparticle: characterization and photo-catalytic activity. Adv Powder Technol 28:2035–2043
14. Biswas MC, Jeelani S, Rangari V (2017) Influence of biobased silica/carbon hybrid nanoparticles on thermal and mechanical properties of biodegradable polymer films. Compos Commun 1(4):43–53
15. Cai H, Chen G, Peng C, Xu L, Zhu X, Zhang Z, Dong Y, Shang G, Ke F, Gao H, Wan X (2017) Enhanced removal of fluoride by tea waste supported hydrous aluminium oxide nanoparticles:

anionic polyacrylamide mediated aluminium assembly and adsorption mechanism. RSC Adv 5(37):29266–29275
16. Carvalho JT, Milani PA, Consonni JL, Labuto G, Carrilho EN (2021) Nanomodified sugarcane bagasse biosorbent: synthesis, characterization, and application for Cu (II) removal from aqueous medium. Environ Sci Pollut Res 4744–55
17. Chakravarty A, Ahmad I, Singh P, Sheikh MU, Aalam G, Sagadevan S, Ikram S (2022) Green synthesis of silver nanoparticles using fruits extracts of Syzygium cumini and their bioactivity. Chem Phys Lett 795:139493
18. Chums-ard W, Fawcett D, Fung CC, Poinern GE (2017) Biogenic synthesis of gold nanoparticles from waste watermelon and their antibacterial activity against Escherichia coli and Staphylococcus epidermidis. Int J Res Med Sciences 7(7):2499–2505
19. Dang H, Fawcett D, Poinern GEJ (2019) Green synthesis of gold nanoparticles from waste macadamia nut shells and their antimicrobial activity against Escherichia coli and Staphylococcus epidermis. Int J Res Med Sci 7:1171–1177
20. Das M, Smita SS (2018) Biosynthesis of silver nanoparticles using bark extracts of Butea monosperma (Lam.) Taub. and study of their antimicrobial activity. Appl Nanosci 8:1059–1067
21. Devra V (2022) Plant and agri-waste-mediated synthesis of metal nanoparticles. In: Agri-Waste and Microbes for Production of Sustainable Nanomaterials. Elsevier, pp, 47–77
22. Doan VD, Luc VS, Nguyen TL, Nguyen TD, Nguyen TD (2020) Utilizing waste corn-cob in biosynthesis of noble metallic nanoparticles for antibacterial effect and catalytic degradation of contaminants. Environ Sci Pollut Res 6148–62
23. Donar YO, Bilge S, Sınağ A, Pliekhov O (2018) $TiO_2$/Carbon materials derived from hydrothermal carbonization of waste biomass: a highly efficient, low-cost visible-light-driven photocatalyst. Chem Cat Chem 10(5):1134–1139
24. Elemike EE, Ekennia AC, Onwudiwe DC, Ezeani RO (2022) Agro-waste materials: sustainable substrates in nanotechnology. In: Agri-waste and microbes for production of sustainable nanomaterials. Elsevier, pp 187–214
25. Fang K, Chen J, Zhou X, Mei C, Tian Q, Xu J et al (2018) Decorating biomass-derived porous carbon with $Fe_2O_3$ ultrathin film for high-performance supercapacitors. Electrochim Acta 261:198–205
26. Fuku X, Modibedi M, Mathe M (2020) Green synthesis of Cu/$Cu_2O$/CuO nanostructures and the analysis of their electrochemical properties. SN Appl Sci 2:1–15
27. Gangwar P, Johri P, Datta R, Singh S, Trivedi M (2023) Overview on 1 phytopharmaceuticals and biotechnology of herbal plants. In: Phytopharmaceuticals and biotechnology of herbal plants. CRC Press, pp 1–17
28. Gulia K, James A, Pandey S, Dev K, Kumar D, Sourirajan A (2022) Bio-inspired smart nanoparticles in enhanced cancer theranostics and targeted drug delivery. J Funct Biomaterials 13(4):207
29. Guo D, Zhang L, Song X, Tan L, Ma H, Jiao J, Zhu D, Li F (2018) $NiCo_2O_4$ nanosheets grown on interconnected honeycomb-like porous biomass carbon for high performance asymmetric supercapacitors. New J Chem 42(11):8478–8484
30. Gupta K, Kaushik A, Tikoo KB, Kumar V, Singhal S (2020) Enhanced catalytic activity of composites of $NiFe_2O_4$ and nano cellulose derived from waste biomass for the mitigation of organic pollutants. Arab J Chem 13(1):783–798
31. Gupta G, Paul S, Singh S, Pietramellara G, Pathan SI, Danish S, Jha PN (2022) Exploring functional diversity and community structure of diazotrophic endophytic bacteria associated with Pennisetum glaucum growing under field in a semi-arid region. Land 11(7):991
32. Hu D, Gu X, Si W, Qin W, Jiao J, Hao Y (2019) Biosynthesis of silver nanoparticles using *Bauhinia acuminate* flower extract and their effect to promote osteogenesis of MSCs and improve meniscus injury healing. J Photochem Photobiol B: Biol 197:111536
33. Husen A, Iqbal M (2019) Nanomaterials and plant potential. Springer Nature Publishing
34. Husen A, Rahman QI, Iqbal M, Yassin MO (2019) Plant-mediated fabrication of gold nanoparticles and their application in some cutting-edge areas. In: Husen A, Iqbal M (eds) Nanomaterials and plant potential. Springer Nature, pp 71–110

35. Hussain S, Singh RK, Kumar SS, Kumar N, Kumar G (2022) Synthesis and characterization of crystalline nano silica from rice husk (agricultural waste) and its magnetic composites
36. Ikram M, Javed B, Raja NI, Mashwani ZU (2021) Biomedical potential of plant-based selenium nanoparticles: a comprehensive review on therapeutic and mechanistic aspects. Int J Nanomed 12:249–268
37. Jabasingh SA, Belachew H, Yimam A (2018) Iron oxide induced bagasse nanoparticles for the sequestration of $Cr^{6+}$ ions from tannery effluent using a modified batch reactor. J Appl Polym Sci 135:46683
38. Jabborova D, Davranov K, Jabbarov Z, Bhowmik SN, Ercisli S, Danish S, Datta R (2022) Dual inoculation of plant growth-promoting bacillus endophyticus and funneliformis mosseae improves plant growth and soil properties in ginger. ACS Omega 7(39):34779–34788
39. Jamdagni P, Khatri P, Rana JS, (2018). Green synthesis of zinc oxide nanoparticles using flower extract of *Nyctanthes arbor-tristis* and their antifungal activity. J King Saud Univ Sci 30(2):168–175
40. Joghee S, Ganeshan P, Vincent A, Hong SI (2019) Ecofriendly biosynthesis of zinc oxide and magnesium oxide particles from medicinal plant Pisonia grandis R.Br. Leaf extract and their antimicrobial activity. Bionanoscience 9:141–154
41. Johnson P, Krishnan V, Loganathan C, Govindhan K, Raji V, Sakayanathan P, Vijayan S, Sathishkumar P, Palvannan T (2018) Rapid biosynthesis of Bauhinia variegata flower extract-mediated silver nanoparticles: an effective antioxidant scavenger and α-amylase inhibitor. Artif Cells Nanomedicine Biotechnol 46(7):1488–94
42. Kamran U, Bhatti HN, Iqbal M, Jamil S, Zahid M (2019) Biogenic synthesis, characterization and investigation of photocatalytic and antimicrobial activity of manganese nanoparticles synthesized from *Cinnamomum verum* bark extract. J Mol Struct 1179:532–539
43. Kar A, Ray AK (2014) Synthesis of nano-spherical nickel by templating hibiscus flower petals. J Nanosci Nanotechnol 2:17–20
44. Kaur R, Thakur NS, Chandna S, Bhaumik J (2020) Development of agri-biomass based lignin derived zinc oxide nanocomposites as promising UV protectant-cum-antimicrobial agents. J Mater Chem B 8(2):260–269
45. Khazaei A, Khazaei M, Nasrollahzadeh M (2017) Nano-$Fe_3O_4$@$SiO_2$ supported Pd(0) as a magnetically recoverable nanocatalyst for Suzuki coupling reaction in the presence of waste eggshell as low-cost natural base. Tetrahedron 73:5624–5633
46. Kora AJ, Rastogi L (2018) Green synthesis of palladium nanoparticles using gum ghatti (Anogeissus latifolia) and its application as an antioxidant and catalyst. Arab J Chem 11(7):1097–1106
47. Koul B, Yakoob M, Shah MP (2022) Agricultural waste management strategies for environmental sustainability. Environ Res 15(206):112285
48. Krishnaswamy K, Vali H, Orsat V (2014) Value-adding to grape waste: green synthesis of gold nanoparticles. J Food Eng 142:210–220
49. Kumar B, Smita K, Debut A, Cumbal L (2020) Andean Sacha Inchi (*Plukenetia Volubilis* L.) leaf-mediated synthesis of $Cu_2O$ nanoparticles: a low-cost approach. Bioengineering 7:54
50. Kumar KM, Mandal BK, Kumar KS, Reddy PS, Sreedhar B (2013) Biobased green methotosynthesise palladium and iron nanoparticles using Terminalia chebulaaqueous extract. Spectrochim. Acta A 102:128–133
51. Kumar PV, Kalyani RL, Veerla SC, Kollu P, Shameem U, Pammi SVN (2019) Biogenic synthesis of stable silver nanoparticles via *Asparagus racemosus* root extract and their antibacterial efficacy towards human and fish bacterial pathogens. Mater Res Express 6(10):104008
52. Lakshmanan G, Sathiyaseelan A, Kalaichelvan PT, Murugesan K (2018) Plant-mediated synthesis of silver nanoparticles using fruit extract of Cleome viscosa L.: assessment of their antibacterial and anticancer activity. Karbala Int J Mod Sci 4:61–68
53. Lakshmipathy R, Reddy PB, Sarada NC, Chidambaram K, Khadeer PS (2015) Watermelon rind-mediated green synthesis of noble palladium nanoparticles: catalytic application. Appl Nanosci 5:223–228

54. Le VH, Thuc CNH, Thuc HH (2013) Synthesis of silica nanoparticles from Vietnamese rice husk by sol–gel method. Nanoscale Res Lett 8:58–67
55. Li R, Liang W, Wang JJ, Gaston LA, Huang D, Huang H et al (2018) Facilitative capture of As(V), Pb(II) and methylene blue from aqueous solutions with MgO hybrid sponge-like carbonaceous composite derived from sugarcane leafy trash. J Environ Manage 212:77–78
56. Lopez-Tellez G, Vílchis Néstor AR, Gutierrez-Segura E, Moreno-Marcelino JE, Alcantara-Cobos A, Malvaez-Medina JM, Mejia AC (2018) Green and sustainable synthesis of metal nanoparticles using orange peel pith. In: Green metal nanoparticles: synthesis, characterization and their applications, vol 22, pp 199-215
57. Machado S, Pinto SL, Grosso JP, Nouws HPA, Albergaria JT, Delerue-Matos C (2013) Green production of zero-valent iron nanoparticles using tree leaf extracts. Sci Total Environ 445:1–8
58. Maddala VKS, Singh S (2023) Essential oils from plants and their role in nanomaterial synthesis characterization and applications. In: Secondary metabolites based green synthesis of nanomaterials and their applications. Singapore: Springer Nature, Singapore, pp 191–207
59. Majumdar R, Bag BG, Ghosh P (2016) Mimusops elengi bark extract mediated green synthesis of gold nanoparticles and study of its catalytic activity. Appl Nanosci 6:521–528
60. Mali SC, Dhaka A, Sharma S, Trivedi R (2023) Review on biogenic synthesis of copper nanoparticles and its potential applications. Inorg Chem Commun 25:110448
61. Mathur L, Hossain SS, Majhi MR, Roy PK (2018) Synthesis of nano-crystalline forsterite ($Mg_2SiO_4$) powder from biomass rice husk silica by solid-state route. Boletín de la Sociedad Española de Cerámica y Vidrio 57(3):112–8
62. Mehdizadeh T, Zamani A, Froushani SMA (2020) Preparation of Cu nanoparticles fixed on cellulosic walnut shell material and investigation of its antibacterial, antioxidant and anticancer effects. Heliyon 6:e03528
63. Nagar N, Devra V (2018) Green synthesis and characterization of copper nanoparticles using *Azadirachta indica* leaves. Mater Chem Phys 213:44–51
64. Nagar N, Jain S, Kachhawah P, Devra V (2016) Synthesis and characterization of silver nano-particles via green route. Korea J Chem Eng 33:2990–2997
65. Nagar N, Devra V (2019) Textile dyes degradation from activated peroxomonosulphate by
66. Nakkala JR, Mata R, Sadras SR (2016) The antioxidant and catalytic activities of green synthesized gold nanoparticles from piper longum fruit extract. Process Saf Environ 100:288–294
67. Nilavukkarasi S, Vijayakumar S, Kuma P (2020) Biological synthesis and characterization of silver nanoparticles with capparis zeylanical L. leaf extract for potent antimicrobial and antiproliferation efficiency. Mater Sci Technol 3:371–376
68. Palit S, Hussain C (2021) Green sustainability and the application of polymer nanocomposites—a vast vision for the future. In: Handbook of polymer nanocomposites for industrial applications. Elsevier, pp 733–747
69. Pascoli DU, Dichiara A, Roumeli E, Gustafson R, Bura R (2022) Lignocellulosic nanomaterials production from wheat straw via peracetic acid pretreatment and their application in plastic composites. Carbohyd Polym 295:119857
70. Patani A, Patel A, Prajapati D, Khare N, Singh S (2023) Various agriculture crop plant-based bioactive compounds and their use in nanomaterial synthesis and applications. In: Nanomaterials from agricultural and horticultural products. Singapore: Springer Nature. Singapore, pp 223–241
71. Patel KG, Misra NM, Vekariya RH, Shettigar RR (2018) One-pot multicomponent synthesis in aqueous medium of 1, 4-dihydropyrano[2, 3-c]pyrazole-5-carbonitrile and derivatives using a green and reusable nano-$SiO_2$ catalyst from agricultural waste. Res Chem Intermed 44:289–304
72. Poinern GEJ, Fawcett D (2019) Sustainable utilization of renewable plant-based food wastes for the green synthesis of metal nanoparticles. In: Harnessing nanoscale surface interactions. Contemporary synthesis, applications and theory. Micro and nano technologies, pp 1–39
73. Pushkar B, Sevak PI (2018) Green synthesis of silver nanoparticles using Couroupita guianensis fruit pulp and its antibacterial properties. World J Pharm Res 5:1174–1187

74. Qiu H, Ye M, Zeng Q, Li W, Fortner J, Liu L, Yang L (2019) Fabrication of agricultural waste supported UiO-66 nanoparticles with high utilization in phosphate removal from water. Chem Eng J 360:621–630
75. Rabiee N, Bagherzadeh M, Kiani M, Ghadiri AM, Fatem Etessamifar Jaberizadeh AH, Shakeri A (2020) Biosynthesis of copper oxide nanoparticles with potential biomedical applications. Int J Nanomed 15:3983–3999
76. Rafique M, Sadaf I, Rafique MS, Tahir MB (2017) A review on green synthesis of silver nanoparticles and their applications. Artif Cells Nanomed Biotechnol 45:1272–1291
77. Ramalingam G, Priya AK, Gnanasekaran L, Rajendran S, Hoang TK (2024) Biomass and waste derived silica, activated carbon and ammonia-based materials for energy-related applications–a review. Fuel 355:129490
78. Ramkumar R, Balasubramani G, Raja RK, Raja M, Govindan R, Girija EK, Perumal P (2017) Lantana camara Linn root extract-mediated gold nanoparticles and their in vitro antioxidant and cytotoxic potentials. Artif Cells Nanomedicine Biotechnol 45(4):748–57
79. Rathore A, Devra V (2023) Azadirachta indica leaf mediated synthesis of iron nanoparticles and their catalytic application in methylene blue degradation. Catal Res 3(1):1–12
80. Rovani S, Santos JJ, Corio P, Fungaro DA (2018) Highly pure silica nanoparticles with high adsorption capacity obtained from sugarcane waste ash. ACS Omega 3:2618–2627
81. Salari S, Bahabadi SE, Kermani AS, Yosefzaei F (2019) In-vitro evaluation of antioxidant and antibacterial potential of green synthesized silver nanoparticles using prosopis farcta fruit extract. Iran J Pharm Res 18(1):430–445
82. Sao P, Chand Y, Kumar A, Singh S (2021) Potential drug target identification in porphyromonas gingivalis using in-silico subtractive metabolic pathway analysis. Bangladesh J Med Sci 20(4):887–896
83. Sao P, Parveen R, Khattri A, Sharma S, Tiwari N, Singh S (2022) Understanding the metabolomics of medicinal plants under environmental pollution: challenges and opportunities. Environ Pollut Med Plants 193–205
84. Saratale RG, Saratale GD, Shin HS, Jacob JM, Pugazhendhi A, Bhaisare M, Kumar G (2018) New insights on the green synthesis of metallic nanoparticles using plant and waste biomaterials: current knowledge, their agricultural and environmental applications. Environ Sci Pollut Res 25:10164–10183
85. Sarong MM, Orge RF, Eugenio PJG, Monserate JJ (2020) Utilization of rice husks into biochar and nanosilica: for clean energy, soil fertility and green nanotechnology. Int J Des Nat Eco Dyn 15:97–102
86. Sasikala A, Rao ML, Savithramma N, Prasad TN (2015) Synthesis of silver nanoparticles from stem bark of Cochlospermum religiosum (L.) Alston: an important medicinal plant and evaluation of their antimicrobial efficacy. Appl Nanosci 5:827–835
87. Schrofel A, Kratosová G, Safarík I, Safaríkova M, Raska I, Shor LM (2014) Applications of biosynthesized metallic nanoparticles–a review. Acta Biomater 10(10):4023–42
88. Shaik MR, Ali ZJQ, Khan M, Kuniyil M, Assal ME, Alkhathlan HZ, Al-Warthan A, Siddiqui MRH, Khan M, Adil SF (2017) Green synthesis and characterization of palladium nanoparticles using origanum vulgare L. extract and their catalytic activity. Molecules 22:165–172
89. Shaikh R, Syed IZ, Bhende P (2019) Green synthesis of silver nanoparticles using root extracts of cassia toral L. and its antimicrobial activities. Asian J Green Chem 3:70–81
90. Sharma D, Kanchi S, Bisetty K (2019) Biogenic synthesis of nanoparticles: a review. Arab J Chem 12(8):3576–3600
91. Sharma A, Sharma A, Kashyap P, Dhyani P, Pant M (2023) Wheat straw waste utilization for nanoparticles synthesis and their various applications. In: Nanomaterials from agricultural and horticultural products. Singapore: Springer Nature, Singapore, pp 163–178
92. Siddiqi KS, Husen A (2017) Recent advances in plant-mediated engineered gold nanoparticles and their application in biological system. J Trace Elem Med Biol 40:10–23
93. Siddiqi KS, Husen A, Rao RAK (2018) A review on biosynthesis of silver nanoparticles and their biocidal properties. J Nanobiotechnol 16:1–28

94. Siddiqi KS, Rashid M, Tajuddin Rehman S, Husen A (2019) Synthesis of silver nanoparticles using aqueous leaf extract of diospyros montana Roxb. and their antimicrobial activity against some clinical isolates. Bio Nano Sci 9:302–312
95. Singh A, Sengar RS, Singh AK, Singh S, Kumar A, Ahmad K (2019) Impact of genetic engineering on agriculture food crops. Biotech Today Int J Biol Sci 9(1):17–24
96. Singh S, Datta R, Johri P, Trivedi M (eds) (2022) Phytopharmaceuticals and Biotechnology of Herbal Plants. CRC Press
97. Suganthy N, Ramkumar VS, Pugazhendhi A, Benelli G, Archunan G (2018) Biogenic synthesis of gold nanoparticles from *Terminalia arjuna* bark extract: assessment of safety aspects and neuroprotective potential via antioxidant, anticholinesterase, and antiamyloidogenic effects. Environ Sci Pollut Res 25:10418–10433
98. Sumitha S, Vasanthi S, Shalini S, Chinni SV, Gopinath SC, Anbu P, Bahari MB, Harish R, Kathiresan S, Ravichandran V (2018) Phyto-mediated photo catalysed green synthesis of silver nanoparticles using Durio zibethinus seed extract: antimicrobial and cytotoxic activity and photocatalytic applications. Molecules 23(12):3311
99. Tanase C, Berta L, Mare A, Man A, Talmaciu AI, Roşca I, Mircia E, Volf I, Popa VI (2020) Biosynthesis of silver nanoparticles using aqueous bark extract of Picea abies L. and their antibacterial activity. Eur J Wood Wood Prod 78:281–291
100. Tapan KS, Andrey LR (2009) Nonspherical noble metal nanoparticles: colloid chemical synthesis and morphology control. Adv Mater 21:1–24
101. Thakur BK, Kumar A, Kumar D (2019) Green synthesis of titanium dioxide nanoparticles using Azadirachta indica leaf extract and evaluation of their antibacterial activity. S Afr J Bot 124:223–227
102. Tungare K, Shahu R, Zambare V, Agarwal P, Jobby R, Nisar N, Jha P (2022) Toxicity mitigation of textile dye reactive blue 4 by hairy roots of helianthus annuus and testing its effect in in vivo model systems. Biomed Res Int
103. Verma N, Sao P, Srivastava A, Singh S (2021) Physiological and molecular responses to drought, submergence and excessive watering in plants. In: Harsh environment and plant resilience: molecular and functional aspects, pp 305–321
104. Wang D, Markus J, Wang C, Kim YJ, Mathiyalagan R, Aceituno VC, Ahn S, Yang DC (2017) Green synthesis of gold and silver nanoparticles using aqueous extract of Cibotium barometz root. Artif Cells Nanomed Biotechnol 45(8):1548–1555
105. Xue H, Chen Y, Liu X, Qian Q, Luo Y, Cui M et al (2018) Visible light-assisted efficient degradation of dye pollutants with biomass-supported $TiO_2$ hybrids. Mater Sci Eng C 82:197–203
106. Yadav S, Chauhan M, Mathur D, Jain A, Malhotra P (2020) Sugarcane bagasse-facilitated benign synthesis of $Cu_2O$ nanoparticles and its role in photocatalytic degradation of toxic dyes: a trash to treasure approach. Environ Dev Sustain
107. Yang N, WeiHong L, Hao L (2014) Biosynthesis of Au nanoparticles using agricultural waste mango peel extract and its in vitro cytotoxic effect on two normal cells. Mater Lett 134:67–70
108. Zamani A, Marjani AP, Mousavi Z (2019) Agricultural waste biomass-assisted nanostructures: synthesis and application. Green Process Synth 8(1):421–429
109. Zangeneh MM, Ghaneialvar H, Akbaribazm M, Ghanimatdan M, Abbasi N, Goorani S, Pirabbasi E, Zangeneh A (2019) Novel synthesis of *Falcaria vulgaris* leaf extract conjugated copper nanoparticles with potent cytotoxicity, antioxidant, antifungal, antibacterial, and cutaneous wound healing activities under *in vitro* and *in vivo* condition. J Photochem Photobiol B Biol 197:111556
110. Zayed MF, Mahfoze RA, El-kousy SM, El-Ashkar EA (2020) In-vitro antioxidant and antimicrobial activities of metal nanoparticles biosynthesized using optimized *Pimpinella anisum* extract. Colloids Surf 585:124167
111. Zeng W, Bai H (2014) Swelling-agent-free synthesis of rice husk derived silica materials with large mesopores for efficient $CO_2$ capture. Chem Eng J 251:1–9

112. Zhu J, Yan C, Zhang X, Yang C, Jiang M, Zhang X (2020) A sustainable platform of lignin: from bioresources to materials and their applications in rechargeable batteries and supercapacitors. Prog Energy Combust Sci 76:100788
113. Zuorro A, Iannone A, Miglietta S, Lavecchia R (2022) Green synthesis of silver nanoparticles using spent coffee ground extracts: process modeling and optimization. Nanomaterials 12(15):2597

# Green Synthesis of Nanoparticles Using Plant Extracts

**Chaitanya Metha, Shrutee Pawar, and Vasanti Suvarna**

**Abstract** Nanoparticles have emerged as a significant area of interest because of their distinct physicochemical properties and wide-ranging applications. Plant-derived nanoparticles offer advantages in terms of safety, environmental impact, sustainability, and potential applications compared to conventional methods. This chapter includes synthesis methods, different plant sources, and plant-based products, such as extracts that can stabilize and eliminate agents during the synthesis process. The chapter focuses on the methods and factors affecting the production of nanoparticles, such as reaction circumstances, plant species, and particle properties. Furthermore, applications for plant-derived nanoparticles in antibacterial, antiviral, antidiabetic, and other methods are also explored. This book chapter provides a better understanding of the innovative field of plant-based nanoparticle synthesis by providing an in-depth overview of current developments and challenges.

**Keywords** Metallic nanoparticles · Green Synthesis · Plant sources · Metal oxide nanoparticles

## 1 Introduction

Nanoparticles (NPs), typically 1–100 nm in size, have unique size-dependent properties that have revolutionized diverse fields like electronics, energy, medicine, and environmental remediation. Nanoparticles, characterized by their trivial size and smaller volume-to-surface area ratio, possess superior physicochemical, and optical characteristics, resulting in them being advantageous across various applications. Notably, NPs hold promise for targeted and controlled delivery of therapeutic

C. Metha · S. Pawar
Department of Quality Assurance and Pharmaceutical Analysis, SVKM's Dr. Bhanuben Nanavati College of Pharmacy, Mumbai, Maharashtra, India

V. Suvarna (✉)
Department of Pharmaceutical Analysis, SVKM's Dr. Bhanuben Nanavati College of Pharmacy, Mumbai, Maharashtra, India
e-mail: vasanti.suvarna@bncp.ac.in

 
D. Jabborova et al. (eds.), *Nanomaterials in Agroforestry Systems*, Smart Nanomaterials Technology, https://doi.org/10.1007/978-981-96-1337-3_3

molecules due to their unique characteristics. However, challenges such as potential toxicity and regulatory challenges remain. Their small size facilitates increased absorption and allows them to be used with biomolecules for targeted delivery to specific cells or tissues. Additionally, NPs can enhance their stability, bioavailability, and therapeutic efficacy [19]. Recent advancements in nanomedicine suggested the potential for improved therapeutic efficacy with reduced adverse effects [89].

Semiconductor nanoparticles, particularly quantum dots, exploit size-dependent quantum confinement to show unique electromagnetic and optical properties [80]. Nanoparticles' high surface area, a consequence of their diminutive size, enhances their reactivity and adsorption potential. This characteristic paves the way for their use in effectively mitigating water and air pollution [81]. Functionalized NPs show selective binding to pollutants, enabling their capture, degradation, or removal. Notably, iron NPs have shown effectiveness in remediating contaminated groundwater by selectively removing heavy metals and organic pollutants [27]. Despite promising applications, NPs warrant further investigation regarding their potential human health and environmental risks, as scientific studies highlight concerns about their behavior, toxicity, and long-term effects [53].

NP synthesis with specific properties requires controlled chemical reactions and physical processes using precursors like metal salts or organic compounds [57]. Synthetic methods can precisely control NPs but are usually costly, complex, and hazardous to the environment attributed to the use of toxic chemicals and energy-intensive processes [2]. However, endothermic synthetic routes produce difficult-to-dispose toxic by-products [79]. NP synthesis with a greener approach using materials such as microbes, plant extracts, and biomolecules for reduction and stabilization is an eco-friendly, sustainable option for conventional methods [53]. Green synthesis is cost-effective, and flexible, utilizing renewable resources and less favorable conditions that reduce energy consumption. It produces biocompatible NPs with a low cytotoxicity for biomedical applications [44]. The present chapter summarized various plant-based environment-friendly synthetic routes for the synthesis of NPs and their comparison with conventional chemical methods. Moreover, it analyzes the unique properties and potential applications (medicine, electronics, environmental remediation) of plant-based NPs [62]. Finally, it discusses the challenges and prospects in this mushrooming field, laying the groundwork for further exploration.

## 2 Synthesis Methods

### *2.1 Physical Method*

Green synthesis, a plant-based physical method, uses plant extracts or materials to produce NPs (Fig. 1).

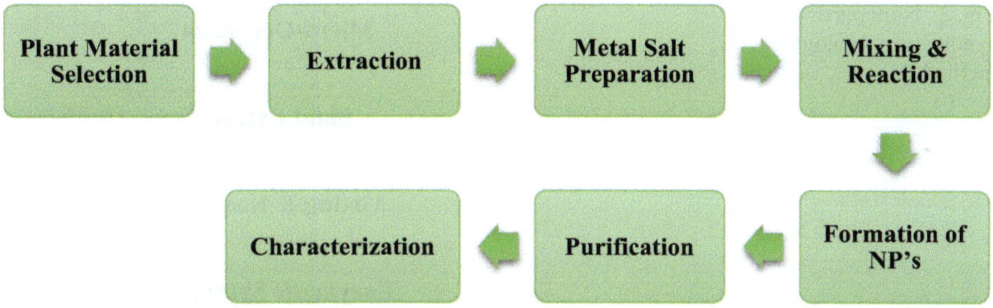


**Fig. 1** Physical synthetic method of nanoparticles

a. **Plant Material Selection**: Selection of a plant species that is rich in bioactive compounds, including but not limited to terpenoids, alkaloids, flavonoids, and phenols. Some of the plants that are often used due to their high concentration of these substances include *Camellia sinensis* (green tea), *Azadirachta indica* (neem), *Aloe barbadensis* (Aloe), and *Curcuma longa* (turmeric) [79].
b. **Extraction**: Plant extracts can be obtained by powdering the plant material and suspending it in a chosen solvent (e.g., water, ethanol, or their mixture). This process can be intensified using heat or ultrasound [50].
c. **Metal Salt Preparation**: To prepare metal salt solutions for NP synthesis, salts were dissolved in appropriate solvents. The concentration should be altered to the desired properties of the final NPs [52].
d. **Mixing and Reaction**: In green synthesis, plant extracts and metal salts were mixed at room temperature, sometimes mildly heated. The extract's bioactive compounds are used as reducing and capping agents, aiding NP synthesis.
e. **Formation of Nanoparticles**: In salt solutions, metal ions reduce to form NPs. Shape, size, and stability of NPs were controlled by adjusting parameters like temperature, pH, and concentration [53].
f. **Purification**: Centrifugation and filtration remove residual plant material and impurities, yielding a purified extract [57].
g. **Characterization**: Characterization of the developed NPs employed diverse techniques (UV spectroscopy, XRD, TEM, DLS) to elucidate composition, morphology, size, and stability, providing a comprehensive understanding of their physicochemical properties [8].

## *2.2 Biological Synthesis*

Biological synthesis, also known as bio-fabrication or green synthesis, uses biological agents like plants, bacteria, or enzymes to produce NPs (Fig. 2).

a. **Microorganisms**: Microorganisms (fungi, bacteria, and yeasts) provide their enzymes and cellular machinery to synthesize NPs through metal ion reduction [56].

**Fig. 2** Nanoparticles synthesis by biological method

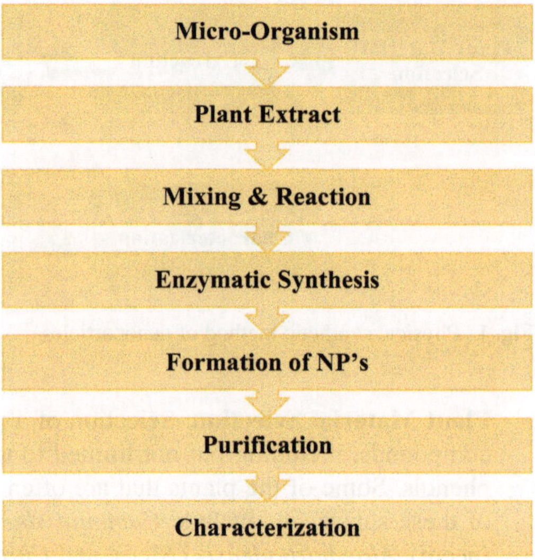


b. **Plant Extracts**: Reducing and stabilizing property of biologically active compounds in herbal extracts such as turmeric, neem, and green tea were used to synthesize NPs. These extracts are prepared through grinding or heating and used to reduce metal ions [58].
c. **Enzymatic Synthesis**: This method uses enzymes from different sources to synthesize NPs. For example, fungal laccases enable controlled NP synthesis of varying sizes, shapes, and compositions [2].
d. **Algae**: Certain algae species serve as stabilizers and reductants, aiding intracellular NP synthesis across strains [71].
e. **Yeasts**: Yeasts such as *Saccharomyces cerevisiae* act as biocatalysts in the formation of many metal and metal oxide NPs [27].
f. **Marine Organisms**: Marine organisms such as diatoms and sponges enable environmentally friendly NP production. Diatoms provide a unique silica exoskeleton for a controlled silica NP, while sponges ease the formation of NPs. Intensive research was conducted in this organic process, and continuous efforts have been made to improve efficiency and accuracy. These bio-derived NPs used in various fields, including electronics, medicine, and environmental remediation [16].

## 2.3 *Chemical Synthesis*

Plant-mediated NP synthesis uses plant extracts or phytochemicals to stabilize and reduce, offering a green sustainable alternative to current methods often exposed to harmful chemicals. This allows control of NP nucleation and growth (Fig. 3).

The synthesis process by chemical methods typically involves the key stages:

Fig. 3 Synthesis of nanoparticles using chemical methods

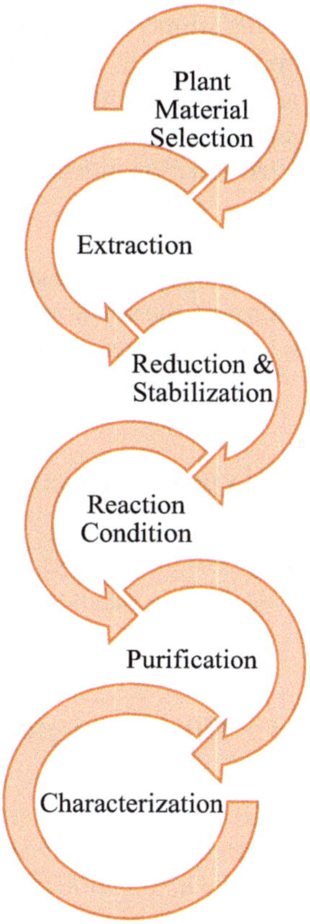


a. **Plant Material Selection**: Plants rich in bioactive compounds like polyphenols, alkaloids, flavonoids, and proteins (e.g., orange, tulsi, neem, etc.) are chosen for NP synthesis due to their potential as capping and reducing agents [96].
b. **Extraction**: Plant extracts are obtained through the processing of various plant parts (leaves, roots, stems, fruits) via grinding, blending, and subsequent solvent or water-based extraction [38].
c. **Reduction and Stabilization**: A precursor solution containing metal or metal oxide salts and plant extract triggers the reduction of metal ions to NPs via phytochemicals. These phytochemicals also used as capping agents, preventing NP aggregation and stabilizing them [92].
d. **Reaction Conditions**: Synthesis of NPs with desired properties requires meticulous optimization of reaction parameters like temperature, time, and pH, influencing NP shape, size, and composition [6].
e. **Characterization**: UV spectroscopy, XRD, SEM, TEM, and FTIR are used to elucidate the shape, size, crystallinity, and surface chemistry of formulated NPs [38, 92].

NPs from plant sources offer a scalable, economical, and ecologically friendly approach due to abundant plant resources. The selection of specific plant species and plant parts plays an important role in the incorporation of phytochemicals which not only facilitate the synthesis process but also instill the resultant NPs with added functionalities, such as antioxidant and antibacterial activities [49]. The NP synthesis process is highly susceptible to several factors, such as plant selection, extraction techniques, and reaction conditions, all of which profoundly affect the morphology, size, and stability of the NPs. As a result, rigorous optimization and strict control of these parameters are necessary for achieving the desired characteristics and performance of NPs [52].

## 3 Types of Metallic Nanoparticles

Plant-based biosynthesis provides a green approach to producing metallic NPs such as silver, gold, iron oxide, zinc oxide, copper, and titanium dioxide NPs.

### *3.1 Silver Nanoparticles*

AgNP, typically 1100 nm, often possess a significant silver oxide content that is attributed to their extensive surface area [23]. Similar to gold NPs, ionic silver finds historical application in yellow glass coloration [95]. Silver NPs find diverse applications in medical products, including incorporation into bone cement, surgical instruments, and masks. In wound therapy, ionic silver offers a potential alternative to silver sulphadiazine [8]. Plant extracts rich in phenolics, flavonoids, and proteins, such as Aloe vera, green tea, neem, and grapefruit, offer a simple one-pot method for synthesizing silver NPs through bioreduction [68, 72]. AgNPs exhibit diverse functionalities (antimicrobial, antibacterial, etc.) influenced by synthesis parameters (shape, size, plant extract, reagents) (Fig. 4) [72, 95]. Gomathi et al. studied the synthesis of AgNPs from *Tamarindus indica* fruit shells, proved their anticancer activity against MCF-7 human breast cancer cells [32]. Spherical AgNPs developed using extracts from *Glochidion lanceolarium, Semecarpus anacardium,* and *Bridelia retusa* exhibited broad-spectrum antibacterial activity against both gram-negative and gram-positive bacteria, including those forming biofilms [54]. Biogenic AgNPs formulated using *Azadirachta indica* and *Fusarium oxysporum* (10–40 nm, spherical) exhibited superior bactericidal activity against *S. aureus* and *E. coli* compared to chemically developed counterparts [73]. However, AgNPs derived from *Murraya koenigii* and *Tradescantia pallida* extracts (98–20 nm) also displayed antibacterial efficacy, with Tradescantia pallida effective at 40 μg/ml [35]. *Murraya koenigii* L.-derived silver nanoparticles (MK-AgNPs) exhibited broad-spectrum efficacy against multidrug-resistant (MDR) bacteria, encompassing both Gram-negative and Gram-positive strains [64]. Fereshteh et al. studied the green synthesis of AgNPs using

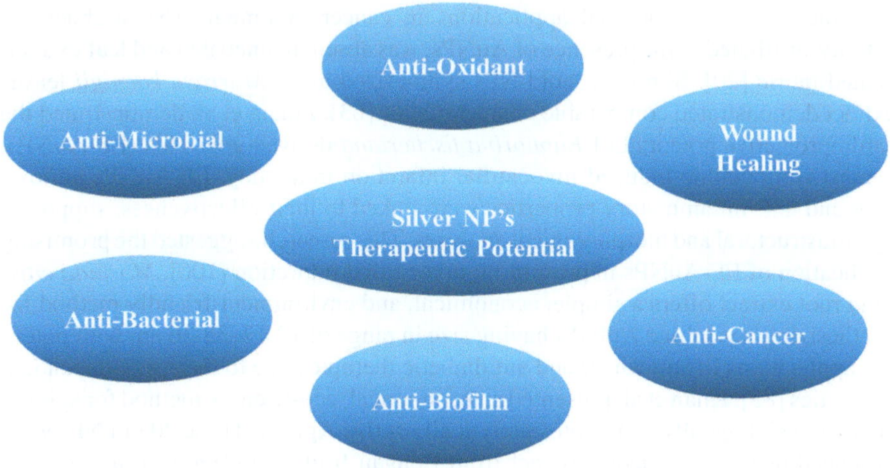


**Fig. 4** Therapeutic potential of silver nanoparticles

various plant extracts, including *Ferula latisecta*, exhibited antimicrobial activity against *S. aureus* and *E. coli*. The resultant AgNPs possessed a mean size of 20 nm [5, 9, 73].

### 3.2 *Gold Nanoparticles*

Gold NPs, also known as colloidal gold, are suspensions having microscopic gold particles. Colloidal solutions, with a rich history extending back to Roman times, were initially used for glass decoration [81]. Modern scientific interest in colloidal gold stems from Michael Faraday's 1850s work, where he observed distinct properties in colloidal gold solutions compared to bulk gold [94]. Herbal extracts rich in phytochemicals like polyphenols, alkaloids, and terpenoids offer a green approach for gold NP synthesis. Extracts from plants like turmeric, green tea, garlic, and aloe vera function as reducing agents, easing the conversion of gold ions into stable NPs [50]. AuNPs demonstrate therapeutic potential in various areas, including antibacterial, antimicrobial, bio-imaging, anticancer, antiproliferative, and antidiabetic effects (Fig. 5). Azri et al. synthesized AuNPs using *Etlingera elatior* extract, showed diverse shapes and sizes with good stability. These AuNPs effectively modified electrodes, enhanced electrochemical current for sensitive Cu(II) detection, comparable to the standard citrate method. This eco-friendly and cost-effective approach presents potential for large-scale AuNP production using *Etlingera elatior* [14]. Boomi et al. studied the synthesis of AuNPs with diverse shapes and sizes using *Coleus aromaticus* leaf extract. These AuNPs displayed crystalline structure, enhanced UV protection on cotton fabric, and showed bacteriocidal activity against *E. coli* (larger inhibition zone) and *S. epidermidis* [49]. The observed cytotoxicity against the $HepG_2$

cell line suggested potential applications in cancer treatment. The antibacterial activity, attributed to the presence of AuNPs, was absent in uncoated and leaf extract-coated fabric [20]. Similarly, gold NPs synthesized using *Murraya koenigii* leaves extract demonstrated comparable characteristics [63]. Zhang et al. demonstrated the cardioprotective potential of *Euphorbia fischeriana*-derived gold NPs (EF-AuNPs) against isoprenaline-induced myocardial infarction in a study. EF-AuNPs antioxidant and anti-inflammatory properties were linked to their effectiveness, supported by ultrastructural and morphological analyses. This research suggested the promising application of EF-AuNPs in preventing myocardial infarction [100]. *Morinda citrifolia* root extract offers a simple, economical, and environment-friendly method for synthesizing crystalline AuNP's having size in range of 12.17–38.26 nm with potential applications in anticancer and antidiabetic therapies due to their size-dependent properties [83]. Khan et al. presented an economical, eco-friendly method for synthesizing physiologically and photo catalytically active AgNPs. These 20 nm NPs were produced using the aqueous extract from Longan fruit peel (*Dimocarpus longan*), acting as a reducing and stabilizing agent. At a concentration of 100 g/ml, these AgNPs demonstrated significant anticancer properties against MCF-7 breast cancer cells, with cytotoxicity reaching 88% [43]. This study proved the superior free radical scavenging and dye degradation of AgNPs at room temperature. Green-synthesized AgNPs hold promise in different fields, including food, pharmaceuticals, textiles, and environmental remediation. However, thorough evaluation of their impact and potential drug delivery applications, including potential cytotoxicity, is necessary before human use [43].

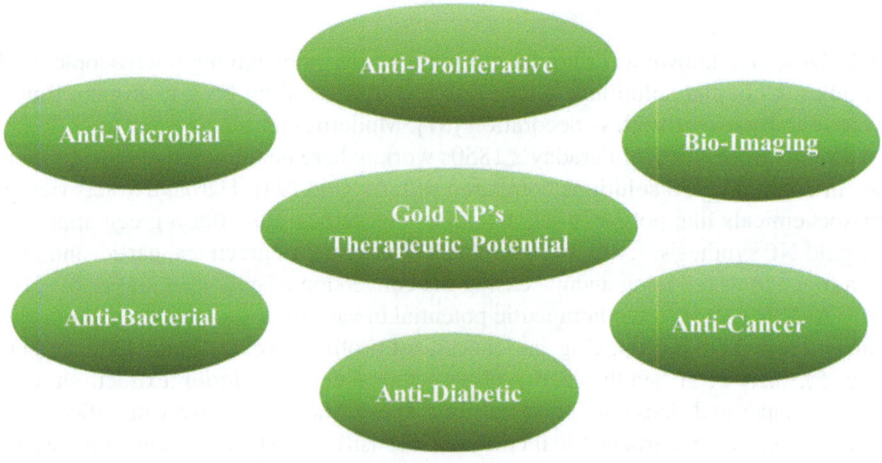


**Fig. 5** Therapeutic potential of gold nanoparticles

### 3.3 *Iron Oxide Nanoparticles*

Iron(III) oxide ($Fe_2O_3$), a reddish-brown paramagnetic compound, is one of the most prevalent iron oxides. The other two principal forms are iron (II) oxide (FeO) and magnetite ($Fe_3O_4$), a naturally occurring superparamagnetic mineral [2, 25]. Superparamagnetic iron oxide NPs (SPIONs) have emerged as versatile tools in biomedicine because of unique properties enabling applications in: Enhanced MRI contrast agents, Targeted drug delivery and imaging, Hyperthermia therapy, Gene therapy, Stem cell tracking, Molecular and cellular level tracking, Magnetic separation technologies, and Early detection of various diseases (inflammation, cancer, diabetes, atherosclerosis) [57]. High magnetization is critical for effective biomedical applications of $Fe_2O_3$NPs, enabling high-resolution MRI. Green synthesis methods using plant extracts, particularly natural polyphenols like tannins, offer a promising approach. These polyphenols function as both reducing and stabilizing agents. Green tea, coffee, and grapefruit extracts were successfully employed for this synthesis. The resulting NPs showed a broad spectrum of activities, including antimicrobial, bactericidal, anticancer, and antifungal properties, along with cytotoxicity (Fig. 6). This diverse functionality highlighted $Fe_2O_3$NPs as a fascinating area for further research [53]. *Rhamnus triquetra* leaves extract mediated the development of $Fe_2O_3$NPs with a mean diameter of 21 nm, proved both antifungal and bactericidal properties [1]. Moreover, *Ruellia tuberosa*-derived iron oxide NPs exhibited antibacterial activity against both Gram-positive and Gram-negative bacteria, additionally demonstrated photocatalytic degradation of crystal violet dye [87]. *Lawsonia Inermis* (henna) leaves extract mediated formation of $Fe_2O_3$NPs which exhibited antimicrobial, antioxidant, and cytotoxic activities, particularly against pathogenic bacteria [24]. Similarly, *Borassus Flabellifer* extract yielded hexagonal iron oxide NPs with size of 35 nm and efficient antimicrobial and antioxidant properties [75]. *Punica Granatum* peel and seed extracts were utilized for the green synthesis of $Fe_2O_3$NPs exhibited anticancer activity against various cancer cell lines and promising photocatalytic dye degradation under UV light [18, 98]. *Centella Asiatica* extract was utilized to synthesize sphere shape iron oxide NPs with a mean diameter of 15.2 nm [46]. This research reviews several studies exploring the development of $Fe_2O_3$NPs using plant extracts [2].

### 3.4 *Zinc Oxide Nanoparticles*

ZnO NP, having a diameter of not more than 100 nm and high surface area, showed significant catalytic activity. Their synthesis method is crucial, influencing both physical and chemical properties [65]. A variety of techniques are available for ZnO NP synthesis, including hydrothermal, laser ablation, and electrochemical techniques. Chemical methods like sol–gel, co-precipitation, and precipitation offer control over properties through parameters like solution concentration, pH, and washing

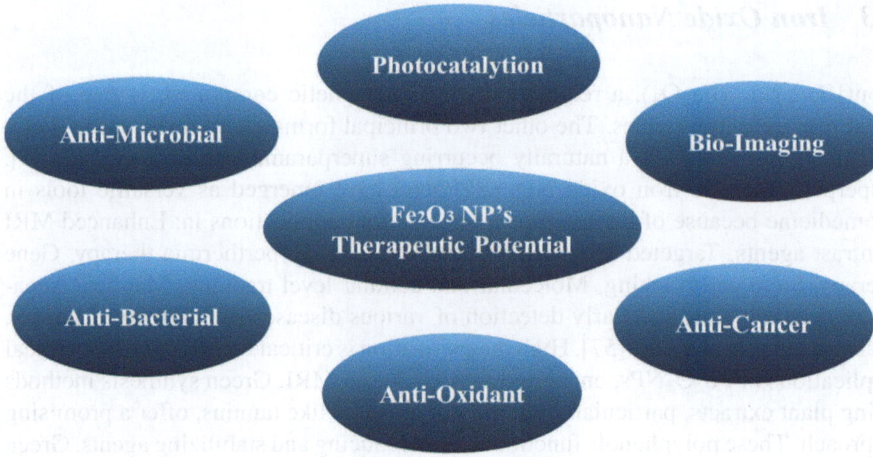


**Fig. 6** Therapeutic potential of iron oxide nanoparticles

conditions. Other notable approaches include thermal decomposition, sonication, and microwave-assisted combustion [95]. ZnO NPs can be synthesized using plant extracts rich in biomolecules like flavonoids, terpenoids, and alkaloids. Common plant sources include green tea, neem, and *Moringa oleifera*. These extracts function as eco-friendly reducing agents, influencing the size and morphology of the resulted NPs [53]. ZnO NPs have a broad spectrum of biological activities (Fig. 7), encompassing antimicrobial, anticancer, antifungal, and antioxidant properties. Notably, Rad et al. showed the formation of ZnO NPs from *Mentha pulegium* L., showing antimicrobial activity against various bacteria (38–49 nm, semi-sphere shape) [61, 65]. Furthermore, studies have shown that ZnO NPs synthesized using plant extracts showed promising biological activities. For example, those derived from *Albizia lebbeck* displayed antimicrobial and cytotoxic properties, while *Crotalaria verrucosa* extracts yielded NPs with strong bactericidal activity against multidrug-resistant bacteria and anticancer potential against specific cancers.

NPs, showing hexagonal and cylindrical rod-like structures and derived from *Xylaria acuta*, were demonstrated to have dimensions within the 35–45 nm range. These NPs exhibited large antimicrobial properties against various pathogens, in addition it showed antifungal and anticancer activities [84]. *Vernonia amygdalina*-derived ZnO NP exhibited antinociceptive and anti-inflammatory effects in mice [47], *Fraxinus rhynchophylla* stem extract-derived compounds showed antinociceptive activity in mice [92]. Furthermore, *Selaginella convolute* leaves extract facilitated synthesis of ZnO NP having size in the range of 40–60 nm and diverse activities, such as muscle relaxation and antinociception [95].

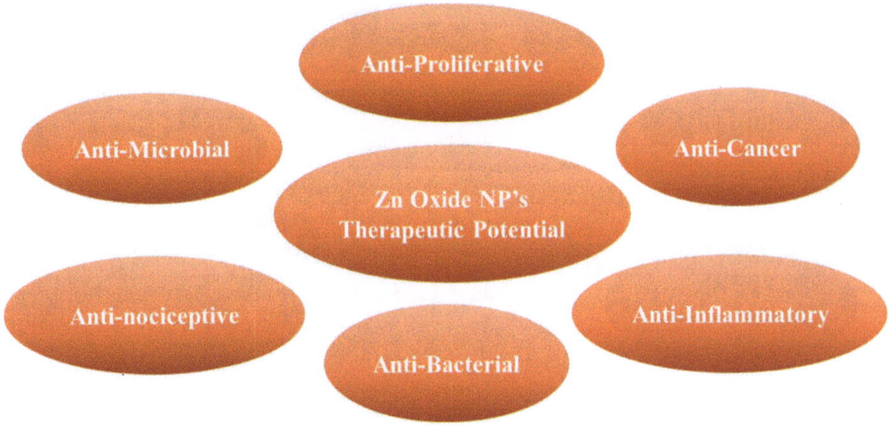


**Fig. 7** Therapeutic potential of zinc oxide nanoparticles

### *3.5 Copper Nanoparticles*

Copper based nanoparticles (CuO NPs), consisting of nanoscale copper and oxygen atoms, have unique properties that have triggered substantial interest across diverse scientific and industrial domains [11]. CuO NPs can be synthesised using different methods, such as thermal decomposition, chemical reduction, and sol–gel processes [61]. These NPs exist in two primary forms: copper (I) oxide ($Cu_2O$) and copper (II) oxide (CuO), each having unique properties and applications [4]. The material proved broad-spectrum biocidal activity against various microorganisms, including viruses, bacteria, and fungi. This property has prompted research into its potential application in antimicrobial coatings for surfaces and medical equipment to reduce the spread of infections [40]. Copper NPs were biologically synthesized using plant extracts rich in phytochemicals with reduced properties, such as neem, onion, and garlic. Flavonoids, phenols, and organic acids in these extracts improved copper ion reduction and stabilization (Fig. 8). The NPs showed various functionalities, like antimicrobial, bactericidal, anticancer, antifungal, antidiabetic, and antioxidant properties [26]. Dhiraj et al. reported the development of Cu NPs using *Plumbago zeylanica* and *Gnidia glauca* leaf extracts which showed potential for antidiabetic therapy. The spherical NPs were ~20 nm in size [40]. Cu NPs synthesized from *Camellia sinensis* exhibited spherical morphology (70–85 nm) and efficiently degraded a dye (83.7%) under sunlight irradiation [4]. Furthermore, *Celastrus paniculatus*-derived Cu NPs exhibited photocatalytic activity and antifungal effects against *F. oxysporum* [51]. Moreover, Das et al. reported Cu NPs synthesized from *Moringa oleifera* leaf extract (sized 35.8–49.2 nm) showed antifungal activity against *Candida* spp., along with antioxidant and antimicrobial properties [26]. Cu NPs derived from *Cissus arnotiana* and *Cissus vitiginea* were sphere shape, with sizes of 60–90 nm and 10–20 nm, respectively, and exhibited both antioxidant and antibacterial activities [69, 93]. *Cissus vitiginea*-derived Cu NPs exhibited enhanced antioxidant and bactericidal activity,

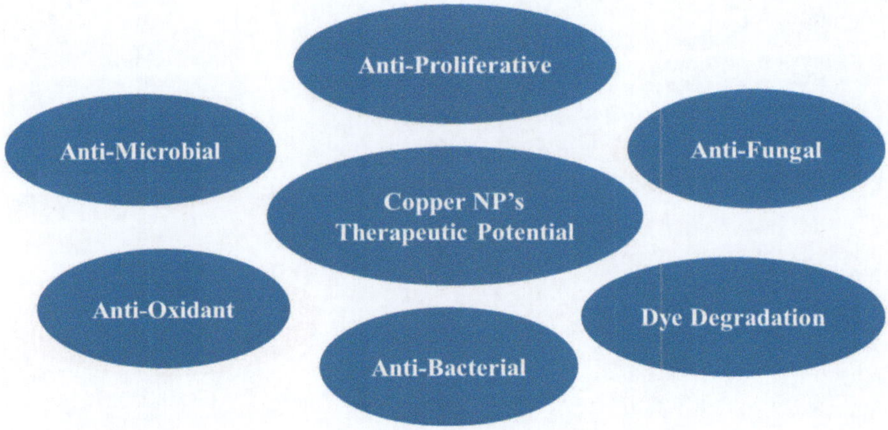


**Fig. 8** Therapeutic potential of copper nanoparticles

effectively targeted DPPH free radicals and UTI pathogens [69]. *Cissus arnotiana*-derived Cu NPs displayed both antioxidant and antibacterial properties, with the strongest antibacterial effect reported against Gram-negative bacteria, particularly E. coli [93]. *Hagenia abyssinica* leaf extract mediated the synthesis of Cu NPs with diverse morphologies (triangular, spherical, hexagonal, and cylindrical) exhibited antimicrobial activity against bacterial pathogens [55]. Additionally, *Cinnamomum Cassia*-derived Cu NPs showed sphericity and a 50 nm size, demonstrated antimicrobial properties [77]. Plant extracts have emerged as a promising route for Cu NPs synthesis, demonstrated their potential across various applications [10].

## 3.6 *Titanium Dioxide Nanoparticles*

Titanium dioxide NPs can be synthesized by many techniques, like hydrothermal, sol–gel, and chemical vapor deposition, using plant extracts rich as reducing agents and stabilizers [48]. Because of their distinct properties, $TiO_2$ NPs exist in 3 crystalline structures (rutile, anatase, and brookite, with rutile and anatase being most prevalent) and have garnered significant interest across diverse scientific and industrial fields [66]. Plant extracts of green tea, aloe vera, and hibiscus were studied for the plant-based synthesis of $TiO_2$NP, acting as reducing and stabilizing agents during the process [3]. These biosynthesized $TiO_2$ NPs showed diverse biological activities, including antimicrobial, antibacterial, and anticancer properties [70]. The recent developments in plant-based synthesis of $TiO_2$ NPs using herbal extracts highlighted their promising applications [90]. Mathiyazhagan et al. synthesized $TiO_2$ NPs using *Coleus aromaticus* leaves extract, showed bactericidal activity against various bacteria and larvicidal activity against *Aedes aegypti* larvae [59]. Ahmad et al. employed *Ocimum sanctum* extract for $TiO_2$ NP synthesis, incorporated them into a 2% chitosan gel for wound healing in diabetic rats. The size of synthesized NPs was in the range of 74–123 nm and spherical, polygonal, and square shape. $TiO_2$ NPs chitosan gel showed substantial wound healing activity in diabetic rats, by wound contraction and histopathological analysis. The research demonstrated the potential of green synthesized $TiO_2$ NPs and their integration into CS gel for wound healing applications [3]. Satti et al. used *Moringa oleifera* extract to synthesize biogenic $TiO_2$ NPs, exhibiting disease-reduction effects in wheat plants, particularly at 40 mg $L^{-1}$ against *Puccinia striiformis* [78]. Rajkumari et al. synthesised $TiO_2$ NPs using *Aloe barbadensis* extract, displaying their ability to inhibit *Pseudomonas aeruginosa* biofilm formation. Characterization revealed spherical, polydispersed $TiO_2$NPs of ~20 nm. $TiO_2$-NPs inhibited *P. aeruginosa* biofilm by 30.76 ± 3.96%, with significant antibiofilm activity at MIC [70]. These findings suggested the broad potential of green-synthesized $TiO_2$ NPs in different fields, including medicine, agriculture, and environmental remediation. Rajkumar et al. synthesised $TiO_2$ NPs using extracts from *Mangifera indica* and *Solanum trilobatum*. The NPs were sphere shape, with sizes of 37.54 nm and 70 nm, respectively [88]. Notably, only NPs from *Solanum trilobatum* exhibited antiparasitic activity against *Pediculus humanus capitis, H. anatolicum*, and *A. subpictus*, while both types displayed larvicidal activity [66, 67]. Furthermore, Narayanan et al. suggested the formulation of $TiO_2$ NPs from *Pouteria campechiana* leaves, exhibited larvicidal and pupicidal activity, which suggested the potential for mosquito control but requiring further development [59]. Zahir et al. developed spherical $TiO_2$ NPs (12.82 nm) from *Euphorbia prostrata* leaf extract, exhibited antileishmanial activity, and suggested their potential applications against leishmaniasis [99]. Plant extracts offer a promising green approach for synthesizing $TiO_2$ NPs with diverse potential, including larvicidal, antibacterial, antiparasitic, anticancer, and antileishmanial activities (Fig. 9 and Tables 1, 2, 3, 4, 5 and 6).

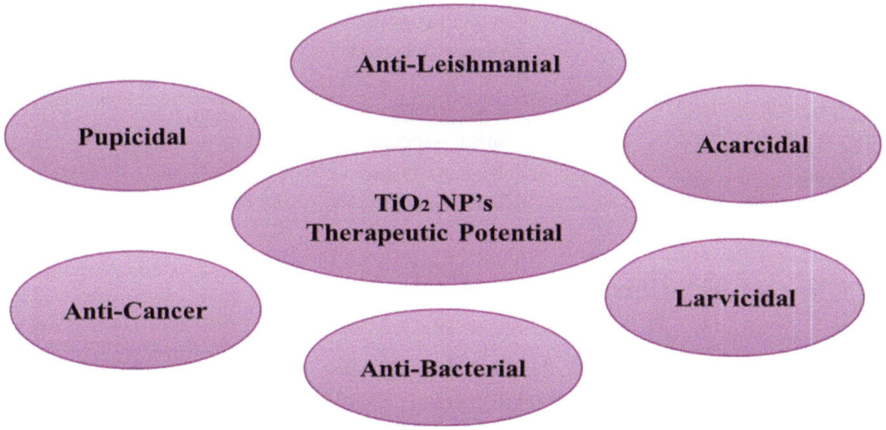


**Fig. 9** Therapeutic potential of titanium oxide nanoparticles

**Table 1** Representative silver nanoparticles, plant, and part of plant used, characteristics, and their activities

| Plant name | Part of plant | Characterization | Conclusion | Ref |
|---|---|---|---|---|
| *Carica papaya* | Peel | Size—16–20 nm<br>Shape—cubic and hexagonal | Antimicrobial, antibacterial | [15] |
| *Ixora henryi*<br>*Rubia cordifolia*<br>*Curcuma longa* | Flowers and roots<br>Stem and roots<br>Roots | Size—8.8–35.4 nm<br>Shape—mostly spherical | Antioxidant, cytotoxic, apoptotic, wound healing | [7] |
| *Semecarpus anacardium*<br>*Glochidion lanceolarium*<br>*Bridelia retusa* | Leaf | Size—350–600 nm<br>Shape—spherical | Antibacterial, anti-biofilm | [54] |
| *Tamarindus indica* | Fruit shell | Size—20–52 nm (SEM)<br>Size—20–30 nm (TEM)<br>Shape—mostly spherical | Anticancer | [32] |
| *Fusarium oxysporum*<br>*Azadirachta indica* | – | Size—10–40 nm<br>Shape—spherical | Antibacterial | [73] |
| *Tradescantia pallida (Setcreasea pallida)* | Leaf | Size—98 nm<br>Shape—spherical | Antibacterial | [35] |
| *Murraya koenigii L* | Leaf | Size—5–20 nm<br>Shape—spherical | Antibacterial | [64] |
| *Ferulago macrocarpa* | Flower | Size—14–25 nm<br>Shape—spherical | Antimicrobial, antibacterial, antifungal | [13] |
| *Tamarind indica* | Fruit | Size—10 nm<br>Shape—spherical | Antibacterial | [5] |
| *Eucalyptus globulus* | Leaf | Size—5–25 nm<br>Shape—spherical | Antibacterial, anti-biofilm | [14] |

## 4 Characterization

Green synthesis uses herbal extracts for the bio-reduction of metal ions to their elemental NP form. This environment-friendly approach offers benefits in simplicity, economics, and minimal environmental impact. Characterization of green-synthesized NPs is achieved through different methods like UV, XRD, FTIR, SEM, and DLS [76].

**Table 2** Representative gold nanoparticles, plant, and part of plant used, characteristics, and their activities

| Plant name | Part of plant | Characteristics | Conclusion | Ref |
|---|---|---|---|---|
| *Etlingera elatior* | Leaf | Size—31.5 ± 0.5 nm Shape—spherical, triangular shapes | Electrochemical, current enhancer | [14] |
| *Coleus aromaticus* | Leaf | Size—80 nm Shape—sphere | Bactericidal, activity | [20] |
| *Panax notoginseng* | Leaf | Size—12–80 nm Shape—oval, and sphere | Antimicrobial and anticancer, activity | [91] |
| *Euphorbia fischeriana* | Root | Size-20–60 nm Shape—spherical | Used in isoprenaline-induced myocardial infarction | [100] |
| *Murraya koenigii* | Leaf | Shape—spherical Size—20 nm | Antibacterial, activity | [63] |
| *Morinda citrifolia L* | Root | Shape—spherical, and hexagonal Size—12.8–38.7 nm | Anticancer, antidiabetic activity | [83] |
| *Dimocarpus longan* | Fruit peel | Avg size—20 nm Shape—sphere | Antiproliferative activity | [43] |
| *Abies spectabillis* | Plant | Shape—spherical Size—20–200 nm | Anticancer activity | [94] |
| *Cassia auriculata* | Leaf | Size—15–25 nm | Antidiabetic activity | [31] |
| *Pholiota adiposa* | Plant | Size—95.07 nm Size—spherical | Anticancer activity | [97] |
| *Syzygium cumini* | Leaf | Size—spherical Size—30–50 nm | Antibacterial activity | [28] |

## 4.1 UV–Visible Spectroscopy

UV–Vis spectroscopy efficiently characterized plant-based NPs by analyzing their light absorption in the UV regions. This technique reveals information about NPs shape, size, and surface plasmon resonance (SPR). The presence and effectiveness of NPs synthesis can be analyzed by the position and intensity of the SPR peak [45].

## 4.2 X-ray Diffraction (XRD)

XRD is a valuable technique for determining the crystalline configuration of NPs synthesized through eco-friendly methods. By identifying both the atomic organization and crystallographic characteristics, XRD facilitates the identification of crystal structure and determining the lattice parameters [22].

**Table 3** Iron oxide nanoparticles, plant, and part of plant used, characteristics, and their activities

| Plant name | Part of plant | Characterization | Conclusion | Ref |
|---|---|---|---|---|
| *Rhamnus triquetra* | Leaf | Size—21 nm<br>Shape—spherical | Antibacterial, antifungal | [1] |
| *Lawsonia inermis (Henna)* | Leaf | Size—150–200 nm<br>Shape—spherical | Antimicrobial, antioxidant, cytotoxic | [24] |
| *Ruellia tuberosa* | Leaf | Size—20–80 nm<br>Shape—hexagonal rods | Antibacterial | [87] |
| *Punica granatum* | Peel | Size—11 nm<br>Shape—spherical | Anticancer | [98] |
| *Punica granatum* | Seed | Size—25–55 nm<br>Shape—semi-spherical | Photocatalytic | [18] |
| *Juglans regia* | Husk | Size—100 nm or less<br>Shape—cubic | Cytotoxicity | [39] |
| *Stevia rebaudiana* | Leaf | Size—100 nm or less<br>Shape—spherical | Antioxidant | [44] |
| *Centella asiatica* | Whole plant | Size—15.2 nm<br>Shape—spherical | Biomedical imaging and therapy | [46] |
| *Laurus nobilis L* | Leaf | Size—8–9 nm<br>Shape—spherical | Antimicrobial | [41] |

**Table 4** Zinc oxide nanoparticles, plant and part of plant used, characteristics, and their activities

| Plant name | Part of plant | Characterization | Biological activity | Ref |
|---|---|---|---|---|
| *Mentha pulegium L* | Leaf | Size—38–49 nm<br>Shape—semi-spherical | Antimicrobial | [65] |
| *Albizia lebbeck* | Stem bark | Size—66.25 nm<br>Shape—hexagonal | Antimicrobial, antioxidant, cytotoxic | [86] |
| *Crotalaria verrucosa* | Leaf | Size—16–38 nm<br>Shape—hexagonal | Antimicrobial, anticancer | [74] |
| *Vernonia amygdalina* | Leaf | Size—20–40 nm<br>Shape—cylindrical | Anti-inflammatory, antinociceptive (Mice) | [47] |
| *Fraxinus rhynchophylla* | Stem bark | Size—100–200 nm<br>Shape—spherical | Antinociceptive (Mice) | [92] |
| *Cucurbita pepo* | Leaf | Size—8 nm<br>Shape—spherical | Cytotoxicity | [36] |
| *Selaginella convolute* | Leaf | Size—40–60 nm<br>Shape—spherical | Antinociceptive | [95] |
| *Xylaria acuta* | Leaf | Size—35–45 nm<br>Shape—hexagonal, cylindrical rod | Anticancer, antifungal, antibacterial | [84] |

**Table 5** Copper nanoparticles, plant and part of plant used, characteristics, and their activities

| Plant name | Part of plant | Characterization | Biological activity | Ref |
|---|---|---|---|---|
| *Cissus vitiginea* | Leaf | Size—10–20 nm<br>Shape—spherical | Antioxidant, antibacterial | [93] |
| *Cissus arnotiana* | Leaf | Size—60–90 nm<br>Shape—spherical | Antioxidant, antibacterial | [69] |
| *Piper retrofractum* | Fruit | Size—2–10 nm<br>Shape—spherical | Antibacterial | [11] |
| *Hagenia abyssinica* | Leaves | Size—34.86 nm<br>Shape—spherical, triangular, hexagonal and cylindrical | Antimicrobial | [55] |
| *Moringea oleifera* | Leaf | Size—35.8–49.2 nm | Antioxidant, antimicrobial, antifungal | [26] |
| *Cinnamomum cassia* | Bark | Size—50 nm<br>Shape—spherical | Antimicrobial | [77] |
| *Camelia sinesis* | Leaf | Size—70–85 nm<br>Shape—spherical | Application in dye degradation | [4] |
| *Vaccinium myrtillus* | Fruit | Size—1.7–5 nm<br>Shape—globular | Antimicrobial | [17] |
| *Celastrus paniculatus* | Leaf | Size—2–10 nm<br>Shape—spherical | Antifungal | [51] |
| *Gnidia glauca*<br>*Plumbago zeylanica* | Leaf | Size—10–30 nm<br>Shape—spherical | Antidiabetic | [40] |

### *4.3 Fourier-Transform Infrared Spectroscopy (FTIR)*

FTIR spectroscopy effectively distinguishes NPs in green synthesis. It identifies the capping agents/biomolecules involved and evaluates NP stability and functionality by analyzing surface functional groups through chemical bond and molecular vibration analysis [30].

### *4.4 Scanning Electron Microscopy (SEM)*

SEM gives high-resolution imaging of NPs, enabling the examination of their dimensions, morphology, and surface structure. This technique, combined with other methods, enhances a comprehensive analysis of green-synthesized NPs, shedding light on their shape, stability, size distribution, and optical properties [37].

**Table 6** Titanium Dioxide nanoparticles, plant and part of plant used, characteristics, and their activities

| Plant name | Part of plant | Characterization | Biological activity | Ref |
|---|---|---|---|---|
| *Morinda citrifolia* | Leaf | Size—15–19 nm<br>Shape—spherical | Antimicrobial | [48] |
| *Ocimum sanctum* | Leaf | Size—75–123 nm<br>Shape—spherical and polyglonal | Diabetic wound healing | [3] |
| *Phyllanthus niruri* | Leaf | Size—20 nm<br>Shape—spherical | Dye adsorption | [60] |
| *Solanum trilobatum* | Leaf | Size—70 nm<br>Shape—spherical and oval | Antiparasitic, larvicidal | [66] |
| *Calotropis gigantea* | Flowers | Size—160–220 nm<br>Shape—spherical | Acaricidal | [74] |
| *Mangifera indica* | Leaf | Size—37.54 nm<br>Shape—spherical | Larvicidal | [67] |
| *Pouteria campechiana* | Leaf | Size—29 nm<br>Shape—sphere | Larvicidal, pupicidal | [59] |
| *Euphorbia prostrata* | Leaf | Size—12.82 nm<br>Shape—spherical | Antileishmanial | [99] |
| *Coleus aromaticus* | Leaf | Size—12–33 nm<br>Shape—hexagonal | Antibacterial, larvicidal, anticancer | [59] |

### *4.5 Dynamic Light Scattering Method (DLS)*

DLS offers a non-invasive method for assessing NP size distribution and hydrodynamic diameter in solution. This technique analyzes fluctuations in scattered light intensity caused by Brownian motion of the particles. DLS data provides beneficial insights into the dimensions, stability, and aggregation behavior of green-synthesized NPs in a liquid medium [82].

### *4.6 Transmission Electron Microscopy (TEM)*

TEM is a powerful tool for nanomaterials characterization, offering exceptional resolution (down to 0.1 nm) that surpasses the atomic scale. This enables direct visualization of individual atoms and the determination of properties like size, shape, crystallinity, and interparticle interactions. Furthermore, the light beam narrows to a diameter of less than 0.3 nm, enables the chemical examination of different nanocrystals [85].

## 5 Toxicity of Synthesized Nanoparticles

NPs can be synthesized using extracts from various plant parts, like leaves, stems, roots, and fruits. These extracts have phytochemicals that function as reducing agents, improving the transformation of metal ions into NPs. Various plants, such as neem, aloe vera, and turmeric, have been utilizing to produce NPs of various dimensions and forms. The potential of these NPs to inflict cellular harm is a significant issue. In vitro experiments have demonstrated that certain plant-derived NPs, such as copper oxide NPs produced from assorted plant extracts, could eliminate human lung epithelial cells. This demonstrated that NPs produced from plants could potentially be hazardous to human health, necessitating comprehensive evaluation prior to their application [50].

The harmfulness of herbal-derived NPs has been explored in living organisms as well. Various animal models have been given NPs orally and via intraperitoneal injection to examine their impact. Xu et al. synthesized silver NPs from neem leaves which indicated potential harm to mice, affecting their kidneys and liver [95]. Similarly, another study on copper NPs made from Aloe vera extract found evidence of liver and kidney toxicity in rats [10]. Borase et al. *used* extract of *J. gossypifolia* to develop SNPs that exhibited amoebic activity. However, these SNPs were found to be non-toxic at the MIC with PBM cells. The most significant inhibition of PBMCs was observed with the SNPs at 50 g/mL concentration, resulting in TGI of 22% [21, 42]. AgNPs have been found to be detrimental in in vitro studies involving diverse cell types such as rat liver cells, human lung epithelial cells, mouse stem cells, and nerve cells. Despite this, AgNPs are recognized for their antibacterial capabilities and their minimal toxicity toward regular mammalian cells [12]. Moreover, it has been demonstrated that AgNP exposure can cause significant mitochondrial dysfunction. Based on the extent of exposure, this can result in either a transient or lasting hearing loss in rat ears. Boomi et al. synthesized minute quantities of AgNPs which are taken up by retinal cells, leading to oxidative stress and subsequent functional and structural harm [20]. Also, several studies were conducted on the biodistribution, and accumulation of NPs synthesized from plants in various organs to comprehend their potential systemic impacts. Investigations on Au NPs obtained from green tea extract revealed their accumulation in the spleen, liver, and lungs of mice following intravenous administration [14]. Similarly, Ag NPs obtained from different plant extracts were discovered to accumulate in the liver, lungs, and kidneys of mice [81]. Factors that influence NP toxicity, such as shape, size, surface charge, and dosage, need to be considered. It has been observed that smaller NPs with volume-to-high surface area ratios are more hazardous than larger ones. Furthermore, surface charge plays an important role in determining the interactions and toxicity of NPs with cells [2, 33].

It is essential to understand the mechanisms of toxicity of NPs synthesized from plants, including cellular uptake, oxidative stress, and inflammatory responses, and establish standardized procedures for toxicity testing, including both in vitro and in vivo tests. Long-term studies are necessary to assess the potential cumulative effects of NPs on organisms [53]. Other studies suggested that factors such as shape, particle size, surface charge, and capping agent, along with the type of cell, influence the noxiousness of NPs [29, 34].

## 6 Future Scope

This book chapter shows a future with immense potential and a multitude of possibilities in green synthesis of NP. The study involves a broad range of plant species that could result in the identification of effective bioactive compounds to synthesize NPs. Recent advances in the medicinal field include advancements in targeted drug transport, bio-imaging, and thermonostics. Applications in the environmental field extend to remediation processes such as the removal of pollutants. The cost-effectiveness and environmental sustainability of this technology could promote its economic feasibility and enable large-scale production. Interdisciplinary research involving several scientific disciplines is an intriguing possibility. However, it is still necessary to conduct comprehensive studies on the environmental impact, human health risks, and legal implications of NPs synthesized using different environmentally friendly methods.

## 7 Conclusion

The NPs synthesis using plant-based methods represents a promising avenue in the field of nanotechnology. The herbal extracts used as reducing agents produced NPs efficiently and sustainably. Numerous scientific studies have successfully produced NPs of gold, iron, zinc, silver, and copper using chemical, physical, and biological processes. Due to their distinct composition and properties, these NPs, which are typically between 5 and 100 nm in size, showed several activities, such as antioxidant, antimicrobial, anti-inflammatory, and antidiabetic effects. The efficacy of these plant-derived NPs can vary depending on the plant source, synthesis method, NP size, and surface chemistry. The integration of these plant-derived NPs into various technological developments has significantly advanced scientific innovation and promoted sustainable development.

## References

1. Abbasi BA, Iqbal J, Zahra SA et al (2020) Bioinspired synthesis and activity characterization of iron oxide nanoparticles made using Rhamnus Triquetra leaf extract. Mater Res Express 6:1250e7. https://doi.org/10.1088/2053-1591/ab664d

2. Agarwal H, Nakara A, Shanmugam VK (2019) Anti-inflammatory mechanism of various metal and metal oxide nanoparticles synthesized using plant extracts: a review. Biomed Pharmacother 109:2561–2572. https://doi.org/10.1016/j.biopha.2018.11.116
3. Ahmad MZ, Alasiri AS, Ahmad J et al (2022) Green synthesis of titanium dioxide nanoparticles using ocimum sanctum leaf extract: in vitro characterization and its healing efficacy in diabetic wounds. Molecules 27:7712. https://doi.org/10.3390/molecules27227712
4. Ahmed A, Usman M, Liu Q-Y et al (2019) Plant mediated synthesis of copper nanoparticles by using *Camelia sinensis* leaves extract and their applications in dye degradation. Ferroelectrics 549:61–69. https://doi.org/10.1080/00150193.2019.1592544
5. Ahmed RH, Mustafa DE (2020) Green synthesis of silver nanoparticles mediated by traditionally used medicinal plants in Sudan. Int Nano Lett 10:1–14. https://doi.org/10.1007/s40089-019-00291-9
6. Ahmed S, Ahmad M, Swami BL, Ikram S (2016) A review on plants extract mediated synthesis of silver nanoparticles for antimicrobial applications: a green expertise. J Adv Res 7:17–28. https://doi.org/10.1016/j.jare.2015.02.007
7. Ahn E-Y, Jin H, Park Y (2019) Assessing the antioxidant, cytotoxic, apoptotic and wound healing properties of silver nanoparticles green-synthesized by plant extracts. Mater Sci Eng C 101:204–216. https://doi.org/10.1016/j.msec.2019.03.095
8. Ahn E-Y, Park Y (2020) Anticancer prospects of silver nanoparticles green-synthesized by plant extracts. Mater Sci Eng C 116:111253. https://doi.org/10.1016/j.msec.2020.111253
9. Akintelu SA, Bo Y, Folorunso AS (2020) A review on synthesis, optimization, mechanism, characterization, and antibacterial application of silver nanoparticles synthesized from plants. J Chem 2020:1–12. https://doi.org/10.1155/2020/3189043
10. Al-Hakkani MF (2020) Biogenic copper nanoparticles and their applications: a review. SN Appl Sci 2:505. https://doi.org/10.1007/s42452-020-2279-1
11. Amaliyah S, Pangesti DP, Masruri M et al (2020) Green synthesis and characterization of copper nanoparticles using Piper retrofractum Vahl extract as bioreductor and capping agent. Heliyon 6:e04636. https://doi.org/10.1016/j.heliyon.2020.e04636
12. Asghar MA, Asghar MA (2020) Green synthesized and characterized copper nanoparticles using various new plants extracts aggravate microbial cell membrane damage after interaction with lipopolysaccharide. Int J Biol Macromol 160:1168–1176. https://doi.org/10.1016/j.ijbiomac.2020.05.198
13. Azarbani F, Shiravand S (2020) Green synthesis of silver nanoparticles by *Ferulago macrocarpa* flowers extract and their antibacterial, antifungal and toxic effects. Green Chem Lett Rev 13:41–49. https://doi.org/10.1080/17518253.2020.1726504
14. Azri FA, Selamat J, Sukor R et al (2019) Etlingera elatior-mediated synthesis of gold nanoparticles and their application as electrochemical current enhancer. Molecules 24:3141. https://doi.org/10.3390/molecules24173141
15. Balavijayalakshmi J, Ramalakshmi V (2017) Carica papaya peel mediated synthesis of silver nanoparticles and its antibacterial activity against human pathogens. J Appl Res Technol 15:413–422. https://doi.org/10.1016/j.jart.2017.03.010
16. Bao Y, He J, Song K et al (2021) Plant-extract-mediated synthesis of metal nanoparticles. J Chem 2021:1–14. https://doi.org/10.1155/2021/6562687
17. Benassai E, Del Bubba M, Ancillotti C et al (2021) Green and cost-effective synthesis of copper nanoparticles by extracts of non-edible and waste plant materials from Vaccinium species: characterization and antimicrobial activity. Mater Sci Eng C 119:111453. https://doi.org/10.1016/j.msec.2020.111453
18. Bibi I, Nazar N, Ata S et al (2019) Green synthesis of iron oxide nanoparticles using pomegranate seeds extract and photocatalytic activity evaluation for the degradation of textile dye. J Market Res 8:6115–6124. https://doi.org/10.1016/j.jmrt.2019.10.006
19. Bobo D, Robinson KJ, Islam J et al (2016) Nanoparticle-based medicines: a review of FDA-approved materials and clinical trials to date. Pharm Res 33:2373–2387. https://doi.org/10.1007/s11095-016-1958-5

20. Boomi P, Ganesan RM, Poorani G et al (2019) Biological synergy of greener gold nanoparticles by using coleus aromaticus leaf extract. Mater Sci Eng C 99:202–210. https://doi.org/10.1016/j.msec.2019.01.105
21. Borase HP, Patil CD, Sauter IP et al (2013) Amoebicidal activity of phytosynthesized silver nanoparticles and their *in vitro* cytotoxicity to human cells. FEMS Microbiol Lett 345:127–131. https://doi.org/10.1111/1574-6968.12195
22. Bunaciu AA, Udriştioiu E, gabriela, Aboul-Enein HY, (2015) X-ray diffraction: instrumentation and applications. Crit Rev Anal Chem 45:289–299. https://doi.org/10.1080/10408347.2014.949616
23. Chand K, Cao D, Eldin Fouad D et al (2020) Green synthesis, characterization and photocatalytic application of silver nanoparticles synthesized by various plant extracts. Arab J Chem 13:8248–8261. https://doi.org/10.1016/j.arabjc.2020.01.009
24. Chauhan S, Upadhyay LSB (2019) Biosynthesis of iron oxide nanoparticles using plant derivatives of Lawsonia inermis (Henna) and its surface modification for biomedical application. Nanotechnol Environ Eng 4:8. https://doi.org/10.1007/s41204-019-0055-5
25. Chouhan PN, Azimov A, Jabborova D, Singh S (2023) Review on the role of indigenous plants and plant derivatives of ayurveda in bone healing. Plant Sci Today 10(sp2):143–151
26. Das PE, Abu-Yousef IA, Majdalawieh AF et al (2020) Green synthesis of encapsulated copper nanoparticles using a hydroalcoholic extract of moringa oleifera leaves and assessment of their antioxidant and antimicrobial activities. Molecules 25:555. https://doi.org/10.3390/molecules25030555
27. Das RK, Gogoi N, Bora U (2011) Green synthesis of gold nanoparticles using Nyctanthes arbortristis flower extract. Bioprocess Biosyst Eng 34:615–619. https://doi.org/10.1007/s00449-010-0510-y
28. Diksha D, Gupta SK, Gupta P et al (2023) Antibacterial potential of gold nanoparticles synthesized from leaf extract of syzygium cumini against multidrug-resistant urinary tract pathogens. Cureus. https://doi.org/10.7759/cureus.34830
29. El Badawy AM, Silva RG, Morris B et al (2011) Surface charge-dependent toxicity of silver nanoparticles. Environ Sci Technol 45:283–287. https://doi.org/10.1021/es1034188
30. Fadlelmoula A, Pinho D, Carvalho VH et al (2022) Fourier transform infrared (FTIR) spectroscopy to analyse human blood over the last 20 years: a review towards lab-on-a-chip devices. Micromachines (Basel) 13:187. https://doi.org/10.3390/mi13020187
31. Ganesh Kumar V, Gokavarapu SD, Rajeswari A et al (2011) Facile green synthesis of gold nanoparticles using leaf extract of antidiabetic potent Cassia auriculata. Colloids Surf B Biointerfaces 87:159–163. https://doi.org/10.1016/j.colsurfb.2011.05.016
32. Gomathi AC, Xavier Rajarathinam SR, Mohammed Sadiq A, Rajeshkumar S (2020) Anticancer activity of silver nanoparticles synthesized using aqueous fruit shell extract of Tamarindus indica on MCF-7 human breast cancer cell line. J Drug Deliv Sci Technol 55:101376. https://doi.org/10.1016/j.jddst.2019.101376
33. Gupta G, Paul S, Singh S, Pietramellara G, Pathan SI, Danish S, Jha PN (2022) Exploring functional diversity and community structure of diazotrophic endophytic bacteria associated with Pennisetum glaucum growing under field in a semi-arid region. Land 11(7):991
34. Hackenberg S, Scherzed A, Kessler M et al (2011) Silver nanoparticles: evaluation of DNA damage, toxicity and functional impairment in human mesenchymal stem cells. Toxicol Lett 201:27–33. https://doi.org/10.1016/j.toxlet.2010.12.001
35. Hasnain MS, Javed MdN, Alam MdS et al (2019) Purple heart plant leaves extract-mediated silver nanoparticle synthesis: optimization by box-behnken design. Mater Sci Eng C 99:1105–1114. https://doi.org/10.1016/j.msec.2019.02.061
36. Hu D, Si W, Qin W et al (2019) Cucurbita pepo leaf extract induced synthesis of zinc oxide nanoparticles, characterization for the treatment of femoral fracture. J Photochem Photobiol B 195:12–16. https://doi.org/10.1016/j.jphotobiol.2019.04.001
37. Inkson BJ (2016) Scanning electron microscopy (SEM) and transmission electron microscopy (TEM) for materials characterization. In: Materials characterization using nondestructive evaluation (NDE) methods. Elsevier, pp 17–43

38. İpek İY, Yüksel S, Kabay N, Yüksel M (2014) Investigation of process parameters for removal of bisphenol A (BPA) from water by polymeric adsorbents in adsorption-ultrafiltration hybrid system. J Chem Technol Biotechnol 89:835–840. https://doi.org/10.1002/jctb.4317
39. Izadiyan Z, Shameli K, Miyake M et al (2020) Cytotoxicity assay of plant-mediated synthesized iron oxide nanoparticles using Juglans regia green husk extract. Arab J Chem 13:2011–2023. https://doi.org/10.1016/j.arabjc.2018.02.019
40. Jamdade DA, Rajpali D, Joshi KA et al (2019) *Gnidia glauca*–and *Plumbago zeylanica*–mediated synthesis of novel copper nanoparticles as promising antidiabetic agents. Adv Pharmacol Sci 1–11. https://doi.org/10.1155/2019/9080279
41. Jamzad M, Kamari Bidkorpeh M (2020) Green synthesis of iron oxide nanoparticles by the aqueous extract of Laurus nobilis L. leaves and evaluation of the antimicrobial activity. J Nanostructure Chem 10:193–201. https://doi.org/10.1007/s40097-020-00341-1
42. Kanipandian N, Kannan S, Ramesh R et al (2014) Characterization, antioxidant and cytotoxicity evaluation of green synthesized silver nanoparticles using Cleistanthus collinus extract as surface modifier. Mater Res Bull 49:494–502. https://doi.org/10.1016/j.materresbull.2013.09.016
43. Khan AU, Yuan Q, Khan ZUH et al (2018) An eco-benign synthesis of AgNPs using aqueous extract of Longan fruit peel: antiproliferative response against human breast cancer cell line MCF-7, antioxidant and photocatalytic deprivation of methylene blue. J Photochem Photobiol B 183:367–373. https://doi.org/10.1016/j.jphotobiol.2018.05.007
44. Khatami M, Alijani HQ, Fakheri B et al (2019) Super-paramagnetic iron oxide nanoparticles (SPIONs): Greener synthesis using Stevia plant and evaluation of its antioxidant properties. J Clean Prod 208:1171–1177. https://doi.org/10.1016/j.jclepro.2018.10.182
45. Passos MLC, Saraiva MLMFS (2019) Detection in UV-visible spectrophotometry: detectors, detection systems, and detection strategies. Measurement 135:896–904. https://doi.org/10.1016/j.measurement.2018.12.045
46. Poka LP, Krishna Mohan G, Venkateswara Rao K, Shanker K (2019) Biosynthesis, characterization and acute oral toxicity studies of synthesized iron oxide nanoparticles using ethanolic extract of Centella asiatica plant. Mater Lett 236:256–259. https://doi.org/10.1016/j.matlet.2018.10.037
47. Liu H, Kang P, Liu Y et al (2020) Zinc oxide nanoparticles synthesised from the *Vernonia amygdalina* shows the anti-inflammatory and antinociceptive activities in the mice model. Artif Cells Nanomed Biotechnol 48:1068–1078. https://doi.org/10.1080/21691401.2020.1809440
48. Sundrarajan M, Bama K, Bhavani M et al (2017) Obtaining titanium dioxide nanoparticles with spherical shape and antimicrobial properties using M. citrifolia leaves extract by hydrothermal method. J Photochem Photobiol B 171:117–124. https://doi.org/10.1016/j.jphotobiol.2017.05.003
49. Maddala VKS, Singh S, Bandi J (2024) Soil properties influencing nutrient signaling in plant soil systems. In: Essential minerals in plant-soil systems. Elsevier, pp 373–393
50. Majoumouo MS, Sharma JR, Sibuyi NRS et al (2020) Synthesis of biogenic gold nanoparticles from terminalia mantaly extracts and the evaluation of their in vitro cytotoxic effects in cancer cells. Molecules 25:4469. https://doi.org/10.3390/molecules25194469
51. Mali SC, Dhaka A, Githala CK, Trivedi R (2020) Green synthesis of copper nanoparticles using Celastrus paniculatus Willd. leaf extract and their photocatalytic and antifungal properties. Biotechnol Rep 27:e00518. https://doi.org/10.1016/j.btre.2020.e00518
52. Manik UP, Nande A, Raut S, Dhoble SJ (2020) Green synthesis of silver nanoparticles using plant leaf extraction of Artocarpus heterophylus and Azadirachta indica. Results Mater 6:100086. https://doi.org/10.1016/j.rinma.2020.100086
53. Mittal AK, Chisti Y, Banerjee UC (2013) Synthesis of metallic nanoparticles using plant extracts. Biotechnol Adv 31:346–356. https://doi.org/10.1016/j.biotechadv.2013.01.003
54. Mohanta YK, Biswas K, Jena SK et al (2020) Anti-biofilm and antibacterial activities of silver nanoparticles synthesized by the reducing activity of phytoconstituents present in the Indian medicinal plants. Front Microbiol 11. https://doi.org/10.3389/fmicb.2020.01143

55. Murthy HCA, Desalegn T, Kassa M et al (2020) Synthesis of green copper nanoparticles using medicinal plant *Hagenia abyssinica (Brace) JF. Gmel.* leaf extract: antimicrobial properties. J Nanomater 1–12. https://doi.org/10.1155/2020/3924081
56. Mustapha T, Misni N, Ithnin NR et al (2022) A review on plants and microorganisms mediated synthesis of silver nanoparticles, role of plants metabolites and applications. Int J Environ Res Public Health 19:674. https://doi.org/10.3390/ijerph19020674
57. Nair GM, Sajini T, Mathew B (2022) Advanced green approaches for metal and metal oxide nanoparticles synthesis and their environmental applications. Talanta Open 5:100080. https://doi.org/10.1016/j.talo.2021.100080
58. Nande A, Raut S, Michalska-Domanska M, Dhoble SJ (2021) Green synthesis of nanomaterials using plant extract: a review. Curr Pharm Biotechnol 22:1794–1811. https://doi.org/10.2174/1389201021666201117121452
59. Narayanan M, Devi PG, Natarajan D et al (2021) Green synthesis and characterization of titanium dioxide nanoparticles using leaf extract of Pouteria campechiana and larvicidal and pupicidal activity on Aedes aegypti. Environ Res 200:111333. https://doi.org/10.1016/j.envres.2021.111333
60. Panneerselvam A, Velayutham J, Ramasamy S (2021) Green synthesis of $TiO_2$ nanoparticles prepared from *Phyllanthus niruri* leaf extract for dye adsorption and their isotherm and kinetic studies. IET Nanobiotechnol 15:164–172. https://doi.org/10.1049/nbt2.12033
61. Parveen R, Jain T, Parveen R, Singh S (2023) Genome-wide transcriptome profiling of crop plants. In: Genomics, transcriptomics, proteomics and metabolomics of crop plants. Academic Press, pp 145–171
62. Patani A, Prajapati D, Shukla K, Patel M, Patani P, Patel A, Singh S (2024) Environmental stress–induced alterations in the micro-and macronutrients status of plant. In: Essential minerals in plant-soil systems. Elsevier, pp 181–195
63. Philip D, Unni C, Aromal SA, Vidhu VK (2011) Murraya Koenigii leaf-assisted rapid green synthesis of silver and gold nanoparticles. Spectrochim Acta A Mol Biomol Spectrosc 78:899–904. https://doi.org/10.1016/j.saa.2010.12.060
64. Qais FA, Shafiq A, Khan HM et al (2019) Antibacterial effect of silver nanoparticles synthesized using *Murraya koenigii* (L.) against multidrug-resistant pathogens. Bioinorg Chem Appl 2019:1–11. https://doi.org/10.1155/2019/4649506
65. Rad SS, Sani AM, Mohseni S (2019) Biosynthesis, characterization and antimicrobial activities of zinc oxide nanoparticles from leaf extract of Mentha pulegium (L.). Microb Pathog 131:239–245. https://doi.org/10.1016/j.micpath.2019.04.022
66. Rajakumar G, Rahuman AA, Jayaseelan C et al (2014) Solanum trilobatum extract-mediated synthesis of titanium dioxide nanoparticles to control Pediculus humanus capitis, Hyalomma anatolicum anatolicum and Anopheles subpictus. Parasitol Res 113:469–479. https://doi.org/10.1007/s00436-013-3676-9
67. Rajakumar G, Rahuman AA, Roopan SM et al (2015) Efficacy of larvicidal activity of green synthesized titanium dioxide nanoparticles using Mangifera indica extract against blood-feeding parasites. Parasitol Res 114:571–581. https://doi.org/10.1007/s00436-014-4219-8
68. Rajasekharreddy P, Usha Rani P, Sreedhar B (2010) Qualitative assessment of silver and gold nanoparticle synthesis in various plants: a photobiological approach. J Nanopart Res 12:1711–1721. https://doi.org/10.1007/s11051-010-9894-5
69. Rajeshkumar S, Menon S, Venkat Kumar S et al (2019) Antibacterial and antioxidant potential of biosynthesized copper nanoparticles mediated through Cissus arnotiana plant extract. J Photochem Photobiol B 197:111531. https://doi.org/10.1016/j.jphotobiol.2019.111531
70. Rajkumari J, Magdalane CM, Siddhardha B et al (2019) Synthesis of titanium oxide nanoparticles using Aloe barbadensis mill and evaluation of its antibiofilm potential against Pseudomonas aeruginosa PAO1. J Photochem Photobiol B 201:111667. https://doi.org/10.1016/j.jphotobiol.2019.111667
71. Raymond C (2020) Plant extracts based nanoparticles, a good perspective in the development of drugs in nanomedicine. Mod Approaches Drug Des 3. https://doi.org/10.31031/MADD.2020.03.000556

72. Roy A (2021) Plant derived silver nanoparticles and their therapeutic applications. Curr Pharm Biotechnol 22:1834–1847. https://doi.org/10.2174/1389201021666201027155708
73. Rozhin A, Batasheva S, Kruychkova M et al (2021) Biogenic silver nanoparticles: synthesis and application as antibacterial and antifungal agents. Micromachines (Basel) 12:1480. https://doi.org/10.3390/mi12121480
74. Sana SS, Kumbhakar DV, Pasha A et al (2020) Crotalaria verrucosa leaf extract mediated synthesis of zinc oxide nanoparticles: assessment of antimicrobial and anticancer activity. Molecules 25:4896. https://doi.org/10.3390/molecules25214896
75. Sandhya J, Kalaiselvam S (2020) Biogenic synthesis of magnetic iron oxide nanoparticles using inedible borassus flabellifer seed coat: characterization, antimicrobial, antioxidant activity and in vitro cytotoxicity analysis. Mater Res Express 7:015045. https://doi.org/10.1088/2053-1591/ab6642
76. Sao P, Chand Y, Kumar A, Singh S (2021) Potential drug target identification in porphyromonas gingivalis using in-silico subtractive metabolic pathway analysis. Bangladesh J Med Sci 20(4):887–896
77. Sarwar N, Bin HU, Kumar M et al (2021) Citric acid mediated green synthesis of copper nanoparticles using cinnamon bark extract and its multifaceted applications. J Clean Prod 292:125974. https://doi.org/10.1016/j.jclepro.2021.125974
78. Satti SH, Raja NI, Ikram M et al (2022) Plant-based titanium dioxide nanoparticles trigger biochemical and proteome modifications in triticum aestivum L. under biotic stress of Puccinia striiformis. Molecules 27:4274. https://doi.org/10.3390/molecules27134274
79. Singh J, Dutta T, Kim K-H et al (2018) 'Green' synthesis of metals and their oxide nanoparticles: applications for environmental remediation. J Nanobiotechnology 16:84. https://doi.org/10.1186/s12951-018-0408-4
80. Singh P, Kim Y-J, Zhang D, Yang D-C (2016) Biological synthesis of nanoparticles from plants and microorganisms. Trends Biotechnol 34:588–599. https://doi.org/10.1016/j.tibtech.2016.02.006
81. Singh P, Mijakovic I (2022) Green synthesis and antibacterial applications of gold and silver nanoparticles from Ligustrum vulgare berries. Sci Rep 12:7902. https://doi.org/10.1038/s41598-022-11811-7
82. Stetefeld J, McKenna SA, Patel TR (2016) Dynamic light scattering: a practical guide and applications in biomedical sciences. Biophys Rev 8:409–427. https://doi.org/10.1007/s12551-016-0218-6
83. Suman TY, Radhika Rajasree SR, Ramkumar R et al (2014) The green synthesis of gold nanoparticles using an aqueous root extract of Morinda citrifolia L. Spectrochim Acta A Mol Biomol Spectrosc 118:11–16. https://doi.org/10.1016/j.saa.2013.08.066
84. Sumanth B, Lakshmeesha TR, Ansari MA et al (2020) Mycogenic synthesis of extracellular zinc oxide nanoparticles from Xylaria acuta and its nanoantibiotic potential. Int J Nanomedicine 15:8519–8536. https://doi.org/10.2147/IJN.S271743
85. Tang CY, Yang Z (2017) Transmission electron microscopy (TEM). In: Membrane characterization. Elsevier, pp 145–159
86. Umar H, Kavaz D, Rizaner N (2018) Biosynthesis of zinc oxide nanoparticles using Albizia lebbeck stem bark, and evaluation of its antimicrobial, antioxidant, and cytotoxic activities on human breast cancer cell lines. Int J Nanomedicine 14:87–100. https://doi.org/10.2147/IJN.S186888
87. Vasantharaj S, Sathiyavimal S, Senthilkumar P et al (2019) Biosynthesis of iron oxide nanoparticles using leaf extract of Ruellia tuberosa: antimicrobial properties and their applications in photocatalytic degradation. J Photochem Photobiol B 192:74–82. https://doi.org/10.1016/j.jphotobiol.2018.12.025
88. Verma N, Sao P, Srivastava A, Singh S (2021) Physiological and molecular responses to drought, submergence and excessive watering in plants. In: Harsh environment and plant resilience: molecular and functional aspects, pp 305–321
89. Vishwakarma SK, Ilyas T, Shahid M, Malviya D, Kumar S, Singh S, Singh HV (2024) Bacillus spp.: nature's gift to agriculture and humankind. In: Applications of bacillus and

bacillus derived genera in agriculture, biotechnology and beyond. Singapore: Springer Nature, Singapore, pp 1–36
90. Vora Z, Pandya J, Vaikuntapu PR, Singh S, Asha S, Purama RK (2023) Genome-wide association of defense hormone crosstalk in plants. In: Hormonal cross-talk, plant defense and development. Academic Press, pp 353–371
91. Wang L, Xu J, Yan Y et al (2019) Synthesis of gold nanoparticles from leaf *Panax notoginseng* and its anticancer activity in pancreatic cancer PANC-1 cell lines. Artif Cells Nanomed Biotechnol 47:1216–1223. https://doi.org/10.1080/21691401.2019.1593852
92. Wang Z, Que B, Gan J et al (2020) Zinc oxide nanoparticles synthesized from Fraxinus rhynchophylla extract by green route method attenuates the chemical and heat induced neurogenic and inflammatory pain models in mice. J Photochem Photobiol B 202:111668. https://doi.org/10.1016/j.jphotobiol.2019.111668
93. Wu S, Rajeshkumar S, Madasamy M, Mahendran V (2020) Green synthesis of copper nanoparticles using *Cissus vitiginea* and its antioxidant and antibacterial activity against urinary tract infection pathogens. Artif Cells Nanomed Biotechnol 48:1153–1158. https://doi.org/10.1080/21691401.2020.1817053
94. Wu T, Duan X, Hu C et al (2019) Synthesis and characterization of gold nanoparticles from *Abies spectabilis* extract and its anticancer activity on bladder cancer T24 cells. Artif Cells Nanomed Biotechnol 47:512–523. https://doi.org/10.1080/21691401.2018.1560305
95. Xu K, Yan H, Cao M, Shao X (2020) Selaginella convolute extract mediated synthesis of ZnO NPs for pain management in emerging nursing care. J Photochem Photobiol B 202:111700. https://doi.org/10.1016/j.jphotobiol.2019.111700
96. Yadi M, Mostafavi E, Saleh B et al (2018) Current developments in green synthesis of metallic nanoparticles using plant extracts: a review. Artif Cells Nanomed Biotechnol 46:336–343. https://doi.org/10.1080/21691401.2018.1492931
97. Yang Z, Liu Z, Zhu J et al (2022) Green synthesis and characterization of gold nanoparticles from *Pholiota adiposa* and their anticancer effects on hepatic carcinoma. Drug Deliv 29:997–1006. https://doi.org/10.1080/10717544.2022.2056664
98. Yusefi M, Shameli K, Ali RR et al (2020) Evaluating anticancer activity of plant-mediated synthesized iron oxide nanoparticles using punica granatum fruit peel extract. J Mol Struct 1204:127539. https://doi.org/10.1016/j.molstruc.2019.127539
99. Zahir AA, Chauhan IS, Bagavan A et al (2015) Green synthesis of silver and titanium dioxide nanoparticles using euphorbia prostrata extract shows shift from apoptosis to $G_0/G_1$ arrest followed by necrotic cell death in leishmania donovani. Antimicrob Agents Chemother 59:4782–4799. https://doi.org/10.1128/AAC.00098-15
100. Zhang T, Dang M, Zhang W, Lin X (2020) Gold nanoparticles synthesized from Euphorbia fischeriana root by green route method alleviates the isoprenaline hydrochloride induced myocardial infarction in rats. J Photochem Photobiol B 202:111705. https://doi.org/10.1016/j.jphotobiol.2019.111705

# Use of Nut Shells in the Production of Nanobiocomposites

**Maria-Beatrice Coltelli, Laura Aliotta, Vito Gigante, and Andrea Lazzeri**

**Abstract** Nut shells are an abundant and underutilized waste of the agro-food sector. Its valorization in the production of nanobiocomposites is a possibility to exploit its renewable content producing advanced bio-based materials with tailored thermomechanical and functional features for high-performance applications. In the present chapter, the most important nut shells were explored in connection with global and local food production. Then the production of biocomposites from the different nut shell micrometric powders was explored considering their importance in applications in furniture, automotive, packaging, and personal care/biomedical applications. This analysis suggested that the use of bio-based and compostable matrices is currently more explored in this latter field. Finally, the use of nut shell in nanobiocomposites was surveyed considering the possibility to exploit nanoparticles coming from nut shell or the possibility to exploit compounds/components obtained by extraction of molecules or conversion to cellulose or lignin of the nut shell waste. This last part revealed, in good agreement with the previous one, that nut shell agro-waste is currently an important source for new highly-technological biorefinery chains in agreement with circular economy and a more sustainable way of producing consumer goods.

**Keywords** Nut · Shell · Walnut · Hazelnut · Biocomposite · Nanobiocomposite · Circular economy

---

M.-B. Coltelli (✉) · L. Aliotta · V. Gigante · A. Lazzeri
Department of Civil and Industrial Engineering (DICI), University of Pisa, Pisa, Italy
e-mail: maria.beatrice.coltelli@unipi.it

Research Unit DICI-UNIPI, National Interuniversity Consortium of Materials Science and Technology (INSTM), Pisa, Italy

 
D. Jabborova et al. (eds.), *Nanomaterials in Agroforestry Systems*, Smart Nanomaterials Technology, https://doi.org/10.1007/978-981-96-1337-3_4

## 1 Types of Shells Used in Nanobiocomposites

Nuts are generally defined as dry fruits containing an edible seed protected by a hard shell and their consumption in human nutrition is known since ancient times. Nuts are nowadays considered superfoods since they are rich in lipids, proteins, vitamins, mineral, and phenolic compounds [38] and it is known that the consumption in the daily diet of nuts has been associated with positive effects on health, above all against cardiometabolic diseases [16, 28]. Nuts production has increased greatly over the past decade, accounting for 4.6 million metric tons in 2019/2020 [57].

Several plants and their respective fruits can be considered as sources of edible nuts because of the presence of many local varieties, with walnuts (*Juglans regia*), almonds (*Prunus dulcis*), hazelnuts (*Corylus avellana*), pistachios (*Pistacia vera*), chestnuts (*Castanea sativa*), and cashews (*Anacardium occidentale*), as the ones with the highest production worldwide [104]. Thus, plants mainly exploited are almond tree, hazelnut tree, pistachio tree, pine walnut tree, and peanut plant (Fig. 1).

Walnuts are produced by the plant *Juglans regia L.* and their yearly global production overcomes 3.7 million tons. The largest producer of walnuts is China, with 1.06 million tons/year. The other major producers of walnuts are Iran, USA, and Turkey

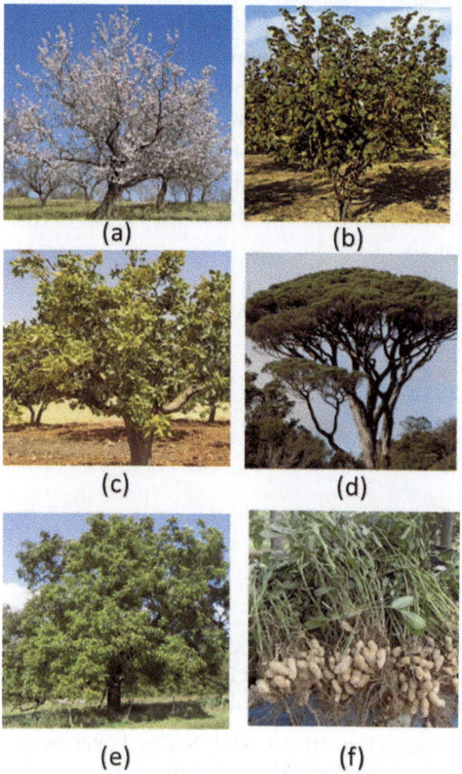


**Fig. 1** The most common plants producing nuts for human consumption: (**a**) almond tree, (**b**) hazelnut tree; (**c**) pistachio tree; (**d**) pine tree; (**e**) walnut tree; (**f**) peanut plant

[52], respectively. Kernels of walnuts, used as food, are very rich in polyunsaturated fatty acids (52–70%) and minerals (1.5–2%). They contain also proteins (12–24%) particularly rich in essential amino acids and a wide variety of flavonoids, polyphenols, and phenolic acids, known to be natural antioxidants. The other parts of the plant, e.g., flowers, leaves, stem, pericarp, bark, and ligneous membranes, are widely exploited in the pharmaceutical or cosmetic industries [50, 84].

Almonds, produced by the almond tree (*Prunus dulcis*), are popular nuts for snack foods and ingredients in many widely diffused industrial foods [16]. According to the INC (International Nut and Dried Fruit Council Foundation), their production accounted for 1.2 million tons/year during the 2017/2018 season. The USA is leader in the almond global production with 81% of the total one, followed by Australia and Spain with 7% and 4%, respectively. Almond by-products consist of their skins and shells that currently are mainly used as livestock feed or exploited for energy production [27]. Thus, the almond processing industries would like to better valorize these by-products. Almond skins, thanks to their flavonoid and phenolic acid content, can be used as an ingredient for limiting oxidative processes in several food products [46]. Almond skins correspond to a significant amount (4–8% by weight) of the total shelled almond [40]. Moreover, almond shells represent over 50% of the dry weight of the almond fruits and they are of ligneous nature. Some authors suggested that they could be exploited in the chemistry industry due to their high xylan content [27].

*P. pinea* L., stone pine, is globally known as a valuable species for the production of wood, but it is certainly better valorized for producing pine kernels. In fact, these kernels have a high market price, because of their delicate and peculiar flavor combined with a high value in terms of nutritive elements. They contain 30% of proteins and 50% of lipids. 80% of these lipids are unsaturated essential fatty acids. Considering these premises, *Pinus pinea* pine nut is considered the most important edible wild seed collected from Mediterranean forests. Pine nut production represents the most profitable and valuable activity for stone pine forests in Spain, Portugal, Italy, and Turkey [102]. In the Iberian Peninsula more than 70% of the pine nut world production is produced [32]. For instance, in Portugal, with an increasing trend of 46% in the period 2005–2010, *P. pinea* is the fifth most important forest species. More recently it was reported that pine nut shells represent over 77% of the weight of the pine nuts [77] and they are ligneous.

Hazelnut world production, from *Corylus avellana* tree, shows an increasing trend from the beginning of the last century, in response to the extensive demand from the confectionery industry [49]. This industry uses and processes large quantities of the harvested nuts [13]. Turkey is reported to be the main producer and exporter of hazelnuts of the species Corylus avellana, with a production of 420.000 tons/year, followed by Italy with 120.572 tons/year. At the third place in hazelnut production is Spain that produces about 15.300 tons/year of hazelnuts [95]. Keeping into account that about 50% of the total hazelnut production corresponds to solid waste, it can be deducted that around 500,000 tons/year of hazelnut shells are produced globally [95] and several studies for its valorization are currently ongoing [29, 93].

The global production of Pistachio nuts, from the plant *Pistacia vera*, in 2017 amounted to 1,115,066 tons [90]. Major producers of pistachios are Iran, Turkey, the United States, and China. Keeping into account that the ratio of the pistachio shell/nut is about 0.45/1, the generation of pistachio shells by-products on a global scale is hundreds of thousands of tons per year. Considering the pistachio shell, the content of biogenic chemical elements was determined to be: oxygen 47.95%, carbon 44.89%, hydrogen 5.66%; sulfur 0.97%; nitrogen 0.53%. Regarding the composition in terms of biopolymers, the cellulose content is 38.1–54.0%, hemicellulose content is 15.2–31.4%, and lignin content is 25.2–29.4% [26].

Peanut, from the plant *Arachis hypogaea*, is a widely diffused grain legume cultivated worldwide with a growing production trend of about 48 million tons [33]. Due to these high production quantities, it seems necessary to consider the waste that peanut processing can generate. In fact, about 25 wt.% of its production is attributable to the shell. Peanut shell contains about 50% of cellulose, 20% of hemicellulose, and 30% of lignin [33]. Lignin makes difficult to digest this by-product and it does not allow it to be used as feedstock for animals. Moreover, its biodegradation is very slow, and severe treatments are thus needed to process this kind of material [103]. As a consequence, some authors suggested that fast pyrolysis seems to be a good alternative to treat and significantly valorize this biowaste [33].

Several other nuts are important in different parts of the world. For its general diffusion chestnut deserves to be mentioned, as it is proposed by studies about valorization of antioxidants like ellagic acid aiming at a better exploitation of its by-products [24]. Moreover, cashew nut, native from south America, currently produced also in Africa and India, deserves to be mentioned. Like for chestnut, the valorization of its by-products is currently considered for granting a better sustainability of its industrial chain [92]. Cashew nuts are incorporated in a shell from which an oil can be extracted. The shell of the nut is approximately 1/8 inch thick. Cashew nut shell liquid (CNSL) is a viscous liquid of dark color. This liquid is present in the honeycomb structure of soft consistency typical of the cashew nuts. It is considered a valuable agricultural by-product of both cashew nut and cashew apple production. Cashew nuts and cashew apples are both produced by the cashew nut tree (*Anacardium occidentale*). CNSL is specifically the pericarp fluid of the cashew nut and it consists of phenolic compounds with aliphatic side chains, and these are 70% anacardic acid, 5% cardanol, and 18% cardol [45]. This liquid is currently considered an important source for present and future biorefinery [66] and is used in surfactants, paints and varnishes, polymer resins, rubber compounding resins, epoxy resins, polyurethane based polymers, cashew cements, and also intermediates for chemical industry.

## 1.1 Composition of Nut Shell Powder

In general, considering the global production of nuts, almonds were the most produced (31%) globally, followed by walnuts (21%), cashews (17%), and hazelnuts (12%). Overall, nuts production value has increased significantly and steadily over the past decade following an average rate of $USD 1.9 billion per year, reaching

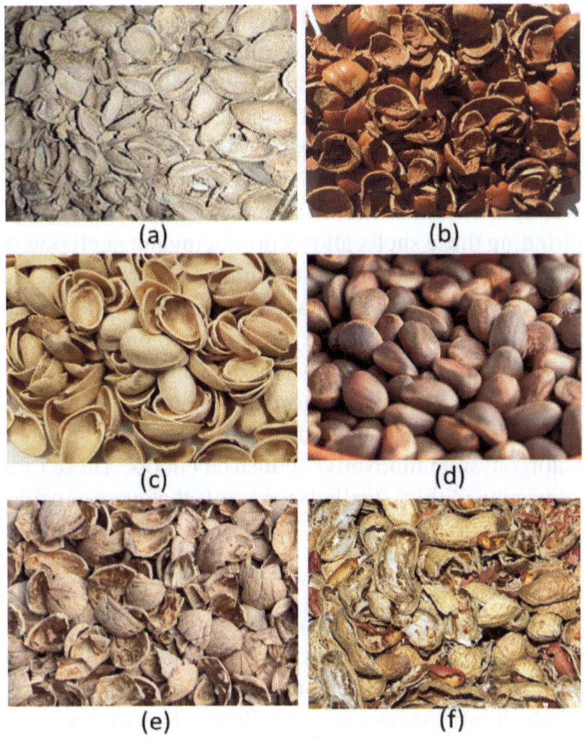


**Fig. 2** Abundant waste of the most common nuts: (**a**) almond shells, (**b**) hazelnut shells; (**c**) pistachio shells; (**d**) pine shells; (**e**) walnut shells; (**f**) peanut shells

$USD 35.6 billion for 2019–2020 season [31, 85]. As a result of nut industrialization processes, high amounts of by-products and residues are produced year by year, being stored or burnt as fuel for heaters or discarded as non-valued waste [95]. Shells represent the most abundant residue that should be valorized (Fig. 2), considering the principles of circular economy.

Agroindustry generates huge sources of biomass that are neither sufficiently nor adequately utilized [11]. The use of plant waste materials as raw materials for producing polymeric and composite materials represents a great opportunity for the general development of circular bio-economy and sustainability. In fact, fruit shells and other agricultural wastes are potentially important sources for producing valuable compounds. It can be considered that these plant-based by-products are produced in huge quantities, and crop waste is valuable in terms of their composition because they are rich in diverse nutritional components, enabling various uses. As a consequence, recently, the use by pharmaceutical and food manufacturers of these by-products was increased to produce valuable compounds from such sectors. As yet evidenced, due to their diverse uses within the food industry, nuts are one of the most important agricultural products. As a consequence, walnut shells have great potential in the production of new bio-based materials due to their production in large quantities. In the walnut processing industry, large quantities of peel and shell are produced after the kernel is separated from the external parts of the fruit. It should be considered that peel and shell are the major part (over 60%) of the nut fruit and they are currently discarded or burned as fuel without any useful high-value application. In particular, this by-product is generally directly burned in situ for heating purposes. On the other hand, it could be better exploited for the production of high value-added chemicals and for the preparation of composites. Therefore, it is needed to find other better uses for nut shells. The composition of nut shell is very similar to that of other woody biomass because it is mainly based on lignin, hemicellulose, and cellulose. Grinding these shells allows producing nut shell powder (NSP) of different sizes and morphologies. Regarding the amount, Barbu et al. [14] reported that shell residues, only derived from walnut and hazelnut, comprises amount of 650 K t/year and 350 K t/year respectively. So, they proposed to produce new composites materials made by walnut and hazelnut shells powder [82] embedded in a thermoset resin.

The composition in terms of chemical elements of walnut, almond, and pine nut shells was determined by different analytical techniques [77] in view of their valorization in innovative industrial chains. These three different shells were mainly consisting of thick-walled stone cells that were considered those conferring its typical brittleness to the material [70]. The authors reported that walnut shells contain 10.6% extractives, 30.1% lignin, and 49.7% polysaccharides, almond shells contain 5.7% extractives, 28.9% lignin, and 56.1% polysaccharides,and pine nut shells contain 4.5% extractives, 40.5% lignin, and 48.7% polysaccharides. We can observe that a high variability in terms of the different fractions can be found in the different shells, with polysaccharides accounting about half of the shell weight. All the examined nut shells showed a high content in lignin. The percentage of hydroxyphenyl (H), guaiacyl (G), and syringyl (S) lignin-derived products were separately summed by the authors, so that the S/G ratio and the H/G/S relation were calculated. The results of this study showed that walnut and almond shells have a SG lignin and pine nut shells have a G lignin. Significant chemical differences were also found in the polysaccharide composition, hemicellulosic profile and in the content of extractives. In particular, extractives were mainly polar with moderate antioxidant properties [93].

As already highlighted in the previous sections, the knowledge of chemical composition of the nut shells indicates as promising the potential valorization of hemicelluloses and lignin as main components on one side. On the other side several authors have explored the possibility of extracting by hydroalcoholic extraction [43] polyphenols (flavonoids and tannins) from nut shells, thus exploiting these compounds in antioxidant products (cosmetics, polymers, biomedical, etc…). In the case of walnuts, the shredding of the shells into very small particles and the use of ultrasound during the extraction process allowed the yield to be increased from 20.6 mg Gallic acid equivalent/g of dry weight to 52 Gallic acid equivalent/g of dry weight [41]. Hydroalcoholic extracts show antioxidant activities due to the presence of gallic acid, tyrosol, gallocatechin, quercetin, vanillin, etc. [43]. Shell extracts could be valorized as natural antioxidants for fossil and bio-based plastics, acting as thermal and photooxidative stabilizers for different types of polymers, including PLA [1]. For example, PLA films containing pecan nut extracts have been prepared which showed good antioxidant properties with a reduction in the intensity of the UV band characteristic of DPPH > 60% in less than 30 min and a delay in the browning of apple smoothies [60]. Furthermore, in other studies, it is shown that the addition of walnut shell powder in quantities varying from 5 to 20% by weight in both PLA and PHA allows for obtaining light biocomposites, in some cases with improved thermal and mechanical properties, with better biodegradability than that of the matrix and a lower cost [113].

The chemical decomposition of powder with production of specific chemical is also considered by several authors. For instance, Serafin et al. [88] prepared highly microporous activated carbons for $H_2$ and $CO_2$ storage. These activated carbons were based on walnut shell biomass. Roquia et al. [81] attempted the synthesis and characterization of carbon nanotubes by exploiting the waste of Juglans regia (walnut) shells. Ngo et al. [19] studied the possible production of activated carbons from nut shells.

## 2 Nut Shell Powder Reinforced Biocomposites

A biocomposite is a composite material formed by a matrix (resin) and a reinforcement of natural fibers [37]. Biocomposites [3] are widely used in several industrial sectors. In the building sector [51, 87], in furniture [25], and in automotive [73] sectors, composites can be used in both structural and aesthetic applications thanks to their unique properties combining a high stiffness with a reduced density. Morever, in packaging [6] and personal care/cosmetic applications [7], biocomposites are considered because of their enhanced biodegradability, low cost, and circularity.

The most important polymeric matrices used for such applications are based on polypropylene (PP) or other polyolefins, mainly used in the structural applications, or biopolyesters. The most important biopolyesters, especially in the packaging [80] and personal care/cosmetic/biomedical sector [22], are poly(lactic acid) (PLA), polyhydroxyalcanoates (PHA) and polybutilenesuccinate (PBS) and its copolymers like polybutylenesuccinate-co-adipate (PBSA) (Fig. 3). In fact, all these polymers have the advantage of being both renewable and compostable.

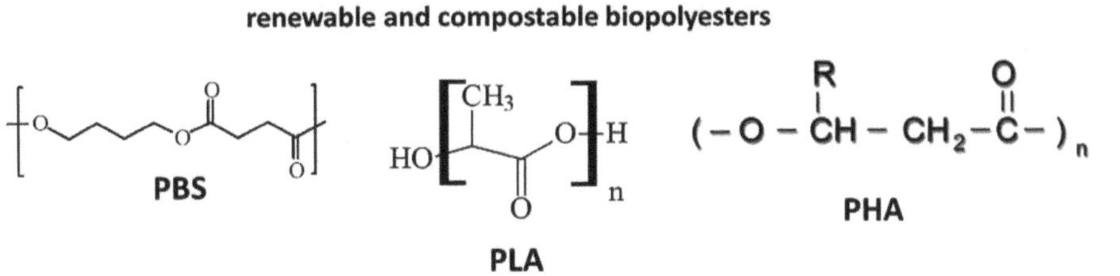


**Fig. 3** Chemical structure of poly(butylene succinate) (PBS), poly(lactic acid) (PLA), and general structure for polyhydroxyalcanoates (PHA), synthesized by bacteria

## 2.1 Walnut Shell Powder Biocomposites

Regarding the use of walnut shell powder (WSP) in composites, Yu et al. [110] have produced a material suitable for additive manufacturing, to be used in selective laser sintering (SLS) by mechanically mixing the powder with a hot-melt copolyester. The maximum amount of WSP incorporated was 40%. Compared to the use of copolyester alone, the properties of the material obtained from the walnut powder were improved and the density of the pieces decreased.

Akincioglu et al. [2] prepared brake pads that integrated up to 7% walnut shell powder in phenolic resin along with other metallic, ceramic, and elastomeric reinforcers.

Pradhan et al. [75] used walnut shell powder to produce polyester thermosetting matrix composites, carefully studying the thermal conduction aspects of these materials which showed variable densities with the geometry of the fillers. An important contribution to thermal resistance is given by the interface between matrix and reinforcing fiber. The study also showed that the glass transition temperature tends to increase with the addition of nut shell powder. Furthermore, the coefficient of thermal expansion tends to decrease. These aspects are interesting for use in the production of objects for the composites sector, for applications in the construction or vehicle furnishing sector and in packaging. However, composites of this type are not recyclable and are not from renewable sources as the thermosetting resin is of fossil origin [35].

Paczkowski [68] investigated an unsaturated polyester resin based on post-consumer recycled poly (ethylene terephthalate) reinforced with WSP. The filler incorporation induced a decrease in gloss and mechanical properties. On the contrary, the flexural strength and modulus resulted significantly improved by increasing the filler amount in the composite. Toluene, distilled water, 1% sodium hydroxide, and acetone were used in chemical resistance test carried out by the immersion, having a duration of 49 days, in solvents. No significant effects were evidenced for the pure resin after the immersion in water, but a plasticizing effect was observed for its composites. All specimens showed resistance toward toluene, but in acetone, the resin and its composite did not resist as well as is an alkaline environment, where a decrease in mechanical properties and optical properties (gloss) was observed.

Interestingly, in the thermoset composites sector, the addition of WSP to epoxy resins allowed the production of structural composites with improved wear resistance [94].

Sowinska-Baranowska et al. [98] added walnut shells that were previously ground and corn starch in different weight compositions as bio-based fillers for biocomposites with a natural rubber (NR) matrix. Additionally, 1-butyl-3-methylimidazolium chloride (BmiCl) and (3-aminopropyl)-triethoxysilane (APTES) ionic liquids were added for increasing the activity of bio-based fillers and for improving the curing features of the natural rubber based composites. BmiCl and APTES efficiently supported the vulcanization and enhanced the dispersion of bio-based fillers in the natural rubber elastomeric matrix. The obtained vulcanizates containing starch showed improved tensile properties thanks to the higher crosslinking density. Natural rubber reinforced with walnut shells powder demonstrated improved resistance to thermo-oxidative aging. This effect was attributed to lignin present in walnut shell that may have an antioxidant activity.

Completely renewable, recyclable, and potentially compostable thermoplastic composites could be of broad interest for countless applications that also consider the end of life of the materials as well as performance. The use of walnut shell powder to obtain these composites has so far been little reported in the literature. Sarsari et al. [86] added walnut shell powder (WSP) to thermoplastic starch (TPS), and nanoclay to prepare biocomposites. The composite samples were formed in a Colin extruder and then they were injection molded. The addition of up to 40% WSP greatly improved the tensile strength, flexural strength, and elasticity modulus of the composite. Also, the composites made with higher WSP contents had increased thickness swelling and water absorption. The incorporation of nanoclay (0–5%) greatly improved the tensile properties. Soil burial degradation experiments showed that biodegradation was accelerated by the increase of starch in the composite mixtures. The study showed that WSP can be successfully utilized for the manufacture of composites, resulting in materials showing useful physical and mechanical properties.

Shaik et al. [89] used agricultural wastes to prepare bioplastic composites: eggshell powder and walnut shell powder in PLA plasticized with 5 wt.% of Epoxidized Soybean Oil. The properties of plasticized PLA reinforced with eggshell powder composite resulted better than the composite reinforced with WSP.

Montava-Jordà et al. [62] prepared by melt compounding a blend consisting of two polymers: polylactide (PLA) and poly(ε-caprolactone) (PCL) at a ratio 4/1 by weight. The blend contained also walnut shell flour (WSF). The content of WSF was in the 10–40 wt.% range. In order to counterbalance the low compatibility between the filler and the biopolymeric matrix, maleinized linseed oil (MLO) was added at 5 parts per hundred (phr) of composite. The MLO-containing composites filled with up to 20 wt.% WSF showed an improved ductility and a more balanced thermo-mechanical response, despite the addition of WSF tended to reduce the mechanical strength and thermal stability of PLA/PCL. The observed improvement of properties was attributed to the plasticization of the biopolymer blend combined with an enhancement of the interfacial adhesion achieved by the extrusion in the presence of MLO.

Song et al. [97] modified nut shell powder through alkaline attack with NaOH solution and subsequent modification with silanes, in particular 3-amino propyl triethoxy silane. The walnut shell powder having a diameter of approximately 20–45 microns and the poly(lactic acid) (PLA) powder of 500 microns in size were mixed in a ball mill and then extruded in a single screw extruder to obtain filaments for Fused Deposition Modeling 3D printing (FDM). The specimens to test the properties were produced by FDM 3D printing. The authors noted an increase in melt fluidity with decreasing powder diameter and increasing silane content. The addition of fiber determines an increase in the tensile modulus. The tensile modulus is lower with the treated fiber compared to the untreated fiber, while the compressive modulus improves. Increasing the fiber content from 5 to 15% results in a decrease in tensile modulus and an increase in tensile strength. Overall this work demonstrated that these composites are suitable for FDM. Interestingly, in the thermoset composites sector, the addition of WSP to epoxy resins allowed the production of structural composites with improved wear resistance [94].

## 2.2 *Hazelnut Shell Powder Biocomposites*

Hazelnut shell powder (HSP) was also added to bio-based matrices for producing light biocomposites that, in specific cases, showed improved thermomechanical properties and enhanced biodegradability with respect to the pure matrices [96]. In addition, another important aspect is that the incorporation of HSP into a biopolymeric matrix certainly contributes to the reduction of the overall biocomposite cost [94]. Since currently the bio-based plastic is still expensive (because often produced in more limited industrial scale than fossil commodities), this aspect is very significant for producing consumer goods at an acceptable price for the market. However, in using agricultural waste and by-products for producing lignocellulosic composites some drawbacks must be mentioned like absence of industrialized processing, unstable fiber availability over the year and the need for big storage facilities and different necessary pretreatments [13]. Aliotta et al. [5] investigated the production by twin screw extrusion of composites consisting of a PLA matrix and a HSP reinforcement. The authors used two hazelnut shell powders (HSPs) characterized by different average sizes and size distributions. To obtain these powders, empty hazelnut shells were ground by an impact mill (Fig. 4).

PLA-based composites including hazelnut shell powder (HSP) were successfully prepared at the semi-industrial scale. The scaled-up composites showed improved mechanical properties in comparison to the lab-scaled produced composites (Fig. 5). The prepared biocomposites investigation suggested that it was possible to achieve an optimized balance between the valorization of a significantly high HSP content and the improvement of mechanical properties. In a more recent work, Aliotta et al. [4] studied the potentialities of HSP in 3D printing, showing the capability of this powder added at 10% to increase the density of the 3D printed specimens.

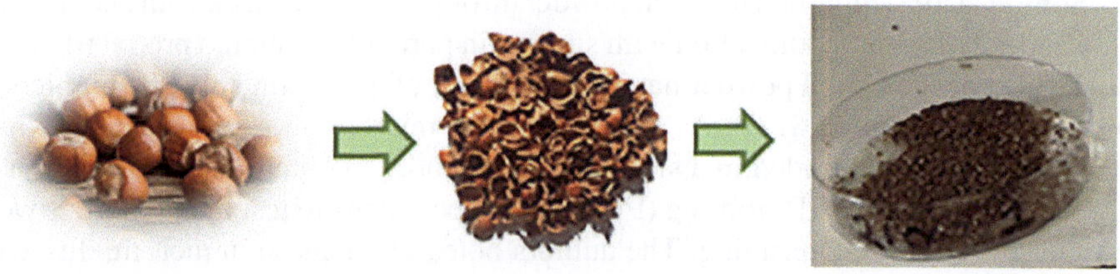

**Fig. 4** Production of empty hazelnut shells as waste and their transformation into a micrometric powder

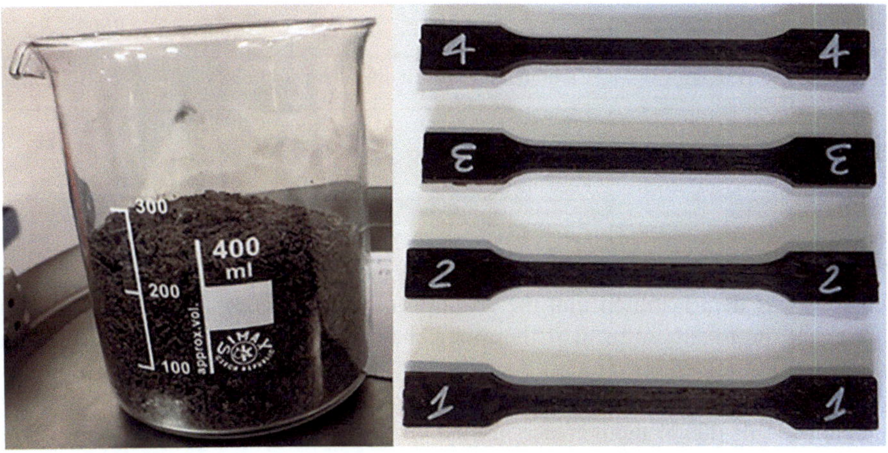


**Fig. 5** Granules and injection molded specimens containing 20% of HSP

Furthermore, in the same research group, Panariello et al. [69] produced biocomposites by extrusion by reinforcing a PLA/PBSA 60/40 blend [6] with HSP. A bio-based chain extender consisting of epoxidized soybean oil (ESO) and a dicarboxylic acid—malic acid (MA) or succinic acid (SA) [23]—was added to limit in the biocomposites the chain scission of PLA that could result in a decrease in melt viscosity during melt extrusion. Melt viscosity studies showed that the ESO/MA and ESO/SA had a modest effect as a chain extender in these biocomposites. The authors evidenced that the best result was obtained by using ESO/MA, but only at a low concentration and considering the finest HSP dimension explored. Chemical reactions involving HSP were revealed thanks to the analysis of band intensity changes in IR spectra recorded before and after the crosslinking reaction.

Interestingly, in this work the authors noticed that HSP biocomposites resulted less degraded by a chain scission mechanism than bran-based ones [23]. However, interestingly, in bran-based biocomposites the ESO/SA chain extension system resulted in more effective in a wider concentration range than in HSP composites. Moreover, in HSP biocomposites MA was more effective than SA. The observed differences in reactivity can be tentatively ascribed to the different compositions of the two fillers [34, 59] (Table 1) being the wheat bran richer in starch, that can be considered a more reactive biopolymer, capable of better inducing chain scission in biopolyesters. On the other hand, the high lignin content of HSP makes it highly stable.

More recently, Ceraulo et al. [21] prepared starch-based Mater-Bi (MB) composites filled with hazelnut shell powder (HSP) by using a co-rotating twin-screw extruder. They also processed their composites by both injection molding and compression molding. Thanks to the investigation carried out through rheological tests, it was possible to evidence that the addition of HSP increased the viscosity of composites. These composites showed a non-Newtonian behavior at low frequencies. It revealed a scarce interfacial adhesion between the matrix and the filler. Moreover,

**Table 1** Comparison between composition of wheat bran and HSP

| Biopolymers | Wheat bran | HSP |
|---|---|---|
| Carbohydrates (excluding starch) | 38 | 30–59 |
| Lignin | 6 | 40–51 |
| Starch | 19 | 0.3 |
| Proteins | 18 | 10–20 |

HSP could promote the crystallization of biocomposites behaving like a nucleating agent. It was demonstrated that the addition of HSP in composites resulted in a significant improvement in their thermomechanical stability. In both compression and injection-molded specimens, a significant improvement in the elastic modulus and impact strength was observed when the content of HSP was 10%. With a higher content of HSP, due to the increase in melt viscosity, the processability in injection molding became more difficult.

### 2.3 Almond Shell Powder Biocomposites

By using polypropylene (rPP) from recycled sources and almond shell including hull, Lewis et al. [54] produced ecocomposites. Virgin PP and an elastomeric polyolefin were used to control the processability and the ductility of the material. In the composite, a finely ground almond shell powder (ASP) was added as a reinforcement to produce the composites at 20 wt.% filler content. The authors evidenced that the particle–matrix interaction was improved thanks to the addition of a compatibilizer consisting of 3% maleic anhydride grafted polypropylene. This improved particle–matrix interfacial adhesion allowed that the tensile and impact strengths of ecocomposites were increased by 17% and 15%, respectively. A similar work was performed to prepare Linear low density polyethylene (LLDPE) reinforced with ASP [18]. A maximum amount of 20% of ASP could be used, because a higher amount resulted in filler agglomeration.

Ramos et al. [79] prepared biopolyester-based biocomposites containing ASP at 10 and 25 wt.% contents with and without two different compatibilizers: maleinized linseed oil and a polyepoxidic oligomer (Joncryl ADR 4400®). Biocomposites were produced by melt blending in an extruder, followed by injection molding. In this paper, the authors investigated the effects of fine (125–250 μ) and coarse (500–1000 μ) milling sizes of ASP onto biocomposites properties. An increase in elastic modulus was observed thanks to the addition of both fine and coarse ASP at 25 wt.%. Moreover, it was evidenced that the addition of maleinized linseed oil and Joncryl produced at low filler contents with some compatibilizing effect. Some decrease in biocomposites thermal stability was shown, but counterbalanced by the reactive additives. In conclusion it was suggested that the developed biocomposites could be used as compostable materials at high filler contents.

Quiles-Carrillo et al. [78] produced green composites by injection molding using polylactide (PLA) filled with almond shell powder (ASP) at a constant content of 25 wt.%. With the aim of increasing the interfacial adhesion between the biopolymer and the fillers, three different compatibilizers were considered in this work: multi-functional epoxy-based styrene-acrylic oligomer (ESAO), aromatic carbodiimide (AC), and maleinized linseed oil (MLO). It was possible to observe that all these compatibilizers showed a good influence on both the thermal stability and the thermomechanical performance of the green composite items. However, they showed a scarce impact on their water uptake profile. ESAO and MLO resulted in the composites characterized by the highest mechanical strength and ductility, respectively.

Liminana et al. [55] used the ASP at 30% by weight to reinforce PBS. Different compatibilizers were added, based on epoxy, maleic anhydride, and acrylic groups. In this work, the authors used epoxidized linseed oil (ELO) and epoxidized soybean oil (ESO), two maleic anhydride-derived compatibilizers, namely, maleinized linseed oil (MLO) and dodecenyl succinic anhydride (DDSA). Two acrylic monomers, namely methyl methacrylate (MMA) and acrylic acid (AA) were also considered. The obtained results suggested that all the compatibilizers derived from vegetable oils (ELO, ESO, and MLO) resulted in a remarkable increase in ductility. However, a scarce compatibilization was observed in these biocomposites by using the acrylic monomers.

Ibanez-Garcia et al. [36] investigated the development of several biodegradable biocomposites based on starch polymer (Mater-Bi DI01A) filled with 30 wt.% ASP. In order to study the influence of almond features on the properties of injected biodegradable items, ASP was obtained from different almond varieties (Desmayo Rojo, Largueta, Marcona, Mollar, and a commercial mixture of varieties). The biocomposites were prepared in a twin-screw extruder. Despite differences in the chemical composition of the selected varieties with respect to the commercial mixture being observed, the results of the mechanical characterization did not show significant differences. Thus, it was concluded that the most sustainable option was to work with the commercial averaged mixture of almond shell varieties. Successively Ibanez-Garcia et al. [44] studied the effect of the reprocessing cycles on the mechanical, thermal, and aesthetic properties of the biocomposites based on thermoplastic starch reinforced with 20 wt.% ASP and epoxidized linseed oil (ELO) as a compatibilizing additive. With the aim of understanding this correlation, the biocomposite was twin-screw extruded and then it was injection molded. The results showed that thermoplastic starch and biocomposites properties underwent changes progressively after each reprocessing cycle. Moreover, the addition of ASP intensified these effects on thermoplastic starch. It was found technically feasible to reprocess the material at least three times without any necessity of incorporating virgin material.

## 2.4 Pistachio Nut Shell Powder Biocomposites

Celik et al. [20] used powders having a size of 0–300 μm, 300–600 μm, and 600–850 μm obtained from pistachio, hazelnut, and apricot kernel shells. Composites were produced by adding 0, 10, 20, and 30% by weight of these powders to the polyester matrix material (Poliber brand cast type thermoset resin). The addition of the powder particles to the polyester adversely affected the tensile strength. On the contrary, the addition of the powder to the matrix significantly improved bending and compressive strength.

Balasunder et al. [12] considered the valorization of pistachio shell powder (PISSP), having a thermal stability and degradation temperature of 240.6 and 274.2 °C, respectively. Regarding the porosity and surface properties, the pores size and pore diameters are 38 $mm^3g^{-1}$ and 3.626 nm respectively,the surface area, determined by calculations, resulted in 0.392 $m^2g^{-1}$. PISSP particle characterization showed properties allowing its use as bio-filler in the polymer matrix to improve the biocomposite properties. PIISSP may be effectively used to develop automobile application such as car dashboard and doors.

Thiagarajan et al. [101] investigated the effect of Pistachio shell powder on the mechanical behavior of chopped glass fiber/epoxy polymer composite. The lamination of composite was carried out by using the method of vacuum assisted resin infusion molding (VARIM). The concentration of filler material of pistachio shell particles was varied up to 3 wt.% respectively. In order to intimately incorporate the pistachio shell particles into the epoxy resin, a high-speed mechanical stirrer was used. It was reported that the flexural strength was increased by 14% by the addition of only 1 wt.% of PISSP. Moreover, the addition of PISSP improved both the tensile and flexural strength of these laminates.

Sutivisedsak et al. [99] examined the possibility of using nut shells powder (mixture of almond, walnut, and pistachio) as fillers in bio-based and compostable poly(lactic acid) and in low density polyethylene. For investigating these aspects, the nutshells were ground, and blended in the melt with the polymer. Successively, the obtained materials were injection molded with final content varying from 10 to 40% by weight. The authors explained that the addition of fillers was detrimental for mechanical properties. However, thermal properties were only slightly affected. The addition of maleic anhydride and peroxide with the fillers produced a negative effect on poly(lactic acid) but, on the contrary, a slightly positive effect on the stiffness of polyethylene was observed. As evidenced by the authors, the analysis of the results suggests that polymer-nutshell composites can be suitable for applications where two different aspects are present: (1) the cost is a concern and (2) some reductions in mechanical properties are acceptable.

By melt functionalization, Altun et al. [8] prepared poly(lactic acid) (PLA)/pistachio shell powder (PISSP) Biocomposites. They adopted a one-step compatibilization process in varying PISSP filler rates (0–30%). In order to significantly increase interfacial adhesion, an alkaline-silane pre-treatment was carried out onto

PISSP, and, additionally, PLA was radically modified by grafting with maleic anhydride (MA). The tensile and flexural properties investigation showed that composites with the best mechanical properties were obtained by blending with maleated PLA 20% of pretreated PISSP. Tensile/flexural strength and modulus for biocomposites were determined by using a universal testing machine. The composites obtained using maleated PLA and pretreated PISSP showed a significantly improved adhesion between the biofiller and the matrix.

## 2.5 *Peanut Shell Powder Biocomposites*

Mandala et al. [56] highlighted in a review paper that peanut shell-based polymer composites have significant attention as sustainable and cost-effective materials for the development and utilization of composites and biocomposites for various applications with potential applications as food packaging films, ceiling tiles, insulation panels, supercapacitors, and electrodes in various industries like the packaging industry, construction, furniture, and electronics.

Yang et al. [108] focused on the use of peanut shell powder (PEASP) as filler in natural rubber (NR). Modified with an alkali treatment (NaOH) and unmodified PEASP were used to obtain composites with varying particle size and filler amount by open mill mixing. The performances of these composites were investigated by analyzing several properties of the vulcanizates: tensile strength, tear strength, and hardness. The results showed that the PEASP is an effective filler in NR at 10 parts per hundred (phr) loading. It was found that the filler reinforcement ability of modified PSP resulted in improvement if compared with unmodified PEASP, then, the best mechanical properties were observed for PSP-NR composites.

Oulidi et al. [67] incorporated different amounts of PEASP, from 5 to 20% by weight, in polyamide 6. The addition of PEASP did not affect the density of PA6. Its crystallinity was not influenced by the addition of up to 15% of PEASP, while it slightly decreased after the addition of 20% PEASP. The matrix kept its structural properties after adding a PEASP concentration of up to 15%. Instead, a higher amount of added PEASP resulted in a peculiar morphological structure.

Prabhakar et al. [74] prepared thermoset composites by adding waste peanut shell powder (PEASP) as a natural filler into epoxy resin matrix. The natural filler was subjected to alkali treatment with the concentrations of 2, 5, and 7 w/v%. The composites were fabricated by varying the weight fractions of filler in the range of 5–15 wt.%. The study revealed that the tensile strength and tensile modulus increased by increasing the bio-filler content. The highest mechanical properties were obtained for 7% alkali treated PEASP loaded Epoxy composite at biofiller content of 15 wt.%.

Zaaba and Ismail [111], focusing on a bio-based and compostable matrix, adopted three different blending sequences to prepare PEASP- PLA/thermoplastic corn starch (TPCS) biocomposites. The blending sequences can be summarized as S1: PLA was added, followed by TPCS and PEASP,S2: PLA was added, followed by PEASP and TPCS,S3: TPCS was added, followed by PLA and PEASP. Various contents (from 0 to 40 wt.%) of PEASP were considered. The results obtained by these experiments showed that S1 system was the best blending sequence for preparing PLA/TPCS biocomposites. In fact, it showed the lowest torque, better tensile strength, elongation at break, and thermal stability. Scanning electron microscopy analysis of S1 sample revealed better adhesion between filler and the matrix. Increment of PEASP content caused an increase in torque and tensile modulus but in a decrease in tensile strength, elongation at break, and thermal stability of the investigated biocomposites. SEM analysis carried out on the tensile fractured surface allowed holes and cavities to be detected. This effect was attributed to the very scarce adhesion between filler and matrix.

## 2.6 *Pine Nut Shell Powder Biocomposites*

A less extensive literature can be found for pine nut shell powder reinforced biocomposites. Gorar et al. [39] explored green composites made from alkali-treated pine nut shell particles (TPS). The modified TPS was then used as reinforcement of fully bio-driven benzoxazine (VB) and epoxy (EP) copolymer. It was reported that the reinforcement with varying weight percent (wt.%) of the modified bio-based TPS enhanced the mechanical properties of composites. In particular, it was demonstrated that the obtained composites can resist to higher temperatures, and for this reason they can be classified as flame-retardant materials. In addition, the dynamic mechanical analysis (DMA) confirmed that composites exhibited a high storage modulus. In particular, the storage modulus was increased up to 77.6% compared to the unfilled copolymer. Finite element analysis (FEA) was proposed by the authors for the prepared composites suggesting a model for mechanical properties. Interestingly, FEA outcomes agreed with experimental findings, suggesting the validity of the proposed model.

## 2.7 *Other Nut Shell Powder Biocomposites*

Ground chestnut shell waste was used by Barczewski et al. [15] as a filler for poly(lactic acid) composites. In this work, the amount of filler incorporated in the biocomposites was ranging from 2.5 to 30 wt.%. The prepared biocomposites were characterized by high stiffness but a lowered impact resistance. It could be concluded that the prepared biocomposites containing different amounts of non-reactive natural waste filler showed acceptable mechanical and thermal properties. Following the author's opinion, these composites could be certainly used as eco-friendly and biodegradable materials, but mainly in low-demanding applications.

Innovative biocomposites based on polylactic acid (PLA) reinforced with argan nut shells powder were explored by Laaziz et al. [53]. The effect of powder chemical surface treatments was investigated making a comparison between three chemical treatments, consisting alkali, bleaching, and silane treatments. Two different filler concentrations (8 and 15% wt.) were also considered. It was found that the highest tensile modulus improvement (16%) was obtained for the biocomposite with 15% of bleached argan nut shell powder, while the highest improvements for tensile strength (1%) and strain at yield (8.5%) were obtained for the Biocomposites made by considering the silane treatment. These results were correlated with good interfacial adhesion and distribution of argan nut shell powder in the matrix. Nevertheless, a lower thermal stability for all the biocomposites was observed with respect to pure PLA. The results about water absorption and water contact angle suggested a better resistance of the biocomposites when a surface treatment was applied to powder.

Macadamia nutshell is a lignocellulosic agricultural waste coming from the macadamia nut production. This production accounts globally for about 44,000 metric tons per year. Pezzana et al. [72] exploited the use of a bio-based monomer, isosorbide, for the production of bio-based resins for coatings. The isosorbide was functionalized to introduce epoxy groups. Macadamia nutshell powder (MAC) bio-based filler was selected for preparing composites for coating and a significant increase in hardness was observed when coatings were prepared including 30 wt.% of MAC. For these coatings, the hardness reached 72 Shore D, whereas the unreinforced bio-based epoxy resin showed a value of 19 Shore D. Moreover, the addition of MAC resulted in a noticeable increase of the glass transition temperature, from 24 °C for the pristine resin to 39 °C for the coating with 20 wt.% of filler.

An investigation based on Design of Experiments was carried out by 29 about mechanical properties of Macadamia nutshell powder/PLA biocomposites. Both stiffness and strength were dependent on the weight content of Macadamia nutshell powders. The elastic modulus increased only 9.8% when the Macadamia nutshell powder content was 40%. Both flexural and tensile strengths decreased with increasing Macadamia nutshell powder content. The hardness resulted independent on the weight content of nutshell powders.

Noè et al. [65] prepared composites consisting of a matrix of acrylated soybean oil reinforced with micro-particles of macadamia nut-shell powder as reinforcing agent. In this work, different formulations were prepared by varying the content of macadamia nut shell. By the successful printing of complex 3D structures with a high resolution, the formulated material was considered suitable for digital light processing (DLP) 3D-printing. By increasing the powder contents, it was found that higher glass transition temperatures, ranging from 25 to 46 °C, and higher elastic modulus, ranging from 15 to 100 MPa, were obtained, respectively. Cytotoxicity as well as cell adhesion and cell proliferation tests with human fibroblast cells were carried out. These tests were performed for assessing the possibility to produce scaffolds for bioengineering purposes. The results envisaged good potentialities in the biomedical field for these fully bio-based composites.

Tamarind nut shell powder was used by Sahayaraj et al. [83] to reinforce jute and hemp plant fibers reinforced composites based on a thermoset epoxide resin by varying weight % of fibers. The composites are fabricated by compression molding. The hybrid composite samples 40:0 (jute: hemp), containing only jute) showed the highest tensile, flexural, impact strengths as well as interlaminar shear strength values.

Coconut shell powder, an agricultural waste, was blended [48] with waste plastic (PP) to form a biocomposite using maleinated PP as coupling agent. In this work, in order to optimize both material and processing, the optimum filler content and the effect of coconut shell ball milling time on the final properties of the composites were studied. Thanks to these investigations, it was possible to deduct that the optimum performance of biocomposite was obtained at 30/70 wt.% ratio plastic waste to coconut shell. Thus, 70 wt.% was the highest coconut shell content that can be achieved in these composites. Moreover, in composites containing 30 wt.% of polypropylene the performances of biocomposite improved significantly by increasing the milling time. This result was attributed to the enhanced interaction between filler and matrix. In fact, it was observed that, as the milling time was increased from 0 to 40 h, the composites density increased, their swelling decreased as well as porosity decreased. The flexural strength, flexural modulus increased and also compressive strength significantly increased. Considering thermogravimetric investigations, it was found that the degradation temperature of biocomposite increased when the milling duration was prolonged. The melting temperature also increased significantly from 160 to 170 °C by prolonging the milling duration. It was observed that the depolymerization occurred at 350 °C. The depolymerization temperature was also found to increase by increasing milling duration. Interestingly, this study revealed that the performance of biocomposite improved significantly by decreasing the filler size.

## 2.8 General Perspectives in Nut Shell Powder Biocomposites

The literature survey regarding nut shell powder biocomposites was analyzed considering a scheme including the bio-based or fossil origin of the matrix and its thermoplastic or thermoset feature (Fig. 6).

In general, the analysis of published works about biocomposites showed that about half of the explored papers was dedicated to biocomposites having a bio-based thermoplastic matrix. PLA is the most explored matrix, but also thermoplastic starch and PBS were considered. The reason is the selection of matrices that are both renewable and compostable, to have products suitable for applications with a sustainable life cycle. This is particularly important in packaging and personal care applications. On the other hand, fossil thermoplastic and thermoset accounted for the other half of papers, dedicated to applications that should be more durable, mainly addressed to the furniture or automotive sectors. Interestingly, WSP was more studied in fossil matrices, whereas ASP mainly in bio-based thermoplastic matrices and HSP only in bio-based thermoplastic matrices. As the walnut tree wood is well known for its good mechanical resistance, probably the use of the walnut shell powder is

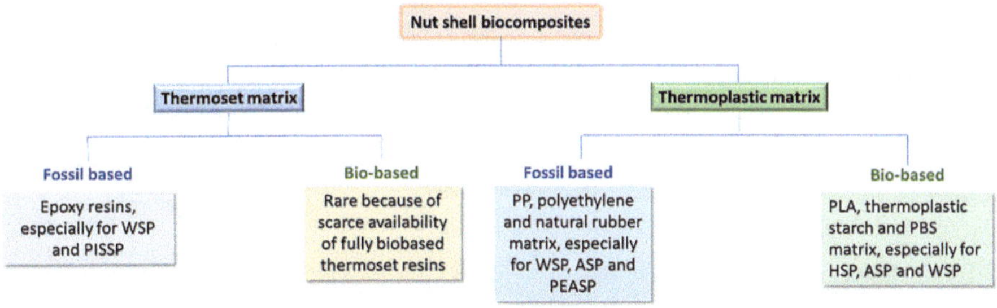


**Fig. 6** Scheme about Nut shell Biocomposites on the basis of literature survey

mainly addressed at durable applications. However, on the basis of literature results, all the nuts shell micrometric powder can be suitable for durable as well as for short life cycle applications.

## 3 Nut Shell-Based Nanobiocomposites

The Biocomposites described in the previous section were obtained by grinding the nut shell and by dispersing this powder in a thermoset or thermoplastic polymer matrix. This grinding operation, carried out in a sustainable way, generally results in a powder having a micrometric dimension. Hence the obtained composites cannot be defined nanocomposites. In fact, a nanocomposite is defined as a composite with a dispersed phase with at least one dimension below 100 nm. Hence dispersed phases in the form of nanoparticles, nanofibrils or nanoplatelets can be used to obtain nanocomposites.

Several methodologies can be adopted for preparing nanobiocomposites, as summarized by Ioregbu and Ray [47]. Nevertheless, for obtaining bionanocomposites from nut shell it is necessary to adopt one of the following strategies: (1) grinding or other techniques allowing to reach a size of the powder in the nanometric range, (2) decomposing the nut shell in submicrometric components and compounds such as cellulose, lignin, and hemicellulose to exploit them as nanometric and sub-nanometric components in materials (Fig. 7).

The first technique results in a solid nanoproduct, often with specific functional properties, that can be used for the production of nanocomposites; the second strategy results in the production of simpler components of the nut shell, controlling them at the molecular level.

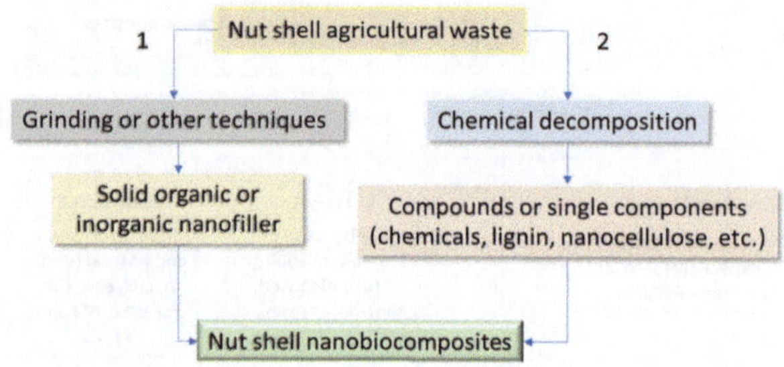


**Fig. 7** Scheme regarding the production of nanobiocomposites from nut shells

## 3.1 *Nanobiocomposites by Production of Specific Nanofillers*

Additive manufacturing is addressed at using functional bionanocomposites from renewable sources and with a reduced impact onto environment. Yin et al. [109] investigated compostable, low-cost, high-efficiency photothermal conversion materials for producing, by additive manufacturing techniques, complex geometrical structures by the photothermal conversion technologies. In their work, a bio-based filament for fused filament additive manufacturing technology was prepared by incorporating hazelnut shell carbon (HSCs) in a polylactic acid (PLA) matrix. The selected fillers, HSCs, were obtained by pyrolysis at temperatures ranging between 300 and 900 °C and it was evidenced that pore structure, morphology, degree of graphitization, particle size, and surface functional groups of HSCs much depended on the selected pyrolysis temperature. Moreover, it was evident that the three-dimensional (3D) printability of PLA-HSC composite filaments and the photothermal performance of the printed structures were also affected by the pyrolysis temperature of HSCs. The analysis of the performed tests showed that PLA-HSC filaments were suitable for 3D printing when HSC was pyrolyzed above 300 °C. Interestingly, the melt fluidity of the composites increased with the pyrolysis temperature of HSCs, suggesting an effect on PLA degradation. Regarding the final properties of the PLA-HSC filaments, it was found that the mechanical properties and the thermal stability showed opposite trends. Regarding photothermal behavior, it was found that in the wavelength range of 250–2500 nm, with HSCs pyrolyzed at 700 and 900 °C, the 3D printed PLA-HSC parts showed excellent photothermal performance with a light absorption intensity of around 93%. Overall, HSCs pyrolyzed at 700 °C resulted in the most cost-effective candidate for the preparation of PLA-based filament for photothermal conversion components. The authors reported that, in the framework of this work, a brine evaporation crystallizer was 3D printed with the aim to demonstrate the application of this novel filament.

With the aim of checking their response against acne, Atif et al. [10] obtained different forms of carbon particles (CP) from walnut shells. The surface chemistry of CPs was modified first, by thermal or oxidative-thermal treatment, and second, by biochemical treatment by using the drugs triamcinolone acetonide (TA) or hydrocortisone sodium succinate (HSS) at pH 4 and 7. Some samples exhibited the highest oil absorption capacities of 0.137 g/0.05 g. The specific anti-inflammatory response has been checked against P. acnes. It was observed, among various prepared samples, that some of them exhibited the most significant levels of anti-inflammatory activity, at 94.19%. Thermally modified samples, additionally, have shown an interesting magnetic behavior. Despite this paper was not dedicated to nanocomposites, the obtained carbon nanoparticles showed interesting functional properties to be exploited in cosmetic and personal care products.

Qadri et al. [76] obtained nanoparticles of aluminum nitride from a thermal treatment above 1450 °C in a nitrogen atmosphere of a mixture of aluminum oxide ($Al_2O_3$) and shells of almond, cashew, coconuts, pistachio, and walnuts. The authors demonstrated that by selecting the appropriate ratios of each nut powder to $Al_2O_3$, stoichiometric aluminum nitride can be produced by carbo-thermal reduction in nitrogen atmosphere consisting of a pure wurtzite phase. Interestingly in the field of nanotechnology, transmission electron microscopy investigations suggested the formation of nanoparticles and in some cases nanotubes of AlN.

Taghizadeh and Rad-Moghadam [100] studied the biosynthesis of copper nanoparticles (CuNPs) that were immobilized on the surface of waste pistachio shell (PS). In this work, the pistachio shell was selected as an environmentally benign support. Moreover, pistachio hull extract (PHE) was used as a reducing and stabilizing agent. The innovative biosynthesis was carried out through an easy, versatile, and inexpensive one-pot procedure. Moreover, the synthesis was carried out without employing any capping agents or toxic reductants. It was demonstrated that these novel CuNPs and copper/pistachio shell nanocomposite could be employed at ambient temperature as efficient catalysts in the reduction of 4-nitrophenol (4-NP), methylene blue (MB), rhodamine B (RhB), and methyl orange (MO). Hence, these nanoparticles can be exploited in nanobiocomposites for depollution membranes.

Wongcharee et al. [107] studied nanosorbents that are increasingly used for targeted contaminant removal. However, they stated that handling and separation of spent sorbents from treated water remains a challenge. To find a solution for this issue, a hybrid magnetic nanosorbent was prepared from waste macadamia nut shell and magnetite nanoparticles. This novel nanosorbent showed a primarily meso- and macroporous structure with 70 $m^2g^{-1}$ specific surface area. In order to quantitatively test their effectiveness, batch sorption tests using methylene blue model pollutant were performed. These tests revealed sorption capacities increasing from 33 to 42 mg $g^{-1}$ with temperature in the 25–45 °C range. Elaborations by nonlinear regression analyses highlighted that process kinetics was successfully and accurately described by a fractal-like pseudo first-order model. The isotherms showed excellent fits to the Langmuir model and reasonably suggested a monolayer adsorption mechanism.

The thermodynamic parameters confirmed that the process was spontaneous, endothermic, and involved physisorption. The ferrimagnetic sorbent had 48 emu $g^{-1}$ saturation and 0.65 emu $g^{-1}$ remanence that allowed easy handling and rapid separation by magnetic field. Spent sorbents were effectively regenerated by acidic wash for subsequent reuse over four cycles. The intrinsic characteristics of the magnetite/carbon nanosorbent were found suitable for water and wastewater treatment applications.

Morifi et al. [63] investigated the synthesis of a polypyrrole (Ppy) composite based on Macadamia nutshells (AMN) and binary metal oxides (Mn-Cu oxide). These innovative materials were investigated to be used for the selective removal of Cr(VI) from aqueous solution. Ppy/AMN-MnCu oxide nanocomposite was prepared via in-situ oxidative polymerization of pyrrole monomer in the presence of AMN-Mn-Cu oxide composite by using $FeCl_3$ as an oxidant. It was found that the adsorption of Cr(VI) mainly depended on the pH of the solution and, under optimized conditions, a maximum adsorption capacity of 199.2 mg/g was achieved. The adsorbent resulted in selective Cr(VI) adsorption also in the presence of co-existing ions. AMN-Mn-Cu oxide-Ppy nanocomposite resulted recyclable. In fact it was successfully reused for six adsorption–desorption cycles without losing its original adsorption capacity.

Mohan et al. [61] used Walnut Shell Powder (WSP) in the synthesis of silver nanoparticles. WSP was immersed in 5 (milli Molar) mM Silver Nitrate solution. The solution was maintained at 80 °C for a day to ensure in-situ generation of silver nanoparticles with the aid of the one step hydrothermal method. It was observed by electron microscopy that the modified WSP had on its surface spherical AgNPs with an average size of 85 nm. Antibacterial studies have showed that there are no inhibition zones formed on WSP. On the contrary, on modified WSP, an excellent inhibition was revealed against both gram negative and gram-positive bacteria. This work suggested that modified WSP can represent a low-cost filler for producing polymer composites for both medical and food packaging applications.

Wang et al. [105] prepared electromagnetic absorption materials. For this purpose, they used NiO decorated biomass porous carbon derived from pine nut shells as a promising microwave absorbing material. The NiO/biomass porous carbon (BPC) is thermally converted from $Ni(OH)_2$/BPC with BPC as the base for precipitation. It was observed that NiO nanoflakes were uniformly self-assembled on the surface of the activated carbon. The authors suggested that the improved microwave absorption properties reasonably originated from the electric/dielectric polarization of the NiO decorated BPC structures.

Blessy Rebecca et al. [17] reported in their review the use of macadamia nut shells to prepare graphene by adopting a hydrothermal method applied to peanut shell, by activation and mechanical exfoliation. They also reported the preparation of graphene tin oxide nanohybrids using sources of coconut shell and wood charcoal.

Sharahi et al. [91] prepared nanoparticles from walnut shells via physical milling followed by a chemical treatment. Lignocellulosic nanoparticles having an average dimension of 560 nm and a crystallinity of 28% were produced. Nanoparticles were then co-electrospun together with a biopolyester (polycaprolactone (PCL)) and a biopolymer (gelatin). Nanoparticles increased the average diameter of PCL and Gel nanofibers from 250 and 300 nm to about 600 and 550 nm, respectively. Moreover, it was found that the moduli of coaxially electrospun PCL-Gel membranes significantly increased passing from 11.9 to 16.6 MPa, while, on the contrary, their thermal stability decreased. PCL-Gel nanofibers loaded with 2% WSP were considered by the authors the best formulation because of their excellent mechanical properties. Additionally, the scaffolds obtained by using these fibers showed excellent viability, proliferation, and growth of mesenchymal stem cells.

## 3.2 Nanobiocomposites from Compounds and Components Coming from Nut Shell

Movva et al. [64] investigations were focused on the extraction of cellulose from pistachio shell. In this work, a partially degradable nanocomposite with extracted cellulose and a polyester matrix was prepared. The extraction methodology resulted efficient in obtaining 95% crystalline cellulose. Reinforced composites showed a significant increase in tensile and flexural strengths of 43 and 127 MPa, at a weight percent of 5%. Thus, cellulose from pistachio shells has great potential for manufacturing promising green materials in the future.

Anand Raj et al. [9] focused on evaluating the potential of cellulose agar bionanocomposite films in food packaging applications. Cellulose microfiber was extracted from peanut shell powder. Three steps of treatments were adopted in the isolation process for microcellulose: (1) enzymatic pretreatment, (2) chemical treatment, and (3) ultrasonic treatment. For the prepared cellulose/agar nanobiocomposites the physico-mechanical properties (tensile strength (TS), Young's modulus (YM), and elongation at break (E)) resulted increased thanks to the addition of cellulose microfiber (CMF). In particular, TS was increased from $38.8 \pm 3.2$ to $49.4 \pm 4.3$ and about a 6% increase in the elongation at break was also observed. CMF films showed a $54 \pm 0.2\%$ water solubility, a 1.304 opacity, and a $1.71 \pm 0.07$ GPa elasticmodulus, respectively. Furthermore, the bionanocomposite film showed decreased swelling property and an increased soil degradation rate, suggesting the useful application of these materials in food packaging.

With the aim of developing cellulose reinforced starch films, Harini et al. [42] extracted cashew nut shell (CNS) starch and walnut shell cellulose (WNC). Moreover, the extraction and characterization of pomegranate peel extract was investigated for using the obtained extract in the functionalization of films. CNS starch was examined to be a moderate amylose starch with $26.32 \pm 0.43\%$ amylose content. Thermal degradation temperature of CNS starch was found to be 310 °C. Walnut shell cellulose showed a high crystallinity index of 72% and two thermal degradation temperatures of 319 °C and 461 °C. CNS starch films reinforced with 2% of WN were found to have good oxygen transfer rate, and good mechanical and physical properties. Thermal degradation temperature of films was found to be in the range of 298–302 °C. Surface roughness of films was found to increase by increasing the cellulose concentration in films. The major active compounds found in pomegranate peels extract were Hydroxymethylfurfurole, Benzene, 2-methoxy-1,3,4-trimethyl and 1,2,3-Propanetriol, 1-acetate. 2% WN cellulose reinforced starch films functionalized with hydrophilic active compounds of pomegranate peel showed good active packaging properties.

Meng et al. [58] investigated the antioxidant ability of peanut shell and skin extracts and their effects on the physical and structure properties of starch-chitosan film. It was found that the DPPH radical scavenging ability of peanut skin extracts was significantly higher than the one of peanut shell extracts. This interesting result was attributed by the authors to the rich rutin and 4-O-caffeoulquinic acid content in the peanut skin extracts. When the peanut skin and shell extracts were added into the starch-chitosan film, the apparent viscosity of film forming solution decreased. Moreover, water vapor permeability and swelling of film decreased by adding peanut skin and shell extracts. Interestingly, the tensile strength of film increased with the addition of peanut skin extracts. Instead, it decreased by adding the peanut shell extracts. The addition of both extracts resulted in the increase in degradation temperature of the starch-chitosan film. The infrared analysis suggested that the peanut shell and skin extracts disturbed the formation of hydrogen bond in the film matrix.

Wang et al. [106] investigated innovative methodologies for the high-yield recovery of lignin with retention of its native C–O bonded structure. Enzymatic residual lignin isolation, a methodology that leaves the lignin unaltered thanks to enzymatic desaccharification, was mainly considered in this work. Different highly representative lignocellulose sources (walnut, birch, pine shell and reed) were evaluated for lignin isolation, mainly focusing on the effect on the lignin purity and structure. By analyzing the residual saccharides and the structural features of the obtained lignin, the effect of both enzyme content and ball milling duration were studied. A high ball milling time resulted in a higher carbohydrate removal and reduced the need of extra enzyme. The application of two or more steps of enzymatic hydrolysis with higher enzyme content and short ball milling time was shown as an alternative to long ball milling time to achieve similar carbohydrate removal, but avoiding extensive decrease in the lignin molecular weight (MW). The recalcitrance toward increased enzyme hydrolysis activity by ball milling was different for the four representative biomasses and followed an order of walnut shell > reed ≈ pine > birch. In general, the results evidenced a synergy between enzymatic treatment and ball milling efficiency to isolate lignin with high yield, high native linkage content, purity, and minimal MW reduction.

The recovery of value-added compounds from chestnut by-products (shells, leaves, burs) was attempted by Conidi et al. [24] by an effective extraction process followed by a combination, in a sequential procedure, of several membrane operations including ultrafiltration (UF), nanofiltration (NF) and reverse osmosis (RO). This integrated process allowed different classes of bioactive compounds (gallic, ellagic, and tannic acids) to be separated and purified from dried chestnut shell extracts in order to obtain polyphenols through an eco-friendly route: in fact, water was selected for the extraction process. The novel investigated process, based on a circular economy approach, resulted promising for effectively valorizing chestnut shells waste, suggesting a feasible industrial process.

Walnut shell biomass was used by Zaheer [112] for the extraction at room temperature of juglone, a naturally occurring naphthoquinone, by using water as solvent. By the addition of $AgNO_3$ to a dye solution, a transparent pale brown color develops within the reaction time. The characterization by UV–visible spectroscopy revealed the appearance of surface plasmon absorption peak silver nanoparticles (AgNPs). Juglone-surfactant interactions have been studied by using cationic cetyltrimethylammonium bromide. This study showed a significant impact on size, shape, and size distribution of AgNPs. It also catalyzes the $Ag^+$ ions reduction by juglone with a rate enhancement of about 100-fold. The antioxidant activity of juglone was assessed by the scavenging effect on DPPH radical.

Perez-Gutierrez et al. [71] have investigated the preparation of innovative biomedical patches. They used the hydrosoluble hazelnut shell extract (HSE) as the active ingredient of patches prepared by casting. The patches consisted of composites including green clay and highly deacetylated chitosan. In vitro immunomodulatory tests showed that was able to stimulate keratinocyte growth. This is useful for healing purposes. Moreover, microbiological tests showed that the formulation containing HSE could inhibit the growth of *S. aureus*, often responsible for wound infections. The produced patches showed the suitable tensile properties that are necessary for this biomedical application.

## 4 Conclusions

Nut shell waste is an abundant source currently considered in several applications because of the necessity of finding alternative to fossil sources and because of the necessity of extending the circular economy approach. Its good thermal stability makes nut shell powder suitable for preparing biocomposites to be used in several applications ranging from furniture, automotive to packaging and biomedical/personal care applications. In the present chapter, the most abundant nut shells were explored in connection with global and local food production. The production of biocomposites from the different nut shell micrometric powders, considering the different types of nuts, was explored and it was evidenced a general tendency in considering biocomposites with a bio-based and biodegradable matrix, for instance PLA, thermoplastic starch, PBS, and their blends, reasonably linked to the necessity of finding more sustainable alternative for consumer goods with a shorter life cycle because they are those generating a greater amount of waste.

The use of nut shell in nanobiocomposites was investigated considering the possibility to exploit nanoparticles coming from nut shell that can be exploited in nanobiocomposites production. It was evident, from this analysis of the scientific literature, that different synthesis methodologies were explored by researchers, so that nut shell powder can be considered a source of carbon filler (for instance, activated carbons or graphene) or as support or precursor for catalytic metal or ceramic compounds.

The other use of nut shell in nanobiocomposites is linked to the possibility to exploit compounds/components obtained by extraction of molecules or conversion to cellulose or lignin of the nut shell waste. This approach was also explored by several researchers. In fact, cellulose, lignin, or polyphenols can be obtained from nut shell waste and used to produce specific functional nanobiocomposites. In general, it can be concluded that nut shell agro-waste is currently an important source for new sustainable biorefinery-based industrial chains addressed to advanced materials.

## References

1. Agustin-Salazar S, Gamez-Meza N, Medina-Juárez LÁ, Malinconico M, Cerruti P (2017) Stabilization of polylactic acid and polyethylene with nutshell extract: efficiency assessment and economic evaluation. ACS Sustain Chem Eng 5(6):4607–4618. https://doi.org/10.1021/acssuschemeng.6b03124
2. Akıncıoğlu G, Akıncıoğlu S, Öktem H, Uygur İ (2020) Wear response of non-asbestos brake pad composites reinforced with walnut shell dust. J Aust Ceram Soc 56(3):1061–1072. https://doi.org/10.1007/s41779-020-00452-6
3. Aliotta L, Gigante V, Coltelli M-B, Cinelli P, Lazzeri A, Seggiani M (2019) Thermo-mechanical properties of PLA/short flax fiber biocomposites. Appl Sci 9(18). https://doi.org/10.3390/app9183797
4. Aliotta L, Sergi C, Dal Pont B, Coltelli MB, Gigante V, Lazzeri A (2024) Sustainable 3D printed poly (lactic acid) (PLA)/hazelnut shell powder (HSP) biocomposites for design applications: directly from extruded pellets to prototypes. Mater Tod Sust 26:100780. https://doi.org/10.1016/j.mtsust.2024.100780
5. Aliotta L, Vannozzi A, Bonacchi D, Coltelli MB, Lazzeri A (2021) Analysis, development, and scaling-up of poly(lactic)acid (pla) biocomposites with hazelnuts shell powder (hsp). Polymers (Basel) 13(23). https://doi.org/10.3390/polym13234080
6. Aliotta L, Vannozzi A, Canesi I, Cinelli P, Coltelli MB, Lazzeri A (2021) Poly(lactic acid) (PLA)/poly(butylene succinate-co-adipate) (PBSA) compatibilized binary biobased blends: Melt fluidity, morphological, thermo-mechanical and micromechanical analysis. Polymers (Basel) 13(2):1–22. https://doi.org/10.3390/polym13020218
7. Aliotta L, Vannozzi A, Cinelli P, Fiori S, Coltelli MB, Lazzeri A (2022) Wheat bran addition as potential alternative to control the plasticizer migration into PLA/PBSA blends. J Mater Sci 57(30):14511–14527. https://doi.org/10.1007/s10853-022-07534-9
8. Altun M, Celebi M, Ovali S (2022) Preparation of the pistachio shell reinforced PLA biocomposites: effect of filler treatment and PLA maleation. J Thermoplast Compos Mater 35(9):1342–1357. https://doi.org/10.1177/08927057211010880
9. Anand Raj LFA, Shanmugapriya R, Jeslin J (2019) Biosynthesis of cellulose microfibre from peanut shell for the preparation of bio-nanocomposite films for food-packaging application. Bull Mater Sci 42(2):1–9. https://doi.org/10.1007/s12034-019-1751-2
10. Atif M, Mehmood RA, Noor AZ, Shaukat S, Mahmood S, Ali I (2023) Surface modified walnut shell derived carbon particles for anti-acne skin treatment. Diam Relat Mater 140(PA):110394. https://doi.org/10.1016/j.diamond.2023.110394
11. Bala JM, Vennila JJ, Ganesh S, Sachidanand Singh SS (2011) Analysis of active components in Acanthus ilicifolius leaves for their potential chemoprotective activity against hepatocellular carcinoma: an in silico approach
12. Balasundar P, Narayanasamy P, Senthil S, Abdullah Al-Dhabi N, Prithivirajan R, Shyam Kumar R, Ramkumar T, Subrahmanya Bhat K (2019) Physico-chemical study of pistachio (Pistacia vera) nutshell particles as a bio-filler for eco-friendly composites. Mater Res Express 6(10). https://doi.org/10.1088/2053-1591/ab3b9b
13. Barbu MC, Sepperer T, Tudor EM, Petutschnigg A (2020) Walnut and hazelnut shells: untapped industrial resources and their suitability in lignocellulosic composites. Appl Sci 10(18). https://doi.org/10.3390/APP10186340
14. Barbu MC, Reh R, Cavder AD (2017) Non-Wood Lignocellulosic Composites. In: Materials Science and Engineering: Concepts, Methodologies, Tools, and Applications. IGI global, pp 947–977. file:///D:/Dropbox-(Personale)/0-lavoro/1-Ingegneria-Civile-e-Industriale/pubblicazioni/pubblicazioni-2023/book-springer/literature/intro/Preliminary-assessment-of-hazelnut-shell-biomass-as-a-raw-material-for-pellet-production.pdf
15. Barczewski M, Matykiewicz D, Krygier A, Andrzejewski J, Skórczewska K (2018) Characterization of poly(lactic acid) biocomposites filled with chestnut shell waste. J Mater Cycles Waste Manag 20(2):914–924. https://doi.org/10.1007/s10163-017-0658-5

16. Barreca D, Nabavi SM, Sureda A, Rasekhian M, Raciti R, Silva AS, Annunziata G, Arnone A, Tenore GC, Süntar İ, Mandalari G (2020) Almonds (Prunus dulcis Mill. D. A. webb): a source of nutrients and health-promoting compounds. Nutrients 12(3). https://doi.org/10.3390/nu12030672
17. Blessy Rebecca PN, Durgalakshmi D, Balakumar S, Rakkesh RA (2022) Biomass-derived graphene-based nanocomposites: a futuristic material for biomedical applications. ChemistrySelect 7(5). https://doi.org/10.1002/slct.202104013
18. Boujelben M, Abid M, Kharrat M, Dammak M (2021) Production and mechanical characterization of LLDPE biocomposite filled with almond shell powder. Polym Polym Compos 29(4):271–276. https://doi.org/10.1177/0967391120910869
19. Cam Quyen Ngo T, Kim Ngan Tran T, Dung Chau H, Ngoc Hoang B (2023) The material potential and application of activated carbon from nut shells: mini review. Mater Today Proc. https://doi.org/10.1016/j.matpr.2023.03.511
20. Çelik YH, Yalcin R, Topkaya T, Başaran E, Kilickap E (2021) Characterization of hazelnut, pistachio, and apricot kernel shell particles and analysis of their composite properties. J Nat Fibers 18(7):1054–1068. https://doi.org/10.1080/15440478.2020.1739593
21. Ceraulo M, La Mantia FP, Mistretta MC, Titone V (2022) The use of waste hazelnut shells as a reinforcement in the development of green biocomposites. Polymers (Basel) 14(11). https://doi.org/10.3390/polym14112151
22. Coltelli MB, Aliotta L, Vannozzi A, Morganti P, Panariello L, Danti S, Neri S, Fernandez-Avila C, Fusco A, Donnarumma G, Lazzeri A (2020) Properties and skin compatibility of films based on poly(lactic acid) (PLA) bionanocomposites incorporating chitin nanofibrils (CN). J Funct Biomater 11(2):1–23. https://doi.org/10.3390/jfb11020021
23. Coltelli MB, Bertolini A, Aliotta L, Gigante V, Vannozzi A, Lazzeri A (2021) Chain extension of poly(lactic acid) (pla)–based blends and composites containing bran with biobased compounds for controlling their processability and recyclability. Polymers (Basel) 13(18). https://doi.org/10.3390/polym13183050
24. Conidi C, Donato L, Algieri C, Cassano A (2022) Valorization of chestnut processing by-products: A membrane-assisted green strategy for purifying valuable compounds from shells. J Clean Prod 378:134564. https://doi.org/10.1016/j.jclepro.2022.134564
25. Członka S, Strąkowska A, Kairytė A (2020) Effect of walnut shells and silanized walnut shells on the mechanical and thermal properties of rigid polyurethane foams. Polym Test 87. https://doi.org/10.1016/j.polymertesting.2020.106534
26. da Silva JCG, Alves JLF, de Galdino WVA, de Moreira RFPM, José HJ, de Sena RF, Andersen SLF (2018) Combustion of pistachio shell: physicochemical characterization and evaluation of kinetic parameters. Environ Sci Pollut Res 25(22):21420–21429. https://doi.org/10.1007/s11356-017-8945-1
27. de Hoyos-Martínez PL, Erdocia X, Charrier-El Bouhtoury F, Prado R, Labidi J (2018) Multistage treatment of almonds waste biomass: characterization and assessment of the potential applications of raw material and products. Waste Manag 80:40–50. https://doi.org/10.1016/j.wasman.2018.08.051
28. De Souza RGM, Schincaglia RM, Pimente GD, Mota JF (2017) Nuts and human health outcomes: a systematic review. Nutrients 9(12). https://doi.org/10.3390/nu9121311
29. Di Michele A, Pagano C, Allegrini A, Blasi F, Cossignani L, Di Raimo E, Faieta M, Oliva E, Pittia P, Primavilla S, Sergi M, Vicino C, Ricci M, Schirone B, Perioli L (2021) Hazelnut shells as source of active ingredients: extracts preparation and characterization. Molecules 26(21). https://doi.org/10.3390/molecules26216607
30. Dong C, Davies IJ, Fornari Junior CCM, Scaffaro R (2017) Mechanical properties of macadamia nutshell powder and PLA bio-composites. Aust J Mech Eng 15(3):150–156. https://doi.org/10.1080/14484846.2016.1187245
31. Du F, Tan T (2021) Recent studies in mechanical properties of selected hard-shelled seeds: a review. Jom 73(6):1723–1735. https://doi.org/10.1007/s11837-021-04688-w
32. El Khoury Y, Noujeim E, Bubici G, Tarasco E, Al Khoury C, Nemer N (2021) Potential factors behind the decline of pinus pinea nut production in mediterranean pine forests. Forests 12(9):1–11. https://doi.org/10.3390/f12091167

33. Fermanelli CS, Chiappori A, Pierella LB, Saux C (2022) Towards biowastes valorization: peanut shell as resource for quality chemicals and activated biochar production. Sustain Environ Res 32(1). https://doi.org/10.1186/s42834-021-00112-9
34. Fuso A, Risso D, Rosso G, Rosso F, Manini F, Manera I, Caligiani A (2021) Potential valorization of hazelnut shells through extraction, purification and structural characterization of prebiotic compounds: a critical review. Foods 10(6). https://doi.org/10.3390/foods10061197
35. Gangwar P, Johri P, Datta R, Singh S, & Trivedi M. (2023). Overview on 1 phytopharmaceuticals and biotechnology of herbal plants. In: Phytopharmaceuticals and biotechnology of herbal plants. CRC Press, pp 1–17
36. García AI, García AM, Bou SF (2020) Study of the influence of the almond shell variety onthe mechanical properties of starch-basedpolymer biocomposites. Polymers (Basel) 12(9). https://doi.org/10.3390/POLYM12092049
37. Gigante V, Aliotta L, Phuong VT, Coltelli MB, Cinelli P, Lazzeri A (2017) Effects of waviness on fiber-length distribution and interfacial shear strength of natural fibers reinforced composites. Compos Sci Technol 152. https://doi.org/10.1016/j.compscitech.2017.09.008
38. Gonçalves B, Pinto T, Aires A, Morais MC, Bacelar E, Anjos R, Ferreira-Cardoso J, Oliveira I, Vilela A, Cosme F (2023) Composition of nuts and their potential health benefits—an overview. Foods 12(5):1–19. https://doi.org/10.3390/foods12050942
39. Gorar AAK, Zhiyi G, Wang Z, Daham A, Wang J, Liu W Bin, Wang JY, Derradji M (2023) Development of green composites from bio-benzoxazine and epoxy copolymer reinforced with alkali-treated pine nut shell particles. Polym Adv Technol. https://doi.org/10.1002/pat.6245
40. Gupta G, Paul S, Singh S, Pietramellara G, Pathan SI, Danish S, Jha PN (2022) Exploring functional diversity and community structure of diazotrophic endophytic bacteria associated with Pennisetum glaucum growing under field in a semi-arid region. Land 11(7):991
41. Han H, Wang S, Rakita M, Wang Y, Han Q, Xu Q (2018) Effect of ultrasound-assisted extraction of phenolic compounds on the characteristics of walnut shells. Food Nutr Sci 09(08):1034–1045. https://doi.org/10.4236/fns.2018.98076
42. Harini K, Chandra Mohan C, Ramya K, Karthikeyan S, Sukumar M (2018) Effect of Punica granatum peel extracts on antimicrobial properties in walnut shell cellulose reinforced bio-thermoplastic starch films from cashew nut shells. Carbohydr Polym 184:231–242. https://doi.org/10.1016/j.carbpol.2017.12.072
43. Herrera R, Hemming J, Smeds A, Gordobil O, Willför S, Labidi J (2020) Recovery of bioactive compounds from hazelnuts and walnuts shells: quantitative–qualitative analysis and chromatographic purification. Biomolecules 10(10):1–16. https://doi.org/10.3390/biom10101363
44. Ibáñez-García A, Martínez-García A, Ferrándiz-Bou S (2021) Recyclability analysis of starch thermoplastic/almond shell biocomposite. Polymers (Basel) 13(7):1–16. https://doi.org/10.3390/polym13071159
45. Ike DC, Ibezim-Ezeani MU, Akaranta O (2021) Cashew nutshell liquid and its derivatives in oil field applications: an update. Green Chem Lett Rev 14(4):618–631. https://doi.org/10.1080/17518253.2021.1991485
46. Ingegneri M, Smeriglio A, Rando R, Gervasi T, Tamburello MP, Ginestra G, La Camera E, Pennisi R, Sciortino MT, Mandalari G, Trombetta D (2023) Composition and biological properties of blanched skin and blanch water belonging to three sicilian almond cultivars. Nutrients 15(6):1–23. https://doi.org/10.3390/nu15061545
47. Iroegbu AOC, Ray SS (2022) Recent developments and future perspectives of biorenewable nanocomposites for advanced applications. Nanotechnol Rev 11(1):1696–1721. https://doi.org/10.1515/ntrev-2022-0105
48. Ismail I, Aini Q, Jalil Z, Olaiya NG, Mursal M, Abdullah CK, Abdul Khalil HPS (2022) Properties enhancement nano coconut shell filled in packaging plastic waste bionanocomposite. Polymers (Basel) 14(4):1–23. https://doi.org/10.3390/polym14040772

49. Jabborova D, Davranov K, Jabbarov Z, Bhowmik SN, Ercisli S, Danish S, Datta R (2022) Dual inoculation of plant growth-promoting Bacillus endophyticus and Funneliformis mosseae improves plant growth and soil properties in ginger. ACS Omega 7(39):34779–34788
50. Jahanban-Esfahlan A, Ostadrahimi A, Tabibiazar M, Amarowicz R (2019) A comparative review on the extraction, antioxidant content and antioxidant potential of different parts of walnut (juglans regia l.) fruit and tree. Molecules 24(11). https://doi.org/10.3390/molecules24112133
51. Jannat N, Latif Al-Mufti R, Hussien A, Abdullah B, Cotgrave A (2021) Utilisation of nut shell wastes in brick, mortar and concrete: a review. Constr Build Mater 293:123546. https://doi.org/10.1016/j.conbuildmat.2021.123546
52. Jovičić N, Antonović A, Matin A, Antolović S, Kalambura S, Krička T (2022) Biomass valorization of walnut shell for liquefaction efficiency. Energies 15(2). https://doi.org/10.3390/en15020495
53. Laaziz SA, Raji M, Hilali E, Essabir H, Rodrigue D, Bouhfid R, el kacem Qaiss A (2017) Bio-composites based on polylactic acid and argan nut shell: production and properties. Int J Biol Macromol 104:30–42. https://doi.org/10.1016/j.ijbiomac.2017.05.184
54. Lewis R, Weldekidan H, Rodriguez AU, Mohanty AK, Mielewski DF, Misra M (2023) Design and engineering of sustainable biocomposites from ocean-recycled polypropylene-based polyolefins reinforced with almond shell and hull. Compos Part C Open Access 12:100373. https://doi.org/10.1016/j.jcomc.2023.100373
55. Liminana P, Garcia-Sanoguera D, Quiles-Carrillo L, Balart R, Montanes N (2018) Development and characterization of environmentally friendly composites from poly(butylene succinate) (PBS) and almond shell flour with different compatibilizers. Compos Part B Eng 144(January):153–162. https://doi.org/10.1016/j.compositesb.2018.02.031
56. Mandala R, Hegde G, Kodali D, Kode VR (2023) From waste to strength: unveiling the mechanical properties of peanut-shell-based polymer composites. J Compos Sci 7(8):1–22. https://doi.org/10.3390/jcs7080307
57. Manterola-Barroso C, Contreras DP, Ondrasek G, Horvatinec J, Cuicui GG, Meriño-Gergichevich C (2023) Hazelnut and walnut nutshell features, as emerging added value by-products of the nut industry: a review. https://doi.org/10.20944/preprints202309.1563.v1
58. Meng W, Shi J, Zhang X, Lian H, Wang Q, Peng Y (2020) Effects of peanut shell and skin extracts on the antioxidant ability, physical and structure properties of starch-chitosan active packaging films. Int J Biol Macromol 152:137–146. https://doi.org/10.1016/j.ijbiomac.2020.02.235
59. Merali Z, Collins SRA, Elliston A, Wilson DR, Käsper A, Waldron KW (2015) Characterization of cell wall components of wheat bran following hydrothermal pretreatment and fractionation. Biotechnol Biofuels 8(1):1–13. https://doi.org/10.1186/s13068-015-0207-1
60. Moccia F, Agustin-Salazar S, Verotta L, Caneva E, Giovando S, D'Errico G, Panzella L, D'Ischia M, Napolitano A (2020) Antioxidant properties of agri-food byproductsland specific boosting effects of hydrolytic treatments. Antioxidants 9(5). https://doi.org/10.3390/antiox9050438
61. Mohan S, Panneerselvam K (2020) An investigation on antibacterial filler property of silver nanoparticles generated from walnut shell powder by insitu process. Mater Today Proc 39:368–372. https://doi.org/10.1016/j.matpr.2020.07.516
62. Montava-Jord S, Quiles-Carrillo L, Richart N, Torres-Giner S, Montanes N (2019) Enhanced interfacial adhesion of linseed oil
63. Morifi E, Chimuka L, Richards H, Senyolo L, Pillay K (2022) Modified Macadamia nutshell nanocomposite for selective removal of hexavalent chromium from wastewater. South African J Chem Eng 42:176–187. https://doi.org/10.1016/j.sajce.2022.09.001
64. Movva M, Kommineni R (2017) Extraction of cellulose from pistachio shell and physical and mechanical characterisation of cellulose-based nanocomposites. Mater Res Express 4(4). https://doi.org/10.1088/2053-1591/aa6863
65. Noè C, Cosola A, Tonda-Turo C, Sesana R, Delprete C, Chiappone A, Hakkarainen M, Sangermano M (2022) DLP-printable fully biobased soybean oil composites. Polymer (Guildf) 247. https://doi.org/10.1016/j.polymer.2022.124779

66. Nyirenda J, Zombe K, Kalaba G, Siabbamba C, Mukela I (2021) Exhaustive valorization of cashew nut shell waste as a potential bioresource material. Sci Rep 11(1):1–14. https://doi.org/10.1038/s41598-021-91571-y
67. Oulidi O, Nakkabi A, Boukhlifi F, Fahim M, Lgaz H, Alrashdi AA, Elmoualij N (2022) Peanut shell from agricultural wastes as a sustainable filler for polyamide biocomposites fabrication. J King Saud Univ Sci 34(6):102148. https://doi.org/10.1016/j.jksus.2022.102148
68. Pączkowski P (2023) Properties of eco-friendly composites based on post-consumer recycled resin filled with walnut shell powder. Polymers (Basel) 15(22):4389. https://doi.org/10.3390/polym15224389
69. Panariello L, Coltelli MB, Vannozzi A, Bonacchi D, Aliotta L, Lazzeri A (2021) Fully biobased reactive extrusion of biocomposites based on PLA blends and hazelnut shell powders (HSP). Chem 3(4):1464–1480. https://doi.org/10.3390/chemistry3040104
70. Patani A, Patel A, Prajapati D, Khare N, Singh S (2023) Various agriculture crop plant-based bioactive compounds and their use in nanomaterial synthesis and applications. In: Nanomaterials from agricultural and horticultural products. Singapore: Springer Nature, Singapore, pp 223–241
71. Pérez Gutíerrez CL, Di Michele A, Pagano C, Puglia D, Luzi F, Beccari T, Ceccarini MR, Primavilla S, Valiani A, Vicino C, Ricci M, Viseras Iborra CA, Perioli L (2023) Polymeric patches based on chitosan/green clay composites and hazelnut shell extract as bio-sustainable medication for wounds. Pharmaceutics 15(8):1–17. https://doi.org/10.3390/pharmaceutics15082057
72. Pezzana L, Emanuele A, Sesana R, Delprete C, Malmström E, Johansson M, Sangermano M (2023) Cationic UV-curing of isosorbide-based epoxy coating reinforced with macadamia nut shell powder. Prog Org Coatings 185. https://doi.org/10.1016/j.porgcoat.2023.107949
73. Phuong VT, Gigante V, Aliotta L, Coltelli M-B, Cinelli P, Lazzeri A (2017) Reactively extruded ecocomposites based on poly(lactic acid)/bisphenol A polycarbonate blends reinforced with regenerated cellulose microfibers. Compos Sci Technol 139. https://doi.org/10.1016/j.compscitech.2016.12.013
74. Prabhakar MN, Shah AUR, Rao KC, Il SJ (2015) Mechanical and thermal properties of epoxy composites reinforced with waste peanut shell powder as a bio-filler. Fibers Polym 16(5):1119–1124. https://doi.org/10.1007/s12221-015-1119-1
75. Pradhan P, Nanda BP, Satapathy A (2020) Polyester composites filled with walnut shell powder: preparation and thermal characterization. Polym Compos 41(8):3294–3308
76. Qadri SB, Gorzkowski EP, Rath BB, Feng CR, Amarasinghe R (2016) Nanoparticles of wurtzite aluminum nitride from the nut shells. AIP Adv 6(11). https://doi.org/10.1063/1.4967279
77. Queirós CSGP, Cardoso S, Lourenço A, Ferreira J, Miranda I, Lourenço MJV, Pereira H (2020) Characterization of walnut, almond, and pine nut shells regarding chemical composition and extract composition. Biomass Convers Biorefinery 10(1):175–188. https://doi.org/10.1007/s13399-019-00424-2
78. Quiles-Carrillo L, Montanes N, Garcia-Garcia D, Carbonell-Verdu A, Balart R, Torres-Giner S (2018) Effect of different compatibilizers on injection-molded green composite pieces based on polylactide filled with almond shell flour. Compos Part B Eng 147:76–85. https://doi.org/10.1016/j.compositesb.2018.04.017
79. Ramos M, Dominici F, Luzi F, Jiménez A, Garrigós MC, Torre L, Puglia D (2020) Effect of almond shell waste on physicochemical properties of polyester-based biocomposites. Polymers (Basel) 12(4). https://doi.org/10.3390/POLYM12040835
80. Reichert CL, Bugnicourt E, Coltelli MB, Cinelli P, Lazzeri A, Canesi I, Braca F, Martínez BM, Alonso R, Agostinis L, Verstichel S, Six L, De Mets S, Gómez EC, Ißbrücker C, Geerinck R, Nettleton DF, Campos I, Sauter E, Pieczyk P, Schmid M (2020) Bio-based packaging: materials, modifications, industrial applications and sustainability
81. Roquia A, khalfan hamed Alhashmi A, hamed Abdullah alhasmi B (2021) Synthesis and characterisation of carbon nanotubes from waste of Juglans regia (walnut) shells. Fuller Nanotub Carbon Nanostructure 29(11):860–867. https://doi.org/10.1080/1536383X.2021.1900123

82. Rovira M (2021) Advances in hazelnut (Corylus avellana L.) rootstocks worldwide. Horticulturae 7(9). https://doi.org/10.3390/horticulturae7090267
83. Sahayaraj AF (2021) Properties and characterization of tamarind nut shell powder filled jute and hemp fibers reinforced hybrid polymer composites, pp 1–16
84. Sao P, Chand Y, Kumar A, Singh S (2021) Potential drug target identification in porphyromonas gingivalis using in-silico subtractive metabolic pathway analysis. Bangladesh J Med Sci 20(4):887–896
85. Sao P, Vats S, Singh S (2022) Porphyromonas gingivalis resistance and virulence: an integrated functional network analysis. Gene 839:146734
86. Sarsari NA, Pourmousa S, Tajdini A (2016) Physical and mechanical properties of walnut shell flour-filled thermoplastic starch composites. BioResources 11(3):6968–6983. https://doi.org/10.15376/biores.11.3.6968-6983
87. Sathiparan N, Anburuvel A, Selvam VV (2023) Utilization of agro-waste groundnut shell and its derivatives in sustainable construction and building materials—a review. J Build Eng 66:105866. https://doi.org/10.1016/j.jobe.2023.105866
88. Serafin J, Dziejarski B, Cruz Junior OF, Sreńscek-Nazzal J (2023) Design of highly microporous activated carbons based on walnut shell biomass for $H_2$ and $CO_2$ storage. Carbon N Y 201:633–647. https://doi.org/10.1016/j.carbon.2022.09.013
89. Shaik SA, Schuster J, Shaik YP, Kazmi M (2022) Manufacturing of biocomposites for domestic applications using bio-based filler materials. J Compos Sci 6(3). https://doi.org/10.3390/jcs6030078
90. Shaikhiev IG, Kraysman NV, Sverguzova SV (2023) Review of pistachio (Pistacia) shell use to remove pollutants from aqua media. Biointerface Res Appl Chem 13(4):1–11. https://doi.org/10.33263/BRIAC134.389
91. Sharahi M, Hivechi A, Bahrami SH, Hemmatinejad N, Milan PB (2021) Co-electrospinning of lignocellulosic nanoparticles synthesized from walnut shells with poly(caprolactone) and gelatin for tissue engineering applications. Cellulose 28(8):4943–4957. https://doi.org/10.1007/s10570-021-03709-w
92. Sharma P, Gaur VK, Sirohi R, Larroche C, Kim SH, Pandey A (2020) Valorization of cashew nut processing residues for industrial applications. Ind Crops Prod 152:112550. https://doi.org/10.1016/j.indcrop.2020.112550
93. Singh A, Sengar RS, Singh AK, Singh S, Kumar A, Ahmad K (2019) Impact of genetic engineering on agriculture food crops. Biotech Today Int J Biol Sci 9(1):17–24
94. Sivakumar J, Srinivasan SA, Pradeep GM, Sivakandhan C, Hasane Ahammad SK, Maheskumar P (2023) Effect of alkali treatment on wear behaviour of walnut shell reinforced bio-composites. Mater Today Proc 1–11. https://doi.org/10.1016/j.matpr.2023.08.036
95. Solís A, Rocha S, König M, Adam R, Garcés HO, Candia O, Muñoz R, Azócar L (2023) Preliminary assessment of hazelnut shell biomass as a raw material for pellet production. Fuel 333. https://doi.org/10.1016/j.fuel.2022.126517
96. Song X, Guan W, Qin H, Han X, Wu L, Ye Y (2022) Properties of poly(lactic acid)/walnut shell/hydroxyapatite composites prepared with fused deposition modeling. Sci Rep 12(1):1–13. https://doi.org/10.1038/s41598-022-15622-8
97. Song X, He W, Yang S, Huang G, Yang T (2019) Fused deposition modeling of poly (lactic acid)/walnut shell biocomposite filaments-surface treatment and properties. Appl Sci 9(22). https://doi.org/10.3390/app9224892
98. Sowińska-Baranowska A, Maciejewska M, Duda P (2022) The potential application of starch and walnut shells as biofillers for natural rubber (NR) composites. Int J Mol Sci 23(14). https://doi.org/10.3390/ijms23147968
99. Sutivisedsak N, Cheng HN, Burks CS, Johnson JA, Siegel JP, Civerolo EL, Biswas A (2012) Use of nutshells as fillers in polymer composites. J Polym Environ 20(2):305–314. https://doi.org/10.1007/s10924-012-0420-y
100. Taghizadeh A, Rad-Moghadam K (2018) Green fabrication of Cu/pistachio shell nanocomposite using Pistacia Vera L. hull: an efficient catalyst for expedient reduction of 4-nitrophenol and organic dyes. J Clean Prod 198:1105–1119. https://doi.org/10.1016/j.jclepro.2018.07.042

101. Thiagarajan A, Velmurugan K, Sangeeth PP (2020) Synthesis and mechanical properties of pistachio shell filler on glass fiber polymer composites by VARIM process. Mater Today Proc 39:610–614. https://doi.org/10.1016/j.matpr.2020.09.001
102. Torrado I, Dionísio A, Fernandes MC, Roseiro LB, Carvalheiro F, Pereira H, Duarte LC (2023) Production of oligosaccharides from pine nut shells by autohydrolysis. Bioenergy Res. https://doi.org/10.1007/s12155-023-10585-8
103. Tungare K, Shahu R, Zambare V, Agarwal P, Jobby R, Nisar N, Jha P (2022) Toxicity mitigation of textile dye reactive blue 4 by hairy roots of Helianthus annuus and testing its effect in in vivo model systems. Biomed Res Int
104. Verma N, Sao P, Srivastava A, Singh S (2021) Physiological and molecular responses to drought, submergence and excessive watering in plants. In: Harsh environment and plant resilience: molecular and functional aspects, pp 305–321
105. Wang H, Zhang Y, Wang Q, Jia C, Cai P, Chen G, Dong C, Guan H (2019) Biomass carbon derived from pine nut shells decorated with NiO nanoflakes for enhanced microwave absorption properties. RSC Adv 9(16):9126–9135. https://doi.org/10.1039/c9ra00466a
106. Wang Z, Zhu X, Deuss PJ (2021) The effect of ball milling on birch, pine, reed, walnut shell enzymatic hydrolysis recalcitrance and the structure of the isolated residual enzyme lignin. Ind Crops Prod 167:113493. https://doi.org/10.1016/j.indcrop.2021.113493
107. Wongcharee S, Aravinthan V, Erdei L, Sanongraj W (2017) Use of macadamia nut shell residues as magnetic nanosorbents. Int Biodeterior Biodegrad 124:276–287. https://doi.org/10.1016/j.ibiod.2017.04.004
108. Yang Z, Peng H, Wang W, Liu T (2010) Crystallization behavior of poly(ε-caprolactone)/layered double hydroxide nanocomposites. J Appl Polym Sci 116(5):2658–2667. https://doi.org/10.1002/app
109. Yin Q, Kong F, Wang S, Du J, Tao Y, Li P (2023) Hazelnut shell carbon filled polylactic acid composite filaments for 3D printing photothermal structures. J Mater Res Technol 27:3923–3935. https://doi.org/10.1016/j.jmrt.2023.10.299
110. Yu Y, Guo Y, Jiang T, Li J, Jiang K, Zhang H (2017) Study on the ingredient proportions and after-treatment of laser sintering walnut shell composites. Materials (Basel) 10(12). https://doi.org/10.3390/ma10121381
111. Zaaba NF, Ismail H (2020) The Influence of different compounding sequence and peanut shell powder loading on properties of polylactic acid/thermoplastic corn starch biocomposites. J Vinyl Addit Technol 26(4):413–422. https://doi.org/10.1002/vnl.21756
112. Zaheer Z (2019) Eco-friendly walnut shell powder based facile fabrication of biogenic Ag-nanodisks, and their interaction with bovine serum albumin. J Photochem Photobiol B Biol 193:8–17. https://doi.org/10.1016/j.jphotobiol.2019.01.015
113. Zheng H, Sun Z, Zhang H (2020) Effects of walnut shell powders on the morphology and the thermal and mechanical properties of poly(lactic acid). J Thermoplast Compos Mater 33(10):1383–1395. https://doi.org/10.1177/0892705719828801

# Biosynthesis of Nanoparticles from *Jatropha curcas* Latex

**Sagnik Nag, Janardhan Pallavi, H. Soundharya, Shatakshi Mishra, Anamika Mishra, B. Stany, Sourav Mohanto, Vetriselvan Subramaniyan, Faheem Ahmad, B. H. Jaswanth Gowda, and Mohammed Gulzar Ahmed**

**Abstract** Green synthesis or Biosynthesis of nanoparticles refers to synthesizing nanoparticles using environmentally friendly methods and sustainable materials. It aims to reduce hazardous chemicals and energy-intensive processes typically associated with traditional nanoparticle synthesis. Jatropha latex, derived from the *Jatropha curcas* plant, has been studied for its potential use in the synthesis of nanoparticles. The latex of Jatropha contains various compounds, including proteins, enzymes, and other organic molecules, which can serve as reducing agents or stabilizers in nanoparticle synthesis. Utilizing Jatropha latex for nanoparticle synthesis provides a sustainable alternative to conventional chemical methods, reducing the reliance on harsh chemicals and promoting environmentally friendly practices. The synthesis of nanoparticles from Jatropha latex typically involves mixing the latex with a metal ion solution under controlled conditions. The reaction parameters, such as temperature, pH, and incubation time, can influence the resulting nanoparticles' size, shape, and properties. After the synthesis process, the nanoparticles are characterized using various techniques, such as transmission electron microscopy (TEM), scanning electron microscopy (SEM), X-ray diffraction (XRD), or spectroscopic methods. These analyses provide information about the synthesized nanoparticles' size, morphology, crystallinity, and surface chemistry. Researchers continue to explore and optimize

S. Nag · V. Subramaniyan
Jeffrey Cheah School of Medicine and Health Sciences (JCSMHS), Monash University Malaysia, Bandar Sunway, 47500 Selangor, Malaysia

S. Nag · J. Pallavi · H. Soundharya · S. Mishra · A. Mishra · B. Stany
School of Bio-Sciences and Technology (SBST), Vellore Institute of Technology (VIT), Tiruvalam Road, Vellore 632014, Tamil Nadu, India

S. Mohanto · B. H. J. Gowda · M. G. Ahmed
Department of Pharmaceutics, Yenepoya Pharmacy College and Research Centre, Yenepoya (Deemed to Be University), Mangaluru 575018, Karnataka, India

F. Ahmad (✉)
Department of Botany, Aligarh Muslim University, Aligarh 202002, India
e-mail: faheem.bt@amu.ac.in

B. H. J. Gowda
School of Pharmacy, Medical Biology Centre, Queen's University Belfast, Belfast BT9 7BL, UK



D. Jabborova et al. (eds.), *Nanomaterials in Agroforestry Systems*, Smart Nanomaterials Technology, https://doi.org/10.1007/978-981-96-1337-3_5

the biosynthesis of nanoparticles from Jatropha latex, considering factors like eco-friendliness, scalability, and the potential applications of the synthesized nanoparticles in various fields, including medicine, catalysis, and sensing. Thus, this chapter emphasizes plausible outcomes of nanoparticle biosynthetic or green production from Jatropha latex and focuses on its subsequent biomedical, pharmaceutical, and industrial applications.

**Keywords** Nanotechnology · Nanoparticles · Green synthesis · Jatropha latex · Toxicity · Phytocompounds

## 1 Introduction

The biosynthesis of various nanoparticles (NPs) with the aid of Jatropha latex is one of the emerging fields of plant research that acknowledge the usage of natural components to acquire potential theragnostic NPs. The family Euphorbiaceae, to which Jatropha belongs, is renowned for its abundant latex content. Furthermore, latex comprises various proteins, enzymes, and secondary metabolites; all of these stabilizing and reducing agents can be used for NPs biosynthesis [55]. The biosynthesis of NPs from the latex is a two-step process, including the extraction of latex and the green biosynthesis of NPs [88]. The latex can be extracted by tapping the stems and branches of the Jatropha, has a high potential for synthesizing NPs, and is a milky fluid in nature. After purification, the latex is centrifuged to remove impurities and obtain concentrated extract as a precursor for NPs synthesis. In addition, the NPs can be obtained from the precursor by chemical reduction and green or biological synthesis process [57]. Here, the biological or green synthesis method is employed, and further, the depletion and stabilization of the bioactive compound in the latex properties are used in the synthesis of NPs. This synthesis involves using a metal salt precursor (e.g., silver nitrate, gold chloride) to obtain the latex extract, and then the reduction is carried out. The reduction can be accomplished by the usage of enzymes or the reducing property of latex itself. This process constructs various metallic NPs, i.e., gold NPs (AuNPs) and silver NPs (AgNPs), etc., based on the metal salt utilized [83]. The chemical and physical parameters such as length, size, structure, shape, and stability of NPs can be managed by adjusting pH, temperature, metal salt concentration, and reaction time. The synthesized NPs were further analyzed using techniques such as transmission electron microscopy (TEM), X-ray diffraction (XRD), scanning electron microscopy (SEM), UV–visible spectroscopy, and Fourier transform infrared spectroscopy (FTIR) [15, 28].

The current advancements in the synthesis of green NPs by the usage of Jatropha latex have immensely increased its application in various fields. For instance, in the use of NP synthesis by latex in the medical field, AgNPs are used widely as antimicrobial agents and used alongside pathogenic microbes; on the other hand, AuNPs are used in catalysis, sensing, and applications in drug delivery depending on their physiochemical properties [51]. The biological synthesis of the NPs has added more value to their use for living organisms. In addition, the investigation into the green synthesis of the NPs from Jatropha latex is evolving daily,hence, the usage of these NPs is also increasing tremendously. In this area, researchers have shown a rapid and environment-friendly method, called "green synthesis," for the synthesis of AgNPs using latexes from different plant species, such as *Jatropha curcas* (Jc) and *Lannea grandis* (Lg). The emulsions of both plants can be reduced via the capping factor in the NP biosynthesis process. The produced AgNPs demonstrate a distinctive surface plasmon resonance (SPR) band is visible in the produced AgNPs at 440 nm for those synthesized with Jc latex and at 415 nm for those synthesized with Lg latex [47]. The TEM images demonstrate that NPs produced from Lg latex were smaller and more regular in shape than Jc latex-derived NPs [83]. Several researchers also investigated the effects of various synthesis parameters on NP morphology, following latex concentration, reaction time, and metal ion concentration. Investigating the samples' UV–Vis spectra allowed for this to be achieved. More precisely, Jatropha latex was used to create the NPs, the latex was combined with silver nitrate, and the silver ions were reduced to create AgNPs. To describe the produced NPs, a number of methods were used, including UV–vis spectroscopy, TEM, and XRD. The study also examined AgNPs antibacterial activity, highlighting potential uses in biotechnology and medicine. This study shows the potential of jatropha latex as an eco-friendly and sustainable source of NPs synthesis. It offers insightful information into the biosynthesis of AgNPs using this material. We stress the significance of utilizing organic materials, like jatropha latex, in creating environmentally friendly processes for synthesizing NPs [90].

The green biosynthesis of AuNPs from the Jatropha latex and the application and synthesis of palladium and platinum NPs are demonstrated. Utilizing latex extract from *Jatropha curcas* and gold salt solutions, AuNPs are created. The gold salt solutions and latex extract were combined in this case, and the latex's bioactive compounds reduced the metal salt while also aiding in the stabilization of the NPs that were created. The resulting AuNPs are special and have numerous uses in catalysis, electronics, and drug delivery [83]. These instances show the potential of jatropha latex for use in the biosynthesis of NPs. The bioactive components and proteins in latex work as efficient stabilizers and reducers, allowing for the creation of NPs with particular characteristics. It is significant to note that additional investigations are currently being conducted in this area, and these investigations may yield fresh information about the biosynthesis of NPs from Jatropha latex [24, 87].

## 2 Paradigm Shift Towards Green Biosynthesis of NPs

Recently, there has been a notable surge of inquisitiveness in the nanotechnology sector, which focuses on exploiting and investigating nanoscale substances ranging from 1 to 100 nm [62]. Conventional NPs synthesis approaches typically rely on chemical compounds and physical methodologies. However, due to growing apprehensions regarding the potential toxicity of these methods on human well-being and the environment, researchers have been motivated to explore more environmentally friendly alternatives [85]. Green synthesis involves utilizing biological entities, including plants, microorganisms, and their extracts, for synthesizing NPs, further summarized in Fig. 1. This green methodology presents numerous benefits, encompassing diminished toxicity, cost-efficiency, and sustainability. Furthermore, various studies explore the methodologies used to detect the external morphology and characteristics of synthesized NPs [55]. Several enzymes, i.e., amylase and sulfite reductase, have been utilized to stimulate the development of NPs or serve as agents for reduction [26]. In the realm of green NP synthesis, using plant extracts as stabilizing and reducing agents is seen to be a promising strategy. Plant extracts including a variety of biomolecules, such as proteins, phenolic compounds, and flavonoids, have shown potential in the creation of nanoparticles. By acting as reducing agents, these biomolecules help metal ions produce nanoparticles (NPs) [2]. Moreover, it has been shown that fungi, yeasts, and bacteria are among the microorganisms that may produce stable, positively defined NPs [26, 72].

Several potential phytochemicals obtained from plants and algae have demonstrated promising capabilities in synthesizing environmentally friendly NPs [22]. These microorganisms can produce NPs within or outside their cells through metabolic processes. Intracellular synthesis refers to the process by which metal ions are reduced within microbial cells. Extracellular synthesis, on the other hand, takes place when microbially secreted enzymes and metabolites are present [26]. The characterization of the synthesized NPs is crucial in order to gain insights into their morphology and properties. In order to achieve this objective, a range of methodologies are commonly utilized, i.e., UV–visible spectroscopy [81], FTIR [73], XRD [4], SEM [26], and TEM [26]. These methodologies offer significant observations

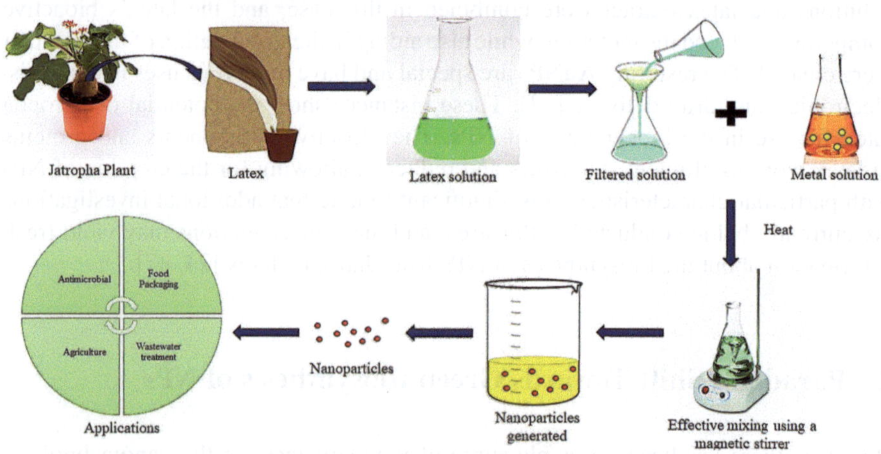


**Fig. 1** Graphical understanding of green synthesis of NPs from Jatropha latex and its applications

regarding the dimensions, morphology, chemical makeup, and crystal lattice arrangement of the NPs, facilitating researchers in comprehending their characteristics and dynamics [26].

In agriculture, the utilization of nanoscale lignocellulosic materials obtained from crops and trees has been observed in various applications, including nano-fertilizers, nano-pesticides, and nano-coatings [78]. AgNPs have been integrated into dental instruments and orthodontic adhesives due to their notable antimicrobial characteristics. Certain NPs derived from green synthesis have demonstrated potent as contrast agents for X-ray imaging due to their notable X-ray absorption coefficient [26]. Moreover, their distinctive optical and physicochemical properties have made them highly valuable in drug delivery systems. The utilization of biological agents and extracts offers a more secure and ecologically sound approach in contrast to traditional chemical and physical methodologies. Green NPs have many applications across diverse fields, i.e., agriculture, dentistry, imaging, and drug delivery systems. These applications offer promising prospects for advancements in these respective domains [26]. In the subject of nanotechnology, green nanotechnology presents viable ways to advance sustainability. The ability of microorganism-mediated synthesis to produce NPs in a regulated and ecologically friendly manner is one of its main advantages [58]. The transition towards utilizing green synthesis methods for the production of NPs is motivated by the growing recognition of the importance of environmental sustainability and the necessity for environmentally friendly manufacturing processes. The transition towards a more sustainable approach in various fields involves several important factors. These include plant-based synthesis, which involves utilizing plants as a source for synthesizing various compounds. Another significant aspect is microorganism-mediated synthesis, which involves harnessing the capabilities of microorganisms to produce desired substances [46]. Additionally, the utilization of bio-waste is crucial in this shift towards sustainability. This involves finding innovative ways to repurpose and utilize waste materials from biological sources, thereby reducing waste and promoting a circular economy. Renewable energy-driven processes, such as solar or wind power, play a significant role in this transition, further reducing reliance on fossil fuels and minimizing the environmental impact of various processes [6]. Furthermore, implementing green solvents and reaction conditions is essential to this shift. Green solvents are environmentally friendly alternatives to traditional solvents, which can harm human health and the atmosphere. Similarly, employing green reaction conditions involves optimizing processes to minimize waste generation and energy consumption. In the subject of nanotechnology, green nanotechnology presents viable ways to advance sustainability. The ability of microorganism-mediated synthesis to produce NPs in a regulated and ecologically friendly manner is one of its main advantages [54].

Green synthesis methods play a pivotal role in promoting sustainable and environmentally conscious production of NPs by harnessing natural resources, minimizing waste, and reducing pollution. The persistent investigation and advancement in this domain are anticipated to result in enhanced and scalable methodologies for green synthesis, thereby facilitating the broader acceptance and implementation of environmentally sustainable NPs fabrication. Green synthesis techniques are useful because they use renewable energy sources, such as wind, hydropower, or solar power, to make it easier to synthesize NPs. The incorporation of renewable energy sources into diverse processes is crucial in order to reduce carbon emissions and the overall environmental impact associated with the manufacture of nanoparticles [54].

## 3 Potential Secondary Metabolites Acquired from *Jatropha Curcas L.*

*Jatropha curcas* is a dense shrub belonging to the genus Jatropha of the family Euphorbiaceae, which comprises various medicinal properties and the potential for biodiesel production. These qualities ultimately come from the numerous phytochemicals that the plant produces. Many secondary metabolites with varied biological functions can be found in the plant. Almost all plant parts create a variety of metabolites that are engaged in various biological processes. The existence of such powerful chemicals has prompted experts to do thorough investigations in order to discover all of the plant's possible attributes. Because of their biological traits, these species have been reported to produce a wide range of metabolites, such as flavonoids, terpenes, steroid use, cyclic peptides, lignin, saponins, tannins, coumarins, and eudemonic acids, which are useful in treating a variety of diseases [77]. The Jatropha genus is notable for producing several secondary metabolites that have medicinal applications [16]. Among various Jatropha species, the parts of *J. curcas*, i.e., leaf, seed oil, fruits, seeds, stem, and latex, have shown major medicinal uses in various health-related issues. The phytochemical investigations of *Jatropha curcas* plant led to the isolation of compounds such as alkaloids, diterpenes, flavonoids, sesquiterpenes, triterpenes, lignans, cyclic peptides, coumarins, phenols, esters, and various fatty acids [69]. These compounds possess several medicinal properties involved in treating a wide variety of health-related conditions. The individual portion of the plant produces different metabolites in different quantities [34]. The concentration of these metabolites depends upon the growth condition of the plant. The various stresses experienced by the plants also trigger the production of additional metabolites and a different concentration of phytochemicals to combat the stress conditions. Table 1 shows the important secondary metabolites obtained from *J. curcas* and its biological functions.

### *3.1 Sterols*

Sterols are bioactive compounds with antiviral, anticarcinogenic, and antioxidant properties. The leaf of *Jatropha curcas* holds the majority of sterol compound production. The steroid components stigmasterol and beta-sitosterol have been found in the leaf extract of *Jatropha curcas*. The presence of stigmasterol, sitosterol,

**Table 1** Biological functions of secondary metabolites obtained from the various parts of *Jatropha curcas L*

| Secondary metabolite | Part of plant | Function | References |
|---|---|---|---|
| Saponins | Leaves, stem barks | Surfactant | [66] |
| Tannins | Ovary walls, leaves | Antimicrobial | [74] |
| Cardiac glycosides | Leaves | Antimicrobial | [64] |
| Terpenoids | Root | Anti-cancer and antimicrobial | [1] |
| Flavonoids | Leaves | Anti-cancer and antimicrobial | [1] |
| Alkaloids | Leaves | Antimicrobial | [64] |
| Steroids | Stem bark | Antimicrobial, larvicidal | [68] |

and other steroid molecules frequently exhibits anti-cancer activities. These sterol compounds have shown cardiovascular protectant properties involving cholesterol-lowering effects. Along with these compounds, there is evidence of the production of metabolites such as phytosterols, tannins, and steroidal sapogenins from the *Jatropha curcas* leaf [69]. The stem bark and roots of Jatropha have also shown an adequate production of β-Sitosterol, which primarily functions as a cholesterol-lowering and antimicrobial agent.

### 3.2 *Terpenoids*

Diterpenoids and triterpenoids are the major terpenes produced by the Jatropha species. Among the several diterpenes produced by the Jatropha species, *Jatropha curcas* has shown a prominent production of diterpenes, i.e., Caniojane, Jatropherol, Curcasone (A, B, C, and D), and Jatrophol with antiplasmodial, insecticidal, anti-invasive effect in tumor cells, cytotoxic rodenticidal along with antibacterial properties, respectively [17]. The triterpenes play a key role in the oxidative reactions when exposed to certain circumstances. There have been reports suggesting that *J. curcas* stem bark and seeds contain triterpenes, including amyrin, phytosterols, lupeol, and pentacyclic triterpenes like ursolic acid, botulinic acid, and oleanolic acid. It has been revealed that the pentacyclic triterpenes produced by *J. curcas* have anti-HIV, anti-tumor, and anti-inflammatory properties [89].

### 3.3 *Flavonoids*

The most widely produced secondary metabolites, flavonoids, primarily have a scavenging effect on free radicals. Depending on the unfavorable environmental stress factors, different flavonoids have different concentrations. The leaves of the plant are where most flavonoids are discovered to be produced, including vitexin, isovitexin, apigenin, and vicenin II. As part of the plant's defensive mechanism, a network of flavonoids makes up the antioxidant complex network, which regulates development and stress tolerance [30, 40]. The flavonoid compounds such as kaempferol, quercetin, and rutin from the *J. curcas* leaves possess anti-inflammatory properties and have been reported to exhibit protective properties against chronic diseases [38]. The oil-rich seeds and the stem bark of Jatropha contain a certain adequate concentration of flavonoids, which exhibit antioxidant properties and other potential health-promoting properties. Several flavonoids, i.e., rhiofolin, isoorientin, and isoquercetin of *J. curcas* of Egyptian origin have reported potential antidiabetic properties [13].

## 3.4 Alkaloids

Alkaloids are bioactive compounds that act as a protective agent for plants against insects and herbivores. The alkaloid compounds are rarely non-toxic to humans, but a few rare compounds have shown potential health benefits. The majority of the functions of alkaloid compounds include growth regulation, detoxification, and source of nitrogen for plants. The two prominent alkaloids produced by *J. curcas* are 5-hydroxypyrrolidin-2-one and pyrimidine-2, 4-dione, which possess antimicrobial properties. The latex of Jatropha has also been reported to contain alkaloids with anticancer properties. Some alkaloid compounds, i.e., curcin produced in the seeds, are unsuitable for human consumption. Meanwhile, an alkaloid, i.e., jatrophine produced from the latex of Jatropha has shown anti-cancerous and disinfectant properties [13, 84].

## 3.5 Coumarins and Cyclic Peptides

*J. curcas* often produces the phytochemicals coumarins and coumarinolignoids. Together with UV-absorbing qualities, the chemical compounds actively defend against herbivores and plant infections and protect the plant from damage brought on by excessive UV radiation. Marmesin, jatrophin, and 5-hydroxy-6,7-dimethoxycoumarin have all been shown to be produced in significant quantities by the roots of the Jatropha plant. Cyclic peptides, on the other hand, are a different category of secondary metabolites produced by Jatropha species. These substances primarily serve as antibacterial agents that prevent the proliferation of harmful microorganisms that destroy plants. According to several reports, the cyclic peptide compounds show characteristics of signaling molecules regulating specific physiological processes connected to growth, development, stress retaliations, etc. As shown in Fig. 2, the three main cyclic peptide substances discovered in *J. curcas* are curcacyclin A, B, and jatrophidin. The isolated Jatrophidin I from the latex

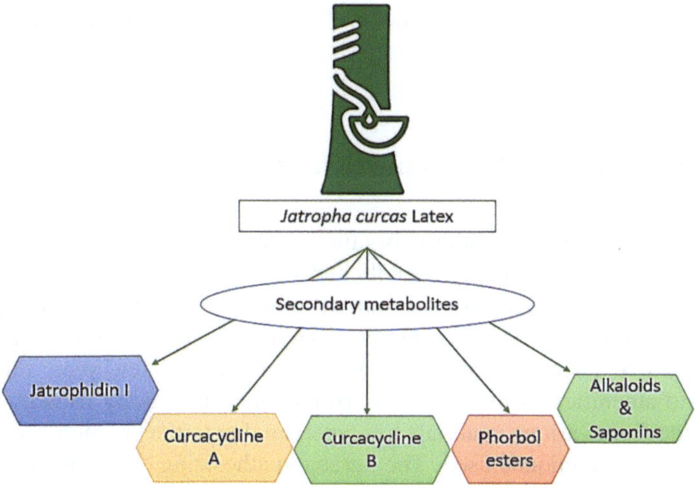


**Fig. 2** Potential secondary metabolites obtained from the latex of *Jatropha curcas L*

of the Jatropha plant has prominently demonstrated antimicrobial, antifungal, and antioxidant effects [13, 69].

### *3.6 Saponins and Tannins*

The two most significant secondary metabolites of *Jatropha curcas* are saponins and tannins. These substances perform various biological tasks and play various roles in regulating plant metabolism. Typically, the leaves and seeds of the *Jatropha curcas* plant contain both of these substances. When agitated in aqueous solutions, saponins and glycosides with hydrophilic and hydrophobic regions generate foam resembling detergent-like properties. The 2,3-dihydro-2,5-dihydroxy6-methyl-4 h-pyran-4-one factor of hydroperoxide molecule of saponins eliminates free radicals. These substances are, therefore, well recognized for their antioxidant properties. Tannins, on the other hand, are polyphenolic substances that can cause protein precipitation. Studies on *J. curcas* have revealed that the plant's stem bark and root bark produced tannins, hydrolyzable tannins, and phlobatatannins. These compounds possess antioxidant properties, while some tannins in traditional medicine have demonstrated few medicinal properties, i.e., the ability to heal wounds, reduce diarrhea, and reduce inflammation [12]. Lignans, neolignans, and sesquineolignans, i.e., jatrophasin C and D, isoamericanol A, isoprincepin, princepin, and americanol A are a few other secondary metabolites obtained from the defatted kernel of *J. curcas* which have shown significant cytotoxicity effect and antioxidant properties [13]. Jatropha species have a rich production of other metabolites, such as phorbol esters, which are identified as toxic compounds produced in plant seeds. These compounds are usually carcinogenic and have other biological effects of inducing inflammatory responses [21].

## 4 Green Synthesis of Nanoparticles from Jatropha Latex

The field of green material synthesis is gaining momentum worldwide, as it offers a way to produce environmentally friendly and safe compounds like NPs. Nanotechnology, with its wide-ranging potential applications, plays a vital role in synthesizing and characterizing nanomaterials. Green nanomaterial production using a variety of plant extracts has advanced significantly over the past few years due to their makeup and amenities. A market niche for the environmentally friendly synthesis of NPs made from various materials has emerged due to the creation and alteration of the synthesis techniques used. The "green synthesizing" of synthetic materials or reagents—also called "green synthesis" of biological materials or reagents—has evolved in recent years to emphasize, among other things, the use of safe in-nature precursors that lessen or eliminate hazardous waste that can be released into the environment. Furthermore, no explicit requirements exist for costly equipment or reagents, high temperatures, or pressures for green synthesis methods. The "Bottom Up" method is used in the biological processes that create NPs. This occurs due to the reduction and oxidation of molecules or atoms, which are tiny entities. Different plant species are extracted by microorganisms, which then use biological processes to create NPs. An economical and environmentally benign method of creating NPs is biological synthesis [35]. NPs have frequently been produced via the most popular sol–gel synthesis techniques. There are two primary phases or components that form the basis of this strategy. It is necessary to homogenize the chemicals, reagents, or compounds that will be utilized. Usually, this is done at ambient temperature and stirred often to prevent granules or lumps from forming. This method enables the progressive synthesis of the requisite crystals through the process's synthesis, the nucleation process, and finally, precipitation. One technique for producing NPs involves burning a precursor fluid or vapor with a flame in a process known as flame spray pyrolysis. In order to obtain the NPs, the precursor used during this method is put into a high-pressure furnace. It is a process that may be used to make NPs in large quantities at an affordable cost [70].

### *4.1 Titanium Dioxide ($TiO_2$) NPs*

Based on its beneficial characteristics, the most important metal oxides for successful antimicrobial, antibacterial, and photocatalytic applications are titanium dioxide ($TiO_2$) NPs. Plant extracts are often made from the original plants' stems, flowers, leaves, and roots. Herbs are primarily used in the medicinal industry. Because the active ingredients in the extract are heat-sensitive, the extraction procedure typically occurs at a temperature of not more than 100° C. The kind of titanium precursor, reaction duration, pH, and extraction and precursor concentration are only a few of the crucial synthesis factors [5].

To get rid of any associated dust, the jatropha leaves were cut into little pieces and thoroughly cleaned with DD water. After that, they were exposed to the sunlight to dry. After adding 20 g of jatropha leaves to a liter of DD water, the mixture was heated to 80° C for up to 20 min. The production of extracts from leaves takes forty minutes. The resulting leaf extract was further purified using filter cloths before being employed in the environmentally friendly production of TiO2 NPs. They then allowed it to cool to ambient temperature [39]. In order to produce TiO2 NPs in an environmentally acceptable manner, a volume of 80 ml of 0.50 M titanium chloride and 80 ml of pure leaf extract were continuously combined at room temperature in a 1:1 ratio. After mixing the precursor mixture and leaf extract for 20 min, the liquid solution's color changed from transparent to brownish-white due to a decrease in metal ions (Ti4 + ), indicating the creation of green $TiO_2$ NPs. In order to form the NPs precipitates, 15 ml of ammonia was added by drops to the NPs liquid solution, which was constantly agitated at room temperature. After filtering out the solution, the resultant NP precipitates have been treated using ethyl alcohol in order to get rid of the ionic impurities. After being cleaned, the precipitates were dried and allowed to air evaporate. Next, they were burned for three hours at 450° C in a furnace with a muffle and then pulverized with a crystal pestle and mortar to create the final powder form of $TiO_2$ NPs. Greenly produced TiO2 NPs were characterized, and the phase and crystal structure were ascertained, using powder XRD. The size and physical characteristics of the environmentally produced $TiO_2$ NPs were assessed by employing field-emitting scanning electron microscopy (FE-SEM). X-ray Energy-Dispersive Spectrometry was used to ascertain the composition of the $TiO_2$ NPs made using green synthesis. Additionally, a technique called dynamic scattered light (DLS) was used to analyze the distribution of the size of particles of $TiO_2$ NPs made by green synthesis [27].

NPs are produced via spinning in a device known as a spinning disk; the reactor typically consists of a rotating disk with a configurable heat regulator. A reactor is filled with inert gas; oxygen and nitrogen are continuously drained from it to suppress chemical reactions. Water and additional liquid precursors are pumped into the reactor or container. The solution blow spinning method uses compressed air to produce nanofibers, which are easily scaled up and utilized to produce composites and nanofibers. Titanium isopropoxide solution serves as the precursor. The major source of $TiO_2$ nanofibers is this solution precursor, produced by mixing seven percent polyvinyl pyrrolidone with ethanol and acetic acid solution in a 3:1 ratio. The 10% solution was heated to 60° C, vigorously mixed, and cooled. A nozzle delivers the prepared precursor at a set pressure of air and feed rate into a solution blow spinning equipment feed tube. For the membrane sample, ethylene terephthalate drives the nanofiber collector. To gather composite nanofibers, use this collector. The next step of calcination uses these composite nanofibers to create $TiO_2$ nanofibers [35].

## 4.2 Silver NPs (AgNPs)

Several studies have been accomplished on metallic NPs because of their unique electrical, optical, and catalytic properties. Specific chemical and physical qualities are necessary for optimization and use. AgNPs are made via various processes, including heat evaporation, electrical reduction, chemical reduction, and photochemical reaction reduction. A reaction process involves diluting 1 ml of crude latex into 20 ml of this latex liquid and combining it with 20 ml of 5 M silver nitrates solution in freshwater after 300 ml of purified deionized freshwater is added to make it 3%. The combination was gradually transformed into AgNPs after four hrs. of heating in a bath of oil at 85° C with continuous stirring. The same reactions were also carried out using different $AgNO_3$ and latex concentrations [71]. Using a copper potassium chromatic filter in the 35–80 range and an X-ray analytical diffractometer, the crystalline composition of metallic silver was investigated. Using the JEOL-JEM-2100 apparatus, the highest-resolution TEM (HR-TEM) pictures were captured in order to examine the shape and size of AgNPs. The FTIR measurements were obtained using the spectrophotometer. To reduce the concentration of silver ions, 5 ml of extract of leaves were added to 45 ml of 0.002 M solutions made of $AgNO_3$ in 100 ml bottles that were stored at room temperature. Before the mixture's color changed, a reaction took place in a dimly lit space. The solution's brownish-gray hue served as a catalyst to generate the AgNPs (Jc-AgNPs). The liquid solution's UV spectroscopy (ranging from 300 to 700 nm) was used to track the biological elimination of the silver ions. Before lyophilization, the water-suspended particles had been frozen (–40° C) for 24 h. The frozen samples were lyophilized for two days at –80° C using Allied Frost FD-3. TEM, AFM, SEM, and XRD have all been used to analyze the structure and composition of frozen Jc-AgNPs. The FTIR analysis provided compelling evidence that multiple biological components were involved in the suspension-based Jc-AgNP synthesis and stabilization. Many organic coatings, such as terpenoids, alkaloid compounds, phenolics, digestive enzymes, polymers, and vitamins, are produced by plants to keep AgNPs suspended. The primary benefit of utilizing plants to synthesize AgNPs is this. Recent research indicates that aqueous extracts of J. curcas leaves include a variety of bioactive compounds that are critical for the synthesis of Jc-AgNPs, stabilization/capping, and strong antibacterial activity. The vibrational bands associated with Jc-AgNPs that have been found using FTIR analysis indicate the presence of many compounds, including both amines and alkaloids, that were previously identified for the formation and stability of NPs. Water filtration, antimicrobial coatings and paints based on nanosilver, silver dressings for wound care, and other need-based applications in a variety of industries (healthcare, textiles, etc.) can all benefit from Jc-AgNPs [14]. Because using plants to create AgNPs is more advantageous than using other synthesis techniques, it is also quicker, less expensive, and more practical. Furthermore, a wide variety of complex chemically structured naturally occurring organic compounds, known as phytochemicals, are found in plants, these medicinal plants exhibit great potential for generating AgNPs with desired therapeutic effects. Additionally, a great deal of research has been done on AuNPs, or and AgNPs derived from different plants that are used medicinally, demonstrating both their ability to transport bioactive compounds and their general efficacy in treating a variety of ailments [53].

## 4.3 Zinc Sulfide NPs (ZnS NPs)

Synthesis of green ZnS NPs is created by jatropha latex. Crude latex made of Jatropha is prepared by cutting the plant's green stems, allowing for latex collection. A one-milliliter amount of crude latex was employed to create solutions of approximately 0.15, 0.10 and 0.05% (v/v) using double-distilled water as the solvent. Next, 20 ml of the latex solutions and 2.5 mM of the water-zinc acetate solution were mixed together. A magnetic stirrer aggressively agitated the liquid for 24 h. at the ambient temperature. The mixture was centrifuged at 15,000 revolutions per minute for 15 min to remove unreacted chemicals, and then it was re-dispersed in distilled water that had been deionized. A mixture of 6 ml was divided among ten 10 ml test tubes to qualitatively identify the existence of ZnS NPsTwo milliliters of potassium ferricyanide (III) and a solution containing the following elements: sodium hydroxide, ammonium hydroxide, and lead acetate were added to each tube. The tubes were assessed based on the quantity of precipitate that was found. Analysis of AFM was performed on the mixes to establish their average size in the vicinity of the nanoscale and UV, and the analysis was performed to ascertain their concentration. The photocatalytic degradation experiments employed the product at the maximum concentration. The latex concentration being utilized affects absorption. The product generated had a higher concentration when the latex concentration was increased. Because absorbance directly relates to quantity, FM analysis revealed that the material products were polydisperse, with a standard size of 80 nm. The amount of latex utilized impacted the amount of ZnS NPs. Additionally, the particle size is decided independently of the latex formulation. With a degradation rate of 7.72%, the maximum degradation of the dye was attained in the first 15 min. Using green chemistry, creating ZnS NPs with potential degradation of organic dyes is feasible [7]. At room temperature, ZnS NPs with a typical diameter of 10 nm can be effectively created using jatropha latex material. Since green synthesis is a pollution-less and environmentally beneficial technique to synthesize ZnS NPs, it presents a difficult alternative to chemical synthesis.

In a standard reaction combination, this latex solution was mixed with a 20 ml diluted acetate of zinc solution at a concentration of 2.5 mM. Using distilled deionized water from the faucet as the solvent, 1 ml of raw latex was added to 300 ml to create 0.3%. The mixture was now let to stand at room temperature (27° C) for 24 to 48 h, stirring continuously with a stirrer that was magnetic. After 25 h, it was discovered that the solution had solidified in distinct, yellow-brow aggregates at the bottom inside the glass flask. After 25, 30, and 35 h, the luminescence and UV–visible spectra of ZnS-based NPs were measured. Following the reaction, the end product underwent several distilled water washes before being further examined using X-ray diffraction. Studies focusing on photocatalysis, antimicrobial activity, germination of seeds, and cytotoxicity would benefit more from ZnS NPs produced sustainably [25].

### 4.4 Lead NPs

Lead NPs have distinct qualities and potential applications in various industries and have attracted significant interest, particularly in chemical interactions. Decreases in aqueous lead, microemulsion, micelles and platinum salts, and UV light irradiation are a few of the synthetic processes used to make them. Ionic liquids based on tetrazolium were recently used to create lead NPs. The 3.0 mM aqueous solution of lead acetate was added to twenty milliliters of the latex solution in a typical chemical combined form. Using water with previously purified ionization to make it 0.5%, one milliliter of raw latex was reduced to 500 ml. The combination was now permitted to stand at ambient temperature in a lab environment while constantly shaken within a minute of the latex solution coming into touch with the lead acetate, which spontaneously reduced, resulting in the synthesis of lead NPs. A UV–vis spectrophotometer was used to acquire the lead NPs' UV–visible absorption spectra. An X-ray diffractometer and a Cu-K radiation dosage of 1.5405 were employed. The size and form of lead NPs were investigated using TEM with a JEOL-1200 Cx and a 120 kV accelerating voltage. The distribution of particle sizes was measured using DLS equipment. The elemental makeup of the sample was investigated using the JED-2300 instrument and EDAX [36].

## 5 Overview of Characterization Tools and Techniques for NPs

The characterization of NPs is a crucial process to understand the application of these NPs concerning their physical, chemical, and biological attributes. The preliminary characterization starts with analyzing the physical attributes of the NPs. Starting with the morphological characterization, which is usually performed using electron microscopy, SEM and TEM analysis are performed to evaluate the physical morphological features of NPs. The electron source is utilized to determine a NP's shape, size, structure, and surface morphology. Titanium dioxide and lead NPs obtained from Jatropha latex have been reported to be morphologically characterized using TEM to understand the structure and size of the particle. The provided sample is exposed to high-energy electrons; the way these electrons interact with the material influences both the form and size of the NPs [32]. Moreover, HR-TEM was used to characterize AgNPs from Jatropha latex [9]. Apart from the electron microscopy, DLS is one of the common approaches used to determine the NPs' hydrodynamic particle size and surface properties. Other topographic characterization techniques are used to study further a given NP's molecular and atomic level anatomy, such as XRD and Brunauer–Emmett–Teller (BET). Most of the Jatropha latex-extracted NPs are studied using XRD to potentially investigate the crystallinity, polycrystallinity, and amorphous nature of the NPs. To assess the crystallinity of a sample, the primary basis of X-ray diffraction (XRD) is the beneficial or elastic scattering of monochromatic incident X-rays that are primarily directed to the sample. Depending on the sample's structure, the patterns that the scattered rays create are analyzed to ascertain the sample's crystallinity [28]. Another popular method for morphological characterization that's employed to ascertain the chemical makeup of the NPs is EDX (energy dispersive X-ray) analysis. It is stated that EDX was used to considerably characterize the isolated copper nanoparticles from Jatropha curcas and examine their elemental makeup. The method determines how much X-ray is produced from a certain specimen and correlates this amount with the properties and nature of the element included in the sample. The primary chemical peak of the NPs and the composition percentage of the sample are shown in the EDX spectra. Similarly, in the green production of Cu-NPs of J. curcas, the chemical peak and structure of copper NPs peculiar to the metal copper were investigated [23].

The chemical and physical constitution of these particles determines the stability of the NPs. To investigate the chemical characteristics of the NPs, methods such as zeta potential, FTIR and ultraviolet (UV) spectroscopy, and measurement study are employed. FTIR is the most frequently used method to examine the nature of molecular bonds of NPs. The method measures the quantity of IR radiation that may flow through the sample; while it absorbs some radiation, most of it goes unaffected. We can assess the type of bonding in a molecule by measuring the strength of the absorption and transmission. This information aids in identifying the chemical characteristics of the NPs as well as their composition and quality [3]. According to a paper, FTIR was used to describe the titanium dioxide, silver, and Pb NPs extracted from J. curcas' latex in order to examine their molecular bonding and chemical makeup. Similarly, another method designed to ascertain the NPs' concentration in a particular sample is UV spectroscopy. With the aid of UV spectroscopy, it is simple to determine the amount, aggregate state, and the refractive index of NPs generated in a certain volume of latex, the ability to absorb light of the NPs is correlated with both their concentration and optical activity. Ultraviolet (UV) analysis was used to do the concentration variation investigation of AgNO3 NPs produced from the Jatropha latex [9].

One more important aspect of NPs, which signifies their stability, is the surface charge of these particles in colloidal solutions. The surface charges help in molecular interaction, allowing aggregation of the particles. A thin layer of counterions, known as the Stern layer, is drawn to the surface of NPs due to their surface charge. As the NPs diffuse, this double layer made up of ions travels through the solution with them. Zeta potential is the electric potential generated at the outside edges of these ion double layers. If the zeta potential of NPs is more than + 30 mV and lower than -30 mV, they are considered to be highly stable. As the zeta potential is least stable at the point where it becomes isoelectric, it is zero, compared to the strong both positive and negative zeta potential, which are assumed to be more stable. The zeta potential measuring method was used to examine the charge distribution of AgNPs that were synthesized from J. curcas leaves. Zeta potential measurements of AgNPs in a colloidal suspension were used to assess the NPs' stability. The outcomes validated the particles' high stability in the colloidal suspension. The analysis is used to keep track of surface functionalization and other alterations that influence the stability of NPs in suspension [14].

An additional crucial investigation that needs to be done to look into the biological function of the NPs in both in vitro and in vivo settings is biological characterization. This aids in our comprehension of the NPs' biological stability and permits us to evaluate the effectiveness of their biological characteristics. Among the characterization methods used to evaluate the biological characteristics of the NPs, such as biological compatibility, toxicity, and possible pharmaceutical uses, are in vitro viability of cells, in vivo survival, and microbiological colony viability [43].

The cell viability assays help assess the NPs' cytotoxicity and stability in biological environments. These tests can demonstrate if the NPs influence cell viability and illustrate details associated with their biocompatibility. To assess the antibacterial qualities for the NPs, a number of tests are frequently used, including the minimum bactericidal concentration (MBC) and minimum inhibitory concentration (MIC). Comparable characterization was carried out for the AgNPs produced from the leaf extracts of *J. curcas*. By applying the microdilution method to evaluate the MIC and MBC values against both gram-positive and gram-negative bacteria, AgNPs' antibacterial potential was ascertained. When used against gram-negative bacteria, the NPs demonstrated significant bactericidal potential [14].

## 6 Pharmaceutical and Industrial Applications of NPs Derived from Jatropha Latex

Plant-based NPs synthesis is one method that may be used to produce non-toxic and extremely biocompatible NPs. Functionalized NPs have several applications in catalysis, bioimaging, and bio-separation. In comparison, magnetic and metal NPs are used for drug delivery and biosensors [60]. Researchers have recently examined the possibility of employing NPs obtained from several natural sources for pharmacological uses. Drug delivery methods may benefit from NPs' unique qualities, such as increased surface area and better bioavailability [9]. Most of the AgNPs obtained from the latex of the Jatropha genus tend to possess antimicrobial properties. The bacterial-nanomaterial interaction has been greatly enhanced by the AgNPs' tiny size, high stability, and ease of internalization into the bacterial cells, allowing the NPs to demonstrate their bactericidal impact. AgNPs derived from Jatropha or latex have also demonstrated antiviral characteristics. AgNPs ranging in size from 1 to 10 nm have been shown to adhere to the outer exterior of HIV-1 with ease [19].

Due to the rise in antibiotic resistance among pathogenic bacteria, it is imperative to discover alternative agents that may effectively limit the growth and development of these bacteria in order to stop the spread of diseases. NPs made from plants have shown encouraging possibilities in the fight against harmful microorganisms [45]. Leveraging this property could lead to the development of innovative treatments for health conditions affected by antimicrobial resistance. These particles can also be employed for designing enzyme inhibitors and bio-controlling agents [59]. AgNPs are now successfully used in bactericidal coatings, wrapping, cosmetics, or pharmaceutical products because numerous studies have demonstrated their strong antibacterial efficacy against a variety of bacterial strains. AgNPs made from *Jatropha latex* have demonstrated fungicidal and anti-biofilm properties against C. albicans, an opportunistic pathogenic yeast [44]. Due to its medicinal properties, Jatropha latex-derived NPs can be used as imaging agents for medical diagnosis to provide a clearer view of certain tissues or organs. It is crucial to stress that any possible medicinal use for NPs made from jatropha latex would need extensive preclinical and clinical research to determine their safety and effectiveness in people. Lead NPs are notable for their industrial applications. The green synthesis of lead NPs from the *Jatropha curcas* latex could be used for the creation of NPs with potential applications in catalysis and lead batteries [36].

NPs have gained widespread recognition over time for a variety of commercial and industrial applications, including environmental monitoring equipment, skincare products, technology for communication and information, the field of biotechnology, and structural applications. Specifically, latex, proteins, phytochemicals, etc. can be used to produce metal nanoparticles (NPs) with the advantage of serving as a reducing and capping agent at the same time, preventing particle aggregation. Produced from the sap of the jatropha plants, ZnS and $TiO_2$ NPs have potential applications in agriculture to promote crop growth. These particles can be primarily utilized as nano-fertilizers and nano-pesticides, effectively providing essential nutrients and crop protection [37]. ZnS and $TiO_2$ NPs exhibit catalytic qualities, making them suitable for use in various industrial processes, including the synthesis of chemicals and environmental cleanup. Due to their semiconducting qualities and capacity to transform light energy into electricity, $TiO_2$ NPs have been researched for their potential use in solar cells and other photovoltaic applications. The $TiO_2$ NPs synthesized from *Jatropha curcas* have reportedly been employed in wastewater treatment applications. The studies have shown the photocatalytic photodegradation of tannery wastewater using $TiO_2$ NPs. $TiO_2$ NPs aid in the photocatalytic processes that produce reactive oxygen compounds (ROS), which are essential for boosting the antibacterial capacity and bringing about modifications that make the contaminated water's surface more hydrophilic [82].

Due to their distinctive characteristics and possible benefits in terms of sustainability, NPs produced from plants have shown promise in various industrial applications. They are used in various fields, including wastewater management, agriculture, textiles, cosmetics, food, drink, and bioremediation. The biomedical sector hopes for green synthesized NPs due to their excellent stability, non-toxic chemical makeup, and biocompatibility. If they possess antimicrobial or antibacterial properties, they can be utilized as efficient substitutes for antibiotics and as means of delivering drugs to improve drug solubility and increase the efficacy of targeted medication therapy. The non-toxic, plant-derived NPs can be used in additional biomedical applications, including diagnostics and bioimaging, without compromising the biological specimen. Although plant-derived NPs may have advantages, their successful implementation in various fields requires careful study, testing, and optimization to guarantee their stability, effectiveness, and safety for particular applications. Prior to introducing nanoparticles (NPs) into manufacturing procedures or consumer goods, regulatory concerns and environmental impact evaluations must be taken into account. Additional novel applications might surface as plant-based NPs research continues, boosting environmentally friendly and sustainable industrial techniques.

## 7 Challenges and Toxicities Associated with NPs from Jatropha Latex

One of the key challenges associated with Jatropha latex NPs is the variability of their composition and properties. The next section provides a detailed explanation of the difficulties encountered in the biosynthesis of NPs. Although potentially are other problems, the biggest ones for Jatropha latex NPs are related to the variability in the composition and characteristics of the latex extracted from the plant. The primary challenges faced during the process of biosynthesis of the Nanoparticles are covered in this section. The first issue is variability and composition. The latex's composition depends on several variables, including the plant's genetic diversity, location, climate, and methods of cultivation. The variability can result in variations in the amounts and makeup of the proteins and enzymes that make up the latex's bioactive compounds. This impacts and reduces latex's ability to reduce and stabilize the synthesis of NPs. The uneven makeup of Jatropha latex can make it difficult to produce a repeatable and standardized synthesis of NPs. The variation in latex composition causes changes in the formed NPs' size, shape, surface properties, and stability, another parameter affecting their characteristics. The affinities of the various bioactive substances and proteins for metal ions vary, which can affect the kinetics of NPs formation. These modifications impact the physicochemical characteristics of Jatropha latex NPs, making it challenging to regulate and optimize the latex's unique properties and applications [92].

The reproducibility and scalability are also affected by the variability in Jatropha latex. The composition and reproduction of the synthesis of NPs with consistent properties can be challenging. Careful optimization and standardization of synthetic protocols may be required to achieve batch-to-batch or inter-laboratory reproducibility. Furthermore, the need to maintain a consistent latex composition and ensure the quality and performance of NPs on a larger scale can make it difficult to scale up the synthesis of Jatropha latex NPs for industrial applications. A wide range of characterization techniques, including spectroscopy, microscopy, and other analytical methods, are essential to assess NPs size distribution, morphology, surface chemistry, and stability. The strict quality control measures must be implemented to ensure the consistency and reliability of jatropha latex NPs manufactured for commercial use. A systematic approach is required to address the challenge of variability in jatropha latex NPs. Moreover, the researchers should conduct intensive characterization studies to understand the effects of various components of Jatropha latex on NPs synthesis and properties. Efforts should be made to optimize synthetic protocols, establish standardized procedures, and implement quality control measures to improve reproducibility and consistency. In addition, exploring strategies to modify or manipulate the composition of jatropha latex or selectively extract specific components could help reduce variability and improve control over NPs synthesis [59].

As the various applications and advantages of the NPs are discussed in this chapter, it is of utmost importance to discuss the toxicities associated with these NPs; the following section talks about various toxicities associated with these NPs. The toxicity of NPs is a critical aspect to assess when considering their applications [56]. While Jatropha latex-based NPs have shown promise in various fields, including medicine and catalysis, their potential toxic effects should be thoroughly investigated. NPs can interact with biological systems and potentially induce adverse effects at the cellular and organismal levels. The cytotoxicity and biocompatibility of the NPs synthesized by the Jatropha latex involve the toxicity of these NPs on the living cells, i.e., lung fibroblast cells [50]. The study provides information on the dose-dependent cytotoxic effect of the NPs on cell viability, indicating the need for careful biocompatibility evaluation. The Jatropha latex NPs can pose potential environmental risks when released into ecosystems. Their effects on aquatic organisms, soil microbes, and plants should be evaluated. Recently, the phytotoxicity of the jatropha latex and zinc oxide nanoparticles on tomato seed growth and germination was investigated by Fakruddin et al. They discovered that high NP levels hampered the growth and germination of seeds, suggesting potential environmental effects. The NPs stability and aggregation ensure the stability of Jatropha latex NPs is very important for successful application. Surface modification or encapsulation should be investigated. In another study, Panda et al. studied the stability of jatropha latex AgNPs and observed aggregation of NPs over time, highlighting the importance of increased stability for optimal performance. The standardization and reproducibility are major challenges in NP biosynthesis using Jatropha latex. Natural materials may vary due to geographic location, seasonal changes, and plant growing conditions. Achieving a consistent and reproducible synthetic protocol is critical to reliably produce jatropha latex NPs with consistent properties. The lack of comprehensive toxicity studies has limited the uses and applications of NPs from the Jatropha latex [10].

Further investigation is needed to understand long- and short-term toxic effects such as systemic toxicity, immunotoxicity, and organ-specific toxicity. For safe use, assessing the potential for genotoxicity and oxidative stress is also important. It is important to conduct a thorough toxicity and environmental risk assessment and comprehend in vivo and in vitro studies. In addition, the standardization of synthetic protocols and extensive characterization of jatropha latex NPs contribute to reliable and safe manufacturing. Researchers should conduct intensive characterization studies to understand the effects of various components of the *Jatropha* latex on NPs synthesis and properties. Efforts should be made to optimize synthetic protocols, establish standardized procedures, and implement quality control measures to improve reproducibility and consistency. In addition, exploring strategies to modify or manipulate the composition of jatropha latex or selectively extract specific components could help reduce variability and improve control over NP synthesis [91].

# 8 Recent Advancements and Future Perspectives

Alternative antimicrobial agents are now required due to the emergence of pathogens that are resistant to antibiotics (Seil and Webster 2012). Due to their special qualities, such as a greater smaller size and surface area which enable effective interaction with microbial cells, bio-fabricated NPs have demonstrated promise. Several studies have documented the antibacterial properties of various NP types. There are several mechanisms involved in how NPs fight bacteria. For instance, the antibacterial properties of AgNPs have been the subject of research extensively. They can damage bacterial cell membranes and cellular machinery, resulting in cell death [79]. Additionally, it has been discovered that the usage of AgNPs in conjunction with conventional antibiotics has a synergistic effect. Several studies have shown that the antibacterial effectiveness was increased when antibiotics like ciprofloxacin, nitrofurantoin, and carbenicillin were combined with AgNPs [8]. NPs of other types have also demonstrated antibacterial activities against various pathogens. *Candida albicans* and *Staphylococcus aureus* have been successfully eradicated from bacteria by AuNPs [49]. Bacteria which is Gram-positive, i.e., *Bacillus subtilis*, *Aspergillus niger*, and Gram-negative bacteria *Klebsiella planticola* were all significantly inhibited by $TiO_2$ NPs made from Planomicrobium sp [48]. According to studies, zinc oxide NPs (ZnONPs) have antibacterial properties that combat *Salmonella typhimurium*, *Proteus mirabilis*, *Pseudomonas alcaligenes*, and other disease-causing bacteria [33, 52, 63]. The green synthesized NPs possess more surface area, allowing for more interactions with microbial cell membranes and disrupting DNA replication and metabolic pathways. The NPs which are smaller in size make it easier for them to enter microbial cells. Additionally, studies have shown that using NPs in addition to conventional antibiotics has improved antibacterial efficacy.

In the food industry, the utilization of NPs is widely accepted for different applications, including food processing and packaging [20, 76]. It is interesting to use zinc oxide NPs (ZnO NPs) in polymeric materials for packaging. Packaging materials with ZnONPs have better antibacterial qualities, according to research [20]. These nanocomposite materials for food packaging can make food safer by preventing bacteria from growing. According to studies, ZnONPs can be used to create containers and lids for food packaging [61, 67]. This can help keep food fresh and prevent contamination. Another type of NP that can pass through bacterial biofilms is AgNPs, which have special characteristics. AgNPs are stress-resistant due to this property, which makes them suitable for cleaning and decontamination procedures in food packaging [31]. Nano-fertilizers of the materials which are carbon-based have been investigated for their potential to improve crop productivity, plant growth, and nutrient uptake [86]. They reduce the need for chemical inputs by acting as effective, environmentally friendly fertilizers [11]. Zeolites, nano clay minerals, and nano clay crystals have also demonstrated potential as nano-fertilizers, offered controlled nutrient release mechanisms, and enhanced soil health [18].

In order to promote sustainable agricultural practices, coating potash fertilizers with nanomaterials has also been shown to be successful in reducing nutrient loss and minimizing the overuse of chemical fertilizers [29, 80]. Additionally, NPs can be used to create nano-pesticides, offering fresh methods for pest management in agriculture. Nanoparticles (NPs) can be found in nano-pesticides as metal oxides (inorganic components) in the shape of tiny particles or particles, or as nano polymers (organic constituents). The insecticidal and pesticidal characteristics of metallic nanoparticles (NPs) made of zinc oxide, silver, oxide of aluminum, and $TiO_2$ have demonstrated promise against a range of pests and insects that significantly lower agricultural production [41]. For instance, new nanoemulsion formulations have been created as pesticide carriers, improving their effectiveness and lowering overall usage [65]. NPs can potentially lessen the environmental impact of pesticides while increasing their efficacy. However, significant obstacles to commercializing NPs as pesticides remain, including figuring out the ideal dosage and dealing with potential plant toxicity. For the removal of persistent and xenobiotic water pollutants, which present significant difficulties for wastewater treatment and water quality management, NPs in bioremediation offer potential solutions. NPs can function as adsorbents or catalysts for pollutants due to their larger surface area and smaller size, which increases the efficiency of the pollutants' removal [91]. For example, silver and gold nanoparticles are good catalysts for the breakdown and discoloration of organic dyes. Their biological makeup and catalytic qualities enable them to efficiently eliminate harmful contaminants from the surroundings [75]. Moreover, nanoparticles (NPs) with characteristics that are advantageous for soil bioremediation include iron, titanium dioxide ($TiO_2$), magnetic, bimetallic, the nanoclays, nanosponges, and nanotubes. These resources offer novel approaches to the management of soil and water contamination [42].

## 9 Conclusions

The utilization of nanomaterials is experiencing rapid growth in various fields. A promising avenue for their production involves the biosynthesis of NPs derived from Jatropha latex. Proteins, enzymes, and phytochemicals are among the bioactive constituents in jatropha latex, which possess the potential for NPs synthesis. The utilization of this green synthesis technique obviates the need for deleterious chemicals and energy-intensive procedures, thereby facilitating a more environmentally friendly and sustainable methodology. Potential future directions for the biosynthesis of Jatropha latex NPs involve optimizing the synthesis procedure, enhancing production efficiency, exploring novel applications, surface functionalization, and assessing the environmental implications. The utilization of NPs derived from jatropha latex holds immense potential for advancement and application in multiple domains such as medicine, energy, catalysis, and environmental restoration. These initiatives have made a path for further increment and investigation of jatropha latex NPs in diverse fields. To overcome the challenges and drawbacks related to the biosynthesis of NPs from *Jatropha* latex, more research is required. Understanding the potential toxicity and long-term stability of these NPs, along with their scalability, standardization of synthesis protocols, and characterization techniques, is crucial. The biosynthesis of NPs using Jatropha latex holds significant potential for advancing eco-friendly nanomaterials and exploring novel application domains. Future research and development efforts in this stage should offer considerable benefits in terms of the advancement of environmentally friendly methods for synthesis and the full investigation of the naturally occurring compounds obtained from *jatropha* latex.

## References


1. Abdelgadir HA, Van Staden J (2013) Ethnobotany, ethnopharmacology and toxicity of Jatropha curcas L. (Euphorbiaceae): A review. S Afr J Bot 88:204–218
2. Adelere IA, Lateef A (2016) A novel approach to the green synthesis of metallic nanoparticles: the use of agro-wastes, enzymes, and pigments. Nanotechnol Rev 5:567–587. https://doi.org/10.1515/ntrev-2016-0024
3. Akhtar S, Ali S (2020) Characterization of nanomaterials: Techniques and tools BT—applications of nanomaterials in human health. In: Khan FA (ed). Springer Singapore, Singapore, pp 23–43
4. Anandalakshmi K, Venugobal J, Ramasamy V (2016) Characterization of silver nanoparticles by green synthesis method using Pedalium murex leaf extract and their antibacterial activity. Appl Nanosci 6:399–408
5. Aslam M, Abdullah AZ, Rafatullah M (2021) Recent development in the green synthesis of titanium dioxide nanoparticles using plant-based biomolecules for environmental and antimicrobial applications. J Ind Eng Chem 98:1–16
6. Bala JM, Vennila JJ, Ganesh S, Sachidanand Singh SS (2011) Analysis of active components in Acanthus ilicifolius leaves for their potential chemoprotective activity against hepatocellular carcinoma: an in silico approach
7. Baniaga BAN, Mendoza DVM (2022) Green synthesis of zinc sulfide nanoparticles using jatropha curcas linn. for photocatalytic degradation of methylene blue. Orient J Chem 38:375
8. Banu A, Rathod V, Ranganath E (2011) Silver nanoparticle production by Rhizopus stolonifer and its antibacterial activity against extended spectrum β-lactamase producing (ESBL) strains of Enterobacteriaceae. Mater Res Bull 46:1417–1423. https://doi.org/10.1016/j.materresbull.2011.05.008
9. Bar H, Bhui DK, Sahoo GP, Sarkar P, De SP, Misra A (2009) Green synthesis of silver nanoparticles using latex of Jatropha curcas. Colloids Surf A Physicochem Eng Asp 339:134–139
10. Barabadi H, Damavandi Kamali K, Jazayeri Shoushtari F, Tajani B, Mahjoub MA, Alizadeh A, Saravanan M (2019) Emerging theranostic silver and gold nanomaterials to combat prostate cancer: A systematic review. J Clust Sci 30:1375–1382. https://doi.org/10.1007/s10876-019-01588-7

11. Bisinoti MC, Moreira AB, Melo CA, Fregolente LG, Bento LR, Vitor dos Santos J, Ferreira OP (2019) Chapter 8—Application of carbon-based nanomaterials as fertilizers in soils. In: do Nascimento RF, Ferreira OP, De Paula AJ, de Oliveira Sousa Neto V (eds) Nanomaterials applications for environmental matrices. Elsevier, pp 305–333
12. Bm O, Adepoju EA, Zainab AA, Ahmed AA (2014) Phytochemical profiling of phytoconstituents of grape, Jatropha curcas and Neem (Azadirachta indica) extracts. J Pharmacogn 6:17–23
13. Cavalcante NB, da Conceição Santos AD, da Silva Almeida JRG (2020) The genus Jatropha (Euphorbiaceae): A review on secondary chemical metabolites and biological aspects. Chem Biol Interact 318:108976
14. Chauhan N, Tyagi AK, Kumar P, Malik A (2016) Antibacterial potential of Jatropha curcas synthesized silver nanoparticles against food borne pathogens. Front Microbiol 7:1748
15. Chouhan PN, Azimov A, Jabborova D, Singh S (2023) Review on the role of indigenous plants and plant derivatives of Ayurveda in bone healing. Plant Science Today 10(sp2):143–151
16. Debnath M, Bisen PS (2008) Jatropha curcas L., a multipurpose stress resistant plant with a potential for ethnomedicine and renewable energy. Curr Pharm Biotechnol 9:288–306
17. Devappa RK, Makkar HPS, Becker K (2011) Jatropha diterpenes: a review. J Am Oil Chem Soc 88:301–322
18. Duhan JS, Kumar R, Kumar N, Kaur P, Nehra K, Duhan S (2017) Nanotechnology: The new perspective in precision agriculture. Biotechnol Rep 15:11–23. https://doi.org/10.1016/j.btre.2017.03.002
19. Elechiguerra JL, Burt JL, Morones JR, Camacho-Bragado A, Gao X, Lara HH, Yacaman MJ (2005) Interaction of silver nanoparticles with HIV-1. J Nanobiotechnology 3:1–10
20. Espitia PJP, Soares N de FF, Coimbra dos JSR, de Andrade NJ, Cruz RS, Medeiros EAA (2012) Zinc oxide nanoparticles: Synthesis, antimicrobial activity and food packaging applications. Food Bioproc Tech 5:1447–1464. https://doi.org/10.1007/s11947-012-0797-6
21. Faria-Machado AF, Licurgo FMS, Pires JMF, da Silveira CR, Wilhelm AE, Maria de Lourdes M, Antoniassi R (2019) Method validation for analysis of phorbol esters from Jatropha curcas. Ind Crops Prod 140:111627
22. Gangwar P, Johri P, Datta R, Singh S, Trivedi M (2023) Overview on 1 phytopharmaceuticals and biotechnology of herbal plants. In: Phytopharmaceuticals and biotechnology of herbal plants. CRC Press, pp 1–17
23. Ghosh MK, Sahu S, Gupta I, Ghorai TK (2020) Green synthesis of copper nanoparticles from an extract of Jatropha curcas leaves: Characterization, optical properties, CT-DNA binding and photocatalytic activity. RSC Adv 10:22027–22035
24. Giri AK, Jena B, Biswal B, Pradhan AK, Arakha M, Acharya S, Acharya L (2022) Green synthesis and characterization of silver nanoparticles using Eugenia roxburghii DC. extract and activity against biofilm-producing bacteria. Sci Rep 12:8383. https://doi.org/10.1038/s41598-022-12484-y
25. Gorai S (2019) A review on biogenic synthesis of ZnS nanoparticles and potential applications. J Indian Chem Soc 97:2972–2980
26. Gour A, Jain NK (2019) Advances in green synthesis of nanoparticles. Artif Cells Nanomed Biotechnol 47:844–851. https://doi.org/10.1080/21691401.2019.1577878
27. Goutam SP, Saxena G, Singh V, Yadav AK, Bharagava RN, Thapa KB (2018) Green synthesis of $TiO_2$ nanoparticles using leaf extract of Jatropha curcas L. for photocatalytic degradation of tannery wastewater. Chem Eng J 336:386–396
28. Gowda BHJ, Mohanto S, Singh A, Bhunia A, Abdelgawad MA, Ghosh S, Ansari MJ, Pramanik S (2023) Nanoparticle-based therapeutic approaches for wound healing: A review of the state-of-the-art. Mater Today Chem 27:101319. https://doi.org/10.1016/j.mtchem.2022.101319
29. Guo H, White JC, Wang Z, Xing B (2018) Nano-enabled fertilizers to control the release and use efficiency of nutrients. Curr Opin Environ Sci Health 6:77–83. https://doi.org/10.1016/j.coesh.2018.07.009
30. Gupta G, Paul S, Singh S, Pietramellara G, Pathan SI, Danish S, Jha PN (2022) Exploring functional diversity and community structure of diazotrophic endophytic bacteria associated with Pennisetum glaucum growing under field in a semi-arid region. Land 11(7):991

31. Huang J, Lin L, Sun D, Chen H, Yang D, Li Q (2015) Bio-inspired synthesis of metal nanomaterials and applications. Chem Soc Rev 44:6330–6374. https://doi.org/10.1039/C5CS00133A
32. Hudlikar M, Joglekar S, Dhaygude M, Kodam K (2012) Latex-mediated synthesis of ZnS nanoparticles: green synthesis approach. J Nanopart Res 14:1–6
33. Ibrahim NA, Nada AA, Hassabo AG, Eid BM, Noor El-Deen AM, Abou-Zeid NY (2017) Effect of different capping agents on physicochemical and antimicrobial properties of ZnO nanoparticles. Chem Pap 71:1365–1375. https://doi.org/10.1007/s11696-017-0132-9
34. Jabborova D, Davranov K, Jabbarov Z, Bhowmik SN, Ercisli S, Danish S, Datta R (2022) Dual inoculation of plant growth-promoting Bacillus endophyticus and Funneliformis mosseae improves plant growth and soil properties in ginger. ACS Omega 7(39):34779–34788
35. Jassal PS, Kaur D, Prasad R, Singh J (2022) Green synthesis of titanium dioxide nanoparticles: Development and applications. J Agric Food Res:100361
36. Joglekar S, Kodam K, Dhaygude M, Hudlikar M (2011) Novel route for rapid biosynthesis of lead nanoparticles using aqueous extract of Jatropha curcas L. latex. Mater Lett 65:3170–3172
37. Khalil HPSA, Aprilia NAS, Bhat AH, Jawaid M, Paridah MT, Rudi D (2013) A Jatropha biomass as renewable materials for biocomposites and its applications. Renew Sustain Energy Rev 22:667–685
38. Khare P, Kishore K, Sharma DK (2017) A study on the standardization parameters of Cassia angustifolia. Asian J Pharm Clin Res 10(7):329–332
39. Khare P, Kishore K, Sharma DK, Khare N (2024) Investigation of memory enhancing activity of combination extracts of bauhinia variegata and madhuca longifolia leaves against colchicine: an experimental study and biochemical alterations in mice. Ind J Pharm Edu Res 58(1s):s282–s288
40. Khare P, Kishore K, Sharma DK (2018) Medicinal uses, Phytochemistry and Pharmacological profile of Madhuca longifolia. Asian J Pharm Pharmacol 4(5):570–581
41. Koul B, Poonia AK, Yadav D, Jin JO (2021) Microbe-mediated biosynthesis of nanoparticles: Applications and future prospects. Biomolecules 11. https://doi.org/10.3390/biom11060886
42. Koul B, Taak P (2018) In situ soil remediation strategies bt—biotechnological strategies for effective remediation of polluted soils. In: Taak P (ed) Koul B. Springer Singapore, Singapore, pp 59–75
43. Kumar A, Dixit CK (2017) Methods for characterization of nanoparticles. In: Advances in nanomedicine for the delivery of therapeutic nucleic acids. Elsevier, pp 43–58
44. Kumar S, Bhattacharya W, Singh M, Halder D, Mitra A (2017) Plant latex capped colloidal silver nanoparticles: A potent anti-biofilm and fungicidal formulation. J Mol Liq 230:705–713
45. Kumawat TK, Kumawat V, Sharma V, Pandit A, Sharma B, Nag S, Kumari N, Biyani M (2023) Chapter 1—Overview and summary of antimicrobial wound dressings and its biomedical applications. In: Khan R, Gowri S (eds) Antimicrobial Dressings. Academic Press, pp 1–20
46. Maddala VKS, Singh S (2023) Essential oils from plants and their role in nanomaterial synthesis characterization and applications. In: Secondary metabolites based green synthesis of nanomaterials and their applications. Springer Nature Singapore, Singapore, pp 191–207
47. Maddala VKS, Singh S, Bandi J (2024) Soil properties influencing nutrient signaling in plant soil systems. In: Essential minerals in plant-soil systems. Elsevier, pp 373–393
48. Malarkodi C, Rajeshkumar S, Paulkumar K, Vanaja M, Gnanajobitha G, Annadurai G (2014) Biosynthesis and antimicrobial activity of semiconductor nanoparticles against oral pathogens. Bioinorg Chem Appl 2014:347167. https://doi.org/10.1155/2014/347167
49. Manivasagan P, Alam MS, Kang K-H, Kwak M, Kim S-K (2015) Extracellular synthesis of gold bionanoparticles by Nocardiopsis sp. and evaluation of its antimicrobial, antioxidant and cytotoxic activities. Bioprocess Biosyst Eng 38:1167–1177. https://doi.org/10.1007/s00449-015-1358-y
50. Matinise N, Mayedwa N, Ikpo CO, Hlongwa NW, Ndipingwi MM, Molefe L, Dywili N, Yonkeu ALD, Waryo T, Baker PGL, Iwuoha EI (2016) Bimetallic nanocomposites of palladium (100) and ruthenium for electrooxidation of ammonia. J Nano Res 44:100–113. https://doi.org/10.4028/www.scientific.net/JNanoR.44.100

51. Meddya S, Meshram S, Sarkar D, Datta R, Singh S, Avinash G, Thulasinathan T (2023) Plant stomata: An unrealized possibility in plant defense against invading pathogens and stress tolerance. Plants 12(19):3380
52. Mohammadi FM, Ghasemi N (2018) Influence of temperature and concentration on biosynthesis and characterization of zinc oxide nanoparticles using cherry extract. J Nanostructure Chem 8:93–102. https://doi.org/10.1007/s40097-018-0257-6
53. Mohammed AE, Al-Keridis LA, Rahman I, Alotaibi MO, Suliman RS, Alrajhi AM, Elobeid MM, Alothman MR, Alhomaidi EA, Korany SM (2021) Silver nanoparticles formation by Jatropha integerrima and LC/MS-QTOF-based metabolite profiling. Nanomaterials 11:2400
54. Moulton MC, Braydich-Stolle LK, Nadagouda MN, Kunzelman S, Hussain SM, Varma RS (2010) Synthesis{,} characterization and biocompatibility of "green" synthesized silver nanoparticles using tea polyphenols. Nanoscale 2:763–770. https://doi.org/10.1039/C0NR00046A
55. Nag S, Mitra OPS, Bhattacharjee A, Mohanto S, Gowda BHJ, Kar S, Ramaiah S, Anbarasu A, Ahmed MG (2024a) Exploring the emerging trends in the synthesis and theranostic paradigms of cerium oxide nanoparticles (CeONPs): A comprehensive review. Mater Today Chem 35:101894. https://doi.org/10.1016/j.mtchem.2023.101894
56. Nag S, Mitra O, Tripathi G, Adur I, Mohanto S, Nama M, Samanta S, Gowda BHJ, Subramaniyan V, Sundararajan V, Kumarasamy V (2024) Nanomaterials-assisted photothermal therapy for breast cancer: State-of-the-art advances and future perspectives. Photodiagnosis Photodyn Ther 45:103959. https://doi.org/10.1016/J.PDPDT.2023.103959
57. Parveen R, Khare N, Singh S, Johri P (2023). An in silico outlook for the detection and surveillance of evolving and persistent plant pathogens. In: Detection, diagnosis and management of soil-borne phytopathogens. Springer Nature Singapore, Singapore, pp 17–40
58. Patani A, Patel A, Prajapati D, Khare N, Singh S (2023) Various agriculture crop plant-based bioactive compounds and their use in nanomaterial synthesis and applications. In: Nanomaterials from agricultural and horticultural products. Springer Nature Singapore, Singapore, pp 223–241
59. Patil SV, Borase HP, Patil CD, Salunke BK (2012) Biosynthesis of silver nanoparticles using latex from few euphorbian plants and their antimicrobial potential. Appl Biochem Biotechnol 167:776–790. https://doi.org/10.1007/s12010-012-9710-z
60. Pramanik S, Mohanto S, Manne R, Rajendran RR, Deepak A, Edapully SJ, Patil T, Katari O (2021) Nanoparticle-based drug delivery system: the magic bullet for the treatment of chronic pulmonary diseases. Mol Pharm 18:3671–3718. https://doi.org/10.1021/acs.molpharmaceut.1c00491
61. Prasad R, Kumar V, Prasad KS (2014) Nanotechnology in sustainable agriculture: Present concerns and future aspects. Afr J Biotechnol 13:705–713
62. Rafique M, Sadaf I, Rafique MS, Tahir MB (2017) A review on green synthesis of silver nanoparticles and their applications. Artif Cells Nanomed Biotechnol 45:1272–1291. https://doi.org/10.1080/21691401.2016.1241792
63. Raghupathi KR, Koodali RT, Manna AC (2011) Size-dependent bacterial growth inhibition and mechanism of antibacterial activity of zinc oxide nanoparticles. Langmuir 27:4020–4028. https://doi.org/10.1021/la104825u
64. Rahu MI, Naqvi SHA, Memon NH, Idrees M, Kandhro F, Pathan NL, Sarker MNI, Bhutto MA (2021) Determination of antimicrobial and phytochemical compounds of Jatropha curcas plant. Saudi J Biol Sci 28:2867–2876
65. Rai M, Ingle A (2012) Role of nanotechnology in agriculture with special reference to management of insect pests. Appl Microbiol Biotechnol 94:287–293. https://doi.org/10.1007/s00253-012-3969-4
66. Rai S, Kafle A, Devkota HP, Bhattarai A (2023) Characterization of saponins from the leaves and stem bark of Jatropha curcas L. for surface-active properties. Heliyon 9
67. Rajamanickam U, Viswanathan S, Muthusamy P (2012) Biosynthesis of zinc nanoparticles using actinomycetes for antibacterial food packaging

68. Rampadarath S, Puchooa D, Jeewon R (2016) Jatropha curcas L: Phytochemical, antimicrobial and larvicidal properties. Asian Pac J Trop Biomed 6:858–865
69. Sabandar CW, Ahmat N, Jaafar FM, Sahidin I (2013) Medicinal property, phytochemistry and pharmacology of several Jatropha species (Euphorbiaceae): A review. Phytochemistry 85:7–29
70. Santiago M, Rivera D, Torres A (2023) Green synthesis of titanium oxide nanoparticles using natural extracts. J Mater Sci Chem Eng 11:29–40
71. Sao P, Chand Y, Kumar A, Singh S (2021) Potential drug target identification in porphyromonas gingivalis using in-silico subtractive metabolic pathway analysis. Bangladesh J Med Sci 20(4):887–896
72. Sao P, Parveen R, Khattri A, Sharma S, Tiwari N, Singh S (2022) Understanding the metabolomics of medicinal plants under environmental pollution: Challenges and opportunities. Environ Pollut Med Plants:193–205
73. Shankar S, Rhim J-W (2015) Amino acid mediated synthesis of silver nanoparticles and preparation of antimicrobial agar/silver nanoparticles composite films. Carbohydr Polym 130:353–363. https://doi.org/10.1016/j.carbpol.2015.05.018
74. Sharma AK, Gangwar M, Kumar D, Nath G, Sinha AŚK, Tripathi YB (2016) Phytochemical characterization, antimicrobial activity and reducing potential of seed oil, latex, machine oil and presscake of Jatropha curcas. Avicenna J Phytomed 6:366
75. Sharma K, Singh G, Singh G, Kumar M, Bhalla V (2015) Silver nanoparticles: facile synthesis and their catalytic application for the degradation of dyes. RSC Adv 5:25781–25788. https://doi.org/10.1039/C5RA02909K
76. Shukla K (2014) Nanotechnology and emerging trends in dairy foods: The inside story to food additives and ingredients
77. Singh A, Sengar RS, Singh AK, Singh S, Kumar A, Ahmad K (2019) Impact of genetic engineering on agriculture food crops. Biotech Today: Int J Biol Sci 9(1):17–24
78. Singh S, Datta R, Johri P, Trivedi M (eds) (2022) Phytopharmaceuticals and biotechnology of herbal plants. CRC Press.
79. Sondi I, Salopek-Sondi B (2004) Silver nanoparticles as antimicrobial agent: a case study on E. coli as a model for Gram-negative bacteria. J Colloid Interface Sci 275:177–182. https://doi.org/10.1016/j.jcis.2004.02.012
80. Subbarao ChV, Kartheek GVK, Sirisha D (2013) Slow release of potash fertilizer through polymer coating. Int J Appl Sci Eng 11:25–30
81. Subhapriya S, Gomathipriya P (2018) Green synthesis of titanium dioxide (TiO(2)) nanoparticles by Trigonella foenum-graecum extract and its antimicrobial properties. Microb Pathog 116:215–220. https://doi.org/10.1016/j.micpath.2018.01.027
82. Sunny NE, Mathew SS, Chandel N, Saravanan P, Rajeshkannan R, Rajasimman M, Vasseghian Y, Rajamohan N, Kumar SV (2022) Green synthesis of titanium dioxide nanoparticles using plant biomass and their applications-A review. Chemosphere 300:134612
83. Suriyakala G, Sathiyaraj S, Devanesan S, AlSalhi MS, Rajasekar A, Maruthamuthu MK, Babujanarthanam R (2022) Phytosynthesis of silver nanoparticles from Jatropha integerrima Jacq. flower extract and their possible applications as antibacterial and antioxidant agent. Saudi J Biol Sci 29:680–688. https://doi.org/10.1016/j.sjbs.2021.12.007
84. Thomas R, Sah NK, Sharma PB (2008) Therapeutic biology of Jatropha curcas: a mini review. Curr Pharm Biotechnol 9:315–324
85. Varma RS (2012) Greener approach to nanomaterials and their sustainable applications. Curr Opin Chem Eng 1:123–128. https://doi.org/10.1016/j.coche.2011.12.002
86. Verma N, Sao P, Srivastava A, Singh S (2021) Physiological and molecular responses to drought, submergence and excessive watering in plants. Harsh Environ Plant Resil: Mol Funct Asp:305–321
87. Vishwakarma SK, Ilyas T, Shahid M, Malviya D, Kumar S, Singh S, Singh HV (2024) Bacillus spp.: Nature's gift to agriculture and humankind. In: Applications of bacillus and bacillus derived genera in agriculture, biotechnology and beyond. Springer Nature Singapore, Singapore, pp 1–36

88. Vora Z, Pandya J, Vaikuntapu PR, Singh S, Asha S, Purama RK (2023) Genome-wide association of defense hormone crosstalk in plants. In: Hormonal cross-talk, plant defense and development. Academic Press, pp 353–371
89. Zaragoza-Martínez F, Lucho-Constantino GG, Ponce-Noyola T, Esparza-García F, Poggi-Varaldo H, Cerda-García-Rojas CM, Trejo-Tapia G, Ramos-Valdivia AC (2016) Jasmonic acid stimulates the oxidative responses and triterpene production in Jatropha curcas cell suspension cultures through mevalonate as biosynthetic precursor. Plant Cell, Tissue Organ Cult (PCTOC) 127:47–56
90. Zhang P, Zhang W, Zhang H (2021) A triboelectric nanogenerator based on waste polyvinyl chloride for Morse code generator. Sens Actuators A Phys 322:112633
91. Zhao J, Wu T, Wu K, Oikawa K, Hidaka H, Serpone N (1998) Photoassisted degradation of dye pollutants. 3. Degradation of the cationic dye rhodamine B in aqueous anionic surfactant/ $TiO_2$ dispersions under visible light irradiation: evidence for the need of substrate adsorption on $TiO_2$ particles. Environ Sci Technol 32:2394–2400. https://doi.org/10.1021/es9707926
92. Zhou X, Cao Q, Orfila C, Zhao J, Zhang L (2021) Systematic Review and Meta-Analysis on the Effects of Astaxanthin on Human Skin Ageing. Nutrients 13. https://doi.org/10.3390/NU13092917

88. Vora Z, Pandya J, Valkantapa PB, Singh S, Avelo S, Purohit RK (2023) Genome-wide association of defense hormone crosstalk in plants. In: Hormonal crosstalk, plant defense and development. Academic Press, pp 353–371
89. Zaragoza-Martínez F, Lucho-Constantino GG, Ponce-Noyola T, Esparza-García F, Poggi-Varaldo H, Cerda-García-Rojas CM, Trejo-Tapia G, Ramos-Valdivia AC (2016) Jasmonic acid stimulates the oxidative responses and triterpene production in *Jatropha curcas* cell suspension cultures through mevalonate as biosynthetic precursor. Plant Cell Tissue Organ Cult (PCTOC) 127:47–56
90. Zhang R, Zhang W, Zhang H (2021) A triboelectric nanogenerator based on waste polyvinyl chloride for Morse code generator. Sens Actuators A Phys 332:112633
91. Zhao J, Wu T, Wu K, Oikawa K, Hidaka H, Serpone N (1998) Photoassisted degradation of dye pollutants. 3. Degradation of the cationic dye rhodamine B in aqueous anionic surfactant/$TiO_2$ dispersions under visible light irradiation: evidence for the need of substrate adsorption on $TiO_2$ particles. Environ Sci Technol 32:2394–2400. https://doi.org/10.1021/es9707926
92. Zhou X, Cao Q, Orfila C, Zhao J, Zhang L (2021) Systematic Review and Meta-Analysis on the Effects of Astaxanthin on Human Skin Ageing. Nutrients 13. https://doi.org/10.3390/nu13092917

# Nutrient Management

# Nanomaterials for Soil Carbon Sequestration: Implications in Agroforestry

**Toushif P. K., Savitha Santosh, Balraju Wagmare, Rakesh S., Jadeyegowda Madegowda, Amarendra Nath Dey, and Dinesha S.**

**Abstract** Agroforestry (AF) is a popular farming technique and a perfect scientific approach that can help to manage resources sustainably and reduce greenhouse gas (GHG) emissions. Using an agroforestry system (AFS) greatly increases Soil organic carbon (SOC), and in many cases, it also enhances farm diversity, microclimate, and many other factors. This happens as a result of adding suitable, deeply rooted multipurpose perennial crops to an AFS that efficiently cycles and pumps nutrients, restocking the soil. By using multidisciplinary research in AF, nanotechnology can improve crop, animal, and tree productivity in a sustainable manner. Additionally, it can help with crop post-harvest management, precise virus diagnosis, targeted pesticide delivery, and disease identification. The soil carbon (C) sequestration, tree-based nanomaterial biosynthesis, SOC, and numerous other ecological processes can also be aided by this nanotechnology-assisted AF. The production of green

Toushif P. K.
Department of Forestry, Mizoram University, Aizawl 796004, Mizoram, India

S. Santosh
Central Research Institute for Dryland Agriculture, Santosh Nagar, Hyderabad 500059, Telangana, India

B. Wagmare
Govindh Ballabh Pant National Institute of Himalayan Environment and Sustainable Development, Pangthang, Sikkim 737101, India

Rakesh S.
International Crops Research Institute for Semi-Arid Tropics, Patancheru 502324, Telangana, India

J. Madegowda
College of Forestry, KSN UAHS, Ponnampet, Shivamogga 571216, Karnataka, India

A. N. Dey
Department of Forestry, Uttar Banga Krishi Viswavidyalaya, Pundibari, Cooch Behar 736165, West Bengal, India

Dinesha S. (✉)
Department of Forestry, North-Eastern Hill University, Tura Campus, Tura 796002, Meghalaya, India
e-mail: dinesha@nehu.ac.in

 
D. Jabborova et al. (eds.), *Nanomaterials in Agroforestry Systems*, Smart Nanomaterials Technology, https://doi.org/10.1007/978-981-96-1337-3_6

nanoparticles (NPs) namely iron (Fe) NPs, silver (Ag) NPs, and gold (Au) NPs from AF tree species such as *Albizia adianthifolia, Emblica officianalis, Moringa oleifera, Tamarindus indica,* and *Terminalia chebula* is becoming more significant. This can help with accessibility, dependability, safety, and sustainability issues that nanotechnology is currently facing. Through case studies, this chapter explores the benefits, challenges, and potential uses of nanotechnology in soil C sequestration in AF and other Land use systems (LUS). In addition to its notable effects on crop yield and soil characteristics, more studies can clear up doubts regarding NM's ability to tackle problems that modern-day AF faces, including problems with accuracy, volatility, phytotoxicity, and bioaccumulation.

**Keywords** Agroforestry · Green nanoparticles · Carbon sequestration · Agrobiodiversity · Food security

## 1 Introduction

Climate change has been an important threat to global food production which is adversely affecting agricultural productivity. Monocropping systems have heavily exploited natural resources in several countries through the green revolution [62]. However, since the late 1990s, these systems have begun to lose hope due to stagnant yields, deteriorating soil, water quality, and environmental degradation brought on by non-judicious management of agrochemicals, pesticides, and introduction of exotics, hybrids, and genetically modified (GM) crops [18]. Agriculture is the key source of the global anthropogenic emissions of methane and nitrous oxide (52 and 84%, respectively) [60]. This hastened level of greenhouse gases (GHGs) in the atmosphere is a reason for concern. Among these GHGs, carbon dioxide ($CO_2$) is a key contributor and its increasing concentration in the atmosphere is one of the significant global concerns [30, 60]. Carbon capture and storage emerged as one of the most effective substitute techniques for lowering the atmospheric concentration of $CO_2$ when compared to other technologies [44, 45]. Therefore, to solve these significant concerns appropriate technologies and strategies for managing carbon and its sequestration in soil and other ways are required.

The application of nanotechnology to sequester carbon in soil has attracted more interest recently. It has been reported that the use of nanotechnology, which manipulates matter and creates new materials at the nanoscale, can improve carbon stability and potential soil sequestration [6, 50]. These NMs are produced using either natural or engineered methods and have unique electrical, magnetic, kinetic, and optical properties, which in turn yield unique functionalities [37]. At this nanoscale, gravity would become less important, whereas surface tension and Vander Waal forces would become more important [16]. In addition to its wider application in the fields of electronics, medicine, civil engineering, energy, and health, nanotechnology is also gaining more importance in agriculture and related industries through the use of nanopesticides, nano-fertilizers, nano-phytoremediation, nanocomposite materials,

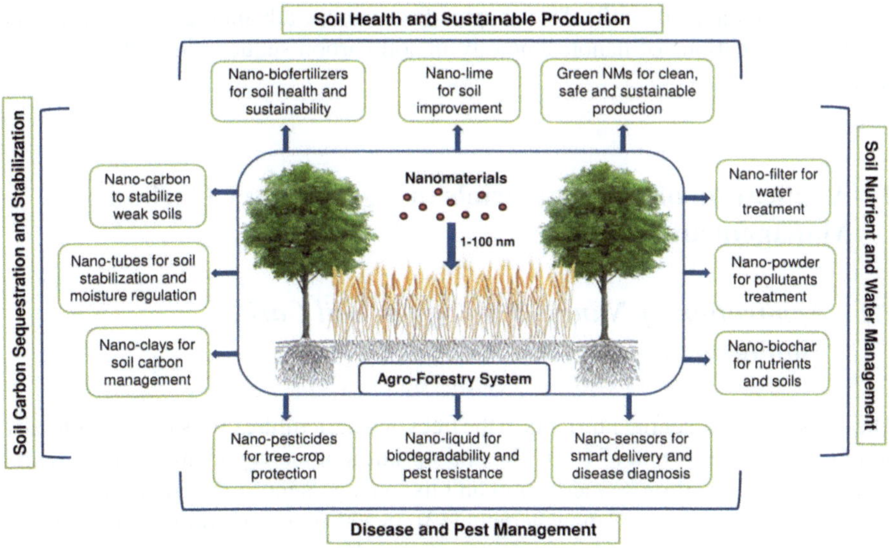


**Fig. 1** Role of nanomaterials in agroforestry soil management

nanosensors, and other products [39]. Its application in agriculture started a few years back while in agroforestry it has been recognized in recent years [38]. Its application is considered as a smart solution for many agroforestry problems (Fig. 1).

Agroforestry (AF) is a trending cultivation practice and an ideal scientific strategy that can potentially mitigate greenhouse gas (GHG) emissions and is helpful in sustainable resource management [10]. The adoption of an agroforestry system (AFS) results in a significant improvement of SOC, increased availability of macro and micronutrients along with ameliorated microenvironment in many instances. Extensive studies have been conducted on the inclusion of suitable deep-rooted perennial crops that provide nutrient enrichment through efficient nutrient cycling and nutrient pumping [19]. Soil carbon sequestration can be enhanced by the application of certain recommended management strategies, such as integrated nutrient management, diversified cropping systems, conservation agriculture, and agroforestry [11]. Nanotechnology can enhance crop, animal, and tree productivity sustainably by applying multidisciplinary research in agroforestry (AF) and other tree-based land use systems (LUS). This technology will be more helpful in developing climate-resilient agroforestry practices for efficient food production and desirable quality timber production. Furthermore, several studies have documented the production of natural and eco-friendly nanoparticles (NPs) namely iron (Fe) NPs, silver (Ag) NPs, and gold (Au) NPs from the AF tree species such as *Albizia adianthifolia, Emblica officianalis, Moringa oleifera, Tamarindus indica,* and *Terminalia chebula* [2, 9]. The nanotechnology-assisted AF can facilitate soil C sequestration, tree-based nanomaterial biosynthesis, and many other ecological functions (Fig. 1). It can also aid in disease identification, accurate virus diagnosis, targeted pesticide delivery, and crop post-harvest management [2]. This chapter discusses the advantages, challenges, and possible applications of nanotechnology in soil carbon sequestration through case studies.

# 2 Application of Nanomaterials in Agroforestry Carbon Management

## *2.1 Application of Nanotechnology in Soil Carbon Management*

The soil supplies essential nutrients to the trees and agriculture crops in AF fields, also acting as a source or sink of $CO_2$. The appropriate soil management practices with a special focus on carbon sequestration and its management in different pools play a pivotal role in ecosystem C management [53]. In addition to adopting certain recommended soil C management strategies, earlier studies have suggested that improved technology and multidisciplinary research in agroforestry are essential for increasing soil carbon [11, 38, 64]. In this view, nanotechnology has more potential in improving soil carbon pools along with the improvement of soil health and the environment. Many studies reported the role of NMs in improving C sequestration in soil [38]. Sequestration of C in soil is governed by various locality factors [55]. In soil, the soil structure and aggregates play a significant part in C storage [5]. Earlier studies have reported the significant effects of NMs such as nano-zeolite, nano-ZnO, and nano-Fe on improving soil structure with respect to mechanical soil properties, and C build-up [47].

NMs are special in terms of their electrical, kinetic, magnetic, and optical properties [37]. Due to their high surface-to-volume ratios and most significant adsorbent activity in the soil, NMs are gaining more importance in soil C Sequestration, regulating nutrients, controlling organic matter (OM) fixation, and stimulating new mineral precipitation [34, 37]. NMs are capable of aggregating and interacting with organic colloids, including humic materials, peptidoglycan, dissolved organic material, and polysaccharides [34]. NMs play a key role in plants by regulating oxygen, nutrient and water transportation, light absorption, improved seed germination, enhanced photosynthetic and respiratory activities, chromosomal and enzymes activities, improved tolerance, enhanced N fixation, and C sequestration (Table 1). This leads to a significant improvement in plant biomass and nutritional status, which raises agricultural productivity [23, 61] which further leads to SOC sequestration and build-up [22].

The amount of fertilizer and pesticide usage can be regulated with the use of nanopesticides and nano-fertilizers [21, 57]. The nano-enhanced products with nano-based smart delivery systems, nano-barcodes, and nano-processing provide nutrients at the specific locations, rate, and time to improve output and solve production-related challenges [22]. Earlier studies reported silicate nanosensors application in pollution

**Table 1** Nanomaterials for improving agroforestry soils

| Nanomaterials | Types | Effects on soil properties | References |
|---|---|---|---|
| Nano-fertilizers | Nano-silica, Nano-zeolite | Enhanced soil microbes and soil physical properties | [17] |
| | NPs of CuO, $Fe_3O_4$, and MgO | Improved soil nitrification, dehydrogenase activity, bulk density, and total biomass carbon | [57] |
| | Nano-ZnO | Application of 0.5 g $kg^{-1}$ significantly increased soil microorganisms | [14] |
| | Nano-$TiO_2$ | Improves soil properties and health | [3] |
| Nano pesticides | NPs encapsulated pesticides | Applied for controlled release, better efficiency, and disease pest management | [21] |
| Nano-lime and nano-dolomite | Nano-CaO and Nano-$CaCO_3$ | Enhanced soil health and the proliferation of soil microorganisms | [15, 49] |
| Nanoclay | nZVInano clays | Improved physical characteristics of the soil that helps in retention of water and liquid agrochemicals | [33, 35] |
| Nano carbon | Carbon nanotube (CNT) and nanofiber | Multiwalled CNTs at 750 μg/mL enhanced the soil moisture and microbial biomass | [1, 8, 26] |
| Nanosensors | Silicate nanosensors | Used in pollution study and plant growth assessment | [24, 25] |
| Nano sheets | Graphene oxide | Improved mechanical properties of the soil | [41] |
| Green NMs | Plant-based NMs | Production of nanocarbon from coconut shell and nanofibers from cotton and wheat residue | [24] |
| | Agroforestry tree-based NMs | Hazardous NMs can be replaced by Iron, silver, and gold NPs, produced from *Moringa oleifera*, and *Emblica officianalis* | [2, 9] |

removal along with the plant growth assessment [24, 25]. Studies reported the positive effects of NMs such as nano clays and hydrous Fe oxides on soil C stabilization [13]. Increasing the chemical recalcitrance of SOC, facilitating organo-mineral interaction, and protecting SOC from microbes and microbial decomposition can all enhance the sequestration of organic C content in soil [4].

## 2.2 *Application of NMs in Microbial Biomass Carbon Management*

The application of NMs on soil microorganisms plays a crucial role in promoting plant growth and nutrient cycling in soils. Studies reported mixed opinions related to NM applications; some researchers reported no harmful effect [14, 46], while others expressed serious concerns related to its toxicity on microorganisms [48, 52]. NMs can influence soil microorganisms through direct toxicity, alterations in toxins, nutrient availability, interactions with natural organic compounds, and many more. NMs are reported to influence significantly soil microbial communities, especially in terms of higher microbial biomass carbon (MBC) content in soil which increases its capacity to sequester carbon in different pools [14, 17]. The zinc nanoparticles have been reported to improve microbial populations in the rhizosphere of *Cyamopsis tetragonoloba* plants [46]. Another study reported increased soil enzyme activities in the rhizosphere between 18 and 283% by the application of Nano-Zn and Nano-Fe [59]. In contrast, some reports indicated that certain NMs can inhibit the growth of plant growth-promoting rhizobacteria (PGPR) such as Pseudomonas and Bacillus spp, as well as nitrifying and denitrifying bacteria [36, 48]. Therefore, further research and scientific approaches are required for the design and development of nanotechnology-based green products and processes that are biodegradable, environmentally friendly, and sustainable [51].

## 2.3 *Biosynthesis of Green NMs and Their Application in Sustainable C Management*

Green nanotechnology is also a promising approach in the design and development of nanotechnology-based products and processes that are biodegradable, environmentally friendly, and sustainable [2, 40]. By incorporating sustainable principles this emerging technology helps in solving global challenges in a responsible and sustainable manner. Most of the green NMs-based approaches are yet to be experimented with at a large scale, and their reproducibility will be a challenging task. Instead of using hazardous metals and toxic chemicals in the synthesis of NM production, green nanotechnology can be used [9, 32]. Globally, many researchers are attempting to create a more reliable and green synthesis of NMs, and numerous studies have documented the use of plant extracts in the creation of biosynthesized NMs [2, 40]. Agroforestry tree species such as *Albizia adianthifolia, Emblica officinalis, Moringa oleifera, Tamarindus indica,* and *Terminalia chebula* yield iron, silver, and gold nanoparticles [2, 9]. These tree species greatly increase SOC in addition to producing green NMs. They also improve the microclimate and farm diversity and support a range of ecological functions [2]. Earlier studies reported that applying biochar significantly increased the amount of C that was retained in soil for a longer time compared to organic waste. This is due to its higher stable structure and long-term stability as compared to organic waste [12]. In this context, nano-biochar, a more advanced form of biochar, can improve soil fertility and sequester C while also absorbing nutrients [27, 43].

## 3 Case Studies

NMs have many potential applications in agroforestry and other LUS crop productivity and soil health [20, 31, 54]. According to a study by [54] iron oxide NPs enhanced the overall growth of AF tree, *Eucalyptus tereticornis*, under extreme salinity stress. A physiological investigation revealed a considerable rise in shoot length and chlorophyll content, while a molecular study revealed that iron oxide NPs up-regulate stress-related genes and improve nutrient availability under stress conditions, suggesting potential applications for NMs in agroforestry interventions [54]. By raising the enzymatic activities, iron oxide NPs functioned as nano-supplements for growth promotion even in non-stressed settings [54]. In tree-based diversified LUS, nano-based products may play a significant role in many ways. Examples of these products include nano filters for waste treatment, nanofluids for optimizing soil health and insect resistance, nano powders for pollutants treatment, and nanotubes for plant and microbial biomass [2, 40].

In a study, Chinnamuthu et al. [7] successfully encapsulated herbicide in a $MnO_2$ core shell shielded with bilayer polymers that open up and exude the active ingredient on receipt of rainfall. Furthermore, this nano herbicide would replace expensive and labor-intensive hand picking and tilling. Nano-fertilizers such as Nano chitosan, Nano-$SiO_2$, Iron Oxide NMs, etc. have significantly improved the growth and yield of many field crops [20, 31]. The study reported that the application of Nano chitosan NPK fertilizer has improved wheat plant growth and yield significantly in sandy soils. Results showed a significant increase in harvest index, crop index, and mobilization index of nano-fertilized wheat plants, as compared with control [56].

Earlier studies reported the reinforcing effect of nano-silica when applied to sandy and clayey soil [17, 24, 25]. Results showed that incorporating nano-silica improved the mechanical properties of both sandy and clayey soil without disrupting the soil's initial chemical environment [33, 58]. Earlier studies reported the successful application of carbon nanotubes in soil stabilization [8, 25]. Another study uses carbon nanotubes as an example of a nano-membrane material to increase $CO_2$ adsorption capability [66]. These smart nanotube materials are also playing an increasingly essential role in the application of smart delivery of nutrients and water under constraints of irrigation or drought conditions. This could consequently enhance contaminant security, storage capacity, and trapping methods [66]. In addition, NPs of $SiO_2$ and $TiO_2$ are shown to be more effective at modifying wettability and lowering interfacial tension in $CO_2$ sequestration.

## 4 Challenges and Ecological Concerns

Some of the challenges and safety concerns of NMs include their entry into the food chain, their long-term effects on human health, unforeseen environmental consequences, high initial costs, the lack of widespread accessibility and affordability of these emerging technologies, and the lack of scientific knowledge on the long-term impacts, interactions with diverse ecosystems, and potential unforeseen challenges [42]. The unregulated production, use, and disposal of NMs-based products may raise serious environmental concerns. Many countries are currently profiting from nanosensors by using this advanced technology in plantations and vineyards to produce superior quality commercial crops [63, 65]. Nevertheless, the study in Aotearoa of New Zealand highlighted the potential risks of other nanotechnological development and adoption in vineyards [52]. Furthermore, the advantageous properties such as nano-size, larger surface area, and reactivity may turn negative and could damage plants and animal health. Hence, it is essential to consider proper approaches to produce NMs with less or no inhibitory impacts on living things.

The impact of metal-based NMs on the functional diversity of soil microorganisms in agricultural systems has threatened the sustainability of the environment and the diversity of beneficial microbial populations [48]. The population of beneficial bacteria and fungi in the soil is negatively impacted by the continuous deposition, low biodegradability, and extended persistence of metal NMs in soils. Some studies reported the toxicity of NMs that affect the microorganisms and inhibit the enzyme's activities in the soil environment and many studies working on this to reduce and prevent the toxicity of NMs on the soil organisms [48, 52]. However, further research and experiment is required on these aspects.

## 5 Policy Framework

The Government of India views nanotechnology as an important area in boosting agricultural productivity at the national level [29]. The National Centre of Excellence for Advanced Research in Agricultural Nanotechnology was established to carry out end-to-end research and harness the benefits of NM-based technologies. Although the use of nanotechnology in agriculture and related fields has grown, there are more concerns over the potential risks to the environment and human health. Luckily, these concerns are monitored and regulated around the world by regulatory bodies through their proper strategies and rules for ensuring the safety and quality of NMs [28]. Many countries have their own regulatory framework for assessing the harmful effects of the NMs used, the possibility of environmental release, and the effect on human health. The International Organization for Standardization (ISO has produced a number of international standards, these have been further improved and applied by the Ministry of Environment, Forests and Climate Change (MoEFCC), the Food

Safety and Standards Authority of India (FSSAI), and the Indian Council of Agricultural Research (ICAR) in India. Some of the important national-level laws and regulations related to Nanotechnology are the Environment Protection Act (EPA-1986), the Food Safety and Standards Act (FSSA-2006), Storage and Import of Hazardous Chemicals Rules-1989, FSSAI Regulations on Food Additives-2011, and ICAR Guidelines on Nanotechnology Research in Agriculture-2010. Furthermore, this evolving technology needs more policy support and regulatory structures to guarantee greater safety and utility.

## 6 Scientific Research and Future Prospects

Nanotechnology has given rise to new opportunities for scientific intervention and strategy creation, enabling us to address a number of issues. The scarcity of studies is a further hint for the additional research on the application of NMs to soil aggregation and SOC sequestration for the long term. The nanofluid technology also holds immense potential in creating NMs with even more precise delivery mechanisms and enhanced biodegradability. Globally further research on novel nanofluid products is going on with broader implications from soil health optimization to pest resistance. Understanding and recognizing potential NMs for improving carbon storage by way of enhanced soil aggregation is further needed. More research is needed to standardize the optimal quantity of NMs application and economic evaluation of natural and manufactured NMs for large-scale application by avoiding any harmful effect on ecosystems.

## 7 Conclusion

Through case studies, this study explored the benefits, challenges, and potential uses of nanotechnology in soil C sequestration in AF. The soil C storage of various tree-based LUS will play a key role in reducing atmospheric $CO_2$ concentrations and mitigating climate change as we strive toward net zero GHG emissions. Tree-based NM biosynthesis, soil carbon sequestration, and numerous other ecological processes can all be facilitated by greening nanotechnology through AF intervention. Numerous issues with accessibility, dependability, safety, and sustainability that nanotechnology is currently facing can be resolved by this AF-assisted green nanotechnology. Improved nanotechnology-based strategies may also remove doubts about NM's ability to address issues that the modern AF faces and have a major impact on sustainability and climate change concerns. When combined, green NM-based technologies and better AF practices could address present problems and enhance crop productivity and soil quality. However, further research is needed to clear up any doubts about phytotoxicity, bioaccumulation, accuracy, and unpredictable outcomes.

## References


1. Alsharef JMA, Taha MR, Firoozi AK, Govindasamy P (2016) Potential of using nanocarbons to stabilize weak soils. Appl Environ Soil Sci 2016:1–9
2. Anand K, Kaviyarasu K, Muniyasamy S, Roopan SM, Gengan RM, Chuturgoon AA (2017) Bio-synthesis of silver nanoparticles using agroforestry residue and their catalytic degradation for sustainable waste management. J Cluster Scien 28:2279–2291
3. Babu S, Joseph S (2016) Effect of Nano materials on properties of soft soil. Inter J Sci Res 5:634–637
4. Barré P, Fernandez-Ugalde O, Virto I, Velde B, Chenu C (2014) Impact of phyllosilicate mineralogy on organic carbon stabilization in soils: incomplete knowledge and exciting prospects. Geoderma 235:382–395
5. Bhattacharyya R, Tuti MD, Kundu S, Bisht JK, Bhatt JC (2012) Conservation tillage impacts on soil aggregation and carbon pools in a sandy clay loam soil of the Indian Himalayas. Soil Sci Soc Am J 76:617–627
6. Calabi-Floody M, Bendall JS, Jara AA, Welland ME, Theng BKG, Rumpel C, Mora ML (2011) Nanoclays from an Andisol: extraction, properties and carbon stabilization. Geoderma 161:159–167
7. Chinnamuthu CR (2010) Nanotechnology in the next generation. In: Invited lecture delivered at the National Seminar on Role of Nanotechnology in The Development of Herbal Medicine-An Update, held during 10-11 February 2010 at the Periyar College of Pharmaceutical Sciences for Girls, Tiruchirappalli, India
8. Correia AAS, Casaleiroa PDF, Rasteiro MGBV (2015) Applying multiwall carbon nanotubes for soil stabilization. Procedia Eng 102:1766–1775
9. Devatha CP, Thalla AK, Katte SY (2016) Green synthesis of iron nanoparticles using different leaf extracts for treatment of domestic wastewater. J Clean Prod 139:1425–1435
10. Dinesha S, Hosur SR, Toushif PK, Bodiga D, Deepthi Dechamma NL, Ashwath MN, Pradhan D (2023) Sustaino-resilient agroforestry for climate resilience, food security and land degradation neutrality. Land Environ Manag For:217–245
11. Dinesha S, Raj A, Bhanusree MR, Balraju W, Rakesh S, Raj WG, Jha RK, Neeraj KK (2022) Agroforestry assisted natural farming in India: Challenges and implications for diversification and restoration of agroecosystem. Int J Environ Clim Chang 12:1053–1069
12. Elbasiouny H, Elbehiry F, El-Ramady H, Hasanuzzaman M (2021) Contradictory results of soil greenhouse gas emissions as affected by biochar application: Special focus on alkaline soils. Int J Environ Res 15:903–920
13. Filimonova S, Kaufhold S, Wagner FE, Häusler W, Kögel-Knabner I (2016) The role of allophane nano-structure and Fe oxide speciation for hosting soil organic matter in an allophanic Andosol. Geoch Cosmochim Acta 180:284–302
14. Ge Y, Priester JH, Van De Werfhorst LC, Walker SL, Nisbet RM, An YJ, Holden PA (2014) Soybean plants modify metal oxide nanoparticle effects on soil bacterial communities. Environ Scien Technol 48:13489–13496
15. Govindasamy P, Taha MR, Alsharef J, Ramalingam K (2017) Influence of nanolime and curing period on unconfined compressive strength of soil. Appl Environ Soil Sci 1017:1–9
16. Gupta G, Paul S, Singh S, Pietramellara G, Pathan SI, Danish S, Jha PN (2022) Exploring functional diversity and community structure of diazotrophic endophytic bacteria associated with Pennisetum glaucum growing under field in a semi-arid region. Land 11(7):991
17. Hareesh P, Vinothkumar R (2016) Assessment of nano materials on Geotechnical properties of clayey soils. In: Proceeding international conference on engineering innovations and solutions held at CMS College of Engineering, Tamil Nadu, India
18. Hazell PB (2010) An assessment of the impact of agricultural research in South Asia since the green revolution. Handb Agric Econ 4:3469–3530
19. Jabborova D, Davranov K, Jabbarov Z, Bhowmik SN, Ercisli S, Danish S, Datta R (2022) Dual inoculation of plant growth-promoting Bacillus endophyticus and Funneliformis mosseae improves plant growth and soil properties in ginger. ACS Omega 7(39):34779–34788

20. Jain R, Bohra N, Singh RK, Upadhyay SK, Srivastava AK, Rajput VD (2022) Nanomaterials for plants: From ecophysiology to signaling mechanisms and nutrient uptake. In: The role of nanoparticles in plant nutrition under soil pollution: Nanoscience in nutrient use efficiency, Springer, pp 183–197
21. Jerobin J, Sureshkumar RS, Anjali CH, Mukherjee A, Chandrasekaran N (2012) Biodegradable polymer based encapsulation of neem oil nanoemulsion for controlled release of Aza-A. Carbohyd Polym 90:1750–1756
22. Jinus SS, Meinam T, Melanglen K, Potsangbam M, Devi AR, Nongthombam L, Bhaigyabati T, Shephrou HD, Tilotama K, Thokchom DS (2021) The climate smart agriculture for carbon capture and carbon sequestration: The challenges and opportunities. Advances in Carbon Capture and Utilization. Springer, Singapore, pp 195–233
23. Kalia A, Kaur H (2019) Nano-biofertilizers: Harnessing dual benefits of nano-nutrient and bio-fertilizers for enhanced nutrient use efficiency and sustainable productivity. In: Pudake RN et al (eds) Nanoscience for sustainable agriculture. Springer Nature Switzerland AG, pp 51–73
24. Kalpana-Sastry R, Rashmi HB, Rao NH, Ilyas SM (2009) Nanotechnology and agriculture in India: the second green revolution. OECD conference on Potential environmental benefits of nanotechnology: fostering safe innovation-led growth 7:15–17
25. Kaur N, Thakur H, Prabhakar N (2016) Conducting polymer and multi-walled carbon nanotubes nanocomposites based amperometric biosensor for detection of organophosphate. J Electroanalyt Chem 775:121–128
26. Keita K, Okafor F, Nyochembeng L, Overton A, Sripathi VR, Odutola J (2018) Plant and microbial growth responses to multi-walled carbon nanotubes. J Nanosci Curr Res 3:2572–2813
27. Khan HA, Naqvi SR, Mehran MT, Khoja AH, Niazi MBK, Juchelková D, Atabani A (2021) A performance evaluation study of nano-biochar as a potential slowrelease nano-fertilizer from wheat straw residue for sustainable agriculture. Chemosphere 285:131382
28. Khare P, Kishore K, Sharma DK, Khare N (2024) Investigation of memory enhancing activity of combination extracts of bauhinia variegata and madhuca longifolia leaves against colchicine: An experimental study and biochemical alterations in mice. Ind J Pharm Edu Res 58(1s):s282–s288
29. Khare P, Kishore K, Sharma DK (2018) Medicinal uses, Phytochemistry and Pharmacological profile of Madhuca longifolia. Asian J Pharm Pharmacol 4(5):570–581
30. Lal R (2009) Challenges and opportunities in soil organic matter research. Euro J Soil Sci. 60:158–169
31. Lohani S, Khati P, Sharma A, Maura J (2023) 5 concepts of nano-based agriculture. Advances in nanotechnology for smart agriculture: Techniques and Applications, p 91
32. Maddala VKS, Singh S (2023) Essential oils from plants and their role in nanomaterial synthesis characterization and applications. In: Secondary metabolites based green synthesis of nanomaterials and their applications. Springer Nature Singapore, Singapore, pp 191–207
33. Majeed ZM, Taha MR, Jawad IT (2014) Stabilization of soft soil using nanomaterials. Res J Appl Sci Eng Technol 8(4):503–509
34. Mani PK, Mondal S (2016) Agrinanotechniques for plant availability of nutrients. In: Kole et al (eds) Plant nanotechnology. Springer, Cham, pp 263–303
35. McMurray TA, Dunlop PSM, Byrne JA (2006) The photocatalytic degradation of atrazine on nanoparticulate $TiO_2$ films. J Photochem Photobiol Chem 182:43–51
36. Mishra VK, Kumar A (2009) Impact of metal nanoparticles on plant growth promoting rhizobacteria. Dig J Nanomater Biostruct 4:587–592
37. Monreal CM, Sultan Y, Schnitzer M (2010) Soil organic matter in nano-scale structures of a cultivated black Chernozem. Geoderma 159:237–242
38. Mukhopadhyay SS (2014) Nanotechnology in agriculture prospects and constraints. Nanotechnol Sci Appl 7:63–71
39. NAAS (2013) Nanotechnology in agriculture: scope and current relevance. Policy paper no. 63, National Academy of Agricultural Sciences, New Delhi, India
40. Nasaruddin RR, Chen T, Yao Q, Zang S, Xie J (2021) Toward greener synthesis of gold nanomaterials: From biological to biomimetic synthesis. Coord Chem Rev 426:213540

41. Naseri F, Irani M, Dehkhodarajabi M (2016) Effect of graphene oxide nanosheets on the geotechnical properties of cemented silty soil. Arch Civil Mech Eng 16:695–701
42. Parveen R, Khare N, Singh S, Johri P (2023) An in silico outlook for the detection and surveillance of evolving and persistent plant pathogens. In: Detection, diagnosis and management of soil-borne Phytopathogens. Springer Nature Singapore, Singapore, pp 17–40
43. Patani A, Patel A, Prajapati D, Khare N, Singh S (2023) Various agriculture crop plant-based bioactive compounds and their use in nanomaterial synthesis and applications. In: Nanomaterials from agricultural and horticultural products. Springer Nature Singapore, Singapore, pp 223–241
44. Rakesh S, Sinha AK, Juttu R, Sarkar D, Jogula K, Reddy SB, Raju B, Danish S, Datta R (2022) Does the accretion of carbon fractions and their stratification vary widely with soil orders? A case study of an Alfisol and an Entisol of sub-tropical eastern India. Land Degrad Dev 33:2039–2049
45. Rakesh S, Sinha AK, Sarkar D, Roy D, Bodiga D, Sahoo S, Jha PK, Dubey PK, Rakshit A (2023) Active and passive carbon fractions in contrasting cropping systems, tillage practices, and soil types. Land 12(2):365. https://doi.org/10.3390/land12020365
46. Raliya R, Tarafdar JC (2013) ZnO nanoparticle biosynthesis and its effect on phosphorus mobilizing enzyme secretion and gum contents in Clusterbean (Cyamopsis tetragonoloba L.). Agric Res 2:48–57
47. Raliya R, Tarafdar JC, Mahawar H, Kumar R, Gupta P, Mathur T, Kaul RK, Kumar P, Kaliya A, Gautam R, Singh SK, Gehlot HS (2014) ZnO nanoparticles induced exopolysaccharide production by B. subtilis strain JCT1 for arid soil application. Inter J Biol Macromol 65:362–368
48. Rastogi S, Sharma G, Kandasubramanian B (2020) Nanomaterials and the environment. The ELSI handbook of nanotechnology: Risk, safety, ELSI and commercialization, pp 1–23
49. Reddy CH, Subramanian KS (2017) Impact of Nano-liming materials on biological properties of acid soils. Int J CurrMicrobiol App Sci 6:451–457
50. Sao P, Chand Y, Kumar A, Singh S (2021) Potential drug target identification in porphyromonas gingivalis using in-silico subtractive metabolic pathway analysis. Bangladesh J Med Sci 20(4):887–896
51. Sao P, Vats S, Singh S (2022) Porphyromonas gingivalis resistance and virulence: An integrated functional network analysis. Gene 839:146734
52. Siimes N, Sharp EL, Lewis N, Kah M (2022) Determining acceptance and rejection of nano-enabled agriculture: A case study of the New Zealand wine industry. Nano Impact 28:100432
53. Singh A, Sengar RS, Singh AK, Singh S, Kumar A, Ahmad K (2019) Impact of genetic engineering on agriculture food crops. Biotech Today: Int J Biol Sci 9(1):17–24
54. Singh D, Sillu D, Kumar A, Agnihotri S (2021) Dual nanozyme characteristics of iron oxide nanoparticles alleviate salinity stress and promote the growth of an agroforestry tree, Eucalyptus tereticornis Sm. Environmental Scien Nano 8:1308–1325
55. Singh M, Sarkar B, Sarkar S, Churchman J, Bolan N, Mandal S, Menon M, Purakayastha TJ, Beerling DJ (2017) Stabilization of soil organic carbon as influenced by clay mineralogy. Adv Agron 148:33–84
56. Singh S, Datta R, Johri P, Trivedi M (eds) (2022) Phytopharmaceuticals and biotechnology of herbal plants. CRC Press
57. Srinivasan R, Maity A, Singh KK, Ghosh PK, Kumar S, Srivastava MK, Kumari B (2017) Influence of copper oxide and zinc oxide nano-particles on growth of fodder cowpea and soil microbiological properties. Range Manag Agrofor 38:208–214
58. Taha MR, Taha OME (2012) Influence of nano-material on the expansive and shrinkage soil behavior. J Nanopart Res 14:1190–1202
59. Tarafdar J, Rathore I, Kaur R, Jain A (2018) Biosynthesis of nanonutrients for agricultural applications. In: Singh B, Katare OP, Souto EB (eds) Emerging trend in nanobiomedicine, nanoagroceuticals and nanophytochemicals. CRC Press, pp 15–30
60. Tian H, Xu R, Canadell JG, Thompson RL, Winiwarter W, Suntharalingam P, Yao Y (2020) A comprehensive quantification of global nitrous oxide sources and sinks. Nature 586:248–256

61. Tungare K, Shahu R, Zambare V, Agarwal P, Jobby R, Nisar N, Jha P (2022) Toxicity mitigation of textile dye reactive blue 4 by hairy roots of Helianthus annuus and testing its effect in in vivo model systems. Biomed Res Int
62. Verma N, Sao P, Srivastava A, Singh S (2021) Physiological and molecular responses to drought, submergence and excessive watering in plants. Harsh Environ Plant Resil: Mol Funct Asp, 305–321
63. Vora Z, Pandya J, Vaikuntapu PR, Singh S, Asha S, Purama RK (2023) Genome-wide association of defense hormone crosstalk in plants. In: Hormonal cross-talk, plant defense and development. Academic Press, pp 353–371
64. Wang D, Behura S, Karim F, Kazi A, Wangila G, Wang S (2021) Nanoscience and nanotechnology for food and agroforestry. ES Food Agrofor 3:1–3
65. Yeshe AS, Vaidya PH, Shinde GU, Gourkhede PH (2022) Application of wireless nano sensors network and nanotechnology in precision agriculture. Int J Adv Agric Scie Tech 9:36–65
66. Youns YT, Manshad AK, Ali JA (2023) Sustainable aspects behind the application of nanotechnology in $CO_2$ sequestration. Fuel 349:128680

# The Effect of Nanoparticles on Nitrogen Fixation by Trees

**Vandana Sahu, Ashwani Kumar Patel, and Faheem Ahmad**

**Abstract** Nitrogen fixation is a vital biological process that plays a crucial role in the nitrogen cycle, contributing to the availability of this essential nutrient for plant growth. The application of nanoparticles in the context of nitrogen fixation by trees has increased major attention owing to their unique physicochemical properties. Nanoparticles (NPs) can penetrate plant tissues and interact with cellular components, influencing key processes involved in nitrogen fixation as nodulation and nitrogenase activity. NPs also act as a carrier for essential nutrients or signaling molecules, promoting nitrogen uptake. Nanoparticle size, concentration, surface charge, and chemical composition can influence their efficacy and potential toxicity. The response of trees to nanoparticles exposure depends on plant species, growth stage, and environmental conditions. Therefore, complete knowledge of the nanoparticles-tree interactions is necessary to optimize their application and minimize potential risks. This chapter provides an overview of the present state of research on the effect of nanoparticles on nitrogen fixation by trees.

**Keywords** Nanoparticles · Plant · Interaction · Nitrogen fixation · Physiological activities

## 1 Introduction

Understanding the connections between plants and their surroundings is essential for tackling climate change and pursuing sustainable environmental practices. Trees are essential to the sequestration of carbon and the cycling of nutrients in terrestrial

---

V. Sahu · A. K. Patel
Department of Mycology and Plant Pathology, Institute of Agricultural Sciences, Banaras Hindu University, Varanasi, Uttar Pradesh, India

F. Ahmad (✉)
Department of Botany, Aligarh Muslim University, Aligarh, India
e-mail: faheem.bt@amu.ac.in

 
D. Jabborova et al. (eds.), *Nanomaterials in Agroforestry Systems*, Smart Nanomaterials Technology, https://doi.org/10.1007/978-981-96-1337-3_7

ecosystems. One important nutrient activity that greatly affects ecosystem productivity is nitrogen fixation. Nitrogen is indispensable for essential biological components like amino acids, proteins, DNA, RNA, chlorophyll, and key cellular molecules [32].

In agriculture, nitrogen serves as a fundamental element for plant development and subsequently influences animal growth and protein production. Maintaining optimal nitrogen levels is crucial for sustaining crop yields, as reduced nitrogen availability leads to decreased productivity. Both traditional and modern agricultural practices are dedicated to ensuring an adequate nitrogen supply for sustained crop production, reflecting the critical role nitrogen plays in agricultural output [22]. Similar to photosynthesis, symbiotic nitrogen fixation is a crucial life mechanism in agroforestry that replenishes nitrogen that is biologically accessible. In agroforestry, the focus is frequently on increasing the ability of rhizobial bacteria to use the energy from tree symbionts to supply nitrogen to related crops. During symbiotic $N_2$-fixation, solar energy from photosynthesis is used to dissolve atmospheric $N_2$ triple bonds. Under tree cover, increasing soil nitrogen is facilitated by the formation of root nodules, which are created by rhizobial bacteria entering $N_2$-fixing legume roots. The processes include root uptake, symbiotic $N_2$-fixation, possible animal-provided nitrogen, and other unknown processes [5] and [9]. Nitrogen fixation cycles in agroforestry begin with a rise in nitrogen availability brought about by symbiotic $N_2$-fixation. Because $N_2$-fixing trees provide nitrogen that benefits annual crops like rubber, annual herbaceous legume cover plants are used to fix nitrogen and improve tree fertilization. Increased yields are the result of this symbiosis, which encourages rubber tree root growth. Ecosystems and agricultural ecosystems have quite different needs for nitrogen [25]. The factors that affect the nitrogen fixation are given in Table 1.

While nanotechnology offers novel avenues for research, its potential impacts on tree-mediated nitrogen fixation remain understudied. Nanoparticles, with unique features, present environmental issues. On the other hand, recent developments in nanotechnology have created new avenues for research into the potential interactions or effects of nanoparticles on nitrogen fixation processes mediated by trees. Polar routes such as stomata, hydathodes, necrotic patches, and trichrome are used by nanoparticles to penetrate plant leaves [4]. As nitrogen fixation enhancers in agricultural and environmental applications, nanoparticles have demonstrated encouraging potential. Because of their special qualities, nanoparticles are a good option to enhance the processes that plants and soil use to fix nitrogen (Table 2).

Integrating trees, particularly nitrogen-fixing trees (NFTs), into agroforestry and silvopastoral systems holds significant potential for enhancing sustainable agriculture. This approach helps safeguard and rejuvenate soil fertility, counteract erosion and desertification, and supply fuel wood. Noteworthy advantages of NFTs encompass their capacity for biological nitrogen fixation (BNF), adaptability to thrive in low-nitrogen soil conditions, and the capability to transfer fixed nitrogen, along with additional organic matter, to neighboring or subsequent crops. [12]. One of the most effective ways to maintain the productivity of agrosystems through the improvement of the soil nitrogen balance, especially in the tropics, is the planting of trees that

**Table 1** Factors that affect the nitrogen fixation

| Factors | Impact on nitrogen fixation |
|---|---|
| Soil nitrogen availability | High nitrogen content reduces reliance on nitrogen fixation. Low nitrogen content increases dependence on nitrogen fixation |
| Soil acidity and pH | Suboptimal pH levels hinder nitrogen-fixing microorganism activity |
| Climate and temperature | Extreme temperatures (hot or cold) decrease nitrogen fixation efficiency |
| Water availability | Drought conditions limit nitrogen-fixing microorganism activity |
| Heavy metal and toxin exposure | Pollution and toxins disrupt nitrogen-fixing microorganism symbiotic relationships |
| Deforestation and land-use changes | Reduction in nitrogen-fixing species leads to decreased fixation rates |
| Air pollution | Pollutants indirectly affect nitrogen fixation by altering atmospheric conditions |
| Loss of biodiversity | Decrease in nitrogen-fixing species reduces overall fixation rates |

**Table 2** Enhancers for nitrogen fixation

| Application | Description |
|---|---|
| Nanoparticle-based fertilizers | Engineered nanoparticles release nitrogen-containing compounds slowly, providing sustained nitrogen supply to plants. Enhances plant growth and development through continuous nitrogen availability |
| Nanoparticles as carriers for microbial inoculants | Serve as carriers for beneficial nitrogen-fixing bacteria, protecting them from environmental stresses. Efficiently deliver microbes to plant root zones, facilitating symbiotic relationships and nitrogen fixation |
| Nano-biochar composites | Combination of biochar with nanoparticles improves nutrient retention, including nitrogen, in the soil. Enhances nutrient availability to plants and supports nitrogen fixation processes |
| Nanoparticles for improved plant–microbe interactions | Modulate plant–microbe interactions positively, promoting growth and colonization of nitrogen-fixing bacteria on plant roots. Enhances efficiency of nitrogen fixation through improved symbiotic relationships |

(continued)

**Table 2** (continued)

| Application | Description |
| --- | --- |
| Nanotechnology-enabled root nodulation | Engineered nanoparticles facilitate formation and development of root nodules, where nitrogen-fixing bacteria reside in symbiosis. Enhances nitrogen fixation by optimizing the symbiotic environment for bacteria and plants |
| Nanoparticles for stress tolerance | Nano-sized nutrients or antioxidants improve stress tolerance in plants undergoing nitrogen fixation processes. Reduced stress leads to increased nitrogen fixation rates and overall plant health |

symbiotically fix atmospheric nitrogen [20]. Rhizobia or Frankia-related trees and shrubs with nitrogen-fixing root nodules are found in 10 plant groups. The status and properties of nodules in herbaceous legumes have been extensively studied; on the other hand, these attributes are unknown for many legume tree species. Among the various adaptations that make them successful is their ability to fix $N_2$ symbiotically. Adaptation to drought and floods, mycorrhizal growth, formation of cluster roots, and defenses against herbivores are a few more [60]. Various NPs were employed to investigate NP uptake, transport, and impacts in plants [17, 27, 61] and [35, 37], NPs in crop plants are well understood, but less is known about how they are absorbed by trees. The purpose of this chapter is to examine the possible advantages and disadvantages of using nanoparticles in the study of nitrogen fixation in trees. We hope to provide light on the complex interplay between nanotechnology and tree-mediated nitrogen fixation through experiments and a review of the literature, with a focus on responsible use for sustainable land-use practices.

## 2 Nanoparticles and Nitrogen Fixation: Mechanisms

### *2.1 Interaction of Nanoparticles with Tree Roots*

The detailed understanding of fundamental nitrogen fixation mechanisms is important, because the more we know the reaction process, the more we can work to improve the nitrogen fixation efficiency with pertinence. For example, Trees have been used for phytoremediation and as biomonitors of air pollution. The exact ways that trees reduce environmental nanoparticle pollution are largely unknown. Ballikaya et al. [49] compared leaf-to-root and root-to-leaf pathways to determine whether two notable tree species, namely European beech (*Fagus sylvatica* L.) and Scots pine (*Pinus sylvestris* L.), demonstrate the ability to uptake and transport gold nanoparticles (Au-NPs) with varying charges into their stems. Both species exhibit absorption of Au-NPs by their roots and leaves, with a small fraction being conveyed to the stem. The transfer of Au-NPs occurred from leaves to roots, but not in the reverse direction, in both species. The interaction of nanoparticles with tree roots is an area of growing interest in environmental science and nanotechnology research. Nanoparticles, due to their small size and unique physicochemical properties, can interact with tree roots in various ways, which may have both positive and negative effects on the trees and the surrounding ecosystem. The interaction of nanoparticles with tree roots is an area of growing interest in environmental science and nanotechnology research. Nanoparticles can be taken up by tree roots and subsequently translocated to other parts of the plant, including leaves and stems. The uptake and translocation mechanisms may vary depending on the nanoparticle properties, such as size, surface charge, and surface coatings [6]. Some nanoparticles may enter the plant cells and tissues, potentially affecting their functions and metabolism [48, 51]. Nanoparticles, particularly those engineered for agricultural applications, can improve nutrient and water absorption in tree roots [55]. Nano-sized fertilizers or nanomaterials with water-retaining properties can enhance nutrient uptake and water retention, promoting tree growth and health [71]. Certain nanoparticles, especially those with metals or other toxic components, may pose risks of toxicity to tree roots. These nanoparticles can induce stress responses and oxidative damage in plants, leading to impaired root growth and functioning [53]. Some studies suggest that exposure to certain nanoparticles can alter root morphology and architecture. For instance, nanoparticles may influence root branching, elongation, and lateral root formation [69]. Nanoparticles may influence the interactions between tree roots and beneficial soil microorganisms. These interactions can have implications for nutrient cycling, nitrogen fixation, and overall soil health [29]. Nanoparticles have been explored for their potential use in phytostabilization and phytoremediation of contaminated soils [50]. Certain nanoparticles can assist trees in sequestering or detoxifying pollutants in the soil through root-mediated processes. Nanoparticles can influence the composition and secretion of root exudates, which are compounds released by roots into the soil. Root exudates play essential roles in plant–microbe interactions and soil nutrient availability. The five following categories best describe the majority of Engineered Nanoparticles (ENPs) that are often found in the environment: Nano polymers, metal oxides, quantum dots, zero-valent metals, and carbonaceous nanoparticles are among the steadily expanding list of items [47]. Depending on the composition, shape, and size of the ENPs as well as the structure of the plant, ENPs may be absorbed by plant roots and delivered to shoots through vascular systems [39]. Since plants are a fundamental component of all ecosystems and ENPs closely interact with their surroundings, interactions with plants, such as uptake and accumulation in plant biomass, will significantly impact the fate and transport of ENPs in the environment (Fig. 1). By [75], the initial report was released. It clearly demonstrated for the first time how pumpkin (*Cucurbita maxima*) roots absorbed iron oxide nanoparticles ($Fe_3O_4$) and transported them through the plant tissues.

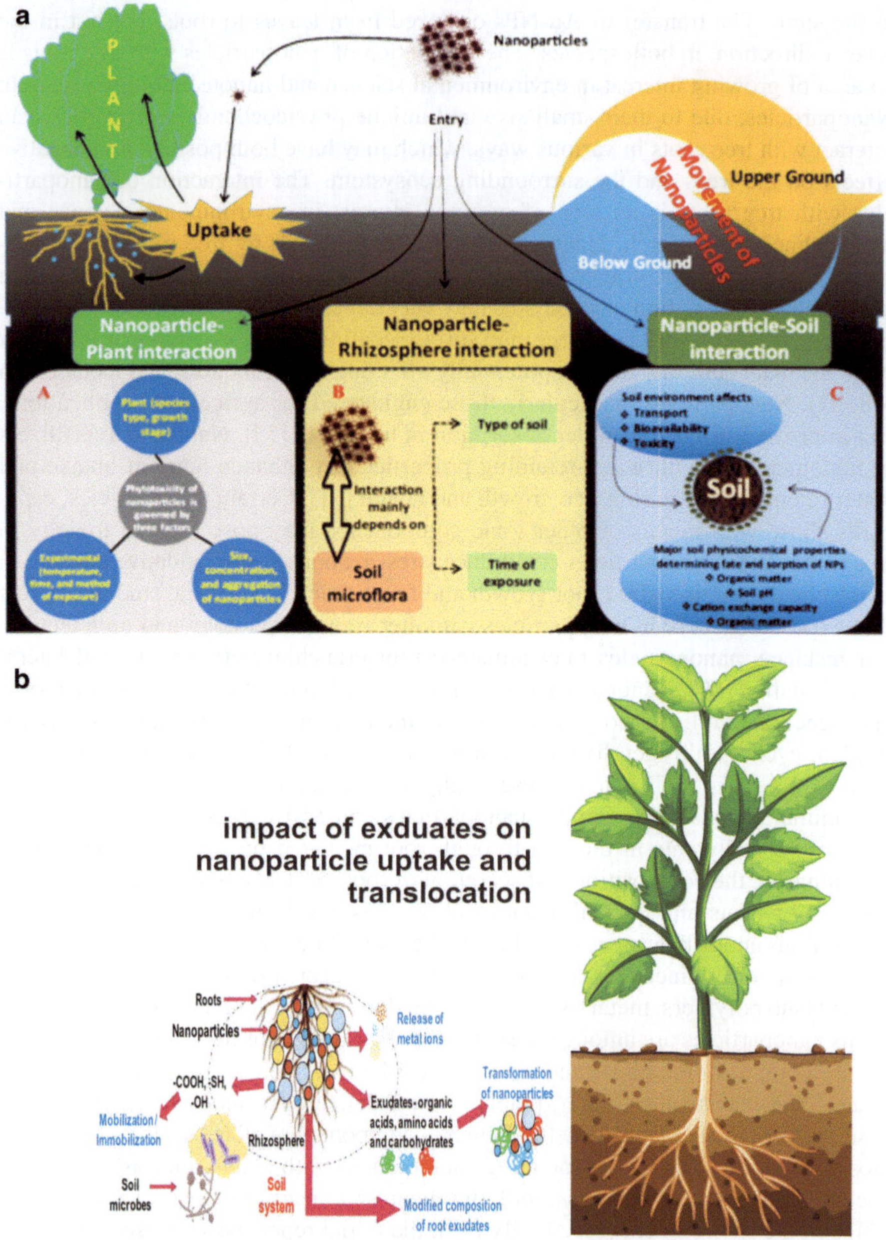


**Fig. 1** The effect of nanoparticles on nitrogen fixation by trees; **a** Nanoparticle interactions with three soil components: plants, soil microflora, and soil itself; **b** Plant root exudates and nanoparticles interact in two ways: (i) Organic acids, amino acids, and carbohydrates found in root exudates cause nanoparticles to change, and (ii) Nanoparticles themselves can change a plant's root exudates pattern, aiding nanoparticles transformation. *Source* Environmental Chemistry Letters (2021) 19:1545–1609

## 2.2 Cellular and Molecular Effects

The cellular and molecular effects of nanoparticles on living organisms, including plants and trees, are of significant interest in environmental science and nanotechnology research. When nanoparticles interact with cells at the molecular level, they can elicit various responses, both beneficial and detrimental, depending on their physicochemical properties, concentration, exposure duration, and the specific biological context [16]. Nanoparticles can be taken up by cells, including plant and tree cells, through various mechanisms such as endocytosis and diffusion. Once inside the cells, nanoparticles can interact with cellular components and influence cell function [69]. Some nanoparticles, particularly those containing metals or having catalytic properties, can generate reactive oxygen species (ROS) within cells. ROS can cause oxidative stress, leading to cellular damage and disruptions in cellular processes. Nanoparticles can trigger specific intracellular signaling pathways in cells. These pathways can regulate various cellular functions, including gene expression, cell proliferation, and responses to environmental stress [1]. Certain nanoparticles have been shown to induce DNA damage in cells, potentially leading to mutations and genotoxic effects. This can have implications for cell division, growth, and development [57]. Nanoparticles can interact with cellular proteins, influencing their function and activity. Enzymes, in particular, may be affected by nanoparticles interactions, altering metabolic pathways and cellular processes. Depending on the type and concentration of nanoparticles, they can influence cell viability and induce cytotoxic effects [68]. High concentrations of certain nanoparticles may lead to cell death or impair cell growth. Nanoparticles can affect the uptake of nutrients and ions by cells. They may enhance or inhibit the uptake of essential elements, influencing cellular metabolism and nutrient utilization. Nanoparticles can impact cellular differentiation and developmental processes. They may alter cell fate and influence tissue development in plants and trees [41]. Nanoparticles can trigger immune responses in cells, including the activation of defense mechanisms and inflammation. These effects can better assess the potential risks and benefits of using nanoparticles in various applications while ensuring responsible and safe nanotechnology practices in the context of environmental and human health [36].

## 2.3 Influences on Nodulation Process

Understanding the influences on the nodulation process is crucial for optimizing nitrogen fixation in agricultural and environmental systems. The nodulation process refers to the formation of specialized structures called nodules on the roots of certain plants, which house nitrogen-fixing bacteria in a symbiotic relationship. This process is essential for biological nitrogen fixation, where atmospheric nitrogen is converted into a form that plants can use for their growth and development [33]. Several factors can influence the nodulation process in plants such as host plant species, rhizobial strain compatibility, soil pH and acidity, soil nitrogen availability, nutrient availability, temperature and moisture, presence of competing microbes, chemical stressors, genetic factors, and age of the plant [44]. Among the critical components of the terrestrial ecosystem, soil microorganisms play a pivotal role in supporting vital ecological processes, including nutrient cycling, organic matter decomposition, and plant growth promotion. Understanding the interactions between nanoparticles and soil microorganisms is crucial for assessing the environmental implications of nanomaterial release into the soil environment. The intricate web of relationships within the soil ecosystem involves a diverse array of microorganisms, including bacteria, fungi, archaea, and viruses. These microbes contribute to the breakdown of organic matter, the release of nutrients, and the stabilization of soil structure. The introduction of nanoparticles into this complex environment has raised questions about their potential effects on soil microbial communities and functions.

## 2.4 Modulation of Nitrogenase Activity

Understanding the factors that modulate nitrogenase activity is crucial for optimizing nitrogen fixation processes in agricultural and environmental applications. It can also help researchers develop strategies to enhance nitrogen fixation efficiency and improve nutrient availability in ecosystems. The activity of nitrogenase, the enzyme responsible for catalyzing the conversion of atmospheric nitrogen ($N_2$) into ammonia ($NH_3$) during nitrogen fixation, can be influenced by various factors. Nitrogenase is a highly sensitive enzyme that requires precise conditions to function efficiently [65]. Nitrogenase is sensitive to oxygen, and its activity is inhibited by the presence of molecular oxygen ($O_2$). Oxygen competes with nitrogen for the active site of the enzyme, leading to the inactivation of nitrogenase. Nitrogen-fixing bacteria have developed strategies to protect nitrogenase from oxygen, such as enclosing it within specialized structures called heterocysts or forming nodules that maintain low oxygen levels [58]. Nitrogenase activity is also influenced by the pH of the environment. Different nitrogen-fixing organisms have specific pH optima for nitrogenase activity. The pH range for optimal activity varies among bacterial species and can also depend on the host plant's root environment [19]. Temperature plays a crucial role in nitrogenase activity. The activity of the enzyme is highly dependent on temperature, and extreme heat or cold can hinder its function. Different nitrogen-fixing organisms have specific temperature optima for nitrogenase activity [46]. Nitrogenase contains metal cofactors, particularly iron and molybdenum, which are essential for its catalytic activity. Adequate molybdenum availability is crucial for nitrogenase synthesis and function [10]. The availability of fixed nitrogen sources, such as ammonia and nitrate, can influence the expression and activity of nitrogenase. In environments with readily available nitrogen, nitrogenase activity may be down regulated to conserve energy. Nitrogen-fixing bacteria that form symbiotic relationships with plants, such as legumes, can modulate nitrogenase activity in response to signals from the host plant. The presence of fixed nitrogen sources from the host may regulate the expression of nitrogenase genes [73]. The availability of carbon and energy sources can impact nitrogenase activity. Nitrogen-fixing bacteria require sufficient energy to carry out the energy-intensive process of nitrogen fixation. The expression and regulation of nitrogenase genes are tightly controlled by various factors, including oxygen levels, fixed nitrogen availability, and specific regulatory proteins. This control ensures that nitrogenase is produced and activated under appropriate conditions for nitrogen fixation [7].

### *2.5 Nanoparticles and Soil-Microbe Interactions*

The fate of nanoparticles in the soil environment is influenced by numerous factors, including soil type, texture, pH, and organic matter content. Nanoparticles may enter the soil through diverse pathways, such as agricultural practices, industrial runoff, and the application of nanomaterial-based products. Once in the soil, nanoparticles may undergo transformations, aggregating into larger structures or interacting with soil components, which can affect their mobility and availability to soil microorganisms. Various studies have investigated the effects of nanoparticles on soil microorganisms, revealing both beneficial and detrimental outcomes. Some nanoparticles have been shown to enhance microbial activity, promoting nutrient cycling and organic matter decomposition, while others may disrupt microbial processes and lead to shifts in microbial community structure. Moreover, interactions between nanoparticles and specific groups of microorganisms, such as nitrogen-fixing bacteria, are of particular interest due to their role in biogeochemical cycles and plant nutrient acquisition. The implications of nanoparticle-soil microbe interactions extend beyond the soil environment, influencing plant health, water quality, and overall ecosystem functioning [15]. Understanding these interactions is vital for making informed decisions regarding the safe use and disposal of nanomaterials, ensuring their sustainable integration into modern technologies without compromising environmental integrity.

## 3 Types of Nanoparticles and Their Effects on Nitrogen Fixation

Nanoparticles, as defined by ISO and ASTM standards, are dimensionally complex particles with a size between 1 and 100 nm. The organic, inorganic, and carbon-based nanoparticles are often categorized as having better qualities than bigger sizes of the corresponding materials. Nanoparticles are measured on the Nano metric scale. Because of their small size, nanoparticles exhibit improved features including high reactivity, strength, surface area, sensitivity, stability, etc. [18]. In comparison to the same particles at higher scales, the nanoparticles display distinct physical, chemical, and biological features at the nanoscale. This phenomenon is caused by a surface area that is comparatively larger than the volume, a chemical process that is more reactive or stable, and improved mechanical strength. The nanoparticles exhibit diverse shapes, sizes, and structures, ranging from spherical, cylindrical, tubular, conical, hollow core, spiral, flat, etc., to irregular forms. Their sizes vary between 1 and 100 nm. The nanoparticle surfaces can be uniform or irregular, featuring surface variations. Some nanoparticles possess crystalline or amorphous structures, existing as single or multi-crystal solids, either in loose form or agglomerated [40]. The nanoparticles are generally classified into the organic, inorganic, and carbon-based. Nanoparticles come in various forms, and their effects on nitrogen fixation can differ based on their physicochemical properties and interactions with nitrogen-fixing organisms. Organic nanoparticles, such as dendrimers, micelles, liposomes, and ferritin, are commonly recognized as organic nanoparticles or polymers. These particles are biodegradable and non-toxic. Some, like micelles and liposomes, feature a hollow core (Fig. 1), referred to as Nano capsules, and are responsive to thermal and electromagnetic radiation, including heat and light [67]. On the other hand, inorganic nanoparticles do not contain carbon. Metal and metal oxide-based nanoparticles fall into this category. Metal-based nanoparticles are synthesized from metals reduced to Nano metric sizes through destructive or constructive methods. Virtually all metals can be synthesized into nanoparticles [54]. Metal oxide-based nanoparticles are created to modify the properties of their respective metal-based counterparts. For instance, iron (Fe) nanoparticles readily oxidize to iron oxide ($Fe_2O_3$) in the presence of oxygen at room temperature, enhancing reactivity compared to iron nanoparticles. The synthesis of metal oxide nanoparticles is primarily driven by the desire to increase reactivity and efficiency [64].Carbon-based-The nanoparticles made completely of carbon are known as carbon-based. They can be classified into fullerenes, graphene, carbon Nanotubes (CNT), carbon nanofibers and carbon black (fig), and sometimes activated carbon in Nano size [8]. Polymeric nanoparticles, such as biodegradable polymers, have been studied for their ability to deliver nutrients or microbial inoculants to plant roots. These nanoparticles can improve the survival and activity of nitrogen-fixing bacteria, potentially leading to enhanced nitrogen fixation. Biochar, a carbon-rich material, can be combined with nanoparticles to form Nano-biochar composites. These composites may enhance nutrient retention in soils, thereby supporting nitrogen fixation in plant root zones.

The effects of nanoparticles on nitrogen fixation can be both positive and negative, depending on several factors, including nanoparticles type, concentration, size, surface chemistry, and the specific nitrogen-fixing organism and host plant involved. While some nanoparticles may enhance nutrient availability, microbial activity, and nodulation processes, others may exert toxic effects on plants or disrupt microbial communities essential for nitrogen fixation. The importance of studying the effects of nanoparticles on nitrogen fixation lies in its potential impact on agricultural practices, ecosystem health, and sustainability. Studying the effects of nanoparticles on nitrogen fixation is crucial to harness their potential benefits in agriculture while also safeguarding the environment, soil health, and ecosystem integrity. A balanced approach is needed to leverage nanotechnology responsibly and sustainably for agricultural and environmental purposes.

## *3.1 Metallic Nanoparticles*

Nanoparticles, including metallic nanoparticles, have been explored for diverse applications in catalysis and environmental processes. Regarding nitrogen fixation, nanoparticles might play a role in catalyzing or facilitating the reaction. Metallic nanoparticles can serve as catalysts in nitrogen fixation reactions [14]. The specific metal and the size of the nanoparticles can influence catalytic activity. Research in catalysis involving metals like iron, cobalt, or molybdenum could be relevant. Metallic nanoparticles could be used as electro-catalysts in processes related to nitrogen fixation, such as electrochemical reduction of nitrogen. These nanoparticles can facilitate the conversion of nitrogen gas to ammonia under milder conditions. The surface properties of metallic nanoparticles, including their composition, structure, and electronic properties, can impact their interactions with reactants in nitrogen fixation reactions. Nanoparticles might enhance reaction kinetics or improve selectivity in nitrogen fixation reactions. Research in this area might explore how nanoparticles modify reaction pathways.

### 3.1.1 Iron Nanoparticles

Iron-based nanoparticles have been investigated for their potential catalytic activity in various reactions, including nitrogen fixation. Iron-based nanoparticles, especially in their more reactive forms like zero-valent iron ($Fe^0$) or iron oxide ($Fe_3O_4$), have been explored for electro-catalytic nitrogen reduction reactions, which involve converting nitrogen gas to ammonia under electrochemical conditions. Such reactions might be facilitated by the unique properties of iron nanoparticles. Hydrogenation reactions, which involve the addition of hydrogen to a molecule, could play a role in nitrogen fixation. Iron nanoparticles might serve as catalysts for these hydrogenation processes, potentially leading to ammonia formation. Iron nanoparticles possess a high surface area and specific surface chemistry that could facilitate interactions with nitrogen molecules, potentially promoting their conversion to ammonia or other nitrogen-containing compounds [72]. Iron nanoparticles could participate in catalytic reactions with various nitrogen species, potentially enabling the formation of ammonia or other products. Iron nanoparticles might be used in combination with other catalysts or materials to create synergistic effects, enhancing their catalytic activity for nitrogen fixation.

### 3.1.2 Silver Nanoparticles

While there might not be direct studies on the effects of silver nanoparticles on nitrogen fixation, here are some general considerations and potential areas of research interest. Silver nanoparticles have been studied for their catalytic activity in various reactions. Research might explore whether silver nanoparticles could influence reactions related to nitrogen fixation or contribute to ammonia synthesis under specific conditions. Silver nanoparticles could potentially be used as electro-catalysts for nitrogen reduction reactions, mimicking aspects of nitrogen fixation. Silver nanoparticles are known for their antimicrobial properties. Research might investigate whether these nanoparticles affect the activity of nitrogen-fixing bacteria or other microorganisms involved in the nitrogen fixation process. The surface chemistry of silver nanoparticles could impact their interactions with nitrogen-containing compounds and potentially influence related chemical reactions. If silver nanoparticles were introduced into soil or water ecosystems, they might interact with nitrogen-fixing organisms and impact nitrogen fixation processes in the environment [24]. Research might explore how nitrogen-fixing plants or organisms respond to the presence of silver nanoparticles, including potential effects on gene expression or enzymatic activity.

## *3.2 Carbon-Based Nanoparticles*

However, carbon-based nanoparticles, especially those with unique catalytic or adsorptive properties, might play a role in related processes or applications. Certain carbon-based nanoparticles, such as doped graphene or carbon nanotubes, might have catalytic properties that could potentially impact reactions related to nitrogen fixation or ammonia synthesis [70]. Carbon-based nanoparticles with specific surface modifications could be used as electro-catalysts for nitrogen reduction reactions, converting nitrogen gas to ammonia under electrochemical conditions. Carbon nanoparticles could serve as supports for other catalysts used in nitrogen fixation processes, enhancing their stability and reactivity. Carbon-based nanoparticles might have adsorption properties that could be relevant to nitrogen fixation, such as adsorbing specific nitrogen-containing molecules or facilitating gas–solid interactions. Carbon nanoparticles could be used as Nano reactors to encapsulate or enhance the activity of catalysts involved in nitrogen fixation reactions. Carbon-based nanoparticles refer to nanoscale structures composed primarily of carbon atoms. These nanoparticles have unique properties due to their small size and can find applications in various fields. Carbon Nanotubes (CNTs) are cylindrical carbon structures with exceptional mechanical, electrical, and thermal properties. Applications include nanocomposites, electronics, sensors, drug delivery, and energy storage. Graphene is a single layer of carbon atoms arranged in a hexagonal lattice. Graphene nanoparticles exhibit excellent electrical and thermal conductivity. Applications include electronics, transparent conductive films, sensors, and supercapacitors.

**Table 3** Other carbon-based Nanoparticles and their applications

| Nanoparticles | Applications |
|---|---|
| Carbon dots | Carbon dots are small carbon nanoparticles with fluorescence properties. They find applications in bio-imaging, drug delivery, and sensors |
| Fullerenes | Fullerenes are spherical carbon molecules, with C60 (buckminsterfullerene) being a well-known example. Fullerenes have potential applications in medicine, electronics, and materials science |
| Nano diamonds | Nano diamonds are carbon structures with diamond-like sp3 carbon bonding. They have applications in drug delivery, biomarkers, imaging, and quantum sensing |
| Carbon Quantum Dots (CQDs) | CQDs are small carbon nanoparticles with quantum confinement effects and unique optical properties. They find applications in bio-imaging, sensors, and photovoltaics |
| Carbon nano spheres and nanoparticles | These are spherical or irregularly shaped carbon structures with various properties. Applications include energy storage, catalysis, and drug delivery |
| Porous carbon nanoparticles | Porous carbon nanoparticles have a high surface area and porosity. They are used in adsorption, catalysis, and energy storage |
| Carbon-based nanocomposites | Carbon nanoparticles can be incorporated into polymers, ceramics, or metals to enhance material properties. Applications include lightweight composites, coatings, and sensors |

### *3.3 Other Carbon-Based Nanoparticles*

Other carbon-based nanoparticles might also play a role in related processes or applications (Table 3).

Carbon-based nanoparticles have diverse applications due to their tunable properties and unique structures. They are extensively studied in materials science, nanotechnology, electronics, energy storage, and biomedicine.

## 4 Factors Influencing Nanoparticle Efficacy

### *4.1 Nanoparticle Size and Surface Area*

Nanoparticle size and surface area can have a significant impact on nitrogen fixation, which is the process by which atmospheric nitrogen ($N_2$) is converted into ammonia ($NH_3$) or other nitrogen compounds that can be used by plants and other organisms

[62]. Nitrogen fixation is a critical biological and chemical process that plays a crucial role in the global nitrogen cycle and is essential for sustaining life on Earth. The effect of nanoparticle size and surface area on nitrogen fixation can be understood in the context of catalysis. Catalysts are substances that increase the rate of a chemical reaction without being consumed in the process. Nanoparticles, due to their small size and high surface area, often exhibit enhanced catalytic properties compared to bulk materials. Smaller nanoparticles have a higher surface area-to-volume ratio compared to larger particles. This increased surface area provides more active sites for chemical reactions to occur. In the context of nitrogen fixation, nanoparticles can act as catalysts to facilitate the conversion of atmospheric $N_2$ into more reactive nitrogen species like $NH_3$. The increased surface area allows more nitrogen molecules to interact with the catalyst; potentially leading to higher nitrogen fixation rates. The high surface area of nanoparticles provides more sites for nitrogen molecules to adsorb onto the catalyst's surface. Adsorption is an essential step in many catalytic processes, as it brings the reactant molecules close to each other, enhancing the chances of reaction. In the case of nitrogen fixation, a higher surface area can promote the adsorption of nitrogen molecules, making them more accessible for subsequent reactions. Nanoparticles often exhibit size-dependent electronic properties due to quantum effects. These electronic properties can influence the adsorption and activation of nitrogen molecules on the nanoparticle's surface. Depending on the nanoparticle size, electronic structure, and composition, the energy required to break the strong nitrogen-nitrogen triple bond in $N_2$ molecules may be lowered, facilitating the nitrogen fixation process. Nanoparticles can undergo surface reconstruction under reaction conditions, leading to the exposure of different crystal facets or surface sites. Some crystal facets may exhibit higher catalytic activity for nitrogen fixation compared to others. The nanoparticle's size and surface area can influence the prevalence of these facets and thus impact the overall catalytic performance. Smaller nanoparticles may also influence the diffusion of reactants and products. Faster diffusion rates around nanoparticles can lead to more efficient utilization of reactants and faster removal of products, contributing to enhanced nitrogen fixation rates.

## 4.2 *Nanoparticle Concentration*

The concentration of nanoparticles can also influence the process of nitrogen fixation, although it's worth noting that the effects can be complex and depend on various factors including nanoparticle size, composition, and the specific reaction conditions [21]. Generally, an increase in nanoparticle concentration can lead to a higher density of catalytic sites available for the nitrogen fixation reaction. This can enhance the overall catalytic activity and potentially lead to increased nitrogen fixation rates. However, there might be an optimal concentration range beyond which adding more nanoparticles might not necessarily result in further improvement due to factors like aggregation, which can reduce the effective surface area of nanoparticles. Nanoparticles can exhibit a tendency to aggregate or clump together at higher concentrations. Aggregation can decrease the available surface area for reactions and alter the accessibility of active sites. To counter this, efforts can be made to ensure proper nanoparticle dispersity and stability at higher concentrations. At high nanoparticle concentrations, mass transport of reactants (e.g., atmospheric nitrogen) to the nanoparticle surface can become a limiting factor. If the reaction is diffusion-limited, increasing nanoparticle concentration might not proportionally increase the reaction rate due to slower diffusion of reactants to the catalytic sites. At higher nanoparticle concentrations, there might be competitive adsorption of reactants on the nanoparticle surfaces. This could lead to increased interactions between nitrogen molecules and the nanoparticle surfaces, possibly promoting nitrogen fixation. However, it could also lead to the blocking of active sites if the adsorption sites are limited. High nanoparticle concentrations can increase the likelihood of particle–particle interactions and surface contamination. This might result in catalyst deactivation or poisoning, where certain sites on the nanoparticle surface become inaccessible or unresponsive to the reaction. Careful control of nanoparticle concentration can help mitigate these issues. The concentration of nanoparticles can influence the reaction mechanisms by altering the likelihood of intermediate species formation and their interactions with the catalyst surface. This can potentially lead to variations in product distribution and selectivity in the nitrogen fixation process. In industrial applications, it's important to consider the scalability of the process. While higher nanoparticle concentrations might be beneficial at the laboratory scale, they might pose challenges in terms of maintaining uniformity, heat and mass transfer, and reactor design when transitioning to larger scales. As with any catalytic process, finding the optimal nanoparticle concentration for nitrogen fixation involves a balance between various factors. It's crucial to conduct systematic experiments and modeling studies to understand the concentration-dependent effects and identify the concentration range that maximizes catalytic efficiency while minimizing potential drawbacks.

## *4.3 Surface Charge and Chemical Composition*

The surface charges and chemical composition of nanoparticles can have a significant impact on the process of nitrogen fixation. These factors influence how the nanoparticles interact with reactants, catalytic sites, and intermediates involved in the nitrogen fixation process.

### 4.3.1 Surface Charges

Nanoparticles can carry positive, negative, or neutral surface charges depending on the pH of the surrounding medium and the nanoparticle's surface properties. Surface charges can affect the adsorption of reactants and intermediates onto the nanoparticle's surface [63]. For nitrogen fixation, charged nanoparticles can attract or repel nitrogen molecules, influencing their interaction with catalytic sites. Charged nanoparticles can alter the adsorption behavior of nitrogen molecules. Electrostatic attraction between the charged nanoparticle surface and the reactants can enhance the adsorption process, potentially leading to a higher concentration of reactants near the catalytic sites and promoting nitrogen fixation. Surface charges can also impact the accessibility of active sites on the nanoparticle surface. Depending on the charge distribution and orientation, certain areas of the nanoparticle might be more accessible to reactants than others. This can affect the reaction pathways and product selectivity in nitrogen fixation. Surface charges can induce changes in the conformation of reactant molecules upon adsorption [59]. This might facilitate the activation of the nitrogen molecules and lower the energy barrier for the nitrogen fixation reaction.

### 4.3.2 Chemical Composition

The chemical composition of nanoparticles determines the types of active sites available for catalysis. Different elements or functional groups on the nanoparticle surface can bind to nitrogen molecules in various ways. The presence of specific chemical moieties can enhance the binding affinity of nitrogen molecules to the nanoparticle, promoting their activation [26]. Certain chemical compositions can impart redox properties to nanoparticles, allowing them to participate in electron transfer reactions. Redox-active nanoparticles can facilitate electron transfer steps in nitrogen fixation reactions, which are often essential for breaking and forming chemical bonds. The chemical composition of the nanoparticle's surface can influence the reaction pathways and intermediate species formed during nitrogen fixation. Different compositions might favor different reaction mechanisms, leading to variations in product distribution and selectivity. The chemical composition of the nanoparticles can also affect their susceptibility to surface contamination or poisoning. Certain compositions might be more resistant to the adsorption of unwanted species that can block active sites and reduce catalytic activity. Nanoparticles with specific compositions can exhibit synergistic effects when combined with other materials or catalysts. These effects can enhance the catalytic performance for nitrogen fixation by promoting cooperative interactions between different components.

The surface charges and chemical composition of nanoparticles play a crucial role in determining their catalytic behavior for nitrogen fixation. These factors influence adsorption, activation of reactants, reaction pathways, and product selectivity [30]. Understanding and controlling these aspects are essential for designing efficient nanoparticle catalysts for nitrogen fixation and other related processes.

## *4.4 Tree Species and Growth Stage*

The effect of tree species and growth stage on nitrogen fixation by nanoparticles is an interesting area of research that explores the interaction between nanomaterials, plants, and the nitrogen cycle.

### 4.4.1 Tree Species

Different tree species have varying root exudates, which are organic compounds released by plant roots into the surrounding soil. These exudates can influence the microbial communities and soil chemistry in the rhizosphere (the region around the roots). Nanoparticles added to the soil can interact with these exudates and microbes, potentially affecting their catalytic properties and their ability to facilitate nitrogen fixation. Different nanoparticles might interact differently with root exudates and microbial populations associated with different tree species. Some nanoparticles might be more effective at promoting nitrogen fixation in association with specific tree species due to the unique biochemical composition of the exudates [52]. Certain nanoparticles can promote the growth of beneficial nitrogen-fixing bacteria (such as rhizobia) around the roots. The choice of tree species might influence the compatibility between nanoparticles and specific nitrogen-fixing microbial strains, leading to enhanced nitrogen fixation.

### 4.4.2 Growth Stage

Root exudation changes during different growth stages of a tree. Young plants might release different exudates compared to mature trees. These changes can influence the interactions between nanoparticles and the root exudates, potentially altering their catalytic behavior and impact on nitrogen fixation. The rhizosphere undergoes changes as plants grow, including shifts in microbial populations and nutrient availability. Nanoparticles introduced at different growth stages might interact with these evolving factors in unique ways, affecting their ability to catalyze nitrogen fixation reactions. Plant metabolism, including the production of secondary metabolites, can change during growth stages. Some of these metabolites might interact with nanoparticles and affect their stability, reactivity, and interaction with nitrogen-fixing microorganisms [42]. The uptake and translocation of nanoparticles within the plant can vary with growth stages. These dynamics can influence how nanoparticles interact with root exudates, rhizosphere microbes, and the plant's nitrogen metabolism, ultimately affecting nitrogen fixation. Changes in plant physiology during growth stages, such as root architecture and nutrient demand, can influence the distribution of nanoparticles in the rhizosphere and their potential to catalyze nitrogen fixation reactions.

## 4.5 Environment Factors

Several environmental factors can influence the process of nitrogen fixation by nanoparticles. These factors interact with nanoparticles, reactants, and biological components in the environment to affect the overall efficiency and effectiveness of nitrogen fixation. The pH of the soil affects the availability of nutrients, the activity of microorganisms, and the surface charge of nanoparticles. Different nanoparticles might have varying catalytic activity under different pH conditions, influencing their ability to facilitate nitrogen fixation. The composition of the soil, including its mineral content and organic matter, can impact the interactions between nanoparticles and other soil components. Certain soil minerals might adsorb nanoparticles or affect their stability, potentially influencing their catalytic properties. Soil contains diverse microbial populations, including nitrogen-fixing bacteria. Nanoparticles can interact with these microbes, either promoting their growth and activity or inhibiting them, depending on nanoparticle properties. The presence and abundance of nitrogen-fixing microbes can significantly influence the nitrogen fixation process. Soil moisture content affects the mobility of nanoparticles, the diffusion of reactants, and microbial activity. Adequate water availability is essential for supporting the growth and activity of microorganisms involved in nitrogen fixation. Temperature affects both chemical reactions and microbial activity. Nanoparticles might have different catalytic properties at different temperatures, and temperature can also influence the rate of microbial processes related to nitrogen fixation. Oxygen availability in the soil affects both the stability of nanoparticles and the activity of nitrogen-fixing bacteria. Some nitrogen-fixing bacteria are sensitive to oxygen, and the presence of nanoparticles could influence the oxygen diffusion and availability around their habitats. Apart from nitrogen, other nutrients like phosphorus and trace elements play a role in supporting the growth of nitrogen-fixing bacteria. Nanoparticles might interact with these nutrients, affecting their bioavailability and microbial utilization. The concentration of nanoparticles in the environment can influence their interactions with reactants and microbial populations. Too high a nanoparticle concentration might lead to aggregation, reduced catalytic activity, or toxicity to microorganisms. Plants release root exudates that can influence microbial communities and the activity of nitrogen-fixing bacteria. Nanoparticles can interact with these exudates, influencing their effects on nitrogen fixation. The physical and chemical properties of nanoparticles, such as size, shape, surface charge, and chemical composition, determine their catalytic activity and interactions with the environment.

Agricultural practices, land use, and land management can all influence the soil environment and microbial communities. These practices can affect the overall conditions for nitrogen fixation and the interactions with nanoparticles.

Understanding the complex interplay between nanoparticles and these environmental factors is crucial for designing effective strategies for using nanoparticles to enhance nitrogen fixation in agricultural and environmental applications. Careful consideration of these factors is necessary to ensure that the use of nanoparticles for nitrogen fixation is sustainable and beneficial without causing unintended consequences.

# 5 Potential Benefits and Challenges

## 5.1 Enhanced Nitrogen Uptake and Assimilation

Enhancing nitrogen uptake and assimilation in plants through the use of nanoparticles is a promising area of research that has the potential to improve agricultural productivity and sustainability. Nitrogen is an essential nutrient for plant growth and is often a limiting factor in crop production. Nanoparticles can be engineered to improve nutrient availability, increase nutrient uptake efficiency, and enhance nitrogen assimilation in plants. Nanoparticles can be designed to carry and release nutrients, including nitrogen, gradually over time. This controlled release can ensure a steady supply of nitrogen to plants, minimizing nutrient leaching and wastage [3]. Nanoparticles can also interact with soil components, improving nutrient retention and availability for plant uptake. Nanoparticles with appropriate surface properties can adhere to root surfaces, increasing the contact area between the roots and nutrient-rich soil. This improved adhesion can enhance the efficiency of nutrient uptake, including nitrogen. Nanoparticles can also influence cell membrane permeability, potentially allowing for easier uptake of nutrients, including nitrogen compounds, through the root cells. This can enhance the overall nutrient absorption rate. Certain nanoparticles can act as growth-promoting agents for roots. Enhanced root growth and branching can lead to increased root surface area, improving nutrient absorption efficiency, including nitrogen. As discussed earlier, nanoparticles can also be used to facilitate nitrogen fixation by promoting the growth and activity of nitrogen-fixing bacteria in the rhizosphere. Some nanoparticles can interact with enzymes involved in nitrogen assimilation pathways, potentially enhancing their activity. This can lead to more efficient conversion of absorbed nitrogen into plant-usable forms. Nanoparticles can help plants cope with abiotic stresses, such as drought and salinity. By reducing stress effects, plants may allocate more resources to nutrient uptake and assimilation, including nitrogen. Nanoparticles can influence gene expression and signaling pathways related to nutrient uptake and metabolism. This can result in improved nitrogen assimilation efficiency and overall plant health. By enhancing nitrogen uptake and assimilation, nanoparticles can lead to improved photosynthetic efficiency and a better balance between carbon fixation and nitrogen assimilation processes in plants.

## 5.2 Nutrient Carriers and Signaling Molecules

Nanoparticles can serve as carriers for nutrients and signaling molecules to enhance nitrogen fixation in plants by improving nutrient availability, promoting beneficial interactions, and modulating plant responses. Nanoparticles can be loaded with nitrogen-containing compounds that gradually release nutrients over time. This controlled release can provide a sustained supply of nitrogen to plants, reducing nutrient leaching and enhancing uptake efficiency [3]. Nanoparticles can be coated with nutrient-rich materials to enhance nutrient availability. Coatings can protect nutrients from being immobilized in the soil and make them more accessible for plant uptake. Nanoparticles can be functionalized to promote the growth of nitrogen-fixing rhizobial bacteria and mycorrhizal fungi in the root zone. This can enhance symbiotic interactions, leading to increased nitrogen fixation and nutrient transfer to plants. Nanoparticles can be coated with molecules that mimic root exudates. These Nano coatings can attract beneficial microorganisms and promote symbiotic interactions, including nitrogen fixation. Nanoparticles can be engineered to release signaling molecules that stimulate the growth and activity of nitrogen-fixing bacteria. These signaling molecules can attract and support the colonization of beneficial bacteria in the rhizosphere. Nanoparticles with antioxidant properties can help plants cope with stress, which can free up resources for nitrogen fixation and enhance overall plant health. Nanoparticles can interact with enzymes involved in nitrogen fixation pathways, enhancing their activity. This can lead to improved conversion of atmospheric nitrogen to ammonia. Nanoparticles can influence gene expression related to nitrogen fixation by delivering signaling molecules or interacting with gene-regulating proteins. This can lead to increased expression of genes involved in nitrogen fixation pathways. Nanoparticles can stimulate root growth and branching, providing more surface area for nitrogen-fixing bacteria and mycorrhizal fungi to colonize and interact with plants. Nanoparticles can be designed to promote a diverse microbial community in the rhizosphere. A diverse microbial community can contribute to various aspects of nutrient cycling, including nitrogen fixation. Some nanoparticles have been shown to facilitate ion transport across cell membranes, potentially enhancing nutrient uptake, including nitrogen.

## 5.3 Eco-Toxicological Concerns

While nanoparticles hold promise for enhancing nitrogen fixation and agricultural productivity, there are also potential eco-toxicological concerns associated with their use (Hai et al. 2013). These concerns arise from the unique properties of nanoparticles, which can lead to interactions with living organisms and ecosystems that differ from those of larger particles or bulk materials. Nanoparticles intended to enhance nitrogen fixation might inadvertently impact beneficial microorganisms, including nitrogen-fixing bacteria and mycorrhizal fungi. Some nanoparticles could inhibit the growth or activity of these organisms, disrupting important ecological interactions. Nanoparticles can have unintended effects on non-target organisms present in the soil and surrounding ecosystems. These effects might include altered growth, reproduction, behavior, and overall health of various organisms, such as earthworms, insects, and other soil-dwelling organisms. Nanoparticles can accumulate in organisms through ingestion or direct contact, potentially leading to their transfer along the food chain. This can pose risks to predators and higher trophic levels, including animals that humans consume. Nanoparticles could influence the diversity and composition of soil microbial communities, potentially disrupting ecosystem functions like nutrient cycling and organic matter decomposition. Nanoparticles might undergo transformations in the environment, changing their properties and potential toxicity. These transformations could impact their interactions with organisms and ecosystems. Nanoparticles applied to soil could potentially leach into groundwater or be carried away by runoff, affecting aquatic ecosystems and water quality. This might lead to unintended exposure of aquatic organisms to nanoparticles and their potential effects. Nanoparticles might affect plant physiology, including nutrient uptake, photosynthesis, and stress responses. While some effects could be beneficial, others might have negative consequences for plant health and ecosystem functioning. The long-term ecological effects of nanoparticle exposure are not well understood. Nanoparticles might have cumulative effects that become apparent over time, affecting ecosystem dynamics and stability. The potential disruption of key ecosystem services, such as nutrient cycling and soil fertility, could have cascading effects on broader ecosystem health and function. Nanoparticles applied to crops could come into contact with pollinators, potentially affecting their behavior, reproductive success, and overall well-being. Nanoparticles could alter soil physical and chemical properties, affecting water retention, nutrient availability, and other factors that influence plant growth and ecosystem dynamics.

## *5.4 Context-Dependent Responses*

The responses of nanoparticles for nitrogen fixation can be context-dependent, meaning that their effects can vary based on specific conditions, including nanoparticle properties, plant species, environmental factors, and application methods. This variability underscores the complexity of using nanoparticles for nitrogen fixation and the importance of considering different contexts in research and applications. Different types of nanoparticles (metallic, metal oxide, organic, etc.) have varying catalytic properties and interactions with plants and microbes. Their effectiveness for nitrogen fixation might depend on their specific surface properties, size, shape, and composition. Different plant species have varying root exudates, microbial communities, and growth patterns. The response to nanoparticles for nitrogen fixation could vary between plant species due to differences in their interactions with the nanoparticles and associated microorganisms. Factors such as soil type, pH, moisture, temperature, and nutrient availability can influence the behavior of nanoparticles and their interactions with plants and microbes. Nanoparticle responses for nitrogen fixation might differ under various environmental conditions. The concentration of nanoparticles applied to the soil can impact their effects. Too high a concentration might lead to negative effects, while an optimal dosage might enhance nitrogen fixation without causing harm. The response to nanoparticles might vary based on the growth stage of plants [45]. Young plants might respond differently from mature plants due to differences in root development, nutrient demand, and physiological processes. The composition and diversity of soil microbial communities can affect the interactions between nanoparticles, plants, and nitrogen-fixing microorganisms. Changes in microbial populations over time can influence nanoparticle responses. Different agricultural practices, such as crop rotation, tillage, and fertilizer management, can influence the effectiveness of nanoparticles for nitrogen fixation. These practices affect the overall soil ecosystem and can impact nanoparticle behavior. The method of applying nanoparticles to the soil or plants (foliar application, seed coating, and soil incorporation) can affect their distribution, interactions, and effectiveness. Within a plant species, genetic variability can lead to different responses to nanoparticles. Some plant genotypes might exhibit enhanced nitrogen fixation with nanoparticles, while others might not respond as positively. Nanoparticles might interact with other chemicals present in the soil, such as pesticides or fertilizers. These interactions can affect nanoparticle stability, behavior, and overall effectiveness. Nanoparticle responses might change over time. Short-term effects might differ from long-term effects due to nanoparticle transformations, microbial community shifts, and plant adaptation. Due to these context-dependent responses, it's important to conduct thorough research in various settings to understand how nanoparticles perform for nitrogen fixation under different conditions. This will help guide responsible and effective nanoparticle-based approaches for enhancing nitrogen fixation while minimizing potential negative impacts.

# 6 Future Directions and Research Needs

## *6.1 Elucidating the Underlying Mechanisms*

Elucidating the underlying mechanisms of nanoparticles in various applications, including nitrogen fixation, involves a comprehensive exploration of how nanoparticles interact with biological systems, catalyze reactions, and influence physiological processes [29]. Understanding these mechanisms is crucial for designing safe, effective, and sustainable nanoparticle-based solutions. Elucidating nanoparticle mechanisms requires a multidisciplinary approach that integrates knowledge from nanotechnology, biology, chemistry, ecology, and other relevant fields. This approach can lead to a comprehensive understanding of how nanoparticles interact with biological systems and contribute to applications like nitrogen fixation.

### 6.2 *Synthesis and Modification Techniques*

Synthesis and modification techniques of nanoparticles involve creating nanoparticles with desired properties for specific applications, including enhancing nitrogen fixation (Nam et al. 2019). These techniques allow control over size, shape, composition, surface chemistry, and other characteristics to optimize nanoparticle performance. These techniques can be tailored to produce nanoparticles optimized for nitrogen fixation and other specific applications. Factors such as precursor choice, reaction conditions, and post-synthesis treatments play crucial roles in controlling nanoparticle properties. It's important to consider scalability, cost-effectiveness, environmental impact, and potential toxicity when selecting synthesis and modification methods for nanoparticle applications [26].

### 6.3 *Long-Term Effects on Tree Growth and Symbiotic Relationships*

The long-term effects of nanoparticles on tree growth and symbiotic relationships, particularly those involving mycorrhizal associations and nitrogen-fixing bacteria, are areas of significant research interest due to the potential implications for forest ecosystems and agricultural practices [66]. While nanoparticles have shown promise for various applications, understanding their long-term impacts on trees and their symbiotic interactions is crucial to ensure sustainability and prevent unintended consequences. Given the complexity of forest ecosystems and the multifaceted nature of nanoparticle interactions, conducting long-term field studies is essential. Researchers should monitor nanoparticle-treated trees over extended periods, assess multiple variables, and consider the cumulative effects on tree health, ecosystem dynamics, and the surrounding environment. It's crucial to strike a balance between harnessing nanoparticle benefits for sustainable tree growth and ensuring the preservation of ecosystem integrity in the long term.

### 6.4 *Assessing Ecological Implications*

Assessing the ecological implications of nanoparticles involves a comprehensive and multidisciplinary approach to understanding their potential impacts on ecosystems, species, and environmental processes [43]. This assessment is crucial to ensure that nanoparticle applications are environmentally safe and sustainable. Considering a variety of perspectives, researchers can gain a better understanding of the ecological implications of nanoparticles and make informed decisions regarding their responsible use in various applications.

# 7 Conclusion

The effect of nanoparticles on nitrogen fixation by trees is an area of research that explores how nanoparticles can potentially influence the process of nitrogen fixation in trees, especially through interactions with nitrogen-fixing microorganisms, such as rhizobia and mycorrhizal fungi. This field of study is still evolving as the promotion of microbial growth, stimulation of symbiotic relationships, facilitation of nutrient uptake, enhanced nutrient cycling, potential toxicity effects, indirect effects on soil properties, influence on plant physiology, competition with native microbes, and interactive effects with other factors and long-term effects. It's important to note that the effects of nanoparticles on nitrogen fixation can vary depending on nanoparticle properties, tree species, soil conditions, and other contextual factors. Research in this area is ongoing, and careful studies are needed to determine the specific mechanisms by which nanoparticles can influence nitrogen fixation in trees and to assess both potential benefits and risks (Fig. 1).

# References

1. Abdal Dayem A, Hossain MK, Lee SB, Kim K, Saha SK, Yang GM, Choi HY, Cho SG (2017) The Role of Reactive Oxygen Species (ROS) in the Biological Activities of Metallic Nanoparticles. Int J Mol Sci 18(1):120. https://doi.org/10.3390/ijms18010120
2. Adhikari T, Kundu S, Biswas AK, Tarafdar JC, Subba Rao A (2015) Characterization of zinc oxide nano particles and their effect on growth of maize (Zea mays L.) plant. Journal of Plant Nutrition, 38(10), 1505–1515. https://doi.org/10.1080/01904167.2014.992536
3. Akhtar N, Ilyas N, Meraj TA, Pour-Aboughadareh A, Sayyed RZ, Mashwani ZU, Poczai P (2022) Improvement of plant responses by nanobiofertilizer: A step towards sustainable agriculture. Nanomaterials (Basel, Switzerland) 12(6):965. https://doi.org/10.3390/nano12060965
4. Avellan A, Yun J, Morais BP, Clement ET, Rodrigues SM, Lowry GV (2021) Critical review: Role of inorganic nanoparticle properties on their foliar uptake and in planta translocation. Environ Sci Technol 55(20):13417–13431
5. Bartholomew WV (1977) Soil nitrogen changes in farming systems in the humid tropics. In: Ayanaba A, Dart PJ (eds) Biological nitrogen fixation in farming systems of the tropics. Wiley-Interscience, Chichester, pp 101–123
6. Behzadi S, Serpooshan V, Tao W, Hamaly MA, Alkawareek MY, Dreaden EC, Brown D, Alkilany AM, Farokhzad OC, Mahmoudi M (2017) Cellular uptake of nanoparticles: journey inside the cell. Chem Soc Rev 46(14):4218–4244. https://doi.org/10.1039/c6cs00636a
7. Bennett EM, Murray JW, Isalan M (2023) Engineering nitrogenases for synthetic nitrogen fixation: From pathway engineering to directed evolution. Biodesign Research, 5:0005. https://doi.org/10.34133/bdr.0005
8. Bhaviripudi S, Mile E, Iii SAS, Zare AT, Dresselhaus MS, Belcher AM, Kong J (2007) CVD Synthesis of single-walled carbon nanotubes from gold nanoparticle catalysts, pp 1516–1517
9. Bormann FH, Likens GE (1979) Pattern and process in a forested ecosystem. Springer-Verlag, New York
10. Burén S, Jiménez-Vicente E, Echavarri-Erasun C, Rubio LM (2020) Biosynthesis of nitrogenase cofactors. Chem Rev 120(12):4921–4968. https://doi.org/10.1021/acs.chemrev.9b00489

11. Cocozza C, Perone A, Giordano C et al (2019) Silver nanoparticles enter the tree stem faster through leaves than through roots. Tree Physiol 39:1251–1261
12. Danso SKA, Bowen GD, Sanginga N (1992) Biological nitrogen fixation in trees in agroecosystems. Plant Soil 141:177–219
13. De Bruijn FJ (2015) The quest for biological nitrogen fixation in cereals: A perspective and prospective. Biological Nitrogen Fixation:1087–1101
14. De Souza-Torres A, Govea-Alcaide E, Gomez-Padilla E, Masunaga SH, Effenberger FB, Rossi LM, Jardim RF (2021) $Fe_3O_4$ nanoparticles and Rhizobium inoculation enhance nodulation, nitrogen fixation and growth of common bean plants grown in soil. Rhizosphere 17:100275
15. Denisse VGJ, Roberto SCC, Hermes PH, Patricio TGA, Andrea PM, Fabián FL (2021) Influence of nanoparticles on the physical, chemical, and biological properties of soils. In: Nanomaterials for soil remediation, pp 151–182
16. Dilnawaz F, Misra AN, Apostolova E (2023) Involvement of nanoparticles in mitigating plant's abiotic stress. Plant Stress, 100280
17. Du W, Tan W, Peralta-Videa JR, Gardea-Torresdey JL, Ji R, Yin Y, Guo H (2017) Interaction of metal oxide nanoparticles with higher terrestrial plants: Physiological and biochemical aspects. Plant Physiol Biochem 110:210–225
18. Ealia SAM, Saravanakumar MP (2017) A review on the classification, characterisation, synthesis of nanoparticles and their application. In: IOP conference series: materials science and engineering, vol 263, no 3, p 032019
19. Frenk S, Hadar Y, Minz D (2014) Resilience of soil bacterial community to irrigation with water of different qualities under Mediterranean climate. Environ Microbiol 16(2):559–569
20. Galiana A, Bouillet JP, Ganry F (2004) The importance of biological nitrogen fixation by trees in agroforestry
21. Garg D, Sridhar K, Stephen Inbaraj B, Chawla P, Tripathi M, Sharma M (2023) Nano-biofertilizer formulations for agriculture: a systematic review on recent advances and prospective applications. Bioengineering (Basel, Switzerland) 10(9):1010. https://doi.org/10.3390/bioengineering10091010
22. Goodwin TW, Mercer EI (1983) Introduction to Plant Biochemistry. Pergamon Press, Oxford
23. Hai Z, Cheng P, Jian-Jun, Y, Ji-yan, S (2013) Eco-toxicological effect of metal-based nanoparticles on plants: Research progress. Yingyong Shengtai Xuebao, 24(3)
24. Huang M, Keller AA, Wang X, Tian L, Wu B, Ji R, Zhao L (2020) Low concentrations of silver nanoparticles and silver ions perturb the antioxidant defense system and nitrogen metabolism in $N_2$-fixing cyanobacteria. Environ Sci Technol 54(24):15996–16005
25. Humphreys LR (1994) Tropical forages: Their role in sustainable agriculture. Longman Scientific & Technical, Essex, England
26. Khan I, Saeed K, Khan I (2019) Nanoparticles: Properties, applications and toxicities. Arab J Chem 12(7):908–931
27. Khan MN, Mobin M, Abbas ZK, AlMutairi KA, Siddiqui ZH (2017) Role of nanomaterials in plants under challenging environments. Plant Physiol Biochem 110:194–209
28. Khan ST, Adil SF, Shaik MR, Alkhathlan HZ, Khan M, Khan M (2021) Engineered nanomaterials in soil: Their impact on soil microbiome and plant health. Plants (Basel, Switzerland) 11(1):109. https://doi.org/10.3390/plants11010109
29. Khanna K, Kohli SK, Handa N, Kaur H, Ohri P, Bhardwaj R, Yousaf B, Rinklebe J, Ahmad P (2021) Enthralling the impact of engineered nanoparticles on soil microbiome: A concentric approach towards environmental risks and cogitation. Ecotoxicol Environ Saf 222:112459. https://doi.org/10.1016/j.ecoenv.2021.112459
30. Kladko DV, Falchevskaya AS, Serov NS, Prilepskii AY (2021) Nanomaterial shape influence on cell behavior. Int J Mol Sci 22(10):5266. https://doi.org/10.3390/ijms22105266
31. Kumar N, Tripathi P, Nara S (2018) Gold nanomaterials to plants: impact of bioavailability, particle size, and surface coating. Nanomaterials in plants, algae, and microorganisms. Academic Press, Elsevier, London, pp 195–220
32. Kumar P, Eriksen RL, Simko I, Shi A, Mou B (2022) Insights into nitrogen metabolism in the wild and cultivated lettuce as revealed by transcriptome and weighted gene co-expression network analysis. Sci Rep 12(1):9852. https://doi.org/10.1038/s41598-022-13954-z

33. Ladha JK, Peoples MB, Reddy PM, Biswas JC, Bennett A, Jat ML, Krupnik TJ (2022) Biological nitrogen fixation and prospects for ecological intensification in cereal-based cropping systems. Field Crop Res 283:108541. https://doi.org/10.1016/j.fcr.2022.108541
34. Leghari SJ, Wahocho NA, Laghari GM, HafeezLaghari A, MustafaBhabhan G, HussainTalpur K, Lashari AA (2016) Role of nitrogen for plant growth and development: A review. Adv Environ Biol 10(9):209–219
35. Liu W, Zeb A, Lian J, Wu J, Xiong H, Tang J, Zheng S (2020) Interactions of metal-based nanoparticles (MBNPs) and metal-oxide nanoparticles (MONPs) with crop plants: a critical review of research progress and prospects. Environ Rev 28(3):294–310
36. Liu Y, Hardie J, Zhang X, Rotello VM (2017) Effects of engineered nanoparticles on the innate immune system. Semin Immunol 34:25–32. https://doi.org/10.1016/j.smim.2017.09.011
37. Lv J, Christie P, Zhang S (2019) Uptake, translocation, and transformation of metal-based nanoparticles in plants: recent advances and methodological challenges. Environ Sci Nano 6(1):41–59
38. Ma X, Quah B (2016) Effects of surface charge on the fate and phytotoxicity of gold nanoparticles to phaseolus vulgaris. J Food Chem Nanotechnol 2(1):57–65
39. Ma X, Geiser-Lee J, Deng Y, Kolmakov A (2010) Interactions between engineered nanoparticles (ENPs) and plants: phytotoxicity, uptake and accumulation. Sci Total Environ 408(16):3053–3061
40. Machado S, Pacheco JG, Nouws HPA, Albergaria JT, Delerue-Matos C (2015) Characterization of green zero-valent iron nanoparticles produced with tree leaf extracts Sci. Total Environ 533:76–81
41. Manke A, Wang L, Rojanasakul Y (2013) Mechanisms of nanoparticle-induced oxidative stress and toxicity. Biomed Res Int 2013:942916. https://doi.org/10.1155/2013/942916
42. Marslin G, Sheeba CJ, Franklin G (2017) Nanoparticles alter secondary metabolism in plants via ROS burst. Front Plant Sci 8:832. https://doi.org/10.3389/fpls.2017.00832
43. Martínez G, Merinero M, Pérez-Aranda M, Pérez-Soriano EM, Ortiz T, Begines B, Alcudia A (2020) Environmental impact of nanoparticles' application as an emerging technology: A review. Materials (Basel, Switzerland) 14(1):166. https://doi.org/10.3390/ma14010166
44. Mendoza-Suárez M, Andersen SU, Poole PS, Sánchez-Cañizares C (2021) Competition, nodule occupancy, and persistence of inoculant strains: key factors in the rhizobium-legume symbioses. Front Plant Sci 12:690567. https://doi.org/10.3389/fpls.2021.690567
45. Mgadi K, Ndaba B, Roopnarain A, Rama H, Adeleke R (2024) Nanoparticle applications in agriculture: overview and response of plant-associated microorganisms. Front Microbiol 15:1354440. https://doi.org/10.3389/fmicb.2024.1354440
46. Morugán-Coronado A, García-Orenes F, McMillan M, Pereg L (2019) The effect of moisture on soil microbial properties and nitrogen cyclers in Mediterranean sweet orange orchards under organic and inorganic fertilization. Sci Total Environ 655:158–167
47. Moulick D, Majumdar A, Choudhury A, Das A, Chowardhara B, Pattnaik BK, Hossain A (2024) Emerging concern of nano-pollution in agro-ecosystem: Flip side of nanotechnology. Plant Physiology and Biochemistry, 108704
48. Nair PM, Chung IM (2014) Physiological and molecular level effects of silver nanoparticles exposure in rice (Oryza sativa L.) seedlings. Chemosphere 112:105–113. https://doi.org/10.1016/j.chemosphere.2014.03.056
49. Paula Ballikaya and others, First evidence of nanoparticle uptake through leaves and roots in beech (*Fagus sylvatica* L.) and pine (*Pinus sylvestris* L.). Tree Physiology, 43(2):262–276
50. Prakash P, Chnadran SS (2023) Nano-phytoremediation of heavy metals from soil: A critical review. Pollutants. 3(3):360–380. https://doi.org/10.3390/pollutants3030025
51. Rastogi A, Zivcak M, Sytar O, Kalaji HM, He X, Mbarki S, Brestic M (2017) Impact of metal and metal oxide nanoparticles on plant: A critical review. Front Chem 5:78. https://doi.org/10.3389/fchem.2017.00078
52. Rehman A, Khan S, Sun F, Peng Z, Feng K, Wang N, Jia Y, Pan Z, He S, Wang L, Qayyum A, Du X, Li H (2024) Exploring the nano-wonders: unveiling the role of Nanoparticles in enhancing salinity and drought tolerance in plants. Front Plant Sci 14:1324176. https://doi.org/10.3389/fpls.2023.1324176

53. Rizwan M, Ali S, Rehman MZU, Riaz M, Adrees M, Hussain A, Zahir ZA, Rinklebe J (2021) Effects of nanoparticles on trace element uptake and toxicity in plants: A review. Ecotoxicol Environ Saf 221:112437. https://doi.org/10.1016/j.ecoenv.2021.112437
54. Salavati-niasari M, Davar F, Mir N (2008) Synthesis and characterization of metallic copper nanoparticles via thermal decomposition. Polyhedron 27:3514–3518
55. Santás-Miguel V, Arias-Estévez M, Rodríguez-Seijo A, Arenas-Lago D (2023) Use of metal nanoparticles in agriculture. A review on the effects on plant germination. Environmental Pollution (Barking, Essex: 1987), 334:122222. https://doi.org/10.1016/j.envpol.2023.122222
56. Sashidhar P, Dubey MK, Kochar M (2019) Sensing soil microbes and interactions: How can nanomaterials help? Microbial nanobionics: Volume 2, Basic Research and Applications, pp 213–236
57. Shukla RK, Badiye A, Vajpayee K, Kapoor N (2021) Genotoxic potential of nanoparticles: Structural and functional modifications in DNA. Front Genet 12:728250. https://doi.org/10.3389/fgene.2021.728250
58. Soto-Urzúa L, Baca BE (2001) Mecanismos de protección de la nitrogenasa a la inactivación por oxígeno [Mechanisms for protecting nitrogenase from inactivation by oxygen]. Rev Latinoam Microbiol 43(1):37–49
59. Spielman-Sun E, Lombi E, Donner E, Howard D, Unrine JM, Lowry GV (2017) Impact of Surface Charge on Cerium Oxide Nanoparticle Uptake and Translocation by Wheat (Triticum aestivum). Environ Sci Technol 51(13):7361–7368. https://doi.org/10.1021/acs.est.7b00813
60. Sprent JI, Parsons R (2000) Nitrogen fixation in legume and non-legume trees. Field Crop Res 65(2–3):183–196
61. Su Y, Ashworth V, Kim C, Adeleye AS, Rolshausen P, Roper C, Jassby D (2019) Delivery, uptake, fate, and transport of engineered nanoparticles in plants: a critical review and data analysis. Environ Sci Nano 6(8):2311–2331
62. Sun H, Lei C, Xu J, Li R (2021) Foliar uptake and leaf-to-root translocation of nanoplastics with different coating charge in maize plants. J Hazard Mater 416:125854. https://doi.org/10.1016/j.jhazmat.2021.125854
63. Sun XD, Yuan XZ, Jia Y, Feng LJ, Zhu FP, Dong SS, Liu J, Kong X, Tian H, Duan JL, Ding Z, Wang SG, Xing B (2020) Differentially charged nanoplastics demonstrate distinct accumulation in Arabidopsis thaliana. Nat Nanotechnol 15(9):755–760. https://doi.org/10.1038/s41565-020-0707-4
64. Tai C Y, Tai C, Chang M and Liu H 2007 Synthesis of Magnesium Hydroxide and Oxide Nanoparticles Using a Spinning Disk Reactor 5536–41
65. Threatt SD, Rees DC (2023) Biological nitrogen fixation in theory, practice, and reality: a perspective on the molybdenum nitrogenase system. FEBS Lett 597(1):45–58. https://doi.org/10.1002/1873-3468.14534
66. Tian H, Kah M, Kariman K (2019) Are Nanoparticles a Threat to Mycorrhizal and Rhizobial Symbioses? A Critical Review. Frontiers in microbiology 10:1660. https://doi.org/10.3389/fmicb.2019.01660
67. Tiwari DK, Behari J, Sen P (2008) Application of nanoparticles in waste. Water Treatment 3 417–33
68. Villanueva-Flores F, Castro-Lugo A, Ramírez OT, Palomares LA (2020) Understanding cellular interactions with nanomaterials: towards a rational design of medical nanodevices. Nanotechnology 31(13):132002. https://doi.org/10.1088/1361-6528/ab5bc8
69. Wang X, Xie H, Wang P, Yin H (2023) Nanoparticles in plants: Uptake, transport and physiological activity in leaf and root. Materials 16(8):3097
70. Xu Y, Li S, Chen M, Zhang J, Rosei F (2022) Carbon-based nanostructures for emerging photocatalysis: $CO_2$ reduction, $N_2$ fixation, and organic conversion. Trends in Chemistry 4(11):984–1004
71. Yadav A, Yadav K, Abd-Elsalam KA (2023) Nanofertilizers: Types, delivery and advantages in agricultural sustainability. Agrochemicals. 2(2):296–336. https://doi.org/10.3390/agrochemicals2020019

72. Yang X, Alidoust D, Wang C (2020) Effects of iron oxide nanoparticles on the mineral composition and growth of soybean (*Glycine max* L.) plants. Acta Physiol Plant 42:1–11
73. Zahran HH (1999) Rhizobium-legume symbiosis and nitrogen fixation under severe conditions and in an arid climate. Microbiol Mol Biol Rev 63(4):968–989. https://doi.org/10.1128/MMBR.63.4.968-989.1999
74. Zhai G, Walters KS, Peate DW, Alvarez PJ, Schnoor JL (2014) Transport of gold nanoparticles through plasmodesmata and precipitation of gold ions in woody poplar. Environ Sci Technol Lett 1:146–151
75. Zhu H, Han J, Xiao JQ, Jin Y (2008) Uptake, translocation, and accumulation of manufactured iron oxide nanoparticles by pumpkin plants. J Environ Monit 10(6):713–717

# Influence of Zinc Oxide (ZnO) Nanomaterials on the Crop: A Perspective Analysis

**Vinaya Tari, Karthik Kannan, Jyoti G. Koliyar-Jatinder Das, K. Gurushankar, and Dwi Kusuma Wahyuni**

**Abstract** Abiotic stresses consequential from climate change can hinder the growth of plants and reduce crop yields, ultimately leading to food scarcity. The cultivation of numerous crops in contaminated environments is currently a major concern for environmentalists. Advanced nanotechnology has a crucial role in enhancing food safety by bolstering food production and sustainability. It aids in optimizing agricultural output through increased input efficiency and minimized losses. This chapter highlights the literature and discusses various methods of zinc oxide synthesis, including physical, chemical, and green synthesis. Various physicochemical and biological properties, as well as the agricultural role of zinc oxide nanomaterials, will be presented. Moreover, this section delves into previous research to illustrate the influence of zinc oxide nanomaterials on mitigating the negative effects of both biotic as well as abiotic stresses. The utilization of zinc oxide nanomaterials stands out as a highly efficacious strategy for substantially improving agricultural

V. Tari (✉) · D. K. Wahyuni
Department of Biology, Faculty of Science and Technology, Universitas Airlangga, Surabaya, East Java 60115, Indonesia
e-mail: drvinaya89@gmail.com

D. K. Wahyuni
e-mail: dwi-k-w@fst.unair.ac.id

K. Kannan
Department of Mechanical Engineering and Advanced Institute of Manufacturing With High-Tech Innovations, National Chung Cheng University, Chiayi County 621301, Taiwan
e-mail: karthikkannanphotochem@gmail.com

J. G. K.-J. Das
Department of Environmental Sciences, SIES (Nerul) College of Arts, Science and Commerce (Autonomous), Thane District, Sector V, Nerul, Navi Mumbai, Maharashtra 400706, India
e-mail: jyotijatinderdas20@gmail.com

K. Gurushankar
Department of General Pathology, Saveetha Dental College and Hospitals, Saveetha University, Saveetha Institute of Medical and Technical Sciences (SIMATS), Chennai, Tamil Nadu 600077, India
e-mail: gurushankar01051987@gmail.com

 
D. Jabborova et al. (eds.), *Nanomaterials in Agroforestry Systems*, Smart Nanomaterials Technology, https://doi.org/10.1007/978-981-96-1337-3_8

productivity on a global scale in challenging environments. Zinc oxide nanomaterials possess the capacity to transform the agricultural and food sectors through the application of diverse cutting-edge methodologies aimed at mitigating oxidative stress manifestations induced by abiotic stressors. This chapter recapitulates the current understanding and impending research possibilities on plant-zinc oxide nanomaterials.

**Keywords** Nanoparticle properties · Biotic stress · Abiotic stress · ZnONPs · Sustainable agriculture

## 1 Introduction

Zinc (Zn) is an imperative element necessary for the development and proper growth of various crops, such as mango, cashew, areca nut, and other rabi and kharif crops [121]. Being classified as a micronutrient, zinc plays multiple roles in plant physiology, encompassing functions like protein synthesis, cell division, defense against environmental stresses by regulating the gene expression in response to abiotic and biotic stressors, tryptophan/auxin pathways, chloroplast functionality, metabolism of biomolecules, maintenance of membrane integrity, and acting as a cofactor for over 300 proteins, including DNA and RNA polymerases, as well as heavy metal finger proteins [54, 62, 70, 84, 120, 122, 127]. Zinc metal is notably involved in regulating the function of six categories of enzymes, which include hydrolases, lyases, ligases, oxidoreductases, isomerases, and transferases as illustrated in Fig. 1.

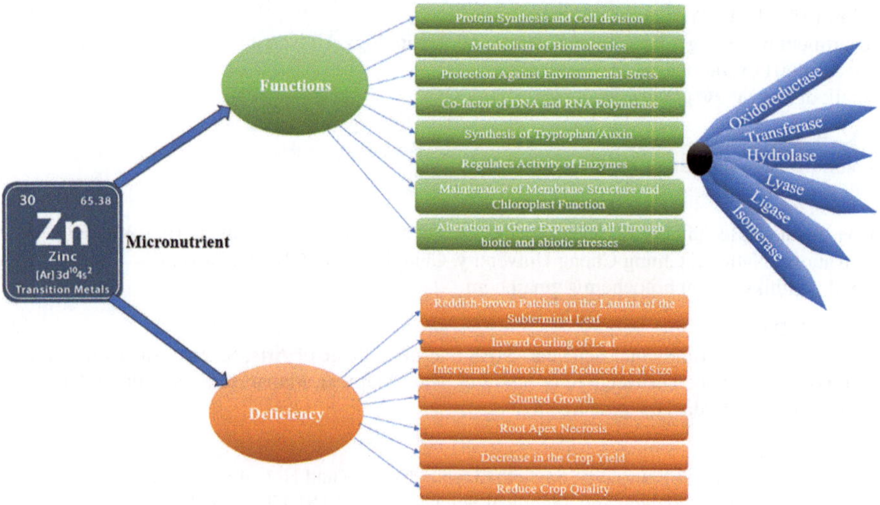


**Fig. 1** Importance of micronutrient "Zinc" for crop

The insufficiency of the essential micronutrient zinc can lead to the appearance of reddish-brown spots on the leaf subterminal lamina, decreased leaf size, inhibited growth, necrosis of root tips, leaf curling, interveinal chlorosis, and a decline in both crop revenue and eminence [122]. Therefore, an adequate supply of zinc is vital for promoting healthy plant development, and optimal crop yield [102].

Nanotechnology has demonstrated notable progress in diverse scientific and technological domains, such as agriculture. The application of nanoparticles (NPs) has exhibited considerable promise in augmenting crop yield, development, and resilience against environmental and biological pressures, along with improving postharvest methodologies [128]. Nanomaterials could alleviate the adverse impacts of chemical pesticides and fertilizers by introducing a natural food source for plants. They have a substantial impact on maintaining plant health, improving soil quality, and managing diseases [131].

Bioengineered nanoparticles composed of different metals like copper (Cu), iron (Fe), silver (Ag), zinc (Zn), and metal oxides such as titanium dioxide ($TiO_2$) and zinc oxide (ZnO) have been identified as promising nano fertilizers within the agricultural sector [2, 61, 90]. On the other hand, zinc compounds and zinc nanoparticles are recognized as fungicides and pesticides.

Moreover, Zn NPs play an imperative role in enhancing plant safeguarding against various pests and pathogens, serving as bacteriostatic agents to safeguard plants from pathogenic infections [94]. According to [111], ZnNPs have the potential to enhance seed germination, radicle and plumule length, and overall seedling vigor.

Numerous metallic nanoparticles are available, with ZnONPs being focused on by researchers and industry professionals because of their unique features such as stability, ionic properties, conductivity, selectivity, surface area, crystal structure, electrochemical properties, antimicrobial features, heat resistance, and catalytic capabilities [48, 52, 83]. ZnONPs have been proven to be innocuous and relatively less toxic compared to other zinc forms like zinc sulfate ($ZnSO_4$) [21]. ZnO plays an imperative role in various physiological and anatomical processes in a plethora of plant species [2]. Furthermore, Zn is a crucial micronutrient for human health, and ZnONPs have demonstrated compatibility with the cells of humans [11, 119, 122]. Additionally, zinc NPs have been linked to enhancing abiotic-stress tolerance in plants, including heavy metals, temperature stress, drought, salinity fluctuations, antioxidant enzyme levels, and metabolites. Zn NPs have shown effectiveness against multidrug-resistant pathogenic microorganisms [55, 111, 113]. Numerous research studies have explored the antimicrobial properties of Zn NPs.

Hence, this chapter critically evaluates the influence of ZnONPs on crops by deployment of current and pertinent literature. The significance of ZnO nanoparticles in the agriculture field and their impacts on biotic and abiotic stresses are also discussed.

## 2 Various Synthesis Methods of ZnO Nanomaterials

Researchers [2] have created different forms of ZnONPs. Although conventional techniques have traditionally been used for producing ZnONPs, recent progress in research and technology has resulted in the emergence of numerous eco-friendly synthesis methods.

### 2.1 *Traditional Method of Synthesis*

Various methods such as the hydrothermal approach, aqueous solution precipitation, vapor deposition, microemulsion precipitation, sol–gel process, and mechanochemical techniques have been utilized for the synthesis of ZnO nanoparticles with several sizes and shapes [88]. Among these methods, hydrothermal processes offer distinct advantages, particularly in terms of operating under low-temperature and low-pressure conditions, facilitating the production of nanoparticles with specific morphologies and sizes, controlled diffusion, and improved crystallinity. The hydrothermal method involves any chemical reaction, whether heterogeneous or homogeneous, taking place in an aqueous solvent over room temperature and pressure exceeding 1 atm within the closed system [14]. When this reaction is carried out using nonaqueous solvents like ethanol or methanol, it is called the solvothermal technique. This approach eliminates the need for organic reagents, ensuring high yield of the final product, good crystallinity of particles, and cost-effectiveness.

The hydrothermal approach facilitates precise temperature control for achieving desired nanoparticle sizes and morphologies. It is a less risky process compared to previous methods, resulting in uniform and monodisperse nanoparticles without the need for complex equipment or catalysts. By controlling the composition, nature, and concentration of chemical starting materials, along with thermodynamic parameters such as reaction time, temperature, and pressure, the hydrothermal method can effectively produce various materials including metal oxides, metals (such as ZnO, Au, $TiO_2$, and Ag nanoparticles), and other luminescent materials.

### 2.2 *Green Synthesis*

Manjunath and Padma in [69] suggest that various techniques, viz. biological, physical, and chemical methods, can be utilized to produce NPs. However, in recent times, the biological approach to nanofabrication has garnered increased attention compared to traditional methods, owing to its biocompatibility, cost-effectiveness, and eco-friendliness [69]. In accordance with the green chemistry principles, the eco-friendly synthesis for metal oxides and metallic NPs ought to encompass 3 preliminary steps: the utilization of non-toxic and biocompatible solvent mediums, environmentally benign reducing agents, and non-toxic materials for NP stabilization [5, 22].

The utilization of plant extracts, bacteria, algae, and fungi in the preparation of NPs renders them more fit for biological applications. Such organic entities and certain phytochemicals derived from plants are used as capping, stabilizing, and reducing agents. Given the abundance of phytochemicals, various plant components such as fruits, leaves, seeds, stems, and roots have been employed in NP production. The stabilizing and reducing effects of these secondary plant compounds enable the large-scale production of nanoparticles that are devoid of added impurities and exhibit enhanced catalytic activity. Contrary to conventional chemical methods which often involve costly processes and necessitate the usage of chemical compounds otherwise organic solvents as reducing agents, which can pose risks and hazards, the "green synthesis" of NPs has appeared as a subject of significant interest [71].

Green chemistry emphasizes waste prevention over waste disposal or treatment by mitigating pollution risks at the source and advocating for the use of environmentally friendly chemicals. The biogenic approach is deemed more profitable and ecologically sustainable compared to traditional techniques, as it is swifter and more accessible for NP synthesis. NPs produced through green methods exhibit heightened catalytic activity, reduced costs, and involve less hazardous chemicals [95, 124]. Tables 2 and 3 delineate the production of ZnONPs by plants and bacteria, algae, and fungi, respectively.

## 3 Various Properties of ZnO Nanomaterials

### *3.1 Physicochemical Properties*

ZnO is classified as the group II–VI semiconductors, exhibiting covalency at the borderline between ionic and covalent semiconductors. ZnO is highly regarded for its potential applications in optoelectronics, electronics, laser technology, and UV light emitting diodes due to its wide direct band gap, i.e., 3.37 eV, substantial excitation binding energy of 60 meV, robust mechanical stability at room temperature, and inherent n-type electrical conductivity [87, 140, 141]. Its distinguished optical absorption in the UV A (315–400 nm) and UV B (280–315 nm) wavelength ranges imparts antibacterial properties, making it a common ingredient in sunscreens and other cosmetic products for protection against ultraviolet radiation. These characteristics play a critical part in the performance of ZnO-based biosensors in nutrition packaging materials.

ZnO crystallizes in three primary forms: rock salt, wurtzite, and zinc blend structures [87, 92, 106, 140]. The hexagonal-shaped wurtzite structure of zinc oxide exhibits lattice parameters, viz. a = 0.325 nm, c = 0.521 nm, and with the c/a ratio of 1.6, closely resembling the ideal hexagonal cell with a c/a ratio of 1.633. ZnO possesses a fully ionic bond structure ($Zn^{2+}$–$O^{2-}$) with approximately 0.140 nm ionic radii for $O^{2-}$ and 0.074 nm that of $Zn^{2+}$. It adopts the hexagonal structure within the space group of P63mc, characterized by interconnected sublattices of $O^{2-}$ and $Zn^{2+}$ ions that form a tetrahedral relationship enhancing polar symmetry throughout the hexagonal axis [72]. This polarity, attributed to properties like spontaneous polarization and piezoelectricity, influences defect formation, crystal growth, and etching processes in ZnO [32, 139].

The wurtzite ZnO crystal exhibits polar (0001), nonpolar (1120) (a-axis), and (1010) faces, each terminating with a uniform number of zinc and oxygen atoms. Under normal conditions, the ZnO structure is thermodynamically constant and is commonly depicted as stacked layers of alternating $Zn^{2+}$ and $O^{2-}$ ions along the c-axis [87]. Synthesis methods can induce stabilization and metastability of the zinc-blende structure in ZnO [112].

## *3.2 Biological Properties*

Innovations in nanotechnology have offered opportunities for exploring a broad range of applications in different sectors. One notable area of focus is the utilization of nanomaterials as antimicrobial agents to combat various pathogenic microorganisms, such as bacteria and viruses. Metal oxides have emerged as a prominent category of nanomaterials due to their inherent stability, biocompatibility, and lack of toxicity, among other favorable attributes. Notably, ZnO, $Fe_2O_3$ [15], $TiO_2$ [35], $SiO_2$-ZnO [13], CdO-NiO-ZnO [49], CdO-ZnO [50], CdO-ZnO-MgO [96], ZnO-$Fe_2O_3$ [116], ZnO-$Y_2O_3$ [115], $Ag_2O$ [6], CaO [46], MgO [8], and CuO [9, 15, 136] have been extensively studied for their efficacy as bactericidal agents. ZnO has garnered significant attention as an n-type semiconductor nanoparticle with promising antibacterial properties. This material is recognized for its non-toxic nature, photostability, and biocompatibility, and has been deemed safe for consumption by the Food and Drug Administration (FDA) in the United States (GRAS) (21CFR182.8991) [36, 64]. ZnO nanoparticles have verified potent antibacterial activity against a range of Gram positive (+ve) and Gram negative (-ve) bacteria, including Staphylococcus aureus, Escherichia coli, Pseudomonas aeruginosa, and, Salmonella enteritidis, among others [86]. The unique characteristics of nanostructured ZnO [30], such as a high excitation binding energy and band gap, enable the reactive oxygen species (ROS) generation upon interaction with water molecules and oxygen, leading to oxidative stress within microbial cells [133]. The antimicrobial efficiency of ZnONPs is closely linked to their surface area, size, and, morphology, as highlighted in various research studies [75, 97].

# 4 The Significance of Zinc Oxide Nanomaterials (ZnONPs) in Agriculture

The most important industry or economic source in the developing world is agriculture. Unfortunately, it continues to face many global challenges, including rapid climate change, urbanization, and environmental problems such as water runoff and pesticide and fertilizer accumulation. Metal oxide nanoparticles have demonstrated positive outcomes in agriculture, promoting effective growth, increased yields, and improved nutrient quality. Additionally, they serve as agents to combat pathogens and safeguard plants. Zinc shows a crucial role in plant systems, contributing to various functions such as stabilizing cell membranes, synthesizing proteins, enhancing plant defense mechanisms, promoting cell elongation, and increasing tolerance to environmental stress [74]. There are other reports found on the beneficial effects of ZnONPs on pearl millet growth and germination [53, 98].

Zinc Oxide NPs have been found to have beneficial impacts on the growth and characteristics of crops such as *Zea mays* and *Triticum aestivum* L. [7]. Zinc Oxide NPs promote chlorophyll production in maize and wheat [73]. The amount of common starch in *Solanum tuberosum* L. increased by using 100 to 500 $mgL^{-1}$ ZnONPs [89]. Lower amounts of Zinc Oxide NPs are essential to promote seed germination [93]. Due to their increased foliar penetration, Zinc Oxide NPs showed improvement in the growth and physiology when applied to coffee (*Coffea arabica* L.) plants compared to Zn ($ZnSO_4$) salt [47]. Zinc Oxide NPs were proven to increase antioxidant and phenolic components during seed germination in *Capsicum annum* L. [63]. In one study, the growth of karanj, milk pine, and neem seedlings was significantly boosted by applying ZnONPs to the leaves during the nursery stage [99]. Additionally, the presence of ZnONPs in MS media has been shown to enhance embryogenesis, plantlet regeneration, and the activity of specific enzymes under biotic stress conditions. In the study on Fagopyrum esculentum, ZnONPs were found to have enhanced antioxidant properties, improved photosynthetic efficiency, and increased proline accumulation, all of which contribute to plant stabilization [28, 42]. With their special physicochemical properties, ZnONPs have been proved as a novel fertilizer to enhance agricultural productivity and food quality [138]. Research on *Nicotiana benthamiana* has demonstrated that ZnONPs can both inhibit the tomato mosaic virus (TMV) and boost the plant's immune response [59]. Other research studies have shown that the use of ZnONPs can lead to higher crop yields, reduced susceptibility to diseases, and increased resistance to various microorganisms [23]. Furthermore, zinc oxide NPs have exhibited strong pesticidal properties against *Artemia salina* larvae [3]. Investigations into the fertility impact of ZnONPs on plants like *Arachis hypogaea* and *Solanum lycopersicum* have shown improvements in seed germination, growth rate, vigor, root development, and flowering, as well as increased protein content [3].

# 5 Influence of Zinc Oxide Nanomaterials Against Biotic Stress

## 5.1 Herbivore

Increased levels of metal ions in the soil or on the plant surfaces can deter, impede, or kill the growth of several herbivores. Consumption of contaminated leaves can expose chewing herbivores to the harmful effects of metals. Herbivores that feed on plant tissues containing high metal concentrations may suffer from toxicity or develop an aversion response. Consequently, insects may acquire the ability to avoid plants with elevated metal levels through a feedback mechanism [68, 79]. Several studies [68, 79, 118] have explored the use of zinc to alleviate herbivore-induced stress. However, caterpillar performance on *Arabidopsis helleri* (Brassicaceae) was inferior on crops grown in zinc-modified soil compared to those cultivated in unamended soil [141]. Hence, there is a need to investigate zinc oxide NPs, a form of particulate zinc. Their slower release in the soil could offer advantages, and foliar application might be more effective as they persist on leaf surfaces for longer periods. This contrasts with ionic zinc, which is rapidly taken up by leaves, thus providing a more enduring protective effect on plants (Fig. 2).

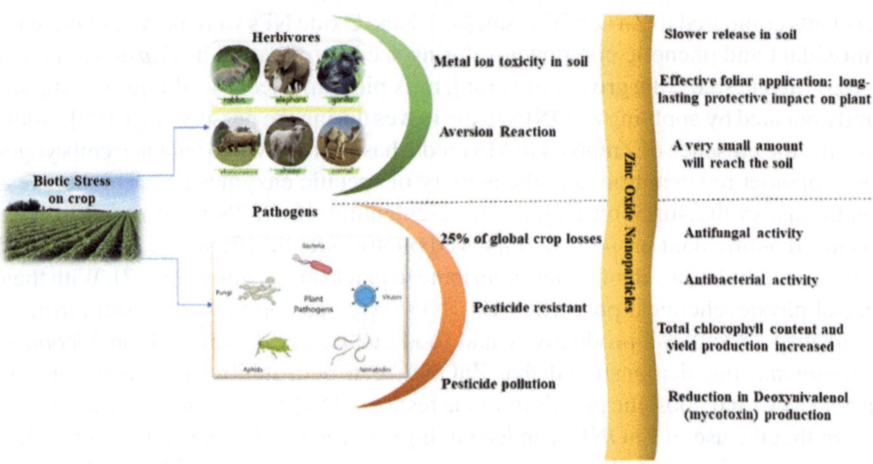


Fig. 2 Role of ZnONPs in countering biotic stress on crop plants

## 5.2 Pathogens

Plant parasites are responsible for causing a minimum of 25% of total crop losses worldwide. Traditional synthetic fungicides are currently the most effective treatments for plant diseases [12, 24, 82]. However, continued exposure to fungicides can bring up pathogen resistance, and the residues of these chemicals pose risks to both the environment as well as human health [114]. Nanoparticles provide a capable solution to this issue by presenting a more environment-friendly substitute to synthetic pesticides. By their distinct physicochemical properties, ZnONPs have demonstrated significant efficacy as antibacterial and antifungal agents against a diverse array of species [77, 114].

Zinc oxide nanoparticles have been proven to impede fungal growth in laboratory settings in a concentration-dependent manner, as reported by Malandrakis et al. in [68]. The nanoparticles displayed increased toxicity during spore germination in contrast to mycelial growth and showed enhanced effectiveness when compared to commercially available fungicides containing copper hydroxide [$Cu(OH)_2$]. Hafez and colleagues [38] investigated the synergistic introduction of the biological agent *Bacillus subtilis* in conjunction with zinc oxide nanoparticles to address powdery mildew affecting cucumber creeper induced by *Podosphaera xanthii.* This kind of application resulted in reduced electrolyte loss, enhanced defense-related enzyme activity, early elevation of reactive oxygen species (ROS) levels, increased chlorophyll content, improved yield production, and enhanced morphological and physiological parameters, including fruit yield. Savi et al. in 2015 investigated the impact of ZnONPs on wheat spikelets infected with *Fusarium graminearum* (*Fg*) during the anthesis stage [80]. The findings indicated a reduction in *Fg* colonies when relevant samples were treated with ZnONPs, leading to decreased deoxynivalenol, i.e., mycotoxin production in the grains. The zinc concentration in the wheat grains remained within acceptable levels for human consumption, and there were no negative impacts observed on the wheat grains because of the zinc oxide nanoparticles treatment. Notably, biologically produced ZnONPs from *Parthenium hysterophorus* exhibited significant inhibition against *Aspergillus niger* and *Aspergillus flavus.* Studies by Rajiv et al. in 2013 and Ingle et al. in 2020 have shown that such small quantities of ZnONPs possess heightened antifungal properties against such fungal infections. Nevertheless, additional research is warranted to optimize the application of ZnONPs in field conditions and to assess their efficacy against a broader spectrum of pathogens [17].

# 6 Influence of Zinc Oxide Nanomaterials Against Abiotic Stress

Abiotic stress factors pose substantial limitations on the growth and progression of plants. These stressors include salinity, drought, heat, metal toxicity, ultraviolet (UV) radiation, and, cold temperatures, all of which are significant challenges for plant survival. Figure 3 provides a visual illustration of the functions of ZnONPs in addressing these stressors. ZnONPs aid in mitigating abiotic stressors by boosting antioxidant activity, facilitating the accumulation of osmolytes, and promoting the availability of stress-responsive amino acids and minerals, as outlined in Table 1.

## *6.1 Heavy Metals*

Due to soil contamination, plants are consistently exposed to high amounts of heavy metals, such as lead (Pb), cadmium (Cd), and arsenic (As), which impede plant growth and development by causing toxicity. Among heavy metals, "Cd" and "As" toxicity is prevalent. Recent literature has shown that Zinc Oxide Nanoparticles (ZnONPs) can mitigate "Cd" toxicity and enhance the growth of *Lycopersicon esculentum* by improving numerous physiological parameters, viz. photosynthetic rate, chlorophyll concentration, antioxidant enzymes, and protein content [31, 132]. Additionally, ZnONPs at a concentration of 500 mg/liter have been found to protect *Zea mays* L. seed germination and growth of seedlings from "Cd" toxicity by preventing the soil from "Cd" uptake and activating the maize seedling's antioxidant defense mechanism, thereby reducing free radical production [51]. Furthermore, ZnONPs at concentrations ranging 10–200 mg/liter have demonstrated efficacy in enhancing rice seed germination and biomass while reducing "As" uptake, thereby conferring resistance to As toxicity [29]. Moreover, ZnONPs have shown promise in alleviating multimetal toxicity induced by As and Cd in rice plants simultaneously [135]. Similarly, in *Leucaena leucocephala* and *Lactuca sativa* L. var. Longifolia, ZnONPs have

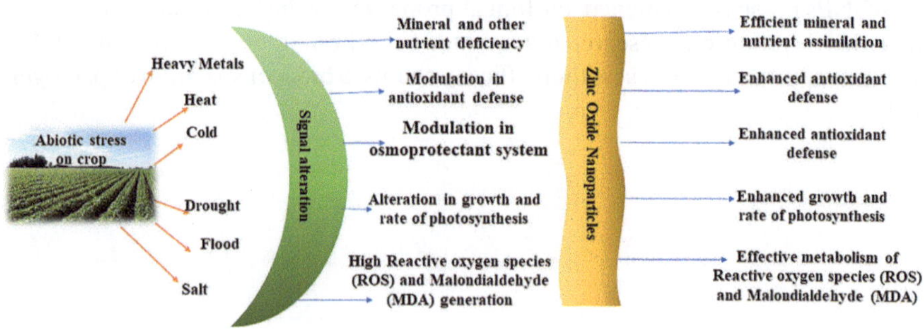


**Fig. 3** Role of ZnO nanoparticles in countering abiotic stress on crop plants

**Table 1** The influence of ZnONPs on plants subjected to various abiotic stressors

| S. no | Plant | Stress | Effects | Refs |
|---|---|---|---|---|
| 1 | *Glycine Max* | Drought | The germination % and rate showed an increase, while there was a decrease in the residual dry and fresh weight of the seeds | [105] |
| 2 | *Triticum aestivum* | Drought | Elevated levels of chlorophyll in leaves, reduced oxidative stress, and heightened activity of superoxide dismutase and peroxidase enzymes in leaves | [1] |
| 3 | *Sorghum bicolor* | Drought | Shoot and root morphology enhancement | [19] |
| 4 | *Leucaena leucocephala* | Heavy metals Cd and Pb | Elevated levels of antioxidant protection enzymes and their associated metabolites | [129] |
| 5 | *Oryza sativa* | Heavy metal "As" | Elevated rate of germination, root and shoot weight, chlorophyll, and biomass were observed with ↑ed conc. in both shoots and roots | [29] |
| 6 | *Gossypium hirsutum* | Heavy metals Cd and Pb | ↑ed shoot, root, and biomass growth in response to "Cd" and "Pb" stress; increased chlorophyll a, b, and carotenoids conc. in leaves | [85] |
| 7 | *Triticum aestivum* | Heat | The wheat crop were induced to enhance their resistance to heat stress | [41] |

(continued)

**Table 1** (continued)

| S. no | Plant | Stress | Effects | Refs |
|---|---|---|---|---|
| 8 | *Arabidopsis thaliana* | Heat | Instability of the genome; transcriptional gene silencing | [29] |
| 9 | *Saccharum officinarum* | Cold | Reduced chlorophyll a, b concentration; increased carotenoids | [25] |
| 10 | *Oryza sativa* L | Water | ↑es in antioxidant activity and growth | [126] |
| 11 | *Helianthus* | Salt | Salt stress was reduced, and SOD activity and shoot dry weight were ↑ed | [123] |
| 12 | *Musa Acuminata* (Banana) | Salt | The protein exhibited a reduction after exposure to salt treatment, while, conversely, there was an observed elevation in protein | [16] |
| 13 | *Solanum lycopersicum* | Salt | Enhanced shoot and root elongation, biomass accumulation, expansion of leaf area, chlorophyll concentration, and photosynthetic characteristics mitigate the deleterious effects of salt | [26] |
| 14 | *Linum usitatissimum* | Salt | Increased growth, carbon and nutrient uptake | [109] |

significantly reduced "Cd" and "Pb" toxicity [107, 129]. Notably, the up-regulation of 24-epibrassinolide brassinosteroids in tomato seedlings in the presence of ZnONPs has been observed, indicating a potential alleviation of stress due to heavy metal [41]. All such findings underscore the potential of ZnO nanoparticles in agriculture to boost crop quality and yield.

## *6.2 Heat*

Plants experience heat stress when exposed to temperatures above the optimal range for an extended period or prolonged intense light, resulting in irreversible damage [27]. Elevated temperatures disrupt the scavenging system for reactive oxygen species [33]. Some studies have examined certain plant's responses to heat stress in the presence of ZnONPs. The introduction of low concentrations of ZnONPs has been found to boost plant genomic stability and induce epigenetic alterations to mitigate heat stress effects [65]. The addition of ZnONPs has been proven to improve overall plant performance and prolong wheat lifespan under heat stress conditions, particularly at the concentration of 10 ppm ZnONPs [110]. This improvement has been linked to elevated levels of several antioxidant enzymes, viz. superoxide dismutase, catalase, peroxidase, and glutathione S-transferase, along with a reduction in the production of the lipid peroxidation process byproduct malondialdehyde [58].

## 6.3 *Cold*

Abiotic stress, such as cold exposure, can significantly impact plant growth and productivity [81]. Cold stress occurs at temperatures ranging 0–15 °C, leading to detrimental effects on plants deprived of the formation of ice crystals in plant tissues. In contrast, frost temperature stress is usually induced at 0 °C which results in the formation of ice crystals within associated plant tissues [60]. Plants under considerable cold stress conditions exhibit various negative outcomes, including solute leakage, membrane fluidity loss, reduced growth, and germination eventually decreasing the crop yield. Additionally, cold stress hampers chlorophyll levels, $CO_2$ absorption, transpiration rate, and Rubisco degradation [40]. Recent research has demonstrated that NPs can mitigate cold stress in plants by enhancing rubisco carboxylation, electron transport rate, chloroplast light absorption capacity, and by inhibiting reactive oxygen species (ROS) production [66]. The use of ZnONPs on plant leaves has been found to reduce in ROS production by boosting the enzymatic activities of catalase, superoxide dismutase, and peroxidase, while also reducing photoinhibition in general [25].

## 6.4 *Drought*

Drought stress arises from insufficient rainfall and reduced groundwater replenishment, leading to limited water availability for crops. Human activities, such as excessive groundwater extraction and deforestation, are the primary contributors to this stress. Drought stress has been observed to impact the composition of subcellular organelles through lipid peroxidation [43], particularly affecting the structure of chloroplasts by disrupting their internal components and reducing starch granule accumulation [137]. This stress has been shown to influence the productivity and nutritional quality of important crops like wheat and soybean [10]. The addition of Zn ions has been found to enhance crop yield. The use of ZnONPs in drought-hassled maize plants has been demonstrated to enhance photosynthetic efficiency, stomatal regulation, and water usage efficiency by increasing the activity of key enzymes like phosphoglucoisomerase, UDP-glucose phosphorylase, and cytoplasmic invertase. ZnONPs indirectly modulate crucial enzymes involved in glucose metabolism to help plants withstand drought stress [117]. Drought stress, as mentioned earlier, alters subcellular structures, leading to the accumulation of malondialdehyde and osmolytes. ZnONPs at a concentration of 100 mg/L stimulate melatonin production and antioxidant defenses in maize, thereby safeguarding cell organelles, mitochondria, and chloroplasts from oxidative harm [101, 117]. The influence of ZnONPs on the physiological responses and growth of *Oryza sativa* under polyethylene glycol (PEG)-induced water stress has also been investigated. ZnO nanoparticles at lower concentrations show promise in mitigating water stress in rice [126]. More research is needed to fully understand the mechanisms by which nanoparticles alleviate water stress [125].

## 6.5 *Flooding*

Floods, like drought, represent a significant form of abiotic stress that can inversely affect plant growth and development, despite their distinct characteristics. They alter the composition of soil, deplete oxygen levels, increase carbon dioxide concentrations, and trigger the anaerobic putrefaction of organic matter. The absence of oxygen in the vicinity of plant roots may lead to severe harm by disrupting several physiological functions. It is believed that plants employ anaerobic respiration through ethanolic fermentation as a crucial mechanism to cope with oxygen deprivation [108]. During periods of flooding stress, the transition from aerobic respiration to anaerobic fermentation is considered a critical process that enables plants to survive under oxygen-deprived conditions [20]. The use of foliar zinc has been shown to enhance the growth of plants, particularly following flooding events, as zinc tends to become less mobile in soil conditions induced by floods [37]. Consequently, the utilization of ZnONPs may serve as an effective approach to delivering zinc to distressed plants [45].

## 6.6 *Salts*

Salinity stress poses a significant concern in arid and semi-arid regions worldwide, disrupting the osmotic balance through ionic imbalance [67]. Research has explored the efficiency of ZnONPs in the mitigation of salinity stress across various crops such as cotton, potato, and millets [76]. In the case of *Trigonella foenum-graecum* L., a semi-arid plant, high concentrations of sodium ion ($Na^+$) under salt stress inhibit the uptake of potassium ion ($K^+$) and calcium ion ($Ca^+$) in shoots and roots, leading to lipid peroxidation. ZnONPs have been found to induce the production of proline, which aids in scavenging reactive oxygen species and free radicals [34]. The effectiveness of ZnONPs on *Trigonella foenum-graecum* under high salt concentrations is affected by factors such as the optimal ZnONP dosage, NaCl concentration, and cultivar type [76]. Priming seeds with ZnONPs at a concentration of 60 mg/L has been recognized as a successful plan for alleviating salt stress, increasing antioxidant enzyme activity, promoting plant growth and development, and increasing phenolic compounds, photosynthetic pigments, and ascorbic acid content [100]. Additionally, ZnONPs have been shown to decrease malondialdehyde (MDA) and salt levels in stressful plants [39, 130]. The application of ZnONPs via foliar treatment has been observed to induce physiological and biochemical alterations in finger millet, activating antioxidant enzymes and enhancing resistance to salt stress. The presence of carotenoids and photosynthetic pigments in finger millet leaves was augmented by ZnONPs supplementation. Moreover, the increased activity of scavenging enzymes like catalase (CAT), superoxide dismutase (SOD), and peroxidase (POX) protects finger millet plants from oxidative damage [56]. In the context of mango trees, the combined application of zinc oxide nanoparticles (ZnONPs) and silicon nanoparticles (SiNPs) demonstrated a beneficial effect under salt stressful conditions [25].

## 7 Conclusion and Outlook

Zinc (Zn) is a crucial micronutrient essential for the optimal growth and development of plants. In instances where the bioavailable concentration of zinc in soils is insufficient, zinc fertilizers are applied to the relevant agricultural regions. However, this doesn't always meet the demand, as zinc is readily bound to unsolvable compounds in the soil. As a result, Zn deficiency persists in crops. Therefore, ZnONPs are used as a substitute to meet the optimal Zn demand of crop plants. Several researchers have already demonstrated that ZnONPs are an efficient nano fertilizer that promotes crop growth and development which protects against various abiotic as well as biotic stresses. Nevertheless, many researchers have reported that ↑er or ↓er concentrations of ZnONPs are toxic to associated crops to some extent. On the other hand, an assessment was conducted on ZnO nanoparticles synthesized through green methods, revealing them to exhibit lower toxicity and greater efficacy in comparison to nanoparticles produced through chemical synthesis. Another aspect that needs considerable attention is the fate of residual nanomaterials, which has recently been termed "nanotoxicity". Effects of residual nanomaterials on soil microbial entities such as microbes, microflora, and microfauna. Therefore, despite the usefulness of ZnO nanomaterials, precautions must be taken in their extensive applications, especially on agricultural land.

**Acknowledgements** The authors (VT and DKW) are thankful to Universitas Airlangga, Indonesia, for providing funding through the APD program.

## References


1. Adrees M, Khan ZS, Hafeez M (2021) Foliar exposure of zinc oxide nanoparticles improved the growth of wheat (Triticum aestivum L.) and decreased cadmium concentration in grains under simultaneous Cd and water deficient stress. Ecotoxicol Environ Saf 208:111627
2. Agarwal H, Venkat KS, Rajeshkumar S (2017) A review on green synthesis of zinc oxide nanoparticles—An eco-friendly approach. Resour Technol 3(4):406–413
3. Ajey Singh NB, Singh SA, Singh T, Hussain I (2018) Zinc oxide nanoparticles: A review of their biological synthesis, antimicrobial activity, uptake, translocation and biotransformation in plants. J Mater Sci 53(1):185–201
4. Singh A, Singh NB, Hussain I, Singh H, Yadav V, Singh SC (2016) Green synthesis of nano zinc oxide and evaluation of its impact on germination and metabolic activity of Solanum lycopersicum. J Biotechnol, 233:84–94
5. Ali A, Ahmed S (2019) Green synthesis of metal, metal oxide nanoparticles, and their various applications. In: Handbook of ecomaterials, vol 4. Springer International Publishing, pp 2281–2325
6. Allahverdiyev AM, Abamor ES, Bagirova M, Rafailovich M (2011) Antimicrobial effects of $TiO_2$ and $Ag_2O$ nanoparticles against drug-resistant bacteria and leishmania parasites. Future Microbiol 6:933–940
7. Singh A, Neelam MK (2019) Physicochemical investigations of zinc oxide nanoparticles synthesized from Azadirachta Indica (Neem) leaf extract and their interaction with Calf-Thymus DNA. Results in Physics 13:102168
8. Azam A, Ahmed AS, Oves M, Khan MS, Habib SS, Memic A (2012) Antimicrobial activity of metal oxide nanoparticles against Gram-positive and Gram-negative bacteria: a comparative study. Int J Nanomed 7:6003–6009
9. Azam A, Ahmed AS, Oves M, Khan MS, Memic A (2012) Size-dependent antimicrobial properties of CuO nanoparticles against Gram-positive and negative bacterial strains. Int J Nanomed 7:3527–3535
10. Bala JM, Vennila JJ, Ganesh S, Sachidanand Singh SS (2011) Analysis of active components in Acanthus ilicifolius leaves for their potential chemoprotective activity against hepatocellular carcinoma: an in silico approach
11. Baybordi A (2005) Effect of zinc, iron, manganese and copper on wheat quality under salt stress conditions. J Water Soil 140:150–170
12. Behmer ST, Lloyd CM, Raubenheimer D (2005) Metal hyperaccumulation in plants: mechanisms of defence against insect herbivores. Funct Ecol 19:55–66
13. Bharathi DS, Boopathyraja A, Nachimuthu S, Kannan K (2022) Green synthesis, characterization and antibacterial activity of $SiO_2$–ZnO Nanocomposite by Dictyota bartayresiana extract and its cytotoxic effect on HT29 cell line. J Clust Sci 33:2499–2515
14. Byrappa K, Namratha K, Byrappa NM (2017) Hydrothermal technology for processing of advanced functional materials. KirkOthmer Encyclopedia of chemical technology; John Wiley & Sons Inc: Hoboken. NJ, USA, pp 1–45
15. Chang YN, Zhang M, Xia L, Zhang J, Xing G (2012) The toxic effects and mechanisms of CuO and ZnO nanoparticles. Materials (Basel) 5:2850–2871
16. Chaudhary D, Basanti B, Singh DJ, Subhash K, Anil P (2018) An insight into in vitro micropropagation studies for banana- review. Int J Agri Sci 10(5):5346–5349
17. Chouhan PN, Azimov A, Jabborova D, Singh S (2023) Review on the role of indigenous plants and plant derivatives of Ayurveda in bone healing. Plant Science Today 10(sp2):143–151
18. Coleman JE Zinc enzymes. Curr Opin Chem Biol, 2:222–234. da Cruz TNM, Savassa SM, Montanha GS (2019) A new glance on root-to-shoot in vivo zinc transport and time-dependent physiological effects of $ZnSO_4$ and ZnO nanoparticles on plants. Scientifc Reports, 9(1998):10416. https://doi.org/10.1038/s41598-019-46796-3
19. Dimkpa CO, Singh U, Bindraban PS (2019) Zinc oxide nanoparticles alleviate drought-induced alterations in sorghum performance, nutrient acquisition, and grain fortification. Sci Total Environ 688:926–934

20. Drew MC (1997) Oxygen deficiency and root metabolism: injury and acclimation under hypoxia and anoxia. Annu Rev Plant Biol 48:223–250. https://doi.org/10.1146/annurev.arplant.48.1.223
21. Du W, Yang J, Xiaoping P, Mao H (2019) Comparison study of zinc nanoparticles and zinc sulphate on wheat growth: From toxicity and zinc biofortifcation. Chemosphere 227:109–116
22. Duan H, Wang D, Li Y (2015) Green chemistry for nanoparticle synthesis. Chem Soc Rev 44(16):5778–5792
23. Tripathi D, Shweta SS, Singh S, Pandey R, Singh VP, Sharma NC, Prasad SM, Dubey NK, Chauhan DK (2017) An overview on manufactured nanoparticles in plants: Uptake, translocation, accumulation and phytotoxicity. Plant Physiol Biochem 110:2–12
24. Eeva T, Lehikoinen E, Ronka M (1998) Air pollution fades the plumage of the Great Tit. Funct Ecol 12:607–612
25. Elsheery NI, Sunoj VSJ, Wen Y, Zhu JJ, Muralidharan G, Cao KF (2020) Foliar application of nanoparticles mitigates the chilling effect on photosynthesis and photoprotection in sugarcane. Plant Physiol Biochem 149:50–60. https://doi.org/10.1016/j.plaphy.2020.01.035
26. Faizan M, Bhat JA, Chen C (2021) Zinc oxide nanoparticles (ZnO-NPs) induce salt tolerance by improving the antioxidant system and photosynthetic machinery in tomato. Plant Physiol Biochem 161:122–130
27. Faizan M, Faraz A, Mir AR (2020) Role of zinc oxide nanoparticles in countering negative effects generated by cadmium in Lycopersicon esculentum. J Plant Growth Regul:1–15
28. Faizan M, Faraz A, Yusuf M, Khan ST, Hayat S (2018) Zinc oxide nanoparticle-mediated changes in photosynthetic efficiency and antioxidant system of tomato plants. Photosynthetica 56(2):678–686
29. Wu F, Fang Q, Yan S, Pan L, Tang X, Ye W (2020) Effects of zinc oxide nanoparticles on arsenic stress in rice (Oryza sativa L.): germination, early growth, and arsenic uptake. Environ Sci Pollut Res 27:26974–26981
30. Forman HJ, Maiorino M, Ursini F (2010) Signaling functions of reactive oxygen species. Biochemistry 49:835–842
31. Gangwar P, Johri P, Datta R, Singh S, Trivedi M (2023) Overview on 1 Phytopharmaceuticals and biotechnology of herbal plants. In: Phytopharmaceuticals and biotechnology of herbal plants. CRC Press, pp 1–17
32. George S, Pokhrel S, Xia T, Gilbert B, Schowalter Z, Ji M, Rosenauer A, Damoiseaux R, Bradley KA, Mädler L, Nel AE (2010) Use of a rapid cytotoxicity screening approach to engineer a safer zinc oxide nanoparticle through iron doping. ACS Nano 4(1):15–29
33. Gowayed S (2017) Impact of zinc oxide nanoparticles on germination and antioxidant system of maize (Zea mays L.) seedling under cadmium stress. J Plant Prod Sci 6(1):1–11
34. Gupta G, Paul S, Singh S, Pietramellara G, Pathan SI, Danish S, Jha PN (2022) Exploring functional diversity and community structure of diazotrophic endophytic bacteria associated with Pennisetum glaucum growing under field in a semi-arid region. Land 11(7):991
35. Gupta K, Singh RP, Pandey A, Pandey A (2013) Photocatalytic antibacterial performance of $TiO_2$ and Ag-doped $TiO_2$ against S. Aureus. P. Aeruginosa and E. Coli. Beilstein J Nanotechnol 4:345–351
36. Hackenberg S, Scherzed A, Technau A, Froelich K, Hagen R, Kleinsasser N (2013) Functional responses of human adipose tissue-derived mesenchymal stem cells to metal oxide nanoparticles in vitro. J Biomed Nanotechnol 9:86–95
37. Hafeez B, Khanif YM, Saleem M (2013) Role of zinc in plant nutrition- a review. Am J Exp Agric 3:374–391. https://doi.org/10.9734/AJEA/2013/2746
38. Hafez YM, Attia KA, Kamel S (2020) Bacillus subtilis as a bio-agent combined with nano molecules can control powdery mildew disease through histochemical and physiobiochemical changes in cucumber plants. Physiol Mol Plant Pathol 111:101489
39. Haripriya P, Stella P, Anusuya S (2018) S. Foliar spray of zinc oxide nanopartcles improves salt tolerance in finger millet crops under glasshouse conditon. SCIOL Biotechnology 1:20–29
40. Hasanuzzaman M, Nahar K, Fujita M (2013) Extreme temperature responses, oxidative stress and antioxidant defense in plants. In: Vahdati K, Leslie C (eds) Abiotic stress—plant responses and applications in agriculture. InTech Open Access Publisher

41. Hassan NS, Salah El Din TA, Hendawey MH, Borai IH, Mahdi AA (2018) Magnetite and zinc oxide nanoparticles alleviated heat stress in wheat plants. Curr Nanomater 3(1):32–43
42. Helaly MN, El-Metwally MA, El-Hoseiny H, Omar SA, El-Sheery NI (2014) Effect of nanoparticles on biological contamination of'in vitro'cultures and organogenic regeneration of banana. Aust J Crop Sci 8(4):612
43. Hu W, Tian S, Di Q, Duan S, Dai K (2018) Effects of exogenous calcium on mesophyll cell ultrastructure, gas exchange, and photosystem II in tobacco (Nicotiana tabacum Linn.) under drought stress. Photosynthetica, 56(4):1204–1211
44. Ingle AP, Biswas A, Vanlalveni C (2020) Biogenic synthesis of nanoparticles and their role in the management of plant pathogenic fungi. In: Pai M, Golinsa P (eds) Microbial nanotechnology, 1st edn. CRC Press, Boca Raton, pp 135–161
45. Jabborova D, Davranov K, Jabbarov Z, Bhowmik SN, Ercisli S, Danish S, Datta R (2022) Dual inoculation of plant growth-promoting Bacillus endophyticus and Funneliformis mosseae improves plant growth and soil properties in ginger. ACS Omega 7(39):34779–34788
46. Jin T, He Y (2011) Antibacterial activities of magnesium oxide (MgO) nanoparticles against foodborne pathogens. J Nanopart Res 13:6877–6885
47. García-López JI, Zavala-García F, Olivares-Sáenz E, Lira-Saldívar RH, Díaz Barriga-Castro E, Ruiz-Torres NA, Ramos-Cortez E, Vázquez-Alvarado R, Niño-Medina G (2018) Zinc oxide nanoparticles boosts phenolic compounds and antioxidant activity of Capsicum annuum L. during germination. Agronomy, 8(10):215
48. Kannan K, Chanda D, Meshesha MM, Yang BeeLyong (2024) Impressive efficiency of zinc oxide-manganese oxide/MAX composite in two-electrode system for photovoltaic-electrolyzer water splitting. Colloids Surf, A 689:133599
49. Karthik K, Dhanuskodi S, Gobinath C, Prabukumar S, Sivaramakrishnan S (2018) Multi-functional properties of microwave assisted CdO–NiO–ZnO mixed metal oxide nanocomposite: enhanced photocatalytic and antibacterial activities. J Mater Sci: Mater Electron 29:5459–5471
50. Karthik K, Dhanuskodi S, Gobinath C, Sivaramakrishnan S (2015) Microwave-assisted synthesis of CdO–ZnO nanocomposite and its antibacterial activity against human pathogens. Spectrochim Acta Part A Mol Biomol Spectrosc 139:7–12
51. Karuppanapandian T, Moon JC, Kim C, Manoharan K, Kim W (2011) Reactive oxygen species in plants: Their generation, signal transduction, and scavenging mechanisms. Aust J Crop Sci 5:709–725
52. Klabunde T, Sträter N, Fröhlich R (1996) Mechanism of Fe (III)–Zn (II) purple acid phosphatase based on crystal structures. J Mol Biol 259(4):737–748
53. Kolenčík M, Ernst D, Komár M, Urík M, Šebesta M, Dobročka E, Černý I, Illa R, Kanike R, Qian Y (2019) Effect of foliar spray application of zinc oxide nanoparticles on quantitative, nutritional, and physiological parameters of foxtail millet (Setaria italica L.) under Field Conditions. Nanomaterials 9(11):1559
54. Lacerda JS, Martinez H, Pedrosa A (2018) Importance of zinc for arabica coffee and its effects on the chemical composition of raw grain and beverage quality. Crop Sci 58(3):1360–1370
55. Lamsal K, Kim SW, Jung J (2011) Application of silver nanoparticles for the control of Colletotrichum species in vitro and pepper anthracnose disease in feld. Mycobiology 39(3):194–199
56. Latef A, Alhmad M, Abdelfattah K (2017) The possible roles of priming with ZnO nanoparticles in mitigation of salinity stress in lupine (Lupinus termis) plants. J Plant Growth Regul 36(1):60–70
57. Laware SL, Raskar S (2014) Influence of zinc oxide nanoparticles on growth, flowering and seed productivity in onion. Int J Curr Microbiol Sci 3(7):874–881
58. Li M, Ahammed GJ, Li C, Bao X, Yu J, Huang C, Yin H, Zhou J (2016) Brassinosteroid ameliorates zinc oxide nanoparticles induced oxidative stress by improving antioxidant potential and redox homeostasis in tomato seedling. Front Plant Sci, 7:615. Limitation Environ Exp Bot 77:25–32

59. Cai L, Liu C, Fan G, Liu C, Sun X (2019) Preventing viral disease by ZnO NPs through directly deactivating TMV and activating plant immunity in Nicotiana benthamiana. Environ Sci.: Nano 6:3653–3669
60. Liu YF, Qi MF, Li TL (2012) Photosynthesis, photoinhibition, and antioxidant system in tomato leaves stressed by low night temperature and their subsequent recovery. Plant Sci 196:8–17. https://doi.org/10.1016/j.plantsci.2012.07.005
61. Liu R, Lal R (2015) Potentials of engineered nanoparticles as fertilizers for increasing agronomic productions. Sci Total Environ 514:131–138
62. Lopez Millan AF, Ellis DR, Grusak MA (2005) Effect of zinc and manganese supply on the activities of superoxide dismutase and carbonic anhydrase in Medicago truncatula wild type and raz mutant plants. Plant Sci 168:1015–1022
63. Rossi L, Fedenia LN, Sharifan H, Ma X, Lombardini L (2019) Effects of foliar application of zinc sulfate and zinc nanoparticles in coffee (Coffea arabica L.) plants. Plant Physiol Biochem 135:160–166
64. Luo Z, Wu Q, Xue J, Ding Y (2013) Selectively enhanced antibacterial effects and ultraviolet activation of antibiotics with ZnO nanorods against E. Coli. J Biomed Nanotechnol 9:69–76
65. Ma X, Sharifan H, Dou F, Sun W (2020) Simultaneous reduction of arsenic (As) and cadmium (Cd) accumulation in rice by zinc oxide nanoparticles. Chem Eng J 384:123802
66. Maddala VKS, Singh S (2023) Essential oils from plants and their role in nanomaterial synthesis characterization and applications. In: Secondary metabolites based green synthesis of nanomaterials and their applications. Springer Nature Singapore, Singapore, pp 191–207
67. Mahmoud AWM, Abdeldaym EA, Abdelaziz SM, El-Sawy MBI, Mottaleb SA (2020) Synergetic effects of zinc, boron, silicon, and zeolite nanoparticles confer tolerance in potato plants subjected to salinity. Agronomy 10(1):19
68. Malandrakis AA, Kavroulakis N, Chrysikopoulos CV (2019) Use of copper, silver and zinc nanoparticles against foliar and soil-borne plant pathogens. 670:292–299
69. Manjunath S, Padma T (2012) Mycobiosynthesis and characterization of silver nanoparticles from aspergillus niger: A soil fungal isolate. Int J Life Sci Biotechnol Pharma Res 1(2):282–289
70. Marschner H (2011) Marschner's mineral nutrition of higher plants. Academic press
71. Mason C, Vivekanandhan S, Misra M, Mohanty AK (2012) Switchgrass (Panicum Virgatum) extract mediated green synthesis of silver nanoparticles. World J Nano Sci Eng 2(2):47–52
72. Moezzi A, McDonagh AM, Cortie MB (2012) Zinc oxide particles: Synthesis, properties and applications. Chem Eng J 15(185):1–22
73. Rizwan M, Ali S, ur Rehman MZ, Adrees M, Arshad M, Qayyum MF, Ali L, Hussain A, Chatha SA, Imran M (2019) Alleviation of cadmium accumulation in maize (Zea mays L.) by foliar spray of zinc oxide nanoparticles and biochar to contaminated soil. Environ Pollut, 248:358–367
74. Nandhini M, Rajini SB, Udayashankar AC, Niranjana SR, Ole S, Lund SHS, Prakash HS (2019) Biofabricated zinc oxide nanoparticles as an eco-friendly alternative for growth promotion and management of downy mildew of pearl millet. Crop Prot 121:103–112
75. Neto V, Lencart J, Dias A, Santos J, Ramos A, Relvas C (2012) The effect of megavoltage radiation on polymeric materials to be used in biomedical devices. J Nanosci Nanotechnol 12:6779–6784
76. Noohpisheh Z, Amiri H, Mohammadi A, Farhadi S (2020) Effect of the foliar application of zinc oxide nanoparticles on some biochemical and physiological parameters of Trigonella foenum-graecum under salinity stress. Plant Biosystems:1–14
77. Noret N, Meerts P, Tolrà R (2005) Palatability of Thlaspi caerulescens for snails: influence of zinc and glucosinolates. New Phytol 165:763–772
78. Padmavathy N, Vijayaraghavan R (2008) Enhanced bioactivity of ZnO nanoparticles—An antimicrobial study. Sci Technol Adv Mater 9(3):035004
79. Pandey S, Giri K, Kumar R (2018) Nanopesticides: opportunities in crop protection and associated environmental risks. Proc Natl Acad Sci India Sect B Biol Sci 88:1287–1308

80. Parveen R, Khare N, Singh S, Johri P (2023) An in silico outlook for the detection and surveillance of evolving and persistent plant pathogens. In: Detection, diagnosis and management of soil-borne phytopathogens. Springer Nature Singapore, Singapore, pp 17–40
81. Patani A, Patel A, Prajapati D, Khare N, Singh S (2023) Various agriculture crop plant-based bioactive compounds and their use in nanomaterial synthesis and applications. In: Nanomaterials from agricultural and horticultural products. Springer Nature Singapore, Singapore, pp 223–241
82. Poschenrieder C, Tolrà R, Barceló J (2006) Can metals defend plants against biotic stress? Trends Plant Sci 11:288–295
83. Pradeeswari K, Venkatesan A, Pandi P, Karthik K, Hari Krishna KV, Mohan KR (2019) Study on the electrochemical performance of ZnO nanoparticles synthesized via non-aqueous sol-gel route for supercapacitor applications. Mater Res Express 6:105525
84. Prasad T, Sudhakar P, Sreenivasulu Y (2012) Effect of nanoscale zinc oxide particles on the germination, growth and yield of peanut. J Plant Nutr 35(6):905–927
85. Priyanka N, Geetha N, Manish T (2021) Zinc oxide nanocatalyst mediates cadmium and lead toxicity tolerance mechanism by differential regulation of photosynthetic machinery and antioxidant enzymes level in cotton seedlings. Toxicol Rep 8:295–302
86. Puzyn T, Rasulev B, Gajewicz A, Hu X, Dasari TP, Michalkova A, Hwang HM, Toropov A, Leszczynska D, Leszczynski J (2011) Using nano-QSAR to predict the cytotoxicity of metal oxide nanoparticles. Nat Nanotechnol 6:175–178
87. Kołodziejczak RA, Jesionowski T, Krysztafkiewicz A (2010) Obtaining zinc oxide from aqueous solutions of KOH and Zn(CH3COO)2. Physicochem Probl Miner Process 44:93–102
88. Radzimska KA, Jesionowski T (2014) Zinc oxide-from synthesis to application: A review. Materials (Basel). 7:2833–2881
89. Raigond P, Raigond B, Kaundal B, Singh B, Joshi A, Dutt S (2017) Effect of zinc nanoparticles on antioxidative system of potato plants. J Environ Biol 38(3):435
90. Raikova OP, Panichkin LA, Raikova NN (2006) Studies on the effect of ultrafine metal powders produced by different methods on plant growth and development. Nanotechnologies and information technologies in the 21st century. In: Proceedings of the international scientific and practical conference, pp 108–111
91. Rajiv P, Rajeshwari S, Venckatesh R (2013) Bio-fabrication of zinc oxide nanoparticles using leaf extract of Parthenium hysterophorus L. and its size-dependent antifungal activity against plant fungal pathogens. Spectrochim Acta Part A Mol Biomol Spectrosc 112:384–387
92. Raliya R, Tarafdar JC (2013) ZnO nanoparticle biosynthesis and its effect on phosphorous-mobilizing enzyme secretion and gum contents in Clusterbean (Cyamopsis Tetragonoloba L.). Agric Res 2(1): 48–57
93. Ramesh M, Palanisamy K, Babu K, Sharma NK (2014) Effects of bulk & nano-titanium dioxide and zinc oxide on physio-morphological changes in Triticum aestivum Linn. J Glob Biosci 3(2):415–422
94. Raskar SV, Laware SL (2014) Effect of zinc oxide nanoparticles on cytology and seed germination in onion. Int J Curr Microbiol Appl Sci 3:467–473
95. Reed SM, Hutchison JE (2020) Green chemistry in the organic teaching laboratory: An environmentally benign synthesis of adipic acid. J Chem Educ 77(12):1627
96. Revathi V, Karthik K (2018) Microwave assisted CdO–ZnO–MgO nanocomposite and its photocatalytic and antibacterial studies. J Mater Sci: Mater Electron 29:18519–18530
97. Rodrigo R, Libuy M, Feliu F, Hasson D (2013) Molecular basis of cardioprotective effect of antioxidant vitamins in myocardial infarction, Biomed Res Int: 437613
98. Sabir S, Arshad M, Chaudhari SK (2014) Zinc oxide nanoparticles for revolutionising agriculture: Synthesis and applications. Sci World J:1–8. https://doi.org/10.1155/2014/925494
99. Chaudhuri S, Malodia L (2017) Biosynthesis of zinc oxide nanoparticles using leaf extract of Calotropis gigantea: Characterisation and its evaluation on tree seedling growth in nursery stage. Appl Nanosci 7(8):501–512

100. Sao P, Chand Y, Kumar A, Singh S (2021) Potential drug target identification in porphyromonas gingivalis using in-silico subtractive metabolic pathway analysis. Bangladesh J Med Sci 20(4):887–896
101. Sao P, Vats S, Singh S (2022) Porphyromonas gingivalis resistance and virulence: An integrated functional network analysis. Gene 839:146734
102. Sarkar D, Rakshit A, Parewa HP, Danish S, Alfarraj S, Datta R (2022) Bio-priming with compatible rhizospheric microbes enhances growth and micronutrient uptake of red cabbage. Land 11(4):536. https://doi.org/10.3390/land11040536
103. Savi GD, Piacentini KC, de Souza SR (2015) Efficacy of zinc compounds in controlling fusarium head blight and deoxynivalenol formation in wheat (Triticum aestivum L.). Int J Food Microbiol 205:98–104
104. Schutzendubel A, Polle A (2002) Plant responses to abiotic stresses: Heavy metal-induced oxidative stress and protection by mycorrhization. J Exp Bot 53(372):1351–1365
105. Sedghi M, Hadi M, Toluie SG (2013) Effect of nano zinc oxide on the germination parameters of soybean seeds under drought stress. Ann West Univ Timişoara Ser Biol XV I(2):73–78
106. Shamsuzzaman MA, Khanam H, Aljawfi RN (2017) Biological synthesis of ZnO nanoparticles using C. Albicans and studying their catalytic performance in the synthesis of steroidal pyrazolines. Arab J Chem 10:S1530–S1536
107. Sharifan H, Ma X, Moore JM, Habib MR, Evans C (2019) Zinc oxide nanoparticles alleviated the bioavailability of cadmium and Lead and changed the uptake of iron in hydroponically grown lettuce (Lactuca sativa L. var. Longifolia). ACS Sustain Chem & Eng, 7(19):16401–16409
108. Singh A, Sengar RS, Singh AK, Singh S, Kumar A, Ahmad K (2019) Impact of genetic engineering on agriculture food crops. Biotech Today: Int J Biol Sci 9(1):17–24
109. Singh P, Arif Y, Siddiqui H (2021) Nanoparticles enhances the salinity toxicity tolerance in Linum usitatissimum L. by modulating the antioxidative enzymes, photosynthetic efficiency, redox status and cellular damage. Ecotoxicol Environ Saf 213:112020
110. Singh S, Datta R, Johri P, Trivedi M (eds) (2022) Phytopharmaceuticals and biotechnology of herbal plants. CRC Press
111. Singh A, Singh NB, Hussain I (2016) Green synthesis of nano zinc oxide and evaluation of its impact on germination and metabolic activity of Solanum lycopersicum. J Biotechnol 233:84–94
112. Sirelkhatim A, Mahmud S, Seeni A, Kaus NHM, Ann LC, Bakhori SKM, Hasan H, Mohamad D (2015) Review on zinc oxide nanoparticles: Antibacterial activity and toxicity mechanism. NanoMicro Lett. 7(3):219–242
113. Soria-Castro M, De la Rosa-García SC, Quintana P (2019) Broad spectrum antimicrobial activity of ca (Zn(OH)3)2•2$H_2O$ and ZnO nanoparticles synthesized by the sol–gel method. J Sol-Gel Sci Technol 89:284–294. https://doi.org/10.1007/s10971-018-4759-y
114. Stolpe C, Krämer U, Müller C (2017) Heavy metal (hyper)accumulation in leaves of Arabidopsis halleri is accompanied by reduced performance of herbivores and shifts in leaf glucosinolate and element concentrations. Environ Exp Bot 133:78–86
115. Suganthi Nachimuthu S, Thangamani C, Thiyagarajulu N, Thangaraj K, Paramasivam D, Thangavel S, Kannan K, Parvathiraja C, Visalakshi VB, Velmurugan P, Chinnathambi A, Alharbi SA, Basavegowda N (2023) Facile synthesis of ZnO-$Y_2O_3$ nanocomposite for photocatalytic and biological applications. Catal Commun 184:106786
116. Suganthi Nachimuthu S, Thangavel KK, Selvakumar V, Muthusamy K, Siddiqui MR, Wabaidur SM, Parvathiraja C (2022) Lawsonia inermis mediated synthesis of ZnO/Fe2O3 nanorods for photocatalysis – Biological treatment for the enhanced effluent treatment, antibacterial and antioxidant activities. Chem Phys Lett 804:139907
117. Sun L, Song F, Guo J, Zhu X, Liu S, Liu F, Li X (2020) Nano-ZnO-induced drought tolerance is associated with melatonin synthesis and metabolism in maize. Int J Mol Sci 21(3):782
118. Sun Q, Li J, Le T (2018) Zinc oxide nanoparticle as a novel class of antifungal agents: current advances and future perspectives. J Agric Food Chem 66:11209–11220

119. Taran N, Storozhenko V, Svietlova N (2017) Effect of zinc and copper nanoparticles on drought resistance of wheat seedlings. Nanoscale Res Lett 12(1):60
120. Tari VS, Patil PY (2015) Study of heavy metals traces observed in mango products from Ratnagiri District, Maharashtra. In: Proceeding of international conference on "Ethical Prospects: Economy, Society and Environment" (ICEPESE-2015), pp 363–367. ISBN no. 978–93–83046–46–1
121. Tari VS, Patil PY (2017a) Challenge of contamination of pesticide for Alphonso in Ratnagiri district, Maharashtra, India. Res J Chem Environ, 21(12):57–67. ISSN: 2278–4527
122. Tari VS, Patil PY (2017b) Transfer factor of Heavy metal in soil to plant from pesticide-contaminated area (Mango orchards), Ratnagiri district, Maharashtra. Res J Chem Environ, 21(1):26–32. ISSN: 2278–4527
123. Torabian S, Zahedi M, Khoshgoftarmanesh A (2016) Effect of foliar spray of zinc oxide on some antioxidant enzymes activity of sunflower under salt stress. J Agric Sci Technol 18:1013–1025
124. Tundo P, Anastas PT (2000) Green chemistry: Challenging perspectives. Oxford University Press
125. Tungare K, Shahu R, Zambare V, Agarwal P, Jobby R, Nisar N, Jha P (2022) Toxicity mitigation of textile dye reactive blue 4 by hairy roots of Helianthus annuus and testing its effect in in vivo model systems. Biomed Res Int
126. Upadhyaya H, Shome S, Tewari S, Bhattacharya MK, Panda SK (2020) Responses to ZnO nanoparticles during water stress in Oryza sativa L. J Stress Physiol & Biochem 16(2):67
127. Upadhyaya HD, Bajaj D, Das S (2016) Genetic dissection of seed-iron and zinc concentrations in chickpea. Sci Rep 6(1):1–2
128. Usman M, Farooq M, Wakeel A (2020) Nanotechnology in agriculture: Current status, challenges and future opportunities. Sci Total Environ 721:137778
129. Venkatachalam P, Jayaraj M, Manikandan R, Geetha N, Eldon R, Rene SNC, Sahi SV (2017) Zinc oxide nanoparticles (ZnONPs) alleviate heavy metal-induced toxicity in Leucaena leucocephala seedlings: A physiochemical analysis. Plant Physiol Biochem 110:59–69
130. Verma N, Sao P, Srivastava A, Singh S (2021) Physiological and molecular responses to drought, submergence and excessive watering in plants. Harsh Environ Plant Resil: Mol Funct Asp:305–321
131. Tari V, Kannan K, Vishwakarma V (2022) "Antimicrobial and antiviral materials: polymers, metals, ceramics, and applications" Chapter 8: Emerging antiviral technologies, 1st edn. CRC Press, Taylor, and Francis Group, pp 137–150. ISBN: 978–03–6769–744–0. https://doi.org/10.1201/9781003143093-8
132. Wahid A, Gelani S, Ashraf M, Foolad MR (2007) Heat tolerance in plants: An overview. Environ Exp Bot 61(3):199–223
133. Wang C, Wang S, Xia Q, He W, Yin J, Fu P, Li J (2013) Phototoxicity of zinc oxide nanoparticles in HaCaT keratinocytes-generation of oxidative DNA damage during UVA and visible light irradiation. J Nanosci Nanotechnol 13:3880–3888
134. Wellings JS, Chaure NB, Heavens SN, Dharmadasa IM (2008) Growth and characterisation of electrodeposited ZnO thin films. Thin Solid Films 516(12):3893–3898
135. Wu J, Wang T (2020) Synergistic effect of zinc oxide nanoparticles and heat stress on the alleviation of transcriptional gene silencing in Arabidopsis thaliana. Bull Environ Contam Toxicol 104(1):49–56
136. Xie Y, He Y, Irwin PL, Jin T, Shi X (2011) Antibacterial activity and mechanism of action of zinc oxide nanoparticles against Campylobacter jejuni. Appl Environ Microbiol 77:2325–2331
137. Xu ZZ, Zhou GS, Shimizu H (2009) Effects of soil drought with nocturnal warming on leaf stomatal traits and mesophyll cell ultrastructure of a perennial grass. Crop Sci 49:1843–1851
138. Yusefi Tanha E, Fallah S, Rostamnejadi A, Pokhrel LR (2020) Zinc oxide nanoparticles (ZnONPs) as nanofertilizer: Improvement on seed yield and antioxidant defense system in soil grown soybean (Glycine max cv. Kowsar). https://doi.org/10.1101/2020.04.13.039644

139. Zgür ÜÖ, Alivov YI, Liu C, Teke A, Reshchikov MA, Doğan S, Avrutin V, Cho SJ, Morkoc HA (2005) Comprehensive, review of ZnO materials and devices. J Appl Phys 98(4):041301
140. Zhang Y, Ram MK, Stefanakos EK, Goswami DY (2012) Synthesis, characterization, and applications of ZnO nanowires. J Nanomater:1–22, Article ID 624520
141. Zhang Z, Jiang W, Jian Q (2015) Residues and dissipation kinetics of triazole fungicides difenoconazole and propiconazole in wheat and soil in Chinese fields. Food Chem 168:396–403

may be generally divided into physical, chemical, and biological ways of synthesis. Each of them has its benefits and drawbacks. While biological approaches have the benefit of being environmentally benign and biocompatible, physical and chemical methods of synthesis are often favored because they produce nanoparticles of uniform size (Mehta et al. 2012). There are already more than 1300 commercial nanoparticles that have several potential uses. In the category of designed nanomaterial, carbon nanotubes and related nanoparticles were first identified in 1985. By 2011, it was anticipated that more than 1000 tonnes of carbon-based nanomaterial were produced annually globally, with certain factories having a capacity of up to 1500 tonnes. These carbon-based nanomaterial may degrade in a variety of environments and be ingested by bacteria, which are then digested by worms, increasing the likelihood that they will enter the food chain [46].

Plants are exposed to the nanoparticles that are discharged into the environment because of their static nature and interaction with soil and air [30]. It's important to take into account the direct contact that plants have with metal and metal oxide nanoparticles. Both positive and negative impacts of nanoparticles on crop development have been shown in recent years. The kind, source, and size of the nanoparticles, the type of plant, and the length of time the nanoparticles were exposed to crops were all factors in these impacts. For instance, iron (Fe) nanoparticles enhanced soybean (*Glycine max L.*) biomass whereas silver (Ag) nanoparticles boosted ascorbate and chlorophyll in the leaves of asparagus (*Asparagus officinalis L.*) [4].

Similar to this, using silica nanoparticles improved the field-grown maize seedlings' seed germination, root and shoot length, photosynthetic rate, and dry weight. In addition, as compared to the control plants, the chickpea (*Cicer arietinum L.*) had less hydrogen peroxide ($H_2O_2$), malondialdehyde (MDA), and electrolyte leakage [41, 68]. Nanoparticles (NPs) have drawn a lot of interest in recent years because of their distinctive characteristics and useful uses in the agricultural and related industries. NPs may be generically categorized as inorganic and organic NPs depending on the primary component. While fullerenes and carbon nanotubes are organic NPs, inorganic NPs include metals (Al, Bi, Co, Cu, Au, Fe, In, Mo, Ni, Ag, Sn, Ti, W, and Zn), metal oxides ($Al_2O_3$, $CeO_2$, CuO, $Cu_2O$, $In_2O_3$, $La_2O_3$, MgO, NiO, $TiO_2$, $SnO_2$, ZnO, and $ZrO_2$), and quantum dots. Metal-based NPs are often utilized, and their harmful effects on the activity, quantity, and variety of flora and animals are closely observed [53].

Forest tree species are critical to the survival of human and animal life because they provide fuelwood, lumber, fruits, medicine, food, fodder, and environmental protection, among other necessities [31]. Furthermore, a multitude of advantageous substances, including flavonoids, phenols, alkaloids, sterols, waxes, lipids, tannins, sugars, gums, suberins, resin acids, and other secondary metabolites, are abundant in these trees [47]. A rising number of people are interested in using certain forest tree species and the chemicals they contain to create nanomaterials (NMs) using a technique called "green synthesis." This procedure is thought to be an easy, economical, and green substitute for traditional chemical and physical production methods.

**Table 1** Metal oxide nanoparticles from forest trees [24]

| Botanical name | Nanoparticles | Application |
|---|---|---|
| *Azadirachta indica* | ZnO | Antibacterial activity |
| *Grewia optiva* | FeO | Antioxidant activity, antibacterial activity |
| *Shorea tumbuggaia* | Ag | Bactericidal, wound healing, and other medical and electronic applications |
| *F. benghalensis* | Au | Antibacterial activity |
| *Pinus* | Pd | Catalytic activity |

Green synthesis of nanoparticles (NPs) has the potential to be a sustainable manufacturing process since it strives to generate desired goods without producing hazardous byproducts (Table 1) [24].

## *1.1 Metal Oxide Nanoparticles*

### 1.1.1 Iron Oxide Nanoparticles

The amount of iron in soil is high, but a significant percentage is attached to soil particles and is inaccessible to plants because it is insoluble ($Fe^{3+}$), while plants only take up $Fe^{2+}$ form from the soil. Iron is a crucial micronutrient for the growth of plants and plays a significant part in a variety of physiological activities, including respiration, redox reactions, and chlorophyll production [70]. In some soils, like calcareous soil, iron is not accessible to plants. As a result, iron nanoparticle applications have surged recently. However, little research has been done on its long-term effects on plant and soil ecosystems. Zero-valent iron nanoparticle use is growing, which poses severe questions about environmental damage. The zero-valent Fe nanoparticles have been employed successfully to address a number of environmental pollutants, increasing the likelihood of their accumulation in the soil ecosystem [77].

### 1.1.2 Zinc Oxide Nanoparticles

Although zinc is a necessary element, too much of it can stunt plant development and produce chlorosis. Zinc nanoparticles have a large specific surface area, are spherical or polished metal particles, and have the chemical formula ZnO. Zinc nanoparticles are used extensively in the glass, cement, rubber, lubricants, paints, ointments, adhesives, plastics, sealants, pigments, food, and battery sectors [65]. ZnO nanostructures, nanoparticles, nanowires, nanorods, nanotubes, nanobelts, and other complex morphologies are created using a variety of techniques. Numerous plants, including soybean, wheat, cucumber, mustard, alfalfa, radish, ryegrass, lettuce, maize, zucchini, spinach, and others, have shown deleterious effects of ZnO nanoparticles on their growth and development [51, 52, 54].

### 1.1.3 Silver Oxide Nanoparticles

When compared to bulk silver, silver nanoparticles (Ag NPs) exhibit several unique physico-chemical characteristics and broad-spectrum antimicrobial effects against all kinds of microbes. Ag NPs are therefore one of the most often utilized designed NPs in a variety of consumer items, and they are predicted to penetrate natural ecosystems, including soil, via a variety of mechanisms. Nevertheless, despite the fact that (i) soil has been recognized as a crucial pathway for NP environmental fate, (ii) it has been strongly advised to include plants (a vital component of all ecosystems) in the development of a thorough toxicity profile for rapidly mounting NPs in various environmental compartments, and (iii) there is a complex relationship between "soil–plant systems" where any change in soil chemical or biological properties is beneficial [5].

### 1.1.4 Magnesium Oxide Nanoparticles

Magnesium oxide nanoparticles (MgO NPs) have attracted a lot of attention over the past ten years due to their distinctive properties, several potential uses in the field of materials science, and availability as non-toxic, reasonably priced materials. MgO NPs can increase plant development and help plants tolerate the toxicity of heavy metals [20]. Due to its nano scale, MgO possesses a variety of unique physical and chemical characteristics. Nanoparticles' small size allows them to be more effectively used by plant cells, promote plant development, and have antibacterial, antifungal, and antiviral effects on pests. Nanoparticles can enter the plant cell because of their tiny size [33].

### 1.1.5 Calcium Oxide Nanoparticles

According to Elmar et al. [16], calcium (Ca) is crucial for sustaining cellular activity and the components of plant tissues. According to Singh et al. [66], calcium ions are also responsible for the regulation of fruit ripening. Because calcium is an immobile element and cannot readily travel from one section of plants to another, its content may be increased in plants by direct contact with calcium more quickly [36]. There are accounts of the use of nano-calcium phosphate on a variety of plants, but to date, no study has been published on the use of nano-calcium on tomato (*S. lycopersicum*) as a nanospray. The current study also includes administering two nano-supplements to plants in combination and seeing how they react. Metal oxide nanoparticles are used in many fields of application, as shown in Fig. 1.

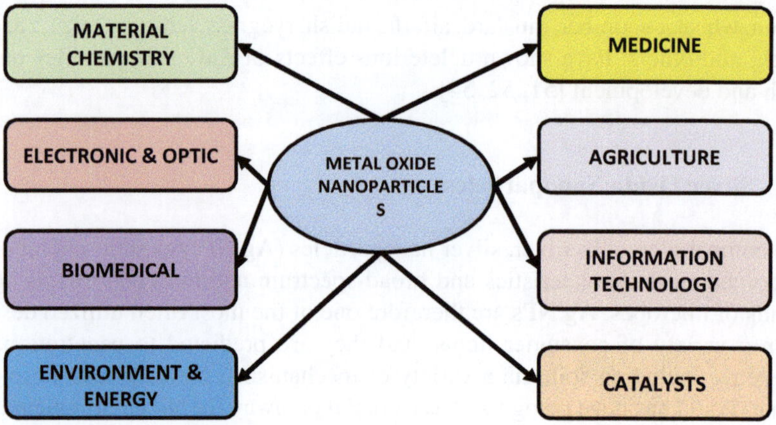


**Fig. 1** Applications of metal oxide nanoparticles

## *1.2 Metal Oxide Nanoparticles: Beneficial Impacts on Soil Agrochemical and Soil Biochemical Properties*

### 1.2.1 Sources of Nanoparticles in Soil

Due to the expanding market for NP-based goods and the subsequent emergence of NPs in many environments, including soil, water, and air, nanoparticle manufacturing is fast rising. One of the primary environmental sinks for NPs is the ocean, followed by soil (e.g., by sludge application to soil). Worldwide, landfills are thought to have received between 63 and 91 percent of all ENPs, which might then be discharged into the soil, water, and environment [5]. Additionally, the deliberate use of NP-based agrochemicals and their emission from industrial sources might result in nanoparticles getting into the soil. Due to the usage of NPs for soil remediation, unintentional releases from manufacturing facilities, irrigation with wastewater, and air fallouts, nanoparticles are getting into the soil [6, 28].

The mobility, toxicity, reactivity, and possible dangers of the released MBNPs and MONPs in agricultural soil are significantly influenced by their environmental behavior. MONPs may aggregate and agglomerate, interact with dissolved organic matter (DOM), hetero-aggregate with inorganic colloids, and change through chemical and dissolving processes after entering the soil matrix [71]. Clay, iron oxides, and other minerals, as well as organic components, make up soil colloids, which are operationally described as having a size between 1 nm and 1 m. Soil colloids are crucial in controlling the behavior, mobility, and destiny of MONPs in soil. DOM is commonly abundant in agricultural soil, and its influence on the aggregation of MONPs is mostly determined by the properties of the MONPs, the DOM, and the environment matrix [11].

### 1.2.2 Effect on Microbial Community

Nanoparticles can infiltrate soil through a variety of channels, including landfills, atmospheric deposition, agricultural sludge additions, and unintentional spills during industrial production [64]. The amount of knowledge currently known on how nanoparticles influence the soil microbial population is insufficient. According to Haris and Iqbal [21], they may have an impact either directly by altering the bioavailability of other toxins and nutrients or indirectly by interacting with natural organic compounds and potentially harmful organic compounds to either enhance or reduce the toxicity of nanoparticles. According to Rajput et al. [51, 52], free radicals produced by nanoparticles and their ions can harm microbial cell membranes, DNA, and mitochondria, ultimately killing microorganisms. By monitoring soil respiration and enzymatic activity, the effect of nanoparticles on microbial activity may be assessed [64]. Metallic nanoparticles may affect changes in the quantity of soil microorganisms and enzymatic activity in the soil. It was proposed that the toxicity of nanoparticles may be significantly influenced by the kinds of soil. Furthermore, the size and makeup of the soil bacterial population depend greatly on the kind of soil and the toxicity of nanoparticles. Ionized nanoparticles are thought to play a crucial factor in the lethality of both pathogenic and helpful microorganisms.

## *1.3 Metal Oxide Nanoparticles: Beneficial Impacts on Germination, Growth, and Yield in Plants*

The term "plant growth and development" is more inclusive and encompasses all phases of a plant's life, from seed germination through senescence [27]. On the growth and developmental processes of plants, such as seed germination, plant growth, and physiology, nanoparticles have been observed to have either positive or negative effects. The effects of metal and metal oxide nanoparticles on plant development have been researched by a number of research teams and have been shown to be positive, negative, and neutral [72, 29]. This might be because of variables including particle size, concentration, physicochemical characteristics, and plant species type. The primary way that metal oxide nanoparticles have an influence on plant growth and development is through increasing or decreasing germination, shoot and root development, biomass production, and biochemical and physiological activities [56, 79].

Additionally, it has been discovered that nanoparticles may be used as nano fertilizers and nano pesticides for nutrient management, plant growth stimulation, genetic enhancement, and disease therapy. The micronutrients for plant growth are provided by nanoparticles in the form of nano fertilizer, while nano pesticides are used to stop insect attacks on crops, reducing agricultural loss. Numerous metals act as micronutrients for plant development, and, as a result, metal nanoparticles have been shown to be beneficial in encouraging plant growth. As growth-promoting compounds for plants, metal oxide nanoparticles are favored above other types of metal nanoparticles. This is due to the simplicity with which they may disperse the metals as micronutrients close to the plant roots, making it simple for the plants to absorb them and carry out additional metabolism [45]. Since many goods that are discharged into the environment contain MONPs, it is important to research how these nanoparticles affect plant physiology and biochemistry. Studies have revealed that NPs have an influence on the physiological and biochemical characteristics of plants in both good and negative ways.

### 1.3.1 Effect on Seed Germination

Depending on the size of the NP, the plant type, and the exposure amount, NPs can either favorably or adversely affect seed germination [57]. Numerous research on seed germination have demonstrated that NP size has an impact on phytotoxicity, the more toxic NPs are to plants, the smaller they are. $TiO_2$ NPs can improve the development of seedlings and shoots at concentrations of 2 and 10 mg/L, respectively [78]. Brassica nigra seed germination and seedling development may be severely inhibited by CuO NPs. The germination of maize and ryegrass seeds was shown to be inhibited by ZnO and Zn NPs when seeds were soaked in 2000 mg/L prior to incubation. As Ag NPs' size increased, the amount of seed germination dropped. However, Yasur and Rani [76] found that Ag NPs (up to 4000 mg/L) had no impact on castor bean (*Ricinus communis* L.) seed germination.

### 1.3.2 Effect on Plant Growth and Root Elongation

MONPs change biochemical, physiological, and genetic features while also being phytotoxic, inhibiting plant development. Reduced root elongation, reduced root biomass, reduced leaf development, decreased yield, and delayed blooming are all symptoms of growth inhibition-related phytotoxicity [69]. NPs have the potential to be employed as nano fertilizers, nano pesticides, and growth stimulators in addition to having detrimental impacts on plant development. For instance, when Arabidopsis thaliana was exposed to a low dose of Ag NPs (2.5 mg/L), plant growth was greatly boosted; yet, when exposed to a larger dose (5 mg/L), plant growth was significantly lowered. Similar to this, wheat plants grew faster thanks to Cu NPs' facilitation of the tri-carboxylic acid cycle, glycolysis, and starch degradation [55].

According to reports, ZnO and $TiO_2$ nanoparticles promote plant development by enhancing nutrient and other necessary element intake. Similar to this, the root apex is discovered to be the most sensitive zone and is the major target of several NPs. According to a study by [32], $Al_2O_3$ NPs were found to decrease root elongation in *Triticum aestivum* (wheat) by 40% (5 mg/ml) and 55% (50 mg/ml), while nZVI (zero valet-iron) increased root elongation by 150–200% by encouraging the OH radical to stimulate the loosening of cell wall. Chickpea and soybean root development is said to be reduced by CuO NPs [75]. Furthermore, maize plants' root development and biomass were unaffected by ZnO NPs at concentrations of 400 and 800 mg/kg, although root elongation in maize and rice has been shown to be inhibited at a higher dose of 2000 mg/L [74].

### 1.3.3 Effect on Pigment Content and Photosynthetic Activity

Terrestrial plants' pigmentation and photosynthetic activity may be influenced by MONPs. In maize (Zea maize), $TiO_2$ NPs increased the pigment content and photosynthesis throughout the reproductive stage. Mung bean (*Vigna radiata L.)* showed adverse effects on the photosynthetic activity and pigment content when exposed to 100 mg/L of CuO NPs for 21 days (Tan et al. 2018a). Similar to ZnO NPs, ZnO NPs (24 3 nm) at 800 mg/kg might decrease photosynthesis and chlorophyll content, while at 400 mg/kg there were no impacts. $Fe_2O_3$ (6 nm) did, however, speed up the photosynthetic rate in *Glycine max.* The production of chlorophyll and photosynthesis was also decreased by Ag NPs in the marine diatom *Thalassiosira weissflogii.* Mn NP solution incubated mung bean (*Vigna radiata*) seedlings demonstrated increased growth and photosynthetic activity [34]. Metal oxide nanoparticles can either positively or negatively affect plants (Table 2).

**Table 2** Metal oxide nanoparticles and their effect on plants [37]

| Metal oxide nanoparticles | Effect on plants |
|---|---|
| Iron oxide nanoparticles | Harms aquaporins<br>*Cucurbita pepo* exhibits cytotoxicity |
| Silver oxide nanoparticles | It causes oxidative stress by causing cells to produce ROS. It causes the electron relay center to malfunction and initiates the synthesis of secondary quinones. It also degrades pigments involved in photosynthetic processes, inhibits electron transport, and throws off the biochemical balance by lowering carbohydrate stores. It also causes chromosomal damage and genotoxicity, which affects the proteome |
| Zinc oxide nanoparticles | It produces ROS within cells, which is harmful to cells and interferes with the expression of genes involved in development. Moreover, it causes cell membranes to become unstable |
| Calcium oxide nanoparticles | It strengthens the biotic stress response of plants and improves nutrition |
| Magnesium oxide nanoparticles | It has several advantages, such as strong antibacterial properties, affordability, nontoxicity, enhanced stability under challenging processing circumstances, and use in a range of sectors |

## 1.4 Metal Oxide Nanoparticles: Beneficial Impacts on Physiological Properties in Plants

### 1.4.1 Iron Oxide Nanoparticles

Due to their powerful magnetic characteristics, iron oxide nanoparticles ($Fe_2O_3$ NPs) are currently receiving a lot of interest from experts all over the world. Rui et al. [58] investigated the efficacy of $Fe_2O_3$ NPs as fertilizer to replace conventional Fe fertilizers, which have a number of drawbacks, in light of these facts. The biomass, chlorophyll content, and total Fe content of peanut plants—a crop that is extremely vulnerable to Fe deficiency—were shown to rise after the addition of $Fe_2O_3$ NPs to the soil. Bombin et al. [7] investigated the impact of positive and negative charged $Fe_2O_3$ NPs at low and high concentrations on the physiology and reproductive ability of A. thaliana. Low concentration-treated plants did not exhibit any appreciable changes in seeding or root length. However, the 25 mg/L treatment decreased the length of the seedlings and the roots. Additionally, a treatment with $Fe_2O_3$ NPs at 3 mg/L resulted in an increase of about 5% in pollen that was aborted, a decrease of 2–6% in pollen viability, and an increase of up to 11% in seed output, depending on the number of treatments. Surprisingly, there were no discernible phenotypic alterations in the general size or structure of the treated plants. This suggests that nanoparticle contamination of the environment may go potentially undetected, which is a cause for alarm. Using a drop of Fe-enriching hematite ($Fe_2O_3$) nanoparticle dispersion, Boutchuen et al. [8] presented a new modified seed presoak technique to increase growth and production in four distinct legume species, including chickpea, green gram, black bean, and red bean. Because of this, it was claimed that this treatment increased plant growth by around 230–830%, with green gram exhibiting the greatest rise. According to Palchoudhury et al. [44], $Fe_2O_3$ NPs can increase root development in legumes by 88–366% at low concentrations. A larger concentration of $Fe_2O_3$ NPs (27.7 mg/L Fe) and hybrid Pt-decorated $Fe_2O_3$ NPs, however, were shown to inhibit root development. This study claims to accurately forecast the huge potential of $Fe_2O_3$ NPs as nano fertilizers because the increase in plant development with $Fe_2O_3$ NPs was seen for many different seed types [48].

### 1.4.2 Silver Oxide Nanoparticles

According to Godfray et al. [18], fungus infections in crop plants result in lower output and significant financial loss. Fungicides that are easily accessible are frequently employed to prevent such agricultural losses. But these fungicides also prevent the growth of helpful organisms, which causes environmental contamination. Therefore, other treatments must be created to stop the spread of dangerous fungus. In this context, silver nanoparticles (Ag NPs) have been shown to be effective against a variety of bacteria and fungi that cause plant diseases. For instance, Ag NPs has reportedly demonstrated antifungal efficacy against *Magnaporthe grisea* and *Bipolaris sorokiana* [26]. On the other hand, *Magnaporthe oryzae* and *Agrobacterium tumefaciens* both exhibited dose-dependent antifungal activity in response to Ag NPs.

Through irrigation, certain soil-born fungus proliferate across the soil ecosystem. As a result, they may readily spread infection to the roots and other plant sections. According to a study led by Mishra et al. [39], foliar application of green synthesized Ag NPs can be effective against soil-borne fungus. *Sclerotium rolfsii*, the cause of chickpea collar rot, *Rhizoctonia solani*, which causes wire stem, root, and collar rot in plants, *Fusarium graminearum*, which causes head blight in wheat and barley, and *Fusarium udum*, which causes wilt disease in pea plants, were all reported to be inhibited by it. Ag NPs have strong antibacterial action in addition to antifungal activity. Because they are very efficient against both Gram positive and Gram negative bacteria, Ag NPs are often favored against bacterial infections. It was discovered that the evenly scattered Ag NPs bind to bacterial surfaces and activate their bactericidal action. At a 400 g/mL concentration, Ag NPs stopped the metabolism of bacterial cells and their capacity to adhere to surfaces. Similar to this, Bacillus cereus produced Ag NPs with a diameter range of 18 to 39 nm, and it was discovered that these Ag NPs inhibited the development of *X. oryzae* [2]. Worldwide, more than 200 plant species, including tomato, potato, olives, and banana, are affected by the bacterial wilt caused by R. solanacearum. According to reports, the biogenic Ag NPs made from *Lantana camara* L. flower extract inhibit the development of this bacteria. Ag NPs also prevent the development of biofilms, inhibit swimming motion, harm cell membranes, and trigger the production of reactive oxygen species (ROS) [13, 73].

### 1.4.3 Zinc Oxide Nanoparticles

Zn is a crucial micronutrient for plant growth and development that regulates the structure, activity, and function of several enzymes [9]. It is widely established in the literature that ZnO NPs promote plant growth and biomass output. For example, Umar et al. (2020) assessed the impact of ZnO NPs applied to the foliar and soil on the growth and development of maize plants and found that the plants' growth, yield, and Zn content had increased. When ZnO NPs were applied topically while the plants were being developed, the fresh weight of the shoot increased by 31% in comparison to the control plants.

Plants treated with ZnO NPs by foliar and soil treatments had higher chlorophyll levels than control plants by 2.6 and 5.2%, respectively. Furthermore, it was shown that, in comparison to control, soil and foliar treatment increased the cob weight by 61 and 51%, respectively. However, Subbaiah et al. [67] looked at the impact of ZnO NPs on the growth and development of maize at concentrations ranging from 50 to 2000 ppm. According to the results, ZnO NPs (1500 ppm) significantly increased the seedling vigor index and germination percentage (80%). Additionally, it was shown that while $ZnSO_4$ totally inhibited seed germination at the same dosage, much greater doses of ZnO NPs (2000 ppm) did not. With ZnO NPs (400 ppm), the highest grain production was 3298 kg/ha.

### 1.4.4 Calcium Oxide Nanoparticles

For development, photosynthesis, stress reduction, and hormone regulation in plants, calcium is essential. Additionally, it is essential for a number of physiological and metabolic processes in plants. Metal oxide nanoparticles are a more effective resource than metal oxide salts in order to enhance the biological roles of numerous species [40]. Nazir et al. [42] looked into the beneficial effects of CaO NPs in reducing the toxicity caused by arsenic stress in the two genotypes of barley (LJZ and Pu-9). They showed that the exogenous application of calcium oxide nanoparticles to both genotypes of barley reduced the harmful effects of As stress, improved plant development, chlorophyll content, and MDA (malondialdehyde) levels, and decreased ROS (reactive oxygen species) generation [62]. Another research on the exogenous use of calcium oxide nanoparticles in reducing cadmium (Cd)-induced oxidative stress in barley seedlings was published by Nazir et al. [43] in the year prior. They discovered that CaO NPs increase photosynthetic rate, antioxidant enzyme activity, plant biomass, and levels of non-enzymatic antioxidants (glutathione and ascorbate), which results in a decrease in $H_2O_2$ (hydrogen peroxide) and MDA in barley seedlings when applied exogenously. The same year, Khalaf and his coworkers demonstrated the function of calcium oxide nanoparticles in Lupinus termis plants grown under cadmium stress, which led to an increase in antioxidant enzyme activity, such as CAT and peroxidase (POD), and an increase in Cd stress tolerance, as well as a decrease in total soluble carbohydrate content in Lupinus plants.

### 1.4.5 Magnesium Oxide Nanoparticles

Magnesium oxide nanoparticles (MgO NPs) have a number of benefits, including biocompatibility, nontoxicity, and affordability, increased stability under difficult processing conditions, potent antibacterial capabilities, and use in a variety of industries. Recent research has shown that MgO NPs have a potent inhibitory effect on the bacteria and fungi that cause phytopathology. MgO NPs made from chamomile flower extract have demonstrated inhibitory action against the bacterial strain of brown stripe disease that affects rice, A. oryzae strain RS-2 [10, 1]. MgO NPs produced from *Rosmarinus officinalis* flowers were assessed by Abdallah et al. (2019) for their antibacterial effectiveness against *X. oryzae* pv. oryzae. But at substantially lower doses, MgO NPs displayed stronger antibacterial action against R. solanacearum. Additionally, MgO NPs (26.74 nm) at doses of 15.36 g/mL fully prevented *F. oxysporum f. sp. lycopersici's* mycelial development, demonstrating effective antifungal action. Regarding the treatment of tobacco black shank and root black rot diseases, MgO NPs may be regarded as one of the cutting-edge substitutes for chemical fungicides. *Phytophthora nicotianae* and *Thielaviopsis basicola*, two soil-borne diseases, were particularly susceptible to the antifungal effects of MgO NPs. It was noted that MgO NPs demonstrated full sporicidal activity and inhibited fungal invasion at a concentration of 500 g/mL [12]. MgO NPs at concentrations of

2, 3, and 100% decreased *A. flavus* growth, whereas MgO NPs at concentrations of 1% inhibited 95% of fungal growth [25].

## 1.5 Conclusions and Future Perspectives

Nanotechnology has demonstrated exciting uses in a variety of fields. However, the use of nanotechnology in the agricultural industry is essential to sustainable development. Numerous kinds of nanoparticles have proven beneficial for this purpose. Some metals and metal oxides are utilized as micronutrients to aid in the development of plants. They can be absorbed by plants when combined with soil. Along the same lines, the respective metal and metal oxide nanoparticles might be beneficial for plant development. The benefit of utilizing nanoparticles of the appropriate metals and metal oxides is that they have a greater effect with a less amount. These nanoparticles can aid in the development of plants. Forest tree extracts are one of the many precursors that may be used in the quick and environmentally friendly synthesis of nanoparticles (NPs). These extracts are becoming more and more known for their potential in the manufacture of NPs. Green synthesis is a simple, economical, and ecologically sustainable method. Forest trees are especially useful for NP production since they are rich providers of phytochemicals and essential carbon sinks. The process, the kind, and concentration of the extract, the reducing agents used, the pH, the incubation period, the temperature, and the amount of light all affect the characteristics and uses of synthesized NPs. The broad range of applications for which NPs generated from different forest tree species have shown promise is indicative of the increased interest in using natural products—in particular, secondary metabolites from different forest tree species—for NP synthesis in recent years. Crop yields are becoming a major source of worry due to the huge production, unrestricted usage of nanoparticles in nano-enabled goods, and their uncontrolled release into ecosystems. When nanoparticles are present in soils, they can readily and quickly infiltrate the intracellular milieu of plant systems due to their nano-size, increased surface area, reactivity, and surface charge. After entrance, the nano-specific characteristics that make nanoparticles so unique and potent might harm human health and agricultural crops through trophic transfer. Nanoparticles ingested by plants (via stomata and roots) bio-accumulate or are transported to different plant organs, such as fruits and grains, as well as subcellular compartments. Some nanoparticles have the potential to influence crop growth, development, and yield, making them ideal for use in agricultural practices. On the other hand, if they are employed in excess of a specific concentration, they may have an impact on the soil ecology, which would therefore limit the growth of both soil microbes and the plants themselves. Therefore, before using nanoparticles for any purpose, it is important to take into account their negative impacts. Collaboration in the fields of material science, plant biology, and toxicity is required for the best utilization of metal oxide nanoparticles for plant growth. The study should concentrate on how to employ nanoparticles most effectively while having the fewest negative consequences on the environment and human health.

## References


1. Abdel-Aziz MM, Emam TM, Elsherbiny EA (2020) Bioactivity of magnesium oxide nanoparticles synthesized from cell filtrate of endobacterium Burkholderia rinojensis against Fusarium oxysporum. Mater Sci Eng 109:110617
2. Ahmed T, Shahid M, Noman M, Niazi MB, Mahmood F, Manzoor I, Zhang Y, Li B, Yang Y, Yan C, Chen J (2020) Silver nanoparticles synthesized by using Bacillus cereus SZT1 ameliorated the damage of bacterial leaf blight pathogen in rice. Pathogens 9(3):160
3. Al-Halafi AM (2014) Nanocarriers of nanotechnology in retinal diseases. Saudi J Ophthalmol 28(4):304–309
4. An J, Zhang M, Wang S, Tang J (2008) Physical, chemical and microbiological changes in stored green asparagus spears as affected by coating of silver nanoparticles-PVP. LWT-Food Sci Technol 41(6):1100–1107
5. Anjum NA, Gill SS, Duarte AC (2013) Silver nanoparticles in soil–plant systems. J Nanopart Res 15:1896
6. Bergeson LL (2010) Nano silver: US EPA's pesticide office considers how best to proceed. Environ Qual Manage 19(3):79–85
7. Bombin S, LeFebvre M, Sherwood J (2015) Developmental and reproductive effects of iron oxide nanoparticles in Arabidopsis thaliana. Int J Mol Sci 16:24174–24193
8. Boutchuen A, Zimmerman D, Aich N (2019) Increased plant growth with hematite nanoparticle fertilizer drop and determining nanoparticle uptake in plants using multimodal approach. J Nanomater: 6890572
9. Brown PH, Cakmak I, Zhang Q (1993) Form and function of zinc plants. In: Zinc in soils and plants, Proceedings of the international symposium on zinc in soils and plants, the University of Western Australia (ed. A.D. Robson). Springer, The Netherlands, pp 93–106
10. Cai L, Chen J, Liu Z (2018) Magnesium oxide nanoparticles: effective agricultural antibacterial agent against Ralstonia solanacearum. Front Microbiol 9. https://doi.org/10.3389/fmicb.2018.00790
11. Chen H (2018) Metal based nanoparticles in agricultural system: behavior, transport, and interaction 591 with plants. Chem Spec Bioavailab 30(1):123–134
12. Chen J, Wu L, Lu M (2020) Comparative study on the fungicidal activity of metallic MgO nanoparticles and macroscale MgO against soil borne fungal phytopathogens. Front Microbiol 11
13. Cheng HJ, Wang H, Zhang JZ (2020) Phytofabrication of silver nanoparticles using three flower extracts and their antibacterial activities against pathogen Ralstonia solanacearum strain YY06 of bacterial wilt. Front Microbiol 11:2110
14. Chouhan PN, Azimov A, Jabborova D, Singh S (2023) Review on the role of indigenous plants and plant derivatives of Ayurveda in bone healing. Plant Science Today 10(sp2):143–151
15. De Lange O, Klavins E, Nemhauser J (2018) Synthetic genetic circuits in crop plants. Curr Opin Biotechnol 49:16–22
16. Elmer PAG, Spiers TM, Wood PN (2007) Effects of pre-harvest foliar calcium sprays on fruit calcium levels and brown rot of peaches. Crop Prot 26(1):11–18
17. FAO, WHO, (2010) Food and Agriculture Organization of the United Nations/World Health Organization: FAO/WHO Expert meeting on the application of nanotechnologies in the food and agriculture sectors: potential food safety implications. Meeting report, Rome
18. Godfray HCJ, Mason-D'Croz D, Robinson S (2016) Food system consequences of a fungal disease epidemic in a major crop. Philos Trans R Soc B: Biol Sci 371:20150467
19. Golinska P, Wypij M, Ingle AP (2014) Biogenic synthesis of metal nanoparticles from actinomycetes: biomedical applications and cytotoxicity. Appl Microbiol Biotechnol 98(19):8083–8097
20. Gupta G, Paul S, Singh S, Pietramellara G, Pathan SI, Danish S, Jha PN (2022) Exploring functional diversity and community structure of diazotrophic endophytic bacteria associated with Pennisetum glaucum growing under field in a semi-arid region. Land 11(7):991

21. Haris Z, Iqbal A (2017) Impact of metal oxide nanoparticles on beneficial soil microorganisms and their secondary metabolites. Int J Life Sci Scienti Res 3(3):1020–1030
22. Hasan MM, Gong L, Nie Z, Feng L, Ahammed GJ, Fang XW (2021) ABA-induced stomatal movements in vascular plants during dehydration versus rehydration. Environ Exp Bot 186:104436
23. Hasan MM, Skalicky M, Jahan MS, Hossain MN, Anwar Z, Nie ZF, Alabdallah NM, Brestic M, Hejnak V, Fang XW, Spermine (2021) Its emerging role in regulating drought stress responses in plants. Cells 10:261
24. Husen A, Jawaid M (eds) (2020) Nanomaterials for agriculture and forestry applications. Elsevier
25. Hussein HZ, Wahbe AA (2020) Assessing the efficacy of certain nano, natural and chemical materials in fungal inhibition and afb1 toxin reduction of Aspergillus flavus isolated from peanut on PDA media. Plant Archives 20:1051–1057
26. Jo YK, Kim BH, Jung G (2009) Antifungal activity of silver ions and nanoparticles on phytopathogenic fungi. Plant Dis 93(10):1037–1043
27. Kanwar MK, Sun S, Chu X, Zhou J (2019) Impacts of metal and metal oxide nanoparticles on plant growth and productivity. In: Nano materials and Plant Potential (eds. A. Husen and M. Iqbal). Springer, Cham
28. Keller S, McFerran A, Lazareva S, Suh (2013) Global life cycle releases of engineered nanomaterials. J Nanopart Res 15:1–17
29. Khan MR, Adam V, Rizvi TF (2019a) Nanoparticle-plant interactions: two-way traffic. Small 15(37)
30. Khare P, Kishore K, Sharma DK (2017) A study on the standardization parameters of Cassia Angustifolia. Asian J Pharm Clin Res 10(7):329–332
31. Khare P, Kishore K, Sharma DK, Khare N (2024) Investigation of memory enhancing activity of combination extracts of Bauhinia variegata and Madhuca longifolia leaves against Colchicine: An experimental study and biochemical alterations in mice. Ind J Pharm Edu Res 58(1s):s282–s288
32. Kim JH, Lee Y, Kim EJ, Gu S, Sohn EJ, Seo YS, An HJ, Chang YS (2014) Exposure of iron nanoparticles to Arabidopsis thaliana enhances root elongation by triggering cell wall loosening. Environ Sci Technol 48(6):3477–3485
33. Koçak R, Okcu M, Haliloğlu K, Türkoğlu A, Pour-Aboughadareh A, Jamshidi B, Janda T, Alaylı A, Nadaroğlu H (2023) Magnesium oxide nanoparticles: An influential element in cowpea (Vigna unguiculata L. Walp.) tissue culture. Agronomy 13(6):1646
34. Liu W, Zeb A, Lian J, Wu J, Xiong H, Tang J, Zheng S (2020) Interactions of metal-based and metal-oxide-based nanoparticles (MBNPs and MONPs) with crop plants: A critical review of research progress and prospects. Environ Rev 28:294–310
35. Maddala VKS, Singh S, Bandi J (2024) Soil properties influencing nutrient signaling in plant soil systems. In: Essential minerals in plant-soil systems. Elsevier, pp 373–393
36. Manganaris GA, Vasilakakis M, Diamantidis G, Mignani I (2005) Effect of calcium additives on physicochemical aspects of cell wall pectin and sensory attributes of canned peach (Prunus persica (L) Batsch cv Andross). J Sci Food Agric 85(10):1773–1778
37. Manna I, Bandyopadhyay M (2018) Physicochemical perturbation of plants on exposure to metal oxide nanoparticle
38. Meddya S, Meshram S, Sarkar D, Datta R, Singh S, Avinash G, Thulasinathan T (2023) Plant stomata: An unrealized possibility in plant defense against invading pathogens and stress tolerance. Plants 12(19):3380
39. Mishra S, Singh BR, Naqvi AH, Singh HB (2017) Potential of biosynthesized silver nanoparticles using Stenotrophomonas sp. BHU-S7 (MTCC 5978) for management of soil-borne and foliar phytopathogens. Scientific Reports 7:45154
40. Modi G, Sharma B, Arora B, Shivani S, Bhardwaj N (2023) Evaluation Of calcium oxide nanoparticles to enhance heavy metal stress tolerance in plants. Int J Adv Agric Sci Technol 10:28–45

41. Mohammadi R, Maali-Amiri R, Mantri NL (2014) Effect of $TiO_2$ nanoparticles on oxidative damage and antioxidant defense systems in chickpea seedlings during cold stress. Russ J Plant Physiol 61:768–775
42. Nazir MM, Li Q, Noman M, Ulhassan Z, Ali S, Ahmed T (2022) Calcium oxide nanoparticles have the role of alleviating arsenic toxicity of barley. Front Plant Sci 13:843795–843795
43. Nazir MM, Noman M, Ahmed T, Ali S, Ulhassan Z, Zeng F (2022) Exogenous calcium oxide nanoparticles alleviate cadmium toxicity by reducing Cd uptake and enhancing antioxidative capacity in barley seedlings. J Hazard Mater 438:129498
44. Palchoudhury S, Jungjohann KL, Weerasena L (2018) Enhanced legume root growth with pre-soaking in alpha-$Fe_2O_3$ nanoparticle fertilizer. RSC Adv 8:24075–24083
45. Panakkal H, Gupta I, Bhagat R, Ingle AP (2021) Effects of different metal oxide nanoparticles on plant growth. Nanotechnol Plant Growth Promot Prot: Recent Adv Impacts:259–282
46. Parveen R, Khare N, Singh S, Johri P (2023) An in silico outlook for the detection and surveillance of evolving and persistent plant pathogens. In: Detection, diagnosis and management of soil-borne phytopathogens. Springer Nature Singapore, Singapore, pp 17–40
47. Patani A, Patel A, Prajapati D, Khare N, Singh S (2023) Various agriculture crop plant-based bioactive compounds and their use in nanomaterial synthesis and applications. In: Nanomaterials from agricultural and horticultural products. Springer Nature Singapore, Singapore, pp 223–241
48. Patani A, Prajapati D, Shukla K, Patel M, Patani P, Patel A, Singh S (2024) Environmental stress–induced alterations in the micro-and macronutrients status of plant. In: Essential minerals in plant-soil systems. Elsevier, pp 181–195
49. Rai M, Yadav A, Gade A (2009) Silver nanoparticles as a new generation of antimicrobials. Biotechnol Adv 27(1):76–83
50. Rajapaksha AU, Ahmad M, Vithanage M, Kim KR, Chang JY, Lee SS, Ok YS (2015) The role of biochar, natural iron oxides, and nanomaterials as soil amendments for immobilizing metals in shooting range soil. Environ Geochem Health 37:931–942
51. Rajput VD, Minkina T, Suskova S (2017a) Effect of nanoparticles on crops and soil microbial communities. J Soils Sediments:1–9
52. Rajput VD, Minkina T, Suskova S, Mandzhieva S, Tsitsuashvili V, Chapligin V, Fedorenko A (2017) Effects of copper nanoparticles (CuO NPs) on crop plants: a mini review. Bio Nano Science. 8:36–42
53. Rajput VD, Minkina TM, Behal A, Sushkova SN, Mandzhieva S, Singh R, Movsesyan HS (2018) Effects of zinc-oxide nanoparticles on soil, plants, animals and soil organisms: A review. Environ Nanotechnol, Monit Manag 9:76–84
54. Rajput VD, Tstitsuashvili VS, Sushkova SN, Nevidomskaya DG (2017c) Effects of ZnO and CuO nanoparticles on soil, plant and microbial community. In: International scientific conference XX Dokoutchaev Youth Readings, St. Petersburg, Russia, p 12
55. Rastogi A, Zivcak M, Sytar O, Kalaji HM, He X, Mbarki S, Brestic M (2017) Impact of Metal and Metal Oxide Nanoparticles on Plant: A Critical Review. Front Chem 5:78
56. Rizwan M, Ali S, Ali B (2019) Zinc and iron oxide nanoparticles improved the plant growth and reduced the oxidative stress and cadmium concentration in wheat. Chemosphere 214:269–277
57. Rizwan M, Ali S, Qayyum MF, Ok YS, Adrees M, Ibrahim M, Zia-ur-Rehman M, Farid M, Abbas F (2017) Effect of metal and metal oxide nanoparticles on growth and physiology of globally important food crops: A critical review. J Hazard Mater 322:2–16
58. Rui M, Ma C, Hao Y (2016) Iron oxide nanoparticles as a potential iron fertilizer for peanut (Arachis hypogaea). Front Plant Sci 7:815
59. Safiuddin M, Gonzalez M, Cao J, Tighe SL (2014) State-of-the-art report on use of nanomaterials in concrete. Int J Pavement Eng 15(10):940–949
60. Sanchez-Dominguez M, Boutonnet M, Solans C (2009) A novel approach to metal and metal oxide nanoparticle synthesis: the oilin- water microemulsion reaction method. J Nanoparticle Res 11:1823–1829
61. Santos CAD, Seckler MM, Ingle AP (2014) Silver nanoparticles: therapeutical uses, toxicity, and safety issues. J Pharm Sci 103(7):1931–1944

62. Sao P, Parveen R, Khattri A, Sharma S, Tiwari N, Singh S (2022) Understanding the metabolomics of medicinal plants under environmental pollution: Challenges and opportunities. environmental pollution and medicinal plants, pp 193–205
63. Sheykhbaglou R, Sedghi M, Shishevan MT, Sharifi RS (2010) Effects of nano-iron oxide particles on agronomic traits of soybean. Notulae Scientia Biologicae 2(2):112–123
64. Simonin M, Richaume A (2015) Impact of engineered nanoparticles on the activity, abundance, and diversity of soil microbial communities: a review. Environ Sci Pollut Res 22:13710–13723
65. Singh A, Sengar RS, Singh AK, Singh S, Kumar A, Ahmad K (2019) Impact of genetic engineering on agriculture food crops. Biotech Today: Int J Biol Sci 9(1):17–24
66. Singh R, Sharma RR, Tyagi SK (2007) Pre-harvest foliar application of calcium and boron influences physiological disorders, fruit yield and quality of strawberry (Fragaria× ananassa Duch.) Sci Hortic 112(2):215–220
67. Subbaiah LV, Prasad TNVKV, Krishna TG (2016) Novel effects of nanoparticulate delivery of zinc on growth, productivity, and zinc biofortification in Maize (Zea mays L.). J Agric Food Chem 64(19):3778–3788
68. Suriyaprabha R, Karunakaran G, Yuvakkumar R, Prabu P, Rajendran V, Kannan N (2012) Growth and physiological responses of maize (Zea mays L.) to porous silica nanoparticles in soil. J Nanopart Res 14:1–4
69. Tripathi DK, Shweta Singh S, Singh S, Pandey R, Singh VP, Sharma NC, Prasad SM, Dubey NK, Chauhan DK (2017) An overview on manufactured nanoparticles in plants: Uptake, translocation, accumulation and phytotoxicity. Plant Physiol Biochem 110:2–12
70. Tungare K, Shahu R, Zambare V, Agarwal P, Jobby R, Nisar N, & Jha P. (2022). Toxicity mitigation of textile dye reactive blue 4 by hairy roots of Helianthus annuus and testing its effect in in vivo model systems. Biomed Res Int
71. Verma N, Sao P, Srivastava A, Singh S (2021) Physiological and molecular responses to drought, submergence and excessive watering in plants. Harsh Environ Plant Resil: Mol Funct Asp:305–321
72. Verma SK, Das AK, Patel MK (2018) Engineered nanomaterials for plant growth and development: a perspective analysis. Sci Total Environ 630:1413–1435
73. Vishwakarma SK, Ilyas T, Shahid M, Malviya D, Kumar S, Singh S, Singh HV (2024) Bacillus spp.: Nature's gift to agriculture and humankind. In: Applications of bacillus and bacillus derived genera in agriculture, biotechnology and beyond. Springer Nature Singapore, Singapore, pp 1–36
74. Yang Z, Chen J, Dou R, Gao X, Mao C, Wang L (2015) Assessment of the phytotoxicity of metal oxide nanoparticles on two crop plants, Maize (Zea mays L.) and Rice (Oryza sativa L.). 1160 Int J Env Res Public Health 12(12):15100–15109
75. Yanik F, Vardar F (2015) Toxic effects of Aluminum Oxide ($Al_2O_3$) nanoparticles on root growth and development in Triticum Aestivum. Water Air Soil Pollut 226(9)
76. Yasur J, Rani PU (2013) Environmental effects of nanosilver: impact on castor seed germination, seedling growth, and plant physiology. Environ Sci Pollut Res 20(12):8636–8648
77. Ye L, Li L, Wang L, Wang S, Li S, Du J (2015) MPK3/MPK6 are involved in iron deficiency-induced ethylene production in Arabidopsis. Front Plant Sci 6:953
78. Zafar H, Ali A, Zia M (2016) CuO nanoparticles inhibited root growth from brassica nigra seedlings but induced root from stem and leaf explants. Appl Biochem Biotechnol 181
79. Zhao L, Lu L, Wang A (2020) Nanobiotechnology in agriculture: use of nanomaterials to promote plant growth and stress tolerance. J Agric Food Chem 68(7):1935–1947
80. Zhou X, Torabi M, Lu J, Shen R, Zhang K (2014) Nanostructured energetic composites: synthesis, ignition/combustion modeling, and applications. ACS Appl Mater Interfaces 6(5):3058–3074

# Pest and Disease Management

# Insights into Defense Mechanisms of Engineered Nanoparticles for Management of Insect Pests and Pathogens

**Sushmita Thokchom, Arindam Pal, Alagesan Keerthana, Priya, Deepika Jeengar, Vyshnavi Sunil, Vinod Kumar Dubey, Sabuj Ganguly, Arati Ningombam, and Laishram Santhalembi**

**Abstract** Nanoparticles have revolutionized agriculture due to their unique properties and paved the way for several branches including pests and disease management. Engineered Nanoparticles (ENPs) can be classified based on their ability to boost the immunity of plants, management of diseases and pests, etc. In this chapter, we discuss the mechanisms and interactions between nanoparticles, pests, and pathogens. How nanoparticles interfere with the defense of plants and immune systems fascinated scientists for a long time. Gold nanoparticles have some negative plant interactions, whereas $TiO_2$NPs have a positive effect on plants and chitosan imparts resistance.

---

S. Thokchom
Department of Entomology, Assam Agricultural University, Jorhat, Assam, India

A. Pal · Priya
Department of Entomology, Post Graduate College of Agriculture, Dr. Rajendra Prasad Central Agricultural University, Samastipur, Pusa, Bihar, India

A. Keerthana
Department of Entomology, Tamil Nadu Agricultural University, Coimbatore, Tamil Nadu, India

D. Jeengar
Department of Entomology, College of Agriculture, Govind Ballabh Pant University of Agriculture and Technology, Pantnagar, Uttarakhand, India

V. Sunil
Department of Entomology, College of Agriculture, Kerala Agricultural University, Vellayani, Thiruvananthapuram, Kerala, India

V. K. Dubey (✉)
Department of Genetics & Plant Breeding, College of Agriculture, Acharya Narendra Deva University of Agriculture and Technology, Ayodhya, Uttar Pradesh, India
e-mail: vkdubeyento@nduat.org

S. Ganguly
BSM&TC (BTSSO), Central Silk Board, Baripada, Odisha, India

A. Ningombam · L. Santhalembi
ICAR Research Complex for North Eastern Hill Region, Manipur Centre, Lamphelpat, Manipur, India

 
D. Jabborova et al. (eds.), *Nanomaterials in Agroforestry Systems*, Smart Nanomaterials Technology, https://doi.org/10.1007/978-981-96-1337-3_10

The factors related to the host that are responsible for the interaction and development of engineered nanoparticles like host cells, biomembrane, proteins, carbohydrates, nucleic acid, and innate immunity were assessed based on their effect. dsRNA-engineered nanoparticles or vectors are novel strategies in the sustainable management of insect pests and belong to several types, like synthetic polymer-based, inorganic, peptide-based, chitosan-based, quantum dots, and liposomal nanoparticles. Despite multiple advantages, there are still concerns about the nanoparticle's impact on the environment. But in terms of future prospects, nanoparticle-mediated control strategies can reduce pesticidal load, overcome environmental stresses, and increase the stability or effectiveness of pesticides. In this chapter, we have tried to encompass the current understanding related to engineered nanoparticles and their relationship with insect pest and pathogen management.

**Keywords** Nanoparticle types · Immune system · Insect pest control · Disease management · Fate and behavior

## 1 Introduction

Nanotechnology engineering focuses on the development and material refinement which are very small scale to be used in physics, chemistry, biology, medicine, environment, and agriculture. In agriculture, nanotechnology acts as the pioneer technology giving accurate data and helping to increase agriculture productivity [136]. With the help of nanotechnology, nanosensors are being established which help in the detection of microbes at levels as less as parts per billion [113]. Moreover, it has the potential to slow down and target release toward the surface area which is large and can replace chemical pesticides with nano pesticides, nano herbicides, genetically modified plants along with animals with the desirable characteristics, and nano plant growth regulators [58, 128]. Nano clay, alumina-silicate, and silicates are found to be applied in packaging food as layers. A nano enzyme has also use in agriculture and shows brilliant properties of antioxidant, i.e., cerium oxide coated with polyacrylic coated cerium oxide (nanoceria) has an effective scavenging of hydroxyl radicals. As a result, a recent worldwide consideration is being given to a biotechnological approach of nano to controlling reactive oxygen species (ROS) homeostasis in plants, and salt tolerance [78]. Recently, nanoparticle-based biosensors or chemo have been proposed and are being commercialized for diagnosis purposes in agriculture [62, 71].

Depending on the mechanism of transduction of the sensory interactions designed, the analytes can easily be recognized by optical characteristics or nanosensors' electrical outputs. The nanomaterial's physical properties help the smaller particles' melting point to be lower. Sometimes the engineered nanomaterial changes its agglomeration, dissolution, and settling when they are exposed, and it becomes difficult to judge their accuracy and efficiency. In agriculture, the use of engineered nanoparticles in crop production as well as in plant protection is under exploration.

More testing has to be done on target pests and, particularly, non-target toxicity needs more attention [143]. Insect pests are the predominant ones in agriculture,hence engineered nanomaterial helps in controlling host pathogens and insect pests. The interactions of engineered nanoparticles could be destructive or valuable and are highly regarded to be used in pathogen control such as fungicides, insecticides, and bactericides along with fertilizers for enhancing plant health. In this chapter, we have discussed the mechanisms and interactions between nanoparticles, pests, and pathogens and how we can manage them effectively by using nanoparticles.

## 2 Different Types of Engineered Nanoparticles

Engineered nanoparticles (ENPs) are increasingly getting important in agriculture because of their potential to enhance nutrient uptake, plant growth, and stress tolerance. A number of engineered nanoparticles has been discovered for their beneficial properties on plants. The nanoparticles based on metals, such as silver AgNPs and CuNPs are shown to improve the growth of plants and increase biotic and abiotic stress resistance. Another type is metal oxide nanoparticles based on metal oxide, including ZnONPs and $TiO_2$NPs, which have demonstrated efficient nutrient delivery to plants and protection against pathogens [74, 131]. Additionally, carbon-based nanoparticles, CNTs and graphene, carbon black, MWCNT, SWCNT, graphene, carbon nanofibers, and carbon onions have shown promise in enhancing photosynthesis and in improving the overall physiology of plants [137]. Another category includes liposomes, micelles, polymers, and dendrimers which are categorized as organic nanomaterials [122, 126]. These examples illustrate various types of potential ENPs in improving plant health and productivity. Quantum dots, sometimes known as "artificial atoms," are the materials which are nanostructured that have captivated the interest of researchers in the field of agriculture due to their unusual features ranging from optical to electrical [43, 44]. The different types of nanoparticles are described in (Fig. 1).

### *2.1 Types of Engineered Nanoparticles to Boost Immunity in Plants*

Boosting plant immunity using engineered nanoparticles is an emerging tool for research that holds a promising future for enhancing crop resistance against various pathogens and environmental stresses. Several types of engineered nanoparticles have been investigated for their potential immune modulatory effects on plants. For instance, some of the engineered nanoparticles known to enhance the immunity in plants are as follows.

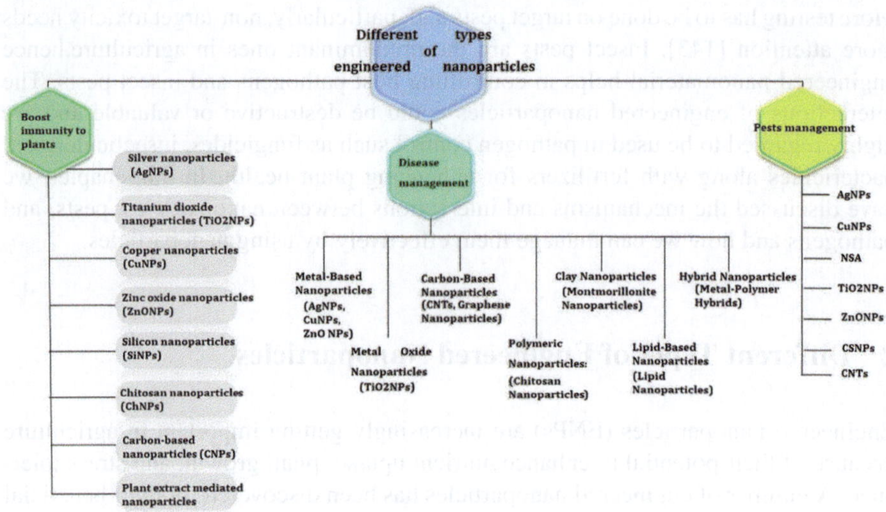


**Fig. 1** Different types of engineered nanoparticles

### 2.1.1 AgNPs

Silver nanoparticles (AgNPs) are extensively studied for having antimicrobial properties. They have been shown to enhance plant immunity by promoting the production of defense-related signaling molecules and proteins, leading to increased resistance against pathogens viz., bacteria, and fungi. Studies have confirmed the efficacy of AgNPs in boosting immunity in crops like rice [146].

### 2.1.2 $TiO_2$NPs

Titanium dioxide ($TiO_2$NPs) nanoparticles have gained attention due to their ability to induce plant defense mechanisms. They can activate the plant's immune system by up-regulating the defense-related gene's expression and enzymes, thereby enhancing resistance against diseases and pests. $TiO_2$ when applied by leaves or roots at lower concentrations was found to improve performance of crop through stimulation of enzymes activity, improving photosynthesis and chlorophyll content, nutrient uptake promotion, stress tolerance strengthening as well as improvement of crop quality, and yield [16].

### 2.1.3 CuNPs

Copper nanoparticles (CuNPs) have been experimented for their potential in combating plant diseases caused by phytopathogens. Copper is known for having antimicrobial properties, and copper-based nanoparticles are used to develop nano pesticides for plant protection. They are considered for their role in inhibiting bacterial and fungal infestations that can threaten crop growth and yield. The interactions between copper nanoparticles and pathogens, as well as their effects on plants, are subjects of research for disease management in plant [61].

### 2.1.4 ZnONPs

Zinc oxide nanoparticles (ZnONPs) are demonstrated as immune modulatory effects on plants by helping to increase the production of ROS and activating antioxidant defense systems. These nanoparticles are shown to give resistance against pathogenic infections in wheat and tomato [110, 130].

### 2.1.5 SiNPs

Silicon nanoparticles (SiNPs) have shown to be beneficial in enhancing plant immunity by inducing the synthesis of defense-related compounds, strengthening the cell wall, and activating plant defense pathways. SiNPs have been utilized to boost the immune response in plants against both abiotic stresses and biotic stresses in resilient agriculture [108].

### 2.1.6 ChNPs

Chitosan nanoparticles (ChNPs) have been deployed for their immune modulatory properties in plants. They can enhance plant resistance by promoting the defense gene's expression and stimulating antimicrobial compound's production. ChNPs have been tested on various crops, including tomato, and finger millet, to develop their immune response against pathogens [53, 114].

### 2.1.7 CNPs

Carbon nanoparticles (CNPs), such as graphene oxide, and carbon nanotubes, have shown potential in boosting plant immunity. These nanoparticles are mentioned to influence the germination of seeds, impact the ratio of shoot-to-root, and affect the growth of seedlings [5, 137]. They can activate defense pathways and improve the defense-related gene's expression, leading to enhanced resistance against pathogens and stressors in crops like *Arabidopsis* and cucumber [41, 69].

#### 2.1.8 Plant Extract-Mediated Nanoparticles

Nanoparticles that are synthesized from plant extracts offer a biologically friendly approach to enhancing plant immunity. Plant-mediated synthesis involves utilizing bioresources to reduce and stabilize metal ions, effectively forming nanoparticles. The nanoparticles that are derived from plant extracts may carry biological properties influenced by the diverse metabolites found in the plants. This approach aims to create nanoparticles that are biocompatible with plant cells and can assist in boosting plant defense against pathogens [1].

## *2.2 Engineered Nanoparticles for Disease Management*

ENPs have gained consideration in recent years for their potential in various fields of agriculture and plant disease management. These nanoparticles can be designed and synthesized to possess specific properties that make them effective in combating plant diseases. Here are some categories of engineered nanoparticles that are explored for plant disease management.

### 2.2.1 Metal-Based Nanoparticles

AgNPs

AgNPs have shown broad-spectrum activity of antimicrobial against pathogens and they can inhibit various plant pathogens' growth by disrupting their cellular structures. Silver nanoparticle is used for the suppression of powdery mildew [64].

CuNPs

CuNPs have been used to control bacterial pathogens and fungi by releasing copper ions that are toxic to microorganisms [105]. Soda-lime glass powder along with CuNPs is antimicrobial to gram-negative and gram-positive fungi, and bacteria.

ZnONPs

ZnONPs possess antimicrobial properties and can be used to control bacterial and fungal diseases in plants [51].

### 2.2.2 Metal Oxide Nanoparticles

$TiO_2$NPs

$TiO_2$NPs have photo-catalytic properties that can contribute to the degradation of pathogens and their spores under UV light exposure [67].

### 2.2.3 Carbon-Based Nanoparticles

CNTs

CNTs can be functionalized with antimicrobial agents or used to deliver bioactive compounds, enhancing their potential for disease management [121].

Graphene Nanoparticles

Graphene and its derivatives have antimicrobial activity and potential for disease management. Graphene oxide has shown bactericidal activity toward bacterium *Xanthomonas oryzae* pv. oryzae [18].

### 2.2.4 Polymeric Nanoparticle

Chitosan Nanoparticles

Chitosan, a natural polymer, can be formulated into nanoparticles with antifungal and antibacterial properties, providing protection against plant pathogens [111].

### 2.2.5 Clay Nanoparticles

Montmorillonite Nanoparticles

These clay nanoparticles have the ability to deliver biopesticides and control parasitic plants and pathogenesis [107].

### 2.2.6 Lipid-Based Nanoparticles

Lipid Nanoparticles

Lipid-based nanoparticles can encapsulate bioactive compounds, such as plant extracts or essential oils, enhancing their stability and efficacy against pathogens [102].

### 2.2.7 Hybrid Nanoparticles

Metal-Polymer Hybrids

Combining metal nanoparticles along with polymers leads to synergistic effects and improved disease management properties [3].

## *2.3 Engineered Nanoparticles for Pest Management*

Different types of engineered nanoparticles used for pest management are summarized in Table 1.

# 3 Innate Immune System and Nanoparticles

When designed ENPs move inside the body, the innate immune system finds them as foreign substances and activates a unique immune response based on their characteristics. Stiffness, size, shape, charge, and hydrophobicity are some of the examples of the physicochemical characteristics that affect how ENPs interact with proteins which are soluble. Neutrophils and APCs in particular have an influence on the downstream signaling that is used to identify pathogens or other immune regulatory processes [36, 81, 91, 100]. Nanoparticles can use the inherent characteristics of monocytes and macrophages for improving their target ability while simultaneously avoiding immune system clearance.

Immune system and nanoparticle interact by affecting neutrophil biomimetic techniques, neutrophil-based drug delivery [140], depleting inflammation-related neutrophils [153], and by modulating neutrophil migration [95]. During inflammation, neutrophils can migrate to lesions which are prevented by designing certain drug-free nanoparticles. When PLG nanoparticles were used to treat mouse models of traumatic primary spinal cord injury (SCI), the amount of neutrophils overall at the injury decreased by four times, and the amount of gliotic scarring and fibrotic against mouse was considerably reduced by three times when compared to the same group

**Table 1** Types of engineered nanoparticles for pest management

| Nanoparticles | Mechanism of action | Targeted insect pests | References |
|---|---|---|---|
| Silver Nanoparticles (AgNPs) | Disrupt cellular membranes, interfere with metabolism | Various insect pests and mosquitoes | [11, 99] |
| Copper Nanoparticles (CuNPs) | Interact with insect cell membranes, biocidal properties | Broad-spectrum insect pests | [22] |
| Nanostructured Alumina (NSA) | Binding on the cuticle and dehydration of the insect | Effective against stored product insect pests | [133] |
| Titanium Dioxide Nanoparticles ($TiO_2$NPs) | Generate reactive oxygen species upon exposure to sunlight | Greenhouse insect pests, crop pests | [46] |
| Zinc Oxide Nanoparticles (ZnONPs) | Penetrate insect cuticle, disrupt cellular processes | Mosquitoes, aphids, fall army worm, and stored product pests | [37, 101, 112] |
| Chitosan Nanoparticles (CSNPs) | Disrupt insect cell membranes, induce apoptosis | Various insect pests | [89] |
| Carbon Nanotubes (CNTs) | Penetrate insect cuticle, physical means of mortality | Various insect pests | [107] |

[95]. Nanoparticles interact with lymphocytes by inducing Th2-related immune tolerance inducing cell expansion of Treg, inducing phenotype tolerogenic in dendritic cells which also induces expansion and differentiation of $FoxP3^+$ Treg cells depleting auto-reactive T cells inhibiting $CD4^+$ T cells, etc.

## 4 How Engineered Nanoparticles Boost the Immune System in Plants

Plants have receptors to sense the invading pathogen which can activate the signaling system to produce the immune response. Receptors of innate immune is present in the plant system intracellular or the plasma membrane which produces a triggered immunity pattern or triggered immunity effector [93]. Many studies based to gold nanoparticle and its exposure to plant growth are reported recently [59]. Spherical gold nanoparticles when treated were not having an effect on barley seed germination, and further deterioration of quality was seen due to gold nanoparticles [30]. When gold nanoparticles enter tobacco plants, they produce toxic symptoms. Epidermal cells were broken and collapsed of cortical cells in barley roots [117].

Numerous investigators have proved that sometimes gold can be gathered, to different degrees, by *Helianthus annuus, Trifolium repens, Brassica juncea,*

*Kalanchoe serratea Sorghum halepense*, *B. campestris,* and *Raphanus sativus* [142]. Spinach growth is accelerated by improved activity of Rubisco activates and increased light absorption due to $TiO_2$NPs [88] whereas in *Ulmus* elongate there growth and it is decelerated by reduced photosynthetic activity [35]. When *Arabidopsis thaliana* leaf cells are exposed to carbon nanoparticles, endocystosis-like structures were formed within the plasma membrane [119]. When *A. thaliana* is treated to gold nanoparticles, the growth, seed germination, and antioxidant metabolic activity are improved [70].

Chitosan is a natural polymer that helps in inducing systemic resistance inside the plants [47]. When chitosan nanoparticles were applied on plant, they increase the accumulation of caffeine, epigallocatechin gallate, gallic acid, epigallocatechin, and epicatechin when compared to the untreated ones. The defense-related gene alterations like thaumatin-like protein (TLP), PAL, β-1, 3-glucanase, and PPO were found in CNP-treated plant cells. CNP showed NO accumulation in treated leaves as compared to control [15].

## *4.1 Interactions*

### 4.1.1 Uptake of ENPs

Usually ENP uptake is hindered in plants by barriers like plasma membrane, cell wall, and cuticle, [115]. ENP can enter the plants either apoplastically or symplastically. *Arabidopsis thaliana* is unable to take up gold nanoparticles of size 4 and 12 nm [31]. AuNPs which are small and positively charged are more efficient than negatively charged and neutral particles [4, 132]. Depending on surface charge, shape, and size, nanoparticles accumulate in the root [68].

### 4.1.2 Effects of AuNPs on Immune Responses

Effect of AuNPs on plants is not by the alteration of receptors but by the environmental factor scavenging or PAMPs that activate responses of defense or clogging of pores [6, 12, 30, 32]. Some studies described increased oxidative stress by AuNPs [42, 123]. Metal response and growth genes were up-regulated, but oxidative stress response gene and immune gene were down-regulated at transcriptome and proteome level [32] indicating the trade-off among immunity and growth are shifted by AuNPs to growth. AuNPs with higher concentration and smaller particle size have injurious effects on plants causing toxicity [124].

# 5 Validation Methods to Boost Engineered Nanoparticles

Engineered nanoparticles are increasingly being developed and adopted in various industries and applications over the few years. However, engineered nanoparticles are found to be associating with potential negative health effects and environmental hazards. These risks must be mitigated through validation methods that are capable of assessing engineered nanoparticles' ability to suppress other nanoparticles, thereby minimizing their unintended releases. So focus on validation methods for evaluating the efficacy of engineered nanoparticles in suppressing engineered nanoparticles is very essential.

## *5.1 Agglomeration*

The agglomeration or aggregation of engineered nanoparticles is the primary mechanism in which nanoparticles suppress one another. As the name implies, aggregation refers to the irreversible formation of large particle clusters, whereas agglomeration refers to the reversible clustering of small particles. Using primary crystallites as blocks of building can facilitate packing of homogenous and rapid sintering. [66] reported that the 3 mol. % yttria-stabilized tetragonal zirconia (3YSZ) which crystallites agglomerated to form secondary particles. By agglomeration, we can suppress the mobility of engineered nanoparticle. A variety of techniques can be used to analyze changes in particle size distribution and determine if there has been agglomeration or aggregation, including (DLS), (NTA), and microscopy.

## *5.2 Sedimentation and Filtration Studies*

ENPs can be evaluated through sedimentation and filtration studies to determine if they settle or are retained by solids. An aggregate's structure influences its fate and behavior, as well as its interaction with contaminants. As aggregates become more porous, and reduces fractal dimension, accelerating faster sedimentation compared to aggregates with advanced fractal dimensions and impermeable spheres [57, 76]. As in natural systems, such as soils and water bodies, these studies simulate the conditions encountered in those systems. The sedimentation or filtration behavior of ENPs is monitored as they are introduced into suspensions or columns. Using sedimentation or filtration to determine whether ENPs can suppress other nanoparticles by facilitating their deposition or retention on solid surfaces can be beneficial.

### 5.3 *Sorption*

As NPs are composed of various properties, including size, purity, structure, pH, and ionic strength, contaminants will be able to attach themselves to them. Compared to materials mainly composed with anatase and additional rutile amount, pure anatase TiO2NPs showed a higher affinity for rutile and with higher sorption of capacity [38]. According to [147] and [19], NP aggregates exhibit adsorption or desorption hysteresis resulting from structural rearrangements of aggregates and finally formation of closed interstitial spaces (which prevent desorption).

### 5.4 *Surface Modification Analysis*

It is essential that engineered nanoparticle surfaces are modified to suppress the interaction of nanoparticles with other nanoparticles. Research into the mechanisms has shown that ENPs bind to and immobilize other nanoparticles that can be gained by studying the surface chemistry and composition of ENPs. Nanoparticle surface modification using polymer surfactant molecules or other modifiers is essential to generating a strong repulsion between them [60]. A variety of techniques can be used to examine the surface properties of ENPs and their potential for suppressing engineered nanoparticles, including (XPS), Fourier-transform infrared spectroscopy (FTIR), and scanning electron microscopy (SEM). These techniques can also be coupled with energy-dispersive X-ray spectroscopy (EDS).

### 5.5 *Mobility and Transport Studies*

For an understanding of their potential to suppress other nanoparticles, it is crucial to assess their mobility and transport. The ability of ENPs to bind to solid matrices and resist transport over porous media is determined through the use of centrifugation, filtration, or sedimentation methods. ENPs may remain in the original state when they are released in the environment, or they undergo some changes due to the environment's action. As they travel through the environment, characteristics of surface changes, reactivity, and structure could be altered. [10] observed that the chemical-physio characteristics (e.g., ionic strength, pH, organic matter) of different environmental media can affect the ENPs' transport. Their ability to suppress other nanoparticles through their reduced mobility and transport in the environment indicates their effectiveness in suppressing them.

### 5.6 *Environmental Fate and Behavior Studies*

For assessing the long-term fate of engineered nanoparticles (ENPs) and whether they are able to suppress other nanoparticles, behavior studies, and fate in the environment are essential. The main purpose of these studies is to monitor the transformation, dissolution, or degradation of ENPs over time under realistic exposure conditions. Tracking the behavior and fate of ENPs can be accomplished using advanced techniques such as Inductively Coupled Plasma-Mass Spectrometry (ICP-MS), High Performance Liquid Chromatography (HPLC), and spectroscopic methods. ENPs can suppress other nanoparticles effectively when we understand how they transform in the environment, and how they interact with other nanoparticles.

So, the development of validating methods for engineered nanoparticles is found to be crucial for assessing whether they suppress other nanoparticles and mitigate risks associated along their unintended release. For evaluating the efficacy of ENPs in suppressing engineered nanoparticles, a number of techniques are essential, including agglomeration and aggregation studies, sedimentation and filtration studies, surface modification studies, mobility and transport studies, and environmental fate and behavior studies. The validation methods can provide insight into nanotechnology's design and application, enabling safe and responsible advancement.

## 6 Host Factor Responsible for Interaction and Development of Engineered Nanoparticles

### 6.1 *Host Cell*

Nanoparticle cell interactions are sometimes affected by the organ from which a cell originates. A cell's shape varies depending on its type. A smooth, spherical shape is exhibited by human erythrocytes, whereas a long, slender shape appears in ependymal cells [7, 92]. These differences lead to differing responses when foreign matter is internalized, such as nanoparticles. Second, the lipid composition of plasma membranes varies among cell types, which influences their physical properties. A third factor is the expression of different membrane receptors by different types of cells. Fourth, nanoparticles can be negatively impacted by different cellular organelles, such as macrophages [54]. Scavenger receptors help macrophages internalize foreign matter non-specifically. A lysosome is an acidic organelle, whereas a cytoplasm is almost neutral in pH. In acidic environments, drug charges are preferably released if they are released from nanoparticles [33]. However, nanoparticles may be degraded in lysosomes, causing release of ions and toxic effects.

## 6.2 *Biomembrane and Nanoparticle Interaction*

Cell membranes are phospholipid bilayer barriers that separate the cell from the environment. Lipopolysaccharides, proteins, and cholesterol are located inside the phospholipid bilayer [109]. These compounds enable for responding the cell to the environment externally and can communicate along with other cells. The transport of solutes across the membrane is mainly done by this communication between surroundings and cells. Engineered nanoparticles can go through the cell membrane via exocytosis without involving interaction of specific receptor-mediated against pests and finally they can also go through the cell membrane through endocytosis [92]. Due to their flexibility, the lipid membranes can be deformed when NP attach to their surface, engulfing and absorbing the NP in its entirety. Nanoparticles can also be absorbed non-specifically into vesicles, suggesting the NP can be taken up solely based on physical interactions. A nanoparticle that does not adhere to a membrane due to weak adhesion energy will undergo Brownian collisions with it. As an alternative, the nanoparticle can be partially covered by the bilayer of lipid at the membrane interface. It is also possible for nanoparticles to completely engulf the membrane in the right conditions, potentially resulting in the detaching of nanoparticles from inside the inner surface by fission, usually leaving a transient pore membrane [148].

## 6.3 *Proteins*

The interaction of proteins with magnetic nanoparticles is the most studied bio-macromolecular groups. Incubation with these molecules can cause them to bind directly to surfaces and to cover them immediately through hydrogen bonds, electrostatic interactions, coordinative bonds, and hydrophobic interactions [75]. With this binding the extent and specificity are determined by a complex interplay of factors. There is evidence that peptides which are positively charged can bond to surfaces which are positively charged, although this occurs due to surface being considerably charged (e.g., +3.7 mV). In close proximity to the IEP, magnetic nanoparticles have heterogeneous surface charges, thereby allowing both types of molecules which are charged (positive and negative) to weakly bind [48].

## 6.4 *Carbohydrates*

Saccharides play a number of roles within the body, including providing structure as well as storage of energy A polysaccharide consists of monosaccharides which are linked by the glycosidic bonds by branched forms or linearly [26]. Since polysaccharides are non-toxic, renewable, biocompatible and contain groups of functional which enable additional functionalization, they are often used to stabilize magnetic nanoparticles all through surface modification and synthesis. Another factor influencing NP interactions is carbohydrate characteristics. A polysaccharide can engage a solid surface through a variety of functional groups, particularly hydrogen-containing groups (hyaluronic acid, alginate and gum arabic) and chitosan [149]. During adsorption, chain length plays an important role. Dextrin is produced by hydrolyzing starch having low molecular weight when compared with starch since it is mainly composed of units of D-glucose bound by the glycosidic bonds. Because of this length, dextrin shows less adsorption capacity since fewer hydroxyl groups are available.

## *6.5 Nucleic Acid*

The adsorption of DNA in NPs is caused by hydrogen bonds and electrostatic interactions. The dehydration process contributes significantly to hydrophobic interactions and hydrogen bonds that are formed during macromolecule adsorption in aqueous systems [87]. The DNA molecule is made soluble by hydrogen bonds formed by phosphate groups with oxygen in its native state thanks to water molecules surrounding it. A hydrogen bond can also be formed with oxygen atoms that are sterically accessible on the surface of nanoparticles, or with silanol groups present in silica coatings. By using agents of chaotropic-like SDS, guanidinium chloride, and urea, chaotropic agents release water molecules and create a hydrophobic environment during dehydration. Additionally, nano-bio interactions develop by hydroxyl group's protonation on charged surfaces which are negative with the creation of hydrogen bonds in between the backbone of phosphate and the surface in solutions of aqueous which have lower pH values. On maghemite nanoparticles with naked surface activity, a genetically encoded plasmid (pDNA) expressing GFP was chemisorbed [82]. Consequently, the bidentate coordination between the charged of negative phosphates from DNA and the surface exposed iron (III), nano bioconjugates are formed.

## *6.6 Innate Immunity*

Engineered nanoparticles interact with the innate immune system in several ways, mostly depending on their characteristics. The response toward foreign materials, the immune system only takes defensive measures if it perceives them as potentially as harmful [86]. As with other borne agents environmentally (such as microorganisms and dust particles), the biological barriers of body and system elimination are generally appropriate to exclude ENPs, and mechanisms of immune recognition will not be triggered. NPs can also elicit an immune reaction that destroys foreign materials in other cases. The cells of effector which involved in the reactions are macrophages of resident tissue, phagocytes, and monocytes of blood-borne and poly-morphonuclear leukocytes, which can eliminate the ENPs by degradation and phagocytosing them.

Once released into an environment, they go through changes of physical and chemical when contact with the innate immune system ("as synthesized").

# 7 dsRNA Engineered Nanoparticles for Insect Pest Control

A recent concern about raising environmental risks due to pesticide residues has repeatedly questioned the sustainability of agro ecosystems. So, the dire need of green alternatives supplemented the innovation of several green strategies like the application of (dsRNA). Exogenous dsRNA application is associated with the RNA interference (RNAi) mechanism which leads to specific gene silencing in insects [52]. RNAi implementation in pest management approaches requires effective delivery and uptake of exogenously applied dsRNA. dsRNA-engineered nanoparticle delivery systems (called Vectors) have been emerged as an efficient solution for the delivery of dsRNA [103].

## *7.1 Synthetic Polymer-Based Delivery Vectors*

Synthetic polymer-based delivery vectors are often requisite for precise polymer chains with accurate narrow molar mass dispersity (Đ), molecular weight, and defined polymer architecture and show tolerance to chemical processes. Several types of synthetic polymers include linear homopolymers, branched polymers, guanidinium-based polymers, conjugated polymer nanoparticles, and dendritic nanocarriers. Types of engineered nanoparticles in RNAi-mediated pest control strategies are depicted in (Fig. 2).

### 7.1.1 Linear Homopolymers

The most simplest polymeric structures, consisting of only one monomer that includes polymer chain of amine groups as backbone or on groups of pendant (+ve charged under their pKa), for example, include poly(L-lysine) (PLL), poly(2-(dimethylamino) ethyl methacrylate) (PDMAEMA), and poly(ethylene imine) (PEI) [2, 13, 20, 65, 80, 144]. These types of polymers are not proficient in complexations and are associated with cell death such as cytotoxicity [138].

### 7.1.2 Branched Polymers

These types of polymers were designed to reduce cytotoxic effects and improve the efficacy of RNAi.

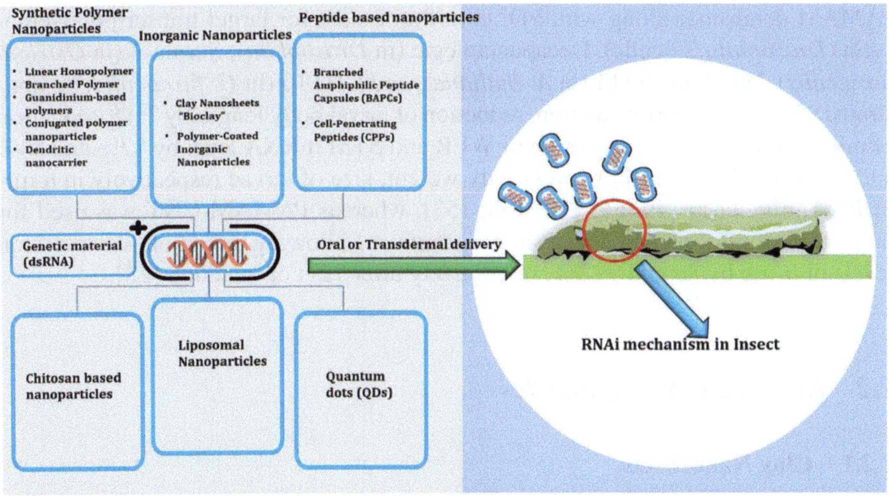


**Fig. 2** Types of engineered nanoparticles in RNAi-mediated pest control strategies

### 7.1.3 Guanidinium-Based Polymers

Guanidinium-based polymeric vectors are developed for protecting dsRNA from the alkaline gut of lepidopteran pest's pH. These show similarity to arginine-rich Cell Penetrating Peptides (CPPs). Christiaens et al. [21] and Parsons et al. [96] both used guanidinium-based polymeric vectors in the case of target transcripts SfV-ATPase (*Spodoptera frugiperda*) and AgCHSB (*Spodoptera exigua*) showing RNAi efficiency of more than 80% knockdown and 53% mortality respectively.

### 7.1.4 Conjugated Polymer Nanoparticles

Conjugated Polymer Nanoparticles (CPNs) consist of polymers including alternating single backbone and double bonds and can create a system conjugate of $\pi$-electrons. Silva et al. [125] used CPNs for target transcript NtCesA-1(in Tobacco BY-2 protoplasts) that showed more than 76% transcript reduction in terms of RNAi efficiency.

### 7.1.5 Dendritic Nanocarriers (Dendrimers)

These are largely polymers architectures branched with a central core, interior structure branched of dimensions defined and a surface which contains groups of functional [97]. They can hold species of active inside the pores which are made by the structure branched on their surface. PAMAM dendrimer for target transcript TCTP (*Bombyx mori* cells) showed higher knockdown at PAMAM concentrations [79].

PAMAM dendrimer along with PDI core fluorescent for target transcripts, Hemocytin (*Drosophila* S2 cells), Decapentaplegic (in *Drosophila*), Serpin-3 (in *Ostrinia furnacalis*), WER and STM (in *A. thaliana*), and CHT10 (in *O. furnacalis*) demonstrated 95.4% transcript reduction, reduction of larval body length by 35%, reduction of mRNA level by 51%, reduction of WER and STM mRNA level by 87% and 84% and reduced CHT10 mRNA level, body weight, size of larvae respectively in terms of RNAi efficiency [49, 56, 120, 145, 153], whereas PAMAM-CNT was used for target transcript α-tub and *Mtpol* (in *T. castaneum*), showing reduction in expression levels of α-tub by 89 and 99.5%, respectively after 72 h of injection [28].

## 7.2 *Inorganic Nanoparticles*

### 7.2.1 Clay Nanosheets

These vectors are composed of layered double hydroxide nanosheet clay (LDH) and used mainly for dsRNA virus-specific delivery [90]. LDH combined with dsRNA forms "Bioclay".

### 7.2.2 Polymer-Coated Inorganic Nanoparticles

Polymer-coated calcium phosphate and polymer-coated gold were used for target transcript luciferase (in luciferase expressing *S. frugiperda* cells) where they showed 35% transcript knockdown and 31% transcript knockdown, respectively [29, 72].

## 7.3 *Peptide-Based Nanoparticles*

Peptide-based nanoparticles are way more ecofriendly than synthetic polymer-based systems in terms of non-toxicity and biodegradability [34].

### 7.3.1 Branched Amphiphilic Peptide Capsules (BAPCs)

BAPCs are mainly developed in the past decade for nano-delivery of nucleic acids. Avila et al. [9] used BAPCs for delivery of dsRNA in insect diet.

### 7.3.2 Cell-Penetrating Peptides (CPPs)

CPPs help the molecule movement across membranes of cell and enhance uptake of dsRNA by cells. CPPs were used for target CHS, YFP and transcripts (in

*Populus tremula* and *A. thaliana)*, GFP and *Renilla luciferase* (in *A. thaliana* and *N. benthamiana*) and AgCHS2 (in *Anthonomus grandis*), showing reduction in YFP by 80%, increased transfection efficiency, and 80% transcript reduction respectively [39, 73, 94].

## 7.4 Chitosan-Based Nanoparticles

Chitosan is a naturally obtained polymer that has been emerged as an efficient medium for delivery of dsRNA. It is a type of polysaccharide in nature. Major successful applications of nanoparticle-mediated RNAi with chitosan based in insects are mentioned in Table 2.

## 7.5 Quantum Dots (QDs)

QDs are used as imaging of biological and probe labeling which are increasing nowadays [129, 152]. Carbon quantum dots were used in case of *Aedes aegypti* for target genes SRC and SNF7 through oral feeding that showed 71 and 40% knockdown for SRC and SNF7 respectively and 75 and 53.33% mortality against SRC and SNF7 respectively [25].

**Table 2** Some of the successful applications of Chitosan-based nanoparticle-mediated RNAi in insects

| Insects | Target gene | Observed effects | References |
|---|---|---|---|
| *Anopheles gambiae* | *AgCHS1* and *AgCHS2* | 62.8% reduction of transcripts | [151] |
| *Aedes aegypti* | Sema1a | 32% reduction of transcripts | [150] |
| *Aedes aegypti* | SNF7 and SRC | 46.7 and 26.7% mortality in case of SNF7 and SRC targeting respectively | [23, 24] |
| *Aedes aegypti* | Vg | 30% mortality | [106] |
| *Aedes aegypti* | IAP | More than 65% mortality | [25] |
| *Aedes aegypti* | DOPAL synthase | ~80% knockdown | [17] |

**Table 3** Some of the successful applications of Liposome-mediated RNAi in insects

| Insects | Target genes | Observed effects | References |
|---|---|---|---|
| *Blattella germanica* | α-tubulin | ~60% knockdown in midgut and ~60% mortality | [77] |
| *Drosophila melanogaster* | V-ATPaseE | 56.2% knockdown and ~65 mortality | [141] |
| *Drosophila suzukii* | Vha26 | 42% knockdown and 42% mortality | [134] |
| *Euschistus heros* | V-ATPaseA and muscle actin | 45 and 42% mortality, respectively | [14] |
| *Spodoptera frugiperda* | IAP | 60% mRNA reduction with 55% mortality | [45] |

### 7.6 *Liposomes*

These are vesicles which are spherical formed by the bilayer of phospholipid and regularly used for delivering dsRNA [98]. Some of the successful applications of liposomal nanoparticle-mediated RNAi in insects are given in Table 3.

## 8 Challenges of Engineered Nanoparticles

Engineered nanoparticles have pioneered a new and innovative road in the domain of pest management. Despite having numerous opportunities and utilities, there are some underlying issues associated with engineered nanoparticles that should be addressed by conducting more studies. The engineered nanoparticle's effects may vary from the other effects which are caused by nanoparticles occurring naturally. There is a possibility that engineered nanoparticles can be proved to be better for evading the body's defenses for the reason of their size and protective coatings [104, 135]. So, the exposure of the environment to engineered nanoparticles needs more study and research.

- The dsRNA-engineered nanoparticle-based pesticides are still not completely declared safe. So, more thorough studies should be conducted for mitigating the concerns.
- Their acceptance in sociological contexts should also be discussed properly.
- Nanoparticles can produce ROS when they interact with bacteria, causing toxicity in several instances. It also affects factors like colony forming unit (CFU), growth, etc. [85]. Some nanoparticles have (especially Ag-NPs) also shown toxicity toward earthworms in soil [50].

- Nanomaterials based on metal oxide and metal have been demonstrated for acting as mediators of damaging DNA in cells of mammalian, bacteria, etc. [8] first reported that nanoparticles based on copper oxide induce damage of DNA in plants (both in grassland and agricultural land).
- Isolation and observation of engineered nanoparticles in environmental matrices may be very hard at times [63].

## 9 Future Prospects

Engineered nanoparticles in insect pests and disease management hold significant promise for revolutionizing agricultural practices. Engineered nanoparticles are specially designed for targeting specific insecticide delivery or antimicrobial agents to pests and pathogens, reducing the need for large-scale spraying and minimizing off-target effects [139]. With enhanced encapsulation techniques and surface modifications, nanoparticles can deliver these agents precisely to affected areas, overcoming pesticide resistance and reducing the environmental impact [84, 127]. Moreover, the advance use of novel nanoparticle-based on formulations may improve the stability and efficacy of pesticides and antimicrobial agents, leading to more sustainable pest management strategies (Shekar et al. 2021, [55]). Nanoparticles can be biomarkers for detection of disease, enabling early diagnosis and monitoring of pathogens in humans, plants, and animals [116]. In precision agriculture, nanoparticles can be integrated into smart farming practices for targeted nutrient delivery and pest control, while in vector control, they can be utilized to combat disease-carrying insects [27]. Furthermore, nanoparticle-mediated gene editing can complement existing gene editing technologies like CRISPR-Cas9, enabling precise modifications in pests and pathogens for effective population control or eradication [83]. Despite these exciting prospects, challenges in regulatory approval, risks of human health, and concerns for environmentals need to be formulate through responsible research and deployment [40, 43, 44]. However, with proper development and implementation, engineered nanoparticles have the potential to transform pest and disease management, contributing to more sustainable and efficient agricultural practices.

## 10 Conclusion

An engineered nanoparticle (ENPs) on plant defense mechanisms is a complex and dynamic area of research that holds both promise and challenges. The application of ENPs has shown to have large potential in agriculture to revolutionize crop protection, nutrient uptake, and overall plant health. However, as with any emerging technology, there are important considerations to be addressed. Studies suggest that ENPs can influence plant defense responses, either by enhancing or suppressing them, depending on factors like nanoparticle type, size, surface properties, and concentration. The manipulation of plant defense pathways through ENP interactions could lead to more resilient crops, capable of withstanding various environmental stressors. Moreover, the targeted delivery of pesticides or growth factors via ENPs can reduce the impact of environmental of conventional agricultural practices. Nonetheless, ethical and ecological concerns must be carefully evaluated. The unintended consequences of ENP exposure on non-target organisms, soil ecosystems, and potential long-term effects on human health require rigorous assessment. Regulation and risk assessment protocols should be established to guarantee the deployment and responsible development of ENP-based technologies.

In conclusion, the interface between engineered nanoparticles and plant defense systems offers exciting opportunities for sustainable agriculture, but it also demands a holistic and precautionary approach. Continued research is essential to elucidate the intricate mechanisms governing ENP plant interactions, and to strike a balance between innovation and safeguarding the environment. Only through comprehensive understanding and responsible practices can we harness the potential benefits of engineered nanoparticles for enhancing plant defense and advancing agricultural practices in a responsible and ethical manner.

## References

1. Adeyemi JO, Oriola AO, Onwudiwe DC, Oyedeji AO (2022) Plant extracts mediated metal-based nanoparticles: Synthesis and biological applications. Biomol 12(5):627. https://doi.org/10.3390/biom12050627
2. Agarwal S, Zhang Y, Maji S, Greiner A (2012) PDMAEMA based gene delivery materials. Mater Today 15(9):388–393. https://doi.org/10.1016/S1369-7021(12)70165-7
3. Alghuthaymi MA, Kalia PR, Bhardwaj AK, Bhardwaj P, Abd-Elsalam KA, Valis M, Kuca K (2021) Nanohybrid antifungals for control of plant diseases: Current status and future perspectives. J Fungi 7(1):48. https://doi.org/10.3390/jof7010048
4. Ali S, Mehmood A, Khan N (2021) Uptake, translocation, and consequences of nanomaterials on plant growth and stress adaptation. J Nanomater 2021:1–17. https://doi.org/10.1155/2021/6677616
5. Aslani F, Bagheri S, Muhd Julkapli N, Juraimi AS, Hashemi FSG, Baghdadi A (2014) Effects of engineered nanomaterials on plants growth: an overview. Sci World J 2014:1–28. https://doi.org/10.1155/2014/641759
6. Asli S, Neumann PM (2009) Colloidal suspensions of clay or titanium dioxide nanoparticles can inhibit leaf growth and transpiration via physical effects on root water transport. Plant, Cell Environ 32:577–584. https://doi.org/10.1111/j.1365-3040.2009.01952.x
7. Asmatulu R, Fakhari A, Wamocha HL, Chu HY, Chen YY, Eltabey MM (2009) Drug-carrying magnetic nanocomposite particles for potential drug delivery systems. J Nanotechnol 2009:1–6
8. Atha DH, Wang H, Petersen EJ, Cleveland D, Holbrook RD, Jaruga P, Nelson BC (2012) Copper oxide nanoparticle mediated DNA damage in terrestrial plant models. Environ Sci Technol 46(3):1819–1827. https://doi.org/10.1021/es202660k
9. Avila LA, Chandrasekar R, Wilkinson KE, Balthazor J, Heerman M, Bechard J, Tomich JM (2018) Delivery of lethal dsRNAs in insect diets by branched amphiphilic peptide capsules. J Controlled Release 273:139–146. https://doi.org/10.1016/j.jconrel.2018.01.010

10. Bannunah AM, Vllasaliu D, Lord J, Stolnik S (2014) Mechanisms of nanoparticle internalizatison and transport across an intestinal epithelial cell model: effect of size and surface charge. Mol Pharm 11(12):4363–4373. https://doi.org/10.1021/mp500439c
11. Barik TK, Kamaraju R, Gowswami A (2012) Silica nanoparticle: a potential new insecticide for mosquito vector control. Parasitol Res 111:1075–1083. 1010.1007/s00436-012-2934-6
12. Barrena R, Casals E, Colon J, Font X, Sanchez A, Puntes V (2009) Evaluation of the ecotoxicity of model nanoparticles. Chemosphere 75:850–857. https://doi.org/10.1016/j.chemosphere.2009.01.078
13. Boussif O, Lezoualc'h F, Zanta MA, Mergny MD, Scherman D, Demeneix B, Behr JP (1995) A versatile vector for gene and oligonucleotide transfer into cells in culture and in vivo: polyethylenimine. Proc Natl Acad Sci 92(16):7297–7301. https://doi.org/10.1073/pnas.92.16.7297
14. Castellanos NL, Smagghe G, Sharma R, Oliveira EE, Christiaens O (2019) Liposome encapsulation and EDTA formulation of dsRNA targeting essential genes increase oral RNAi-caused mortality in the Neotropical stink bug Euschistus heros. Pest Manag Sci 75(2):537–548. https://doi.org/10.1002/ps.5167
15. Chandra S, Chakraborty N, Dasgupta A, Sarkar J, Panda K, Acharya K (2015) Chitosan nanoparticles: a positive modulator of innate immune responses in plants. Sci Rep 5(1):15195. https://doi.org/10.1038/srep15195
16. Chaudhary I, Singh V (2020) Titanium dioxide nanoparticles and its impact on growth, biomass and yield of agricultural crops under environmental stress: A review. Res. J. Nanosci Nanotechno 10:1–8
17. Chen J, Lu HR, Zhang L, Liao CH, Han Q (2019) RNA interference-mediated knockdown of 3, 4-dihydroxyphenylacetaldehyde synthase affects larval development and adult survival in the mosquito Aedes aegypti. Parasites Vect 12(1):1–11. https://doi.org/10.1186/s13071-019-3568-7
18. Chen J, Wang X, Han H (2013) A new function of graphene oxide emerges: inactivating phytopathogenic bacterium Xanthomonas oryzae pv. Oryzae. J Nanopart Res 15:1–14. https://doi.org/10.1007/s11051-013-1658-6
19. Cheng X, Kan AT, Tomson MB (2004) Naphthalene adsorption and desorption from aqueous C60 fullerene. J Chem Eng Data 49(3):675–683. https://doi.org/10.1021/je030247m
20. Cherng JY, Van de Wetering P, Talsma H, Crommelin DJ, Hennink WE (1996) Effect of size and serum proteins on transfection efficiency of poly ((2-dimethylamino) ethyl methacrylate)-plasmid nanoparticles. Pharm Res 13:1038–1042. https://doi.org/10.1023/A:1016054623543
21. Christiaens O, Tardajos MG, Martinez Reyna ZL, Dash M, Dubruel P, Smagghe G (2018) Increased RNAi efficacy in Spodoptera exigua via the formulation of dsRNA with guanylated polymers. Front Physiol 9:316. https://doi.org/10.3389/fphys.2018.00316
22. Cruz LF, Cruz JC, Carrillo D, Mtz-Enriquez AI, Lamelas A, Ibarra-Juarez LA, Pariona N (2021) In-vitro evaluation of copper nanoparticles as a potential control agent against the fungal symbionts of the invasive ambrosia beetle Euwallacea fornicatus. Crop Prot 143:105564. https://doi.org/10.1016/j.cropro.2021.105564
23. Das S, Debnath N, Cui Y, Unrine J, Palli SR (2015) Chitosan, carbon quantum dot, and silica nanoparticle mediated dsRNA delivery for gene silencing in Aedes aegypti: a comparative analysis. ACS Appl Mater Interfaces 7(35):19530–19535. https://doi.org/10.1021/acsami.5b05232
24. Das S, Debnath N, Cui Y, Unrine J, Palli SR (2015) Chitosan, carbon quantum dot, and silica nanoparticle mediated dsRNA delivery for gene silencing in Aedes aegypti: a comparative analysis. ACS Appl Mater Interf 7(35):19530–19535. https://doi.org/10.1021/acsami.5b05232
25. Dhandapani RK, Gurusamy D, Howell JL, Palli SR (2019) Development of CS-TPP-dsRNA nanoparticles to enhance RNAi efficiency in the yellow fever mosquito. Aedes aegypti. Sci Rep 9(1):8775. https://doi.org/10.1038/s41598-019-45019-z
26. Dias AMGC, Hussain A, Marcos AS, Roque ACA (2011) A biotechnological perspective on the application of iron oxide magnetic colloids modified with polysaccharides. Biotechnol Adv 29:142–155. https://doi.org/10.1016/j.biotechadv.2010.10.003

27. Duhan JS, Kumar R, Kumar N, Kaur P, Nehra K, Duhan S (2017) Nanotechnology: The new perspective in precision agriculture. Biotechnol Rep 15:11–23. https://doi.org/10.1016/j.btre.2017.03.002
28. Edwards CH, Christie CR, Masotti A, Celluzzi A, Caporali A, Campbell EM (2020) Dendrimer-coated carbon nanotubes deliver dsRNA and increase the efficacy of gene knockdown in the red flour beetle Tribolium castaneum. Sci Rep 10(1):12422. https://doi.org/10.1038/s41598-020-69068-x
29. Elhaj Baddar Z, Gurusamy D, Laisney J, Tripathi P, Palli SR, Unrine JM (2020) Polymer-coated hydroxyapatite nanocarrier for double-stranded RNA delivery. J Agricul Food Chem 68(25):6811–6818. https://doi.org/10.1021/acs.jafc.0c02182
30. Feichtmeier NS, Walther P, Leopold K (2015) Uptake, effects, and regeneration of barley plants exposed to gold nanoparticles. Environ Sci Pollut Res 22:549–8558. https://doi.org/10.1007/s11356-014-4015-0
31. Ferrari E (2022) Risk assessment of gold nanoparticle in a stable Arabidopsis exposition system. Ph.D. Thesis: University of Tübingen, Tübingen, Germany, pp 76–89. https://doi.org/10.15496/publikation-71666
32. Ferrari E, Barbero F, Busquets-Fite M, Franz-Wachtel M, Ko¨hler HR, Puntes V, Kemmerling B (2021) Growth-promoting gold nanoparticles decrease stress responses in Arabidopsis seedlings. Nanomater 11:3161. https://doi.org/10.3390/nano11123161
33. Gabrielyan L, Hovhannisyan A, Gevorgyan V, Ananyan M, Trchounian A (2019) Antibacterial effects of iron oxide (Fe3O4) nanoparticles: distinguishing concentration-dependent effects with different bacterial cells growth and membrane-associated mechanisms. Appl Microbial Biotechnol 103:2773–2782. https://doi.org/10.1007/s00253-019-09653-x
34. Gangwar P, Johri P, Datta R, Singh S, Trivedi M (2023) Overview on 1 phytopharmaceuticals and biotechnology of herbal plants. In: Phytopharmaceuticals and biotechnology of herbal plants. CRC Press, pp 1–17
35. Gao J, Xu G, Qian H, Liu P, Zhao P, Hu Y (2013) Effects of nano-$TiO_2$ on photosynthetic characteristics of Ulmus elongata seedlings. Environ Pollut 176:63–70. https://doi.org/10.1016/j.envpol.2013.01.027
36. Getts DR, Shea LD, Miller SD, King NJC (2015) Harnessing nanoparticles for immune modulation. Trends Immunol 36:419–427. https://doi.org/10.1016/j.it.2015.05.007
37. Ghidan AY, Al-Antary TM, Salem NM, Awwad AM (2017) Facile green synthetic route to the zinc oxide (ZnONPs) nanoparticles: Effect on green peach aphid and antibacterial activity. J Agricul Sci 9(2):131–138. https://doi.org/10.5539/jas.v9n2p131
38. Giammar DE, Maus CJ, Xie L (2007) Effects of particle size and crystalline phase on lead adsorption to titanium dioxide nanoparticles. Environ Eng Sci 24(1):85–95. https://doi.org/10.1089/ees.2007.24.85
39. Gillet FX, Garcia RA, Macedo LL, Albuquerque EV, Silva MC, Grossi-de-Sa MF (2017) Investigating engineered ribonucleoprotein particles to improve oral RNAi delivery in crop insect pests. Front Physiol 8:256. https://doi.org/10.3389/fphys.2017.00256
40. Gogos A, Knauer K, Bucheli TD (2012) Nanomaterials in plant protection and fertilization: current state, foreseen applications, and research priorities. J Agricul food Chem 60(39):9781–9792. https://doi.org/10.1021/jf302154y
41. González-García Y, López-Vargas ER, Cadenas-Pliego G, Benavides-Mendoza A, González-Morales S, Robledo-Olivo A, Alpuche-Solís ÁG, Juárez-Maldonado A (2019) Impact of carbon nanomaterials on the antioxidant system of tomato seedlings. Int J Mol Sci 20(23):5858. https://doi.org/10.3390/ijms20235858
42. Gunjan B, Sandeep ZMGH, A, (2014) Impact of gold nanoparticles on physiological and biochemical characteristics of Brassica juncea. J Plant Biochem Physiol 2:133. https://doi.org/10.4172/2329-9029.1000133
43. Gupta A, Mehta SK, Kunal K, Mukhopadhyay K, Singh S (2022) Quantum dots as promising nanomaterials in agriculture. In: Agricul Nanobiotechnol. Wood head Publishing, pp 243–296. https://doi.org/10.1016/B978-0-323-91908-1.00016-X

44. Gupta G, Paul S, Singh S, Pietramellara G, Pathan SI, Danish S, Jha PN (2022) Exploring functional diversity and community structure of diazotrophic endophytic bacteria associated with Pennisetum glaucum growing under field in a semi-arid region. Land 11(7):991
45. Gurusamy D, Mogilicherla K, Shukla JN, Palli SR (2020) Lipids help double-stranded RNA in endosomal escape and improve RNA interference in the fall armyworm. Spodoptera frugiperda. Arc Insect Biochem Physiol 104(4):e21678. https://doi.org/10.1002/arch.21678
46. Gutiérrez-Ramírez JA, Betancourt-Galindo R, Aguirre-Uribe LA, Cerna-Chávez E, Sandoval-Rangel A, Ángel ECD, Chacón-Hernández JC, García-López JI, Hernández-Juárez A (2021) Insecticidal effect of zinc oxide and titanium dioxide nanoparticles against Bactericera cockerelli Sulc.(Hemiptera: Triozidae) on tomato Solanum lycopersicum. Agron 11(8):1460. https://doi.org/10.3390/agronomy11081460
47. Hadwiger LA (2013) Multiple effects of chitosan on plant systems: Solid science or hype. Plant Sci 208:42–49. https://doi.org/10.1016/j.plantsci.2013.03.007
48. Harrison E, Hamilton JWJ, Macias-Montero M, Dixon D (2017) Peptide functionalized gold nanoparticles: the influence of pH on binding efficiency. Nanotechnology 28(29):295602. https://doi.org/10.1088/1361-6528/aa
49. He B, Chu Y, Yin M, Müllen K, An C, Shen J (2013) Fluorescent nanoparticle delivered dsRNA toward genetic control of insect pests. Advan Mater 25(33):4580–4584
50. Heckmann LH, Hovgaard MB, Sutherland DS, Autrup H, Besenbacher F, Scott-Fordsmand JJ (2011) Limit-test toxicity screening of selected inorganic nanoparticles to the earthworm Eisenia fetida. Ecotoxicol 20:226–233. https://doi.org/10.1007/s10646-010-0574-0
51. Hernández-Díaz JA, Garza-García JJ, Zamudio-Ojeda A, León-Morales JM, López-Velázquez JC, García-Morales S (2021) Plant-mediated synthesis of nanoparticles and their antimicrobial activity against phytopathogens. J Sci Food Agricul 101(4):1270–1287. https://doi.org/10.1002/jsfa.10767
52. Huvenne H, Smagghe G (2010) Mechanisms of dsRNA uptake in insects and potential of RNAi for pest control: a review. J Insect Physiol 56(3):227–235. https://doi.org/10.1016/j.jinsphys.2009.10.004
53. Ingle PU, Shende SS, Shingote PR, Mishra SS, Sarda V, Wasule DL, Rajput VD, Minkina T, Rai M, Sushkova S, Mandzhieva S (2022) Chitosan nanoparticles (ChNPs): A versatile growth promoter in modern agricultural production. Heliyon 8(2022):e11893. https://doi.org/10.1016/j.heliyon.2022.e11893
54. Ismail RA, Sulaiman GM, Abdulrahman SA, Marzoog TR (2015) Antibacterial activity of magnetic iron oxide nanoparticles synthesized by laser ablation in liquid. Mater Sci Eng C Mater Biol Appl 53:286–297. https://doi.org/10.1016/j.msec.2015.04.047
55. Jabborova D, Davranov K, Jabbarov Z, Bhowmik SN, Ercisli S, Danish S, Datta R (2022) Dual inoculation of plant growth-promoting Bacillus endophyticus and Funneliformis mosseae improves plant growth and soil properties in ginger. ACS Omega 7(39):34779–34788
56. Jiang L, Ding L, He B, Shen J, Xu Z, Yin M, Zhang X (2014) Systemic gene silencing in plants triggered by fluorescent nanoparticle-delivered double-stranded RNA. Nanoscale 6(17):9965–9969. https://doi.org/10.1039/C4NR03481C
57. Johnson CP, Li X, Logan BE (1996) Settling velocities of fractal aggregates. Environ Sci Technol 30(6):1911–1918. https://doi.org/10.1021/es950604g
58. Joshi H, Somdutt PCS (2019) Future prospects of nanotechnology in agriculture. Int J Chem Stud 7(2):957–963
59. Judy JD, Unrine JM, Rao W, Wirick S, Bertsch PM (2012) Bioavailability of gold nanomaterials to plants: importance of particle size and surface coating. Environ Sci Technol 46:8467–8474. https://doi.org/10.1021/es3019397
60. Kango S, Kalia S, Celli A, Njuguna J, Habibi Y, Kumar R (2013) Surface modification of inorganic nanoparticles for development of organic–inorganic nanocomposites-A review. Progress in Polymer Sci 38(8):1232–1261. https://doi.org/10.1016/j.progpolymsci.2013.02.003
61. Khan MR, Siddiqui ZA Fang X (2022) Potential of metal and metal oxide nanoparticles in plant disease diagnostics and management: Recent advances and challenges. Chemosphere 297:134114. https://doi.org/10.1002/etc.2470

62. Khater M, de la Escosura-Muñiz A, Merkoçi A (2017) Biosensors for plant pathogen detection. Biosens Bioelectron 93:72–86. https://doi.org/10.1016/j.bios.2016.09.091
63. Khota LR, Sankarana S, Majaa JM, Ehsania R, Schuster EW (2012) Applications of nanomaterials in agricultural production and crop protection: a review. Crop Prot 35:64–70. https://doi.org/10.1016/j.cropro.2012.01.007
64. Kim HS, Kang HS, Chu GJ, Byun HS (2008) Antifungal effectiveness of nanosilver colloid against rose powdery mildew in greenhouses. Solid State Phenom 135:15–18. https://doi.org/10.4028/www.scientific.net/SSP.135.15
65. Klemm AR, Young D, Lloyd JB (1998) Effects of polyethyleneimine on endocytosis and lysosome stability. Biochem Pharmacol 56(1):41–46. https://doi.org/10.1016/S0006-2952(98)00098-7
66. Kocjan A, Logar M, Shen Z (2017) The agglomeration, coalescence and sliding of nanoparticles, leading to the rapid sintering of zirconia nanoceramics. Sci Rep 7:2541. https://doi.org/10.1038/s41598-017-02760-7
67. Kőrösi L, Pertics B, Schneider G, Bognár B, Kovács J, Meynen V, Scarpellini A, Pasquale L, Prato M (2020) Photocatalytic inactivation of plant pathogenic bacteria using TiO2 nanoparticles prepared hydrothermally. Nanomater 10(9):1730. https://doi.org/10.3390/nano10091730
68. Kranjc E, Mazej D, Regvar M, Drobne D, Remskar M (2018) Foliar surface free energy affects platinum nanoparticle adhesion, uptake, and translocation from leaves to roots in arugula and escarole. Environ Science Nano 5:520–532. https://doi.org/10.1039/C7EN00887B
69. Kumar A, Singh A, Panigrahy M, Sahoo PK, Panigrahi KC (2018) Carbon nanoparticles influence photomorphogenesis and flowering time in Arabidopsis thaliana. Plant cell Rep 37:901–912. https://doi.org/10.1007/s00299-018-2277-6
70. Kumar V, Guleria P, Kumar V, Kumar Yadav S (2013) Gold nanoparticle exposure induces growth and yield enhancement in Arabidopsis thaliana. Sci Total Environ 461:462–468. https://doi.org/10.1016/j.scitotenv.2013.05.018
71. Kwak SY, Wong MH, Lew TTS, Bisker G, Lee MA, Kaplan A, Dong J, Liu AT, Koman VB, Sinclair R, Hamann C, Strano MS (2017) Nanosensor technology applied to living plant systems. Annu Rev Anal Chem 10:113–140. https://doi.org/10.1146/annurev-anchem-061516-045310
72. Laisney J, Gurusamy D, Baddar ZE, Palli SR, Unrine JM (2020) RNAi in Spodoptera frugiperda Sf9 cells via nanomaterial mediated delivery of dsRNA: A comparison of poly-l-arginine polyplexes and poly-l-arginine-functionalized Au nanoparticles. ACS Appl Mater Inter 12(23):25645–25657. https://doi.org/10.1021/acsami.0c06234
73. Lakshmanan M, Kodama Y, Yoshizumi T, Sudesh K, Numata K (2013) Rapid and efficient gene delivery into plant cells using designed peptide carriers. Biomacromol 14(1):10–16. https://doi.org/10.1021/bm301275g
74. Landa P (2021) Positive effects of metallic nanoparticles on plants: Overview of involved mechanisms. Plant Physiol Biochem 161:12–24. https://doi.org/10.1016/j.plaphy.2021.01.039
75. Li J, Pylypchuk I, Johansson DP, Kessler VG, Seisenbaeva GA, Langton M (2019) Self-assembly of plant protein fibrils interacting with superparamagnetic iron oxide nanoparticles. Sci Rep 9:8939. https://doi.org/10.1038/s41598-019-45437-z
76. Li XY, Logan BE (2001) Permeability of fractal aggregates. Water Res 35(14):3373–3380. https://doi.org/10.1016/S0043-1354(01)00061-6
77. Lin YH, Huang JH, Liu Y, Belles X, Lee HJ (2017) Oral delivery of dsRNA lipoplexes to German cockroach protects dsRNA from degradation and induces RNAi response. Pest Manag Sci 73(5):960–966. https://doi.org/10.1002/ps.4407
78. Liu J, Fu C, Li G, Khan MN, Wu H (2021) ROS homeostasis and plant salt tolerance: plant nanobiotechnology updates. Sustain 13 (6):3552. https://doi.org/10.3390/su13063552
79. Lu C, Li Z, Chang L, Dong Z, Guo P, Shen G, Zhao P (2019) Efficient delivery of dsRNA and DNA in cultured silkworm cells for gene function analysis using PAMAM dendrimers system. Insects 11(1):12. https://doi.org/10.3390/insects11010012

80. Lungwitz U, Breunig M, Blunk T, Göpferich A (2005) Polyethylenimine-based non-viral gene delivery systems. Eur J Pharma Biopharma 60(2):247–266. https://doi.org/10.1016/j.ejpb.2004.11.011
81. Luo YH, Chang LW, Lin P (2015) Metal-based nanoparticles and the immune system: Activation, inflammation and potential applications. Biomed Res Int 2015:1–12. https://doi.org/10.1155/2015/143720
82. Magro M, Martinello T, Bonaiuto E, Gomiero C, Baratella D, Zoppellaro G, Vianello, F (2017) Covalently bound DNA on naked iron oxide nanoparticles: Intelligent colloidal nano-vector for cell transfection. Biochim et Biophys Acta (BBA)-Gen Sub 1861(11):2802–2810. https://doi.org/10.1016/j.bbagen.2017.07.025.
83. Manna S, Roy S, Dolai A, Ravula AR, Perumal V, Das A (2023) Current and future prospects of "all-organic" nanoinsecticides for agricultural insect pest management. Front Nanotechnol 4:1082128. https://doi.org/10.3389/fnano.2022.1082128
84. Marella S, Kumar AN, Tollamadugu NP (2021) Nanotechnology-based innovative technologies for high agricultural productivity: Opportunities, challenges, and future perspectives. Recent Develop Appl Microbiol Biochem:211–220. https://doi.org/10.1016/B978-0-12-821406-0.00019-9
85. Maurer-Jones MA, Gunsolus IL, Murphy CJ, Haynes CL (2013) Toxicity of engineered nanoparticles in the environment. Anal Chem 85(6):3036–3049. https://doi.org/10.1021/ac303636s
86. Meddya S, Meshram S, Sarkar D, Datta R, Singh S, Avinash G, Thulasinathan T (2023) Plant Stomata: An Unrealized Possibility in Plant Defense against Invading Pathogens and Stress Tolerance. Plants 12(19):3380
87. Melzak KA, Sherwood CS, Turner RFB, Haynes CA (1996) Driving forces for DNA adsorption to silica in perchlorate solutions. J Colloid Interf Sci 181:635–644. https://doi.org/10.1006/jcis.1996.0421
88. Mingyu S, Liu J, Yin S, Linglan M, Hong F (2008) Effects of nano-anatase on the photosynthetic improvement of chloroplast damaged by linolenic acid. Biol Trace Elem Res 124:173–183. https://doi.org/10.1007/s12011-008-8134-7
89. Mishra KK, Subbanna ARNS, Rajashekara H, Paschapur AU, Singh AK, Jeevan B, Maharana C (2022) Chitosan and chitosan-based nanoparticles for eco-friendly management of plant diseases and insect pests: A concentric overview. In: Role of chitosan and chitosan-based nanomaterials in plant sciences. Academic Press. pp 435–451. https://doi.org/10.1016/B978-0-323-85391-0.00003-4
90. Mitter N, Worrall EA, Robinson KE, Li P, Jain RG, Taochy C, Xu ZP (2017) Clay nanosheets for topical delivery of RNAi for sustained protection against plant viruses. Nat Plants 3(2):1–10. https://doi.org/10.1038/nplants.2016.207
91. Moyano DF, Liu Y, Peer D, Rotello VM (2016) Modulation of immune response using engineered nanoparticle surfaces. Small 12(1):76–82. https://doi.org/10.1002/smll.201502273
92. Na HB, Song IC, Hyeon T (2009) Inorganic nanoparticles for MRI contrast agents. Adv Mater 21:2133–2148. https://doi.org/10.1002/adma.200802366
93. Ngou BPM, Ding P, Jones JDG (2022) Thirty years of resistance: zig-zag through the plant immune system. Plant Cell 34:1447–1478. https://doi.org/10.1093/plcell/koac041
94. Numata K, Ohtani M, Yoshizumi T, Demura T, Kodama Y (2014) Local gene silencing in plants via synthetic ds RNA and carrier peptide. Plant Biotechnol J 12(8):1027–1034. https://doi.org/10.1111/pbi.12208
95. Park J, Zhang Y, Saito E, Gurczynski SJ, Moore BB, Cummings BJ, Shea LD (2019) Intravascular innate immune cells reprogrammed via intravenous nanoparticles to promote functional recovery after spinal cord injury. Proc Natl Acad Sci USA 116(30):14947–14954. https://doi.org/10.1073/pnas.1820276116
96. Parsons KH, Mondal MH, McCormick CL, Flynt AS (2018) Guanidinium-functionalized interpolyelectrolyte complexes enabling RNAi in resistant insect pests. Biomacromol 19(4):1111–1117. https://doi.org/10.1021/acs.biomac.7b01717

97. Parveen R, Khare N, Singh S, Johri P (2023) An in silico outlook for the detection and surveillance of evolving and persistent plant pathogens. In: Detection, diagnosis and management of soil-borne phytopathogens. Springer Nature Singapore, Singapore, pp 17–40
98. Patani A, Patel A, Prajapati D, Khare N, Singh S (2023) Various agriculture crop plant-based bioactive compounds and their use in nanomaterial synthesis and applications. In: Nanomaterials from agricultural and horticultural products. Springer Nature Singapore, Singapore, pp 223–241
99. Pathipati UR, Kanuparthi PL (2021) Silver nanoparticles for insect control: Bioassays and mechanisms. In: Silver nanomaterials for agri-food applications. Elsevier, pp 471–494. https://doi.org/10.1016/B978-0-12-823528-7.00007-X
100. Petrarca C, Clemente E, Amato V, Pedata P, Sabbioni E, Bernardini G, Iavicoli I, Cortese S, Niu Q, Otsuki T, Paganelli R, Di Gioacchino M (2015) Engineered metal based nanoparticles and innate immunity. Clin Mol Allergy 13:1–12. https://doi.org/10.1186/s12948-015-0020-1
101. Pittarate S, Rajula J, Rahman A, Vivekanandhan P, Thungrabeab M, Mekchay S, Krutmuang P (2021) Insecticidal effect of zinc oxide nanoparticles against Spodoptera frugiperda under laboratory conditions. Insects 12(11):1017. https://doi.org/10.3390/insects12111017
102. Prakash B, Kujur A, Yadav A, Kumar A, Dubey SPP, NK, (2018) Nanoencapsulation: An efficient technology to boost the antimicrobial potential of plant essential oils in food system. Food Control 89:1–11. https://doi.org/10.1016/j.foodcont.2018.01.018
103. Pugsley CE, Isaac RE, Warren NJ, Cayre OJ (2021) Recent advances in engineered nanoparticles for RNAi-mediated crop protection against insect pests. Front Agronomy 3:652981. https://doi.org/10.3389/fagro.2021.652981
104. Rai M, Ingle A (2012) Role of nanotechnology in agriculture with special reference to management of insect pests. Appl Microbiol Biotechnol 94:287–293. https://doi.org/10.1007/s00253-012-3969-4
105. Rai M, Ingle AP, Pandit R, Paralikar P, Shende S, Gupta I, da Silva BJK, SS, (2018) Copper and copper nanoparticles: Role in management of insect-pests and pathogenic microbes. Nanotechnol Rev 7(4):303–315. https://doi.org/10.1515/ntrev-2018-0031
106. Ramesh Kumar D, Saravana Kumar P, Gandhi MR, Al-Dhabi NA, Paulraj MG, Ignacimuthu S (2016) Delivery of chitosan/dsRNA nanoparticles for silencing of wing development vestigial (vg) gene in Aedes aegypti mosquitoes. Int J Biol Macromol 86:89–95. https://doi.org/10.1016/j.ijbiomac.2016.01.030
107. Ramezani M, Ramezani F, Gerami M (2019) Nanoparticles in pest incidences and plant disease control. Nanotechnol Agric: Crop Prod & Prot:233–272. https://doi.org/10.1007/978-981-32-9374-8_12
108. Ranjan A, Sinha R, Bala M, Pareek A, Singla-Pareek SL, Singh AK (2021) Silicon-mediated abiotic and biotic stress mitigation in plants: Underlying mechanisms and potential for stress resilient agriculture. Plant Physiol Biochem 163:15–25. https://doi.org/10.1016/j.plaphy.2021.03.044
109. Reddy LH, Arias JL, Nicolas J, Couvreur P (2012) Magnetic nanoparticles: design and characterization, toxicity and biocompatibility, pharmaceutical and biomedical applications. Chem Rev 112(11):5818–5878. https://doi.org/10.1021/cr300068p
110. Rezaei M, Pirsa S, Chavoshizadeh S (2020) Photocatalytic/antimicrobial active film based on wheat gluten/ZnO nanoparticles. J Inorganic Organometallic Polymers Mater 30(7):2654–2665. https://doi.org/10.1007/s10904-019-01407-6
111. Riseh RS, Hassanisaadi M, Vatankhah M, Babaki SA, Barka EA (2022) Chitosan as potential natural compound to manage plant diseases. Int J Biol Macromol 220:998–1009. https://doi.org/10.1016/j.ijbiomac.2022.08.109
112. Sahoo D, Sahoo BR, Sahoo S (2021) Zinc oxide nanostructures as effective pesticide controllers: Sensing and degradation of pesticides. In: Zinc-based nanostructures for environmental and agricultural applications. Elsevier, pp 181–201
113. Sao P, Chand Y, Kumar A, Singh S (2021) Potential drug target identification in porphyromonas gingivalis using in-silico subtractive metabolic pathway analysis. Bangladesh J Med Sci 20(4):887–896

114. Sathiyabama M, Manikandan A (2021) Foliar application of chitosan nanoparticle improves yield, mineral content and boost innate immunity in finger millet plants. Carbohyd Polym 258:117691. https://doi.org/10.1016/j.carbpol.2021.117691
115. Schwab F, Zhai G, Kern M, Turner A, Schnoor JL, Wiesner MR (2016) Barrier pathways and processes for uptake, translocation and accumulation of nanomaterials in plants critical review. Nanotoxicol 10:257–278. https://doi.org/10.3109/17435390.2015.1048326
116. Shanker R, Singh G, Jyoti A, Dwivedi PD, Singh SP (2020) Nanotechnology and detection of microbial pathogens. In: Animal biotechnology. Academic Press, pp 593–611. https://doi.org/10.1016/B978-0-12-811710-1.00026-4
117. Sharma NC, Sahi SV, Nath S, Parsons JG, Gardea-Torresdey JL, Tarasankar P (2007) Synthesis of plant-mediated gold nanoparticles and catalytic role of biomatrix-embedded nanomaterials. Environ Sci Technol 41:5137–5142. https://doi.org/10.1021/es062929a
118. Shekhar S, Sharma S, Kumar A, Taneja A, Sharma B (2021) The framework of nanopesticides: a paradigm in biodiversity. Mater Advan 2(20):6569–6588. https://doi.org/10.1039/D1MA00329A
119. Shen CX, Zhang QF, Li J, Bi FC, Yao N (2010) Induction of programmed cell death in Arabidopsis and rice by single-wall carbon nanotubes. Am J Bot 97(10):1602–1609. https://doi.org/10.3732/ajb.1000073
120. Shen D, Zhou F, Xu Z, He B, Li M, Shen J, An C (2014) Systemically interfering with immune response by a fluorescent cationic dendrimer delivered gene suppression. J Mater Chem B 2(29):4653–4659. https://doi.org/10.1039/C4TB00411F
121. Shoala T (2020) Carbon nanostructures: Detection, controlling plant diseases and mycotoxins. In: Carbon nanomaterials for agri-food and environmental applications. Elsevier, pp 261–277. https://doi.org/10.1016/B978-0-12-819786-8.00013-X
122. Shukla SK, Mishra AK, Arotiba OA, Mamba BB (2013) Chitosan-based nanomaterials: A state-of-the-art review. Int J Biol Macromol 59:46–58. https://doi.org/10.1016/j.ijbiomac.2013.04.043
123. Siddiqi KS, Husen A (2016) Engineered gold nanoparticles and plant adaptation potential. Nano Res Lett 11:400. https://doi.org/10.1186/s11671-016-1607-2
124. Siegel J, Zaruba K, Svorcı'k V, Kroumanova K, Burketova L, Martinec J (2018) Round-shape gold nanoparticles: Effect of particle size and concentration on Arabidopsis thaliana root growth. Nanoscale Res Lett 13:95. https://doi.org/10.1186/s11671-018-2510-9
125. Silva AT, Nguyen A, Ye C, Verchot J, Moon JH (2010) Conjugated polymer nanoparticles for effective siRNA delivery to tobacco BY-2 protoplasts. BMC Plant Biol 10(1):1–14. https://doi.org/10.1186/1471-2229-10-291
126. Silvestre C, Duraccio D, Cimmino S (2011) Food packaging based on polymer nanomaterials. Prog polymer Sci 36(12):1766–1782. https://doi.org/10.1016/j.progpolymsci.2011.02.003
127. Singh A, Sengar RS, Singh AK, Singh S, Kumar A, Ahmad K (2019) Impact of genetic engineering on agriculture food crops. Biotech Today: Int J Biol Sci 9(1):17–24
128. Singh D, Gurjar BR (2022) Nanotechnology for agricultural applications: Facts, issues, knowledge gaps, and challenges in environmental risk assessment. J Environ Manag 322:116033. https://doi.org/10.1016/J.JENVMAN.2022.116033
129. Smith AM, Duan H, Mohs AM, Nie S (2008) Bioconjugated quantum dots for in vivo molecular and cellular imaging. Adv drug delivery Rev 60(11):1226–1240. https://doi.org/10.1016/j.addr.2008.03.015
130. Sofy AR, Sofy MR, Hmed AA, Dawoud RA, Alnaggar AEAM, El-Dougdoug SAM, NK, (2021) Ameliorating the adverse effects of tomato mosaic tobamovirus infecting tomato plants in Egypt by boosting immunity in tomato plants using zinc oxide nanoparticles. Molecules 26(5):1337. https://doi.org/10.3390/molecules26051337
131. Sohail MI, Waris AA, Ayub MA, Usman M, Rehman MZ, Sabir M, Faiz T (2019) Environmental application of nanomaterials: a promise to sustainable future. In Comp Anal Chem 87:1–54. https://doi.org/10.1016/bs.coac.2019.10.002
132. Spielman-Sun E, Avellan A, Bland GD, Tappero RV, Acerbo AS, Unrine JM, Giraldo JP, Lowry GV (2019) Nanoparticle surface charge influences translocation and leaf distribution

in vascular plants with contrasting anatomy. Environ Sci Nano 6:2508–2519. https://doi.org/10.1039/C9EN00626E
133. Stadler T, Buteler M, Valdez SR, Gitto JG (2018) Particulate nanoinsecticides: a new concept in insect pest management. Insectic: Agric Toxicol:83. https://doi.org/10.5772/intechopen.72448
134. Taning CNT, Christiaens O, Berkvens N, Casteels H, Maes M, Smagghe G (2016) Oral RNAi to control Drosophila suzukii: laboratory testing against larval and adult stages. J pest Sci 89:803–814. https://doi.org/10.1007/s10340-016-0736-9
135. Tungare K, Shahu R, Zambare V, Agarwal P, Jobby R, Nisar N, Jha P (2022) Toxicity mitigation of textile dye reactive blue 4 by hairy roots of Helianthus annuus and testing its effect in in vivo model systems. Biomed Res Int
136. Verma N, Sao P, Srivastava A, Singh S (2021) Physiological and molecular responses to drought, submergence and excessive watering in plants. Harsh Environ Plant Resil: Mol Funct Asp:305–321
137. Verma SK, Das AK, Gantait S, Kumar V, Gurel E (2019) Applications of carbon nanomaterials in the plant system: A perspective view on the pros and cons. Sci Total Environ 667:485–499. https://doi.org/10.1016/j.scitotenv.2019.02.409
138. Vora Z, Pandya J, Vaikuntapu PR, Singh S, Asha S, Purama RK (2023) Genome-wide association of defense hormone crosstalk in plants. In: Hormonal cross-talk, plant defense and development. Academic Press, pp 353–371
139. Wang D, Saleh NB, Byro A (2022) Nano-enabled pesticides for sustainable agriculture and global food security. Nat Nanotechnol 17:347–360. https://doi.org/10.1038/s41565-022-01082-8
140. Wang Z, Li J, Cho J, Malik AB (2014) Prevention of vascular inflammation by nanoparticle targeting of adherent neutrophils. Nat Nanotechnol 9:204–210. https://doi.org/10.1038/nnano.2014.17
141. Whyard S, Singh AD, Wong S (2009) Ingested double-stranded RNAs can act as species-specific insecticides. Insect Biochem Mol Biol 39(11):824–832. https://doi.org/10.1016/j.ibmb.2009.09.007
142. Wilson-Corral V, Anderson CWN, Rodriguez-Lopez M (2012) Gold phytomining. A review of the relevance of this technology to mineral extraction in the 21st century. J Environ Manag 111:249–257. https://doi.org/10.1186/s11671-016-1607-2
143. Worrall EA, Hamid A, Mody KT, Mitter N, Pappu HR (2018) Nanotechnology for plant disease management. Agron 8(12):285. https://doi.org/10.3390/agronomy8120285
144. Wu GY, Wu CH (1987) Receptor-mediated in vitro gene transformation by a soluble DNA carrier system. J Biol Chem 262(10):4429–4432. https://doi.org/10.1016/S0021-9258(18)61209-8
145. Xu Z, He B, Wei W, Liu K, Yin M, Yang W, Shen J (2014) Highly water-soluble perylenediimide-cored poly (amido amine) vector for efficient gene transfection. J Mater Chem B 2(20):3079–3086. https://doi.org/10.1039/C4TB00195H
146. Yan X, Chen S, Pan Z, Zhao W, Rui Y, Zhao L (2022) AgNPs-triggered seed metabolic and transcriptional reprogramming enhanced rice salt tolerance and blast resistance. ACS Nano 17(1):492–504. https://doi.org/10.1021/acsnano.2c09181
147. Yang K, Xing B (2007) Desorption of polycyclic aromatic hydrocarbons from carbon nanomaterials in water. Environ Pollut 145(2):529–537. https://doi.org/10.1016/j.envpol.2006.04.020
148. Yun G, Richardson JJ, Capelli M, Hu Y, Besford QA, Weiss AC, Caruso F (2020) The biomolecular corona in 2D and reverse: patterning metal–phenolic networks on proteins, lipids, nucleic acids, polysaccharides, and fingerprints. Adv Func Mater 30(1):1905805. https://doi.org/10.1002/adfm.201905805
149. Zarei M, Aalaie J (2019) Profiling of nanoparticle-protein interactions by electrophoresis techniques. Anal Bioanal Chem 411(1):79–96. https://doi.org/10.1007/s00216-018-1401-3
150. Zhang X, Mysore K, Flannery E, Michel K, Severson DW, Zhu KY, Duman-Scheel M (2015) Chitosan/interfering RNA nanoparticle mediated gene silencing in disease vector mosquito larvae. J Visualized Exp 97:e52523. https://doi.org/10.3791/52523

151. Zhang X, Zhang J, Zhu KY (2010) Chitosan/double-stranded RNA nanoparticle-mediated RNA interference to silence chitin synthase genes through larval feeding in the African malaria mosquito (Anopheles gambiae). Insect Mol Biol 19(5):683–693. https://doi.org/10.1111/j.1365-2583.2010.01029.x
152. Zhang Y, Wang TH (2012) Quantum dot enabled molecular sensing and diagnostics. Theranostics, 2(7):631. 10.7150%2Fthno.4308
153. Zheng Y, Hu Y, Yan S, Zhou H, Song D, Yin M, Shen J (2019) A polymer/detergent formulation improves dsRNA penetration through the body wall and RNAi-induced mortality in the soybean aphid Aphis glycines. Pest Manag Sci 75(7):1993–1999. https://doi.org/10.1002/ps.5313

151. Zhang X, Zhang J, Zhu KY (2010) Chitosan/double-stranded RNA nanoparticle-mediated RNA interference to silence chitin synthase genes through larval feeding in the African malaria mosquito (Anopheles gambiae). Insect Mol Biol 19(5):683–693. https://doi.org/10.1111/j.1365-2583.2010.01029.x
152. Zhang Y, Wang TH (2012) Quantum dot enabled molecular sensing and diagnostics. Theranostics 2(7):631. https://doi.org/10.7150/thno.4308
153. Zheng Y, Hu Y, Yan S, Zhou H, Song D, Yin M, Shen J (2019) A polymer/detergent formulation improves dsRNA penetration through the body wall and RNAi-induced mortality in the soybean aphid Aphis glycines. Pest Manag Sci 75(7):1993–1999. https://doi.org/10.1002/ps.5313

# Potential Effects of Nano Pesticides in Rice-Based Cropping System

**Mohan Ganesh Balaga, K. Sankara Rao, Ajit Kumar Savani, M. Vani Praveena, and Kottam Sushma**

**Abstract** Rice based cropping is one of the most prominent cropping systems followed in different parts of India. During past few decades paddy cropping strategies is governed by certain abiotic (ecological issues) and biotic constraints (insect pests, diseases etc.). Among them, insect pests and disease-causing pathogens viz., fungi, bacteria and viruses are the major biotic constraints accounting for around 10–15% of annual yield losses. In Pertaining to increase in paddy production, insect pest and diseases became as major drivers in harming global food security. So, pesticides became a pivotal source to manage the economic losses due to various pest attack. But, in due course of time i.e., during the mid 1990 the usage of harmful persistent pesticides like organophosphates, carbamates etc. has been increased against the rice cropping system and rice crop addressed as the second most pesticide-consuming crop after cotton. Because of this excessive usage of these conventional pesticides leaded to resurgence and pesticidal resistance against insect pest and diseases which finally caused severe pest outbreak in rice farming system. To overcome the issues due to persistence of conventional pesticides farmers in India required controlled and target-specific pesticidal formulations. Then a new novel concept called Nanotechnology has been entered in minds of the scientific community to develop a nano based formulations known as nano pesticides. Nano pesticides are the micro sized particles which stores agrochemical properties in a nano form. Nano pesticides are controlled release, target specific and slow degradable formulations with enormous

M. G. Balaga (✉)
Assistant Professor, Department of Entomology, Sri Kinjarapu Yerrannaidu College of Agricultural Sciences (SKYCAS), Etcherla, Srikakulam, Andhra Pradesh, India
e-mail: balagaganesh1995@gmail.com

K. Sankara Rao
Department of Entomology, Bihar Agricultural University, Bhagalpur, India

A. K. Savani
ICAR-National Academy of Agricultural Research Management, Hyderabad, Telangana, India

M. Vani Praveena
Acharya N.G. Ranga Agricultural University, Guntur, Andhra Pradesh, India

K. Sushma
Department of Plant Pathology, CoH, Dr YSRHU, Anantharajupeta, Andhra Pradesh, India

 
D. Jabborova et al. (eds.), *Nanomaterials in Agroforestry Systems*, Smart Nanomaterials Technology, https://doi.org/10.1007/978-981-96-1337-3_11

shelf life period. In comparison with harmful persistent pesticides, nanoformulations are environmentally safe and less toxic by increasing the dispersibility and wettability of pesticides.

**Keywords** Rice based cropping system · Conventional pesticides · Nanotechnology · Nano pesticides · Active ingredient · Controlled release

## 1 Introduction

Annually paddy raised with an area of about 162 million hectares and around 755 million tonnes of paddy is harvested throughout the world [32]. Around globe India occupied 2nd Position in paddy cultivation next to China with area and production of 44 million hectares and 118.87 million tonnes, respectively. According to Goyal and Singh [39], by 2030 Indian population is expected to reach 1.53 billion with an estimated requirement of 146 million tonnes of paddy. In India paddy grown in 1/4th of total area with contribution of 40% annual food grain intake for maintaining national food security. West Bengal is leading rice producer, accounting for 13.95% of the country's production. Andhra Pradesh State, widely known as "India's rice bowl", has 25.52 lakh ha of area under rice cultivation annually, ranks 5th among other states with a production of 130.89 lakh tonnes.

There are several biotic and abiotic factors which act as major drivers in harnessing rice production and productivity. Among them, rice is tuned with a loss of 15.1% to certain biotic organisms [94]. Insect pests viz., plant hoppers, leaf folders, and stem borers are the serious biotic attackers in reduction of rice productivity with yield loss of 25% which costs about Rs. 250 billion [26]. To tackle these insect pests and diseases highly persistent conventional pesticides were extensively sprayed in rice agro-ecosystem. One of the bothering issues in India with concern to increase in rice production is the spraying of pesticides injudiciously to manage crop losses [85] which has ultimately caused many environmental and soil health hazards due to the heavy dosage of these toxic pesticides. In ratio of agro chemicals usage applied paddy is second pesticide-consuming crop in India per hectare after cotton [58]. Globally due to this indiscriminate and intensive use of chemical pesticides there is a greatest environmental risk possessed to flora, fauna, human life, bird species and soil health in the rice ecosystem [18]. As there is an urge to solve the problem of impact of conventional pesticides issues on rice ecosystem, a new novel technology called Nanotechnology has been emerged which helps in formulation of nano pesticides with less active ingredients, better efficiency and good controlled released capacity. In this twenty-first century, nanotechnology became a contemporary tool in developing controlled and target-specific chemicals through new methods of formulation and delivery carries of active pesticide ingredients, as well as novel active ingredients, collectively referred to as nanopesticides [44]. Nano pesticides are considered as one of the best alternatives to conventional pesticides that can be applied in a controlled and reduced quantity of pesticides as a stored product [53, 92 104]. Nano is derived from a Greek word called "dwarf" i.e. $10^{-9}$ or one billionth. The evolution of nanoformulation is taken place because nature of its nano scale particles size with 1–100 mm thickness. The nanoscale particles represent molecule size with 100 nm and the differentiation of daily used particles range with nano-sized molecules shown in Table 1. Nanoparticles have been classified into three diameters according to its thickness [98].

(1) >100 nm in diameter- ultrafine sized molecules
(2) between 100 nm to 2.5 μm in diameter- Fine sized molecules
(3) >than 2.5 μm in diameter- Coarse molecules.

Considering particle sizes and biodegradability Keck and Müller [54] separated nano molecules into four different groups:
Group A: >100 nm and renewable,
Group B: >100 nm and unrenewable,
Group C: <100 nm and renewable,
Group D: <100 nm and unrenewable.

Nanoscience dispenses different nanoparticles with various physio-chemical properties. Due to adverse effect of persistent chemicals on mammals and lack of potentially in usage by traditional pest management viz. IPM and ITK'S to counter back against insect pests. Therefore, nanotechnology is an excellent source of green pest for maintaining sustainability and ecofriendly nature in agro ecosystem. Nanopesticides comprise with several agrochemical formulations which cannot categorised into one group. Nano formulations is composed as pellets and molecules with various active ingredients, polymers as organic compounds and metal oxides in inorganic form to increase the apparent solubility soluble ingredients and to release active ingredient in a slow targeted manner by protecting it against degradation.

**Table 1** Differentiation of daily used particles range with nano-sized molecules [118]

| Name of the particle | Nano size range (nm) |
|---|---|
| Water molecule | 0.1 |
| Glucose molecule | 1 |
| Virus | 100 |
| Graphene, dendrimer, fullerene, carbon nanotube | 1–100 |
| Bacteria | $10^3$ |
| Red blood cells | $10^4$ |
| Hair | $10^5$ |
| Ant | $10^6$ |
| Human hand | $10^7$ |
| Baseball | $10^8$ |

## 2 Global Criteria of Nano-Pesticides Under Current Agro Chemicals Era

By 2050, the world population is about to reach 10 billion approximately and the share developing countries will be around 95% in the raised world population [21]. So, there is a much demand in global food requirement and agriculture became one of the major livelihood in the developing countries by engaging in the cultivation of various food, oilseed and horticultural crops with help of contemporary technologies. Although there is rise in food productivity, but the crop is suffering with poor growth yields due to loos of biodiversity, degradation of natural resources and attack of insect pest and diseases [107]. The insect pests are accounting 14% of yield loss in world food production, whereas, biotic agents such insect pests, rodents, birds, plant pathogens and weeds are causing 13% loss with a crop loss of 2000 billion USD per annum [27]. To tackle these losses several conventional pesticides has been inevitably used with higher dosages. Market for pesticides is predicted to increase from $78.16 billion in 2021 to $85.11 billion in 2022 with annual compound rate of 8.9%. By 2026, the pesticidal market is predicted to increase its compound annual growth rate (CAGR) about $105.39 billion with 5.5%. Therefore, pesticides are now a significant component of the agricultural industry in order to minimise financial losses and a decline in crop quality. Due to injudicious application of these pesticides there is drastic reduction in soil and environment health. Currently, the development of innovative formulations has been greatly enhanced by the use of nanotechnology in designing and preparing nanopesticides [89]. Despite improvements in science and technology, crop protection with nanotechnology is still in its infancy [44, 55]. New generation pesticides based on nano particles either act as protectants or nano carriers offers effective substitute for pest management in agriculture [117]. These attributes make nano pesticides eco-green friendly with greater efficiency, dissolution rate, uniform dispersion and smaller volume (Fig. 1).

In 2021, the global market stature of nano formulation was approximately0.6 billion dollars and is expected to reach around 1.9 billion dollars by 2030 with a registered annual growth rate of 13.66%. The highest regional share of nano pesticides during 2022 was recorded in Europe with an annual revenue of 32% followed by Asia Pacific (28%), North America (25%), Latin America, Middle East and Africa (MEA) (6%) as shown in Table 2. During 2022 the nano insecticides contributed highest share with 44% to the global market share by other Agro-chemicals 24%) (Fig. 2). Over the projected period, insecticides are expected to continue their dominance in the worldwide nano pesticides market. Nano pesticides are quite advantageous over conventional pesticides due to its inherited fundamental properties such as stiffness, crystallinity, biodegradability, thermal stability and permeability. Moreover, the toxicity of nano pesticides against non-target organisms is 43.1% which was very less and ecofriendly in nature [113]. According to FAO, around $680 billion USD and $310 billion USD food wastage losses has been recorded in developing and under developed countries, respectively. Increase in food wastage losses and exportation of fresh fruit and vegetable to foreign countries are major driving factors

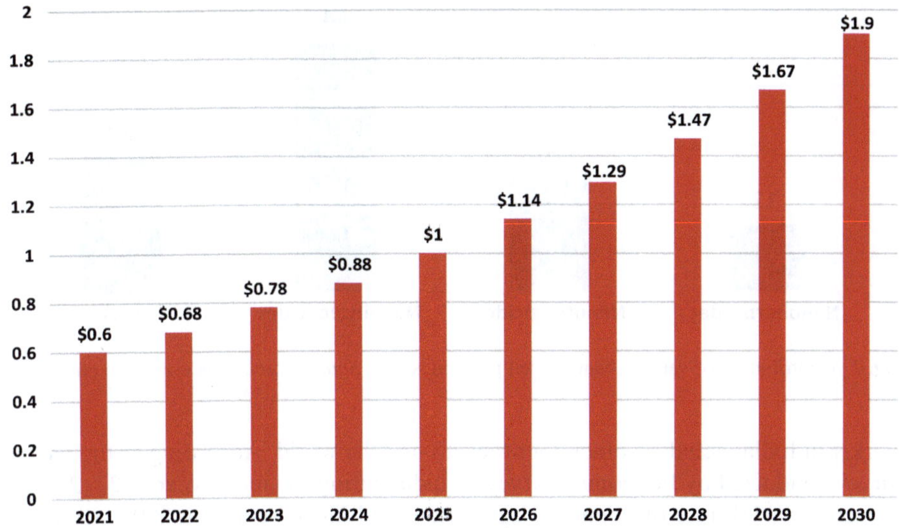


**Fig. 1** Market share of nano pesticides (2021–2030). *Source* (precedenceresearch.com)

**Table 2** Regional wise market size (%) of nano pesticides [117]

| Region | Annual revenue share in 2022 (%) |
|---|---|
| North America | 25 |
| Asia Pacific | 28 |
| Europe | 32 |
| Latin America | 9 |
| Middle East and Africa (MEA) | 6 |

in expanding the growth of nano pesticides market. Hence, continued research for optimizing nanotechnology in plant protection aspects is emerging issue for agriculture development. Research on nano-biopesticides and their concerns to enhance efficiency and environmental safety is also at need of hour.

## 3 Nano Pesticides Versus Conventional Pesticides

In view of enhancing total agricultural productivity in order to safeguard from past few years the usage of harmful persistent pesticides has been increasing in order to gain surplus food with greater sufficiency in concern with raising world population [41]. On an average every year in India approximately 15–25% of food grains lots are been contaminated with various invertebrate and vertebrate pests [47]. From past three financial year (FY14-16) are treated challenging tasks for agro chemicals

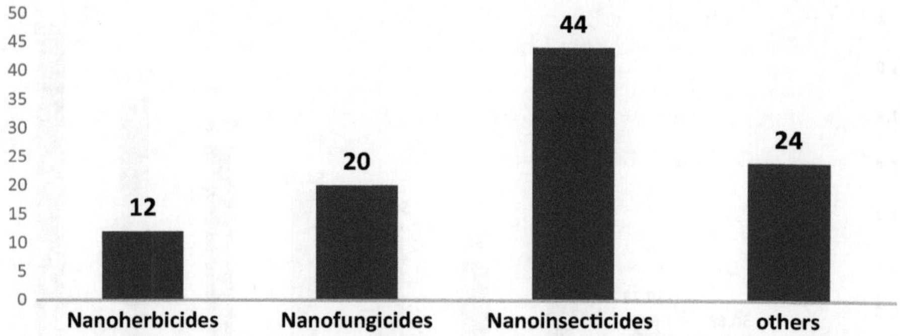


**Fig. 2** Contribution of various Nano based pesticides (%). *Source* (precedenceresearch.com)

market in India including other countries around the world. According to the recent survey conducted by Economic Survey of India during Financial year 2021–22, the expected growth rate of country's agriculture and allied sectors is 3.9% [97]. As the crop yield increases, simultaneously the incidence of pest and pathogen attack is raising which leads to increased demand for pesticides. Agricultural pest and pathogens result in ~90% of the applied pesticides being lost to the air and as run-off, adversely affecting both farmers financially and the environment (Stephenson 2003; [66]). More than 90% of management strategies and control methods which has been applied through pesticides has been lost through.

During 1960's after green revolution the evolution of high yielding verities (HYV'S) been token place, whereas simultaneously the era of pesticides has also been started. In due course of time the indiscriminate usage of these harmful conventional pesticides has been increased and became a barrier for several environmental risks like pesticide poisoning, soil health degradation etc. [79]. The complete overview of environmental risks associated by these harmful conventional agro chemicals is realised by the public during 1960–1975 after initiation of HYV (High Yield Variety) programme [59]. In the current scenario pesticidal toxicity is one of the most researchable problems and several investigations has been carrying out towards the toxic effects associated with the pesticide use against humans, animals by disturbing their ecological balance of life [65]. Out of 100% of applied pesticides it has been noticed that 99% of pesticides entering into surrounding environment in certain ways like spray, soil, seed treatment, etc. Whereas, only 0.1% of sprayed agro chemicals is striking to the specific target which ultimately unbalancing the ecosystem by polluting the soil and groundwater levels [38, 64]. Also the extensive use of these nonselective persistent pesticides will leads to extinction of species by destroying beneficial soil microbial flora, natural enemies, insect pollinators, and birds. As water is the universal solvent so it is the excellent soluble medium to mix many pesticides but its solubility is very poor in water [116]. Organic compounds are another medium for equal dispersion of pesticides [76, 101]. Sometimes, crops suffered with phytotoxicity symptoms due to the interactions incompatible interactions between two

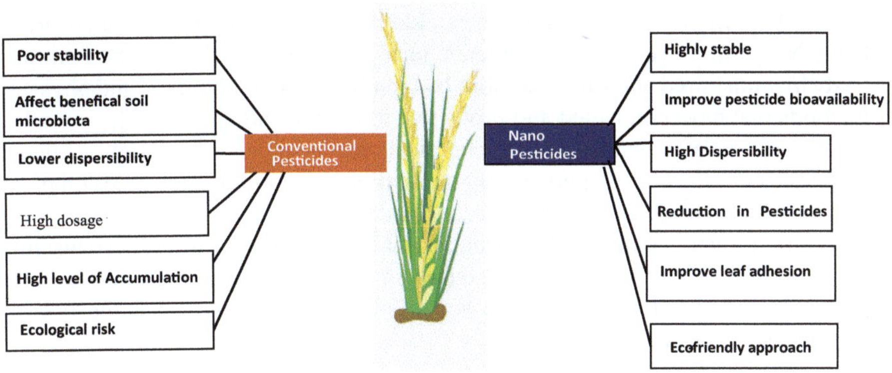


**Fig. 3** Comparison of nano pesticides with conventional pesticides [118]

mixtures of pesticides [86]. To overcome the issues due to persistence of conventional pesticides farmers in India required a controlled and target specific pesticidal formulations. Then a new branch science called Nanotechnology has been striped to the minds of scientific community to develop a nano based formulations known as nano pesticides. Nano pesticides are the minute engineered structure which stores pesticidal properties such as active ingredient (a.i) in a nano form [33]. Nano pesticides are controlled release, target specific and slow degradable formulations with prolonged shelf life period. Comparison with persistent agro chemicals nano formulations are environmentally safe and less toxic by increasing the dispersibility and wettability of pesticides. The brief pictorial comparison of nano pesticides over conventional pesticides has been visualized in Fig. 3.

## *3.1 Benefits of Nano Pesticides in Comparison with Conventional Pesticides*

- In this current 21st century nanotechnology is one of the contemporary tool in developing the nano-pesticide formulations which are target specific and eco-friendly [90].
- Nano pesticides are characterized in a motto to improve the dispersibility with excellent intermingling nature of different chemical compounds (Margulis-Goshen and Magdassi 2013).
- Compared to conventional pesticides lesser dose of insecticidal compounds is enough to deliver nano biocides effectively with a long-lasting period (Fig. 1). Nano formulations act as farmer friendly formulations by decreasing their dose of pesticide application, cultivation cost, harmful effects and phytotoxicity [108].
- Due to its target specific delivery and controlled released formulation nature it not only slow down the rate of pesticide usage and application rate but it also

a best alternative for reducing the pesticide residue and pollution related problems. Nano-microcapsule, nanospheres, nanogels, and micelles are the continuously manufactured nano-formulations by blending various chemical and physical methods that have controlled and protective release formulations [77].

- In comparison with persistent agro chemicals nano-pesticide formulations helps in improving adhesion, dispersion and bio-activity of pesticide molecules on plant surface to decrease losses caused through drift
- To promote sustainability and environmental friendly in agricultural ecosystems nano pesticides are the excellent source in terms of their small size,droplet producibility, wettability and target specific absorption which rises the overall crop protection efficiency [67].

### 3.2 *Restrictions in Association with Nano-Pesticides*

- Lack of complete description and understand related nano-pesticides risk association with interference to environment and animal health
- Act as pathway and source in polluting the environment by contaminating soils and water in ground level as nano-pesticides risk association levels high in terms toxicity and persistence when compared to pesticides
- Therefore better understanding related to cause and effect of nano-pesticides is necessary aspect where all the essential [70].

## 4 Source and Characterization of Nano-Insecticides

Nanoscience is a novel combination of various branches in science like chemistry, physics, biology, medicine and engineering. In nanotechnology, the size of molecule is designed in a nanometre level with distinctive characters like greater surface tension, target specific and controlled release formulation [23]. By using one atom, one molecule theory the physical attributes related to nano-insecticidal particles like solubility, persistence and durability can be manipulated in an diameter 1 and 100 nm irrespective of either natural or man-made [49].

### 4.1 *Source of Nano Pesticides*

In nano emulsions either the liquid or solid active ingredients will be dissolved in little amount of organic solvent whereas in nano dispersions the solid or liquid pesticides will be entrained into an inert matrix [40].

### 4.1.1 Polymer Based Nano Pesticides

In nano emulsions, polymer-based pesticides serve as nano carriers which increase the dispersion of pesticide in liquids towards target specific in a controlled manner. Naeini et al. [72] used ABA-type copolymer with combination of PCA and PEG compounds to achieve target release of the insecticide imidacloprid. Hydrogel nanoparticles also known as polymeric nanogels absorb water in large quantities due to hydrophilic groups [36]. Protonation of amino acids will release the active ingredient copper due to acidification or chitosanolytic enzymatic action by the pathogen [20, 75]. Because of their special qualities of layered double hydroxides (LDHs), biomolecules can be intercalated between the layers, where they are protected from deterioration and released more easily into the soil (Park et al. 2010).

### 4.1.2 Solid Based Nano Pesticides

It makes sense to utilise silica encapsulated nano molecules for managing insect pest as well as diseases as silicon can help plants be more resilient to biotic and abiotic challenges Compared to bulk silica nano encapsulated silica molecules controlled effectively against paddy root weevil [13]. Diatomous earth (DE) is commonly used to get rid from stored grain insects which primarily consists of porous silica particles made from preserved phytoplankton. Enhancing DEs with other pesticides has been the subject of recent research. For example, *Rhyzopertha dominica*, a grain pest, was tested using a mixture of DE and the plant extract bitterbarkomycin and the dosage rate was observed at 150 ppm [11]. Layered double hydroxide (LDHs), also known as anionic clays, are the group of these organic compounds that is believed to be most potential. They have already been employed as carriers for the herbicide 2, 4-dichlorophenoxyacetate and the plant growth regulator-naphthalene acetate [17].

### 4.1.3 Metal Nanoparticles

Because of their effectiveness against bacteria and viruses, less phytotoxicity, charge durability, greater surface tension, crystalline module and adaptation in different compounds. In comparison to conventional pesticides, silver coated nano insecticides are able to deliver larger dosages chemicals to harmful pests and ecofriendly nature to beneficial natural enemies. As a result, they are regarded as environmentally safe [109]. The target organism's acetylcholinesterase activity is decreased by silver nano pesticides, which affects antioxidants and detoxification-related enzymes thus ultimately results in cell death. The effectiveness of silver nanoparticles against the pathogenic fungus *Phytopathogen raffaelea* was examined by Kim et al. [57] and observed cell wall damage and supressed fungal growth in a dose-dependent manner.

There is an immense potential to create powerful, eco-green zinc oxide nanoparticles which can be used in biomedical and agricultural research. It is also possible, affordable and safe to make zinc oxide nanoparticles using various plant extracts [7].

ZnO nanoparticles have been used effectively to control the storage pests namely *T.castaneum*, *S.oryzae* and *C. maculatus*. High mortality of *T. castaneum* and *T. granarium* is caused by Zn–Cu nanoparticles combined with leaf powder of *Jatropha curcas*, *Citrus paradise* and *Ricinus communis* [42].

Nano formulations of insecticides based on titanium oxide are highly sustainable and ecofriendly against storage pests since they have negligible adverse effects on unintended organisms [122]. High mortality of Maize weevil and red flour beetle was observed using titanium dioxide nanoparticles in lab conditions. Cu based nanoparticles can be used to create nanopesticides, nanoherbicides, and nanofertilizers since they have the ability to control insect pest attacks. Pesticides delivered to their intended targets using copper nanoparticles, and their antibacterial action can be increased by stabilising them with polyvinyl pyrrolidone. The comparison of the antifungal effects of Cu-based nanoparticles (11–55 nm) and other commercial agrochemicals on tomato plants (Solanum lycopersicum) infected with *Phytophthora infestans* by Giannousi et al. [35] led to the conclusions that at low concentrations, Cu-based nanoparticles are more active than commercial agrochemicals.

Nano structured aluminium (NSA) has powerful insecticidal properties leading to double action technique that uses electrostatic and physical mechanisms. These negative electrostatic binds into insect's cuticle, which has a positive electrostatic charge, when it comes into contact with NSA. These nanoparticles then abrade the cuticle, degrade the wax, which cause asphyxiation and finally lead to death of insect. The effectiveness of NSA at a dose of 400 mg/kg was studied by Belhamel et al [15] and reported 79% mortality in red flour beetle, 80% mortality in saw tooth beetle and 100% mortality in drug store beetle. Due to their unique physiological attributes properties like form, shape and porosity is easily controlled where silica nanoparticles (SiNP) are considered as good nanocarriers for agrochemicals. They can be built using a range of chemicals by binding with polymeric compounds to develop unique nanoinsecticides since they are extremely stable at high temperatures. Similarly, NSA, silicon dioxide nanoparticles interfere with insect's cuticle, which causes the insect to become dehydrated and eventually die. Lethal effect of $SiO_2$ nanoparticles on *Callosobruchus maculates* was reported by Rouhani et al. [87]. SiNPs effect the insect biological process by interacting with spiracle constriction, tracheal constriction and adsorption of cuticular waxes.

Green synthesis of nanoparticles relies on the elimination of hazardous wastes, utilization of sustainable processes and usage of eco-friendly renewable materials and solvents. Green nanotechnology relies on biotic organisms such as algae, bacteria, enzymes and botanical compounds which were most commonly used eco-friendly alternatives to commercially used chemical pesticides [45]. As physical and chemical procedures became more expensive, need for biosynthesis of nanoparticles was felt important. Research was conducted to find the applicability of using microorganisms and plant extracts for manufacturing nanoparticle in an effort to find less expensive methods. Biosynthesis of metal nanoparticles using plant extracts like *Azadirachta indica, Emblica officinalis,* mango steen leaf, *Chenopodium* have already been reported. The biomolecules viz., phenols, proteins and flavonoids not only reduce the particle size to nano scale also act as crucial thing in shaping nano molecules into different formulations [106].

### 4.1.4 Characterization of Nanoparticles

Nano particles comprised with various important physiological parameters like (1) Nano molecule size, shape and dispersion. (2) Particle stiffness and roughness. (3) Greater surface area and tension. (4) Agglomeration and aggregation. (5) Purity. (6) Reactivity and hydrophobicity.

Stability and dispersion of the nanoparticles influenced through average particle diameter, size, distribution and charge. The performance of the polymer dispersion, its physical stability and dispensability are both impacted by the surface charge of the nanoparticles. The three most crucial factors in characterisation of nanoparticles include particle size, distribution and shape. Dynamic light scattering (DLS) was recently emerged technique as it is the quickest and most popular method of detecting the particle size. By using brownian nanoparticles in colloidal suspensions can be sized down to the nano and submicron range. A Doppler shift occurs when monochromatic light (such as a laser) is passed through a solution of nanoparticles striking a moving particle, which alter the wavelength of the incoming light [61] (Table 3).

With direct visualization of particles using electron microscopy, physio-chemical structure of particles can be worked out. Nano emulsions is initially transformed into dust formulation for SEM characterization, that deposited on a sample catcher which later coated with a gold foil. Ultra high resolution of nano molecules thickness is assessed based on physical structure of the particles with the help of atomic force microscopy to generate topographical map of the sample by scanning its surface

**Table 3** Techniques to characterize nano-particles

| Properties of nano particles | Technique used for various attributes |
|---|---|
| Morphology (shape/size) | Dynamic light scattering, electron microscopy (scanning/ transmission) and atomic force microscopy |
| Topography (surface) | X-ray diffraction, BET |
| Chemical | UV–visible spectroscopy, electron dispersive x-ray spectroscopy, Fourier transform infrared spectroscopy or attenuated total reflection |
| Electrical | Electrokinetics (zeta/cyclic voltammetry studies) |
| Optical | Microscopy, double photon correlation spectroscopy, Raman spectroscopy and surface plasmon resonance |
| Biological | In vitro cell viability and in vivo microbial colony viability |

area in contact or non-contact mode [71]. Ponarulselvum et al. [78] synthesised eco-friendly Ag coated nano molecules (*Catharanthus roseus*) using ultra violet spectrophotometry. The findings demonstrated face-centered cubic AgO based nanoparticles of 37–55 nm mean thickness were successfully synthesized. Banerjee et al. [12] used SEM to characterize green-synthesized silver nanoparticles and observed particle thickness between 35 and 55 nm and crystalline nature of the particles was confirmed by X-ray diffraction (XRD). Thiruvengadam et al. [103] characterized the silver nanoparticles using X-Ray diffraction, Fourier-transform infrared spectroscopy and high-resolution transmission electron microscopy and observed the particle size to be 18.31 nm. The crystalline morphology in face-centered cubic structure was observed using TEM.

## 5 Scope and Utility of Nano-Insecticides

The pests and pathogens that infect plants in nature led to stunted growth and reduced production. Farmers use a variety of techniques to prevent pest and pathogen attacks to overcome enormous crop losses, yet none of them provide complete all-around disease management. To increase the effectiveness of disease management modules, innovative and sophisticated methods must be combined with traditional ways. Gao et al. [34] prepared CNAP-HMS-PDAAM nanopesticide formulation to control *Chilo suppressalis* and *Cnaphalocrocis medinalis* and noticed long lasting potentiality because of its greater adhesiveness. Nanoaluminia as insecticidal dust has been recommended to effectively control *S.oryzae* which led to more than 95% mortality @ 1 gm/kg, while 100% mortality was observed within 14 days @ 2 gm/kg [3]. Kar et al. [52] studied the effect of silica nano-particle of 30 nm size against rice weevil at five different concentrations and observed 80 and 98% mortality at 0.5 g/kg of rice. SEM studies revealed that one time washing is sufficient for rice in terms consumption purpose which is treated with silica encapsulated nano particles prior to cooking. Kumar et al. [62] characterized and evaluated fipronil based nano formulation against brown plant hopper during milking stage at the rate of 30, 45, 60 and 90 g a.i./ha. Results showed that treated plot with an dosage of 60 g a.i./ha noticed highest per cent (93.4%) reduction of BPH population and effect of silver nano coated metal particles like $AgO_2$ $ZnO_2$ and $TiO_2$ to manage root weevil in paddy was studied by Goswami et al. [37]. They have reported 86%, 95% and 70% mortality using hydrophobic, hydrophilic and lipophilic silver nanoparticles while 100% mortality was observed with aluminium oxide nano particles. Similarly, 100% mortality of *Corcyra cephalonica* (rice moth) was reported by Vani and Brindhaa [105] using silica nanoparticle. Aluminium nano particles was found prominent in increasing the mortality rate of brown plant hopper in positive relationship with concentration and time of application. Abou El-Ela et al. [4] highlighted the nanoparticle synthesize using phytohormones would be eco-friendly and effective in controlling BPH in rice. To manage sheath blight in rice caused by *Rhizoctonia solani,* a laboratory experiment has been conducted by Siddhartha et al. [95] and developed nano-formulations based on chloro halogenated compounds. The particle size of developed nano-formulation confirmed using transmission electron microscopy ranged from 1 to 100 nm. The drawback related to issues caused due to effect of AgO nanoparticles on *sheet rot (R.solani)* under both laboratory and field conditions was conducted by Soltani Nejad et al. [99]. Behera et al. [14] noticed the efficacy of nano coated silver molecules that is formulated with the help of *Pseudomonas fluorescens* to effectively control sheath blight in rice and reported 69.90% fungal growth inhibition in comparison with the control. Nanoparticles containing active ingredient derived from *Chaetomium cochliodes* was tested by Song et al. [100] to manage rice blast disease caused by *Magnaporthe oryzae* isolate PO1. Significant inhibition *M. oryzae* in 12 days was observed when nanoparticles derived from *Chaetomium cochliodes* were used at concentrations ranging from 3 to 15 ppm. Also field experimental studies revealed per cent disease reduction was noticed with 37.8% by applying nanoformulation at dosage of 10 ppm. During 2015 an extensive study is conducted by Kalboush et al. [50] to identify the antifungal properties with zinc oxide encapsulated nanoparticles towards blast and brown spot in paddy cropping system. Whereas, observation revealed that spraying of zinc oxide based nano particles five days before inoculation with a spore suspension of *P. grisea* gave the best effect in controlling rice blast disease.

# 6 Nanopesticides for the Management of Rice Insect Pests and Nematodes

Nanoscience is quickly evolving into a highly sought-after method for controlling pests and delivering pesticides [10, 120]. This technology is highly capable in addressing the issues that have been emerged as a result of current pest management tactics [93]. Advances in Nanoscience, may change the process of pesticide development, pesticide formulation and delivery mechanisms. Different nano formulations have been developed as a result of research in nanotechnology. Nanopesticides made of solid nanoparticles are also being explored. Additionally, nano materials can also be employed in effective gene delivery systems [48].

## *6.1 Nano Formulations*

There have been several nano formulations of pesticides, including (i) nano suspensions, (ii) nano emulsions, and (iii) nano capsules or nano encapsulation [62].

### 6.1.1 Nano Suspensions

Particle size of nanosuspension is uniform, and are better than microsuspensions [92, 96]. Beside enhancing solubility and dissolution rate, nanosuspensions increase its stability and efficiency [22, 62] found use of nano formulated fipronil molecules against rice BPH led to a 30% increase in insecticidal activity compared to the commercial formulation. Nano suspensions of Indoxacarb and imidacloprid (200–400 nm) were tested on second instar of cotton leaf worm, *Spodoptera littoralis* (Boisduval) and showed low LC50 values of 2.9 and 15.9 ppm, as opposed to 34.3 and 66.5 ppm, respectively, in conventional formulation. In comparison to commercial products, these were 12 and 4 times more effective [88]. Rahwanudin et al. [81] observed 46% more toxicity of spinetoram nano suspension (<100 nm) against the DBM insect pest in cabbage than particles of conventional suspension concentrate (2299 nm).

### 6.1.2 Nano Emulsions

At present, reducing organic solvent amount in pesticide formulations has become the key interest. As alternatives to emulsifiable concentrates (EC), micro emulsions and emulsions are developed with the less use of organic solvent. However, these products were also facing the drawbacks like low pesticide loading, relatively large droplet size (200 nm to 200 μm), droplet aggregation and Ostwald ripening [9]. The use of nanoemulsions can solve a lot of the issues with emulsifiable concentrates, micro emulsions, and emulsions. The three varieties of formulated nanoemulsions are oil in water (O/W), water in oil (W/O), and, bi-continuous. The more prevalent nano-emulsion is the oil-in-water (O/W) emulsion, which disperses the chemical's active ingredient as nanosized droplets in water while confining surfactant molecules to the pesticide-water interface [112].

Adak et al. [5] prepared oil in water nanoemulsions of Eucalyptus oil using Tween 80 as surfactant and observed the lower $LC_{50}$ of 0.56 and 1.11 $\mu L/cm^2$ on Rice Weevil, *Sitophilus oryzae* (L.) and red flour beetle, *Tribolium castaneum (Herbst), respectively. Whereas,* $LC_{50}$ of eucalyptus oil was 0.795 and 4.178 $\mu L/cm^2$ against *S. oryzae, T. castaneum*, respectively. Imbrahim et al. [46] also tested the Eugenol Nano emulsion (EO-NE) against *S. oryzae* and recorded the high fumigant toxicity with least $LC_{50}$ value (14.40 μl/L air) and more persistence (>12.46%) in nano emulsion treated wheat grains compared to eugenol alone. Nano emulsions also found to reduce the nematode population in soil. Djiwanti et al. [28] recorded the significant suppression of java tea root knot nematode i.e., 99.33%, 97.65%, respectively with use of bio-silica nanoemulsion (2% solution), citronella oil nanoemulsion after three months of application.

### 6.1.3 Nano Encapsulation

The process of nanoencapsulation involves encasing solid, liquid, or gaseous nanoparticles, inside secondary substance, also known as the matrix or shell [68]. Encapsulation helps in controlled release of active ingredient and provide the resistance to harsh environments like temperature and radiation [74]. Overall, they provide excellent protection against the pests at low application rates [114]. Adak et al. [6] observed high efficacy of nano micelle of Imidacloprid for controlling sucking pests beside commercial formulation Gaucho 600 FS in soyabean. Similarly, Pradhan et al. [80] found the 100% mortality of *Spodoptera litura* (Fabricius) and *Oligonychus coffeae* (Nietner) by the application of nano micelle of Acephate shielded with poly ethylene glycol when used at 300 ppm within 7 days and 5 days, respectively. The nanocapsule of *Rosmarinus officinalis* essential oil-loaded formulation was reported to be efficient against *T. castaneum* [56]. Nano gels are much use full for controlled release of pheromones. Methyl Eugenol immobilized in nanogel acted as an effective formulation compared to ME alone for the pest management of *B. dorsalis* [16]. Abd El-Wahab [1] observed significantly a greater number of Rhinoceros beetle, *Rhynchophorus ferrugineus* (Olivier) of (55 number/trap) adults with nanogel as compared to control (35 number/trap) adults/trap.

## 6.2 Nanoparticles as Nano-Pesticides in Rice

Nano particles with insecticidal properties can be directly used as pesticides. Nano copper composite), aluminium (Al NPs), magnesium oxide (MgONPs) and magnesium hydroxide (MgOH NPs) possess insecticidal properties [91]. Silica nano particles ($SiO_2$ NPs) are identified as potential candidates against many bacterial, fungal [31] and insect pests [29, 102]. Debnath et al. [25] found substantial mortality (>90%) of *S. oryzae* in nano silica (13–15 nm) treated bins in comparison to bulk silica treated bins (25%). Borei et al. [19] recorded the adverse effect of silica nanoparticles (20 nm) on biology of *S. littoralis* and found that mortality was dose dependent with the high mortality (>60%) at concentrations above 225 ppm [8]. Further, Thabet et al. [102] found that the efficacy of nano silica differed depending on the feeding habits of the insects. They recorded the lower doses of nano silica to manage the externally feeding insects than internal feeders.

## 6.3 Nanoparticles as Vectors for the Delivery of Genetic Engineering Tools

For delivering gene products such as DNA, RNA, proteins in a self-sufficient manner, efficient delivery methods are required [121]. There are some widely used oldest delivery vehicles like Agrobacterium-mediated transformation, polyethylene glycol (PEG)-mediated delivery, biolistic particle bombardment, and viral transfection but one of major drawback for their poor efficiency is genotype dependence, rapid in vivo degradation and difficult cellular uptake in plants [2, 119]. Nanomaterials such as mesoporous silica particles (MSNs), gold nano particles (AuNPs), carbon nanotubes (CNTs), liposomes and layer double hydroxides (LDHs), have emerged as promising vectors for the delivery of genome engineering tools to plants in a species-independent manner with high efficiency. The novel genome editing tool, clustered regularly interspaced short palindromic repeats (CRISPR)/Cas9 system in combination with nano delivery systems may revolutionize to create ideal genotypes resistant to biotic and abiotic stresses [30]. Wang et al. [114] identified carbon quantum dot as the most efficient carrier for inducing systemic RNAi in stem borer pests like *Chilo supressalis* walker.

## 7 Nanopesticides for the Management of Rice Diseases

About 60% of the global population is relied on Rice (*Oryza sativa* L.) which is considered as one of predominant cereal crop. Being a rainfed crop with mean sea level ranging from 250 to 2500 m above mean sea level (MSL) it can be adapted and grown in different agro ecological and climatic conditions [84]. The production of paddy subjected several biotic agents under different climatic situations by accounting 20–25% huge crop losses [60]. The Indian scientists and professors are in serious concern to develop a novel eco-friendly technique, where nanotechnology is one such type of environmentally safe tool to provide sustainability in agro system [51]. Recent investigations has given an idea for the research community about nanoscience in the management of various important diseases of rice such as blast and sheath blight considered to be major havoc for the farmers. Various studies has elucidated the potential role of nano particles in the disease management i.e., nanoparticles generated by ionic gelation by interaction of chitosan and sodium triphosphate found to inhibit the blast fungus under detached leaf condition [69]. Sheath blight of rice caused by *Rhizoctonia solani* is an important biotic hurdle for the rice production at global level to its instable QTL loci. It is interesting to note that green synthesis of silver nano-particles (Ag NP) from the rice leaf exhibited inhibition of mycelium (81.07–96.78%) at 10 μg/mL, whereas with increase in concentration of Ag Np (20 μg/mL) cent per cent inhibition of the mycelium growth was observed coupled with positive correlation in seed vigour index [60].

## 8 Statutory Issues and Risks Related to Nano Pesticides

In previous times nano-science received a lot of awareness in application of various branches in agriculture in special reference in the field of plant protection and created a novel contemporary pathway in the management insect pests and diseases [82]. Under supervision of current issues we already discussed essentiality of nano-technology and its potential source of green nano materials coupled with the plant growth promotion activities. It became a much debated issue on the effect of nano-encapsulated pesticide formulation in the soil system [110].

As per the European perspective "Very little known regarding background of nanoscience unaware about risks and thinks nano-technology encapsulated formulation is to be adapted" (European Commission 2012). Similarly, without an understanding of the scope and possibility of any potential dangers, these statements cannot support the deployment of nano-scale applications. The balance between benefits and risks is crucial from an ethical standpoint. To minimise risk to customers, animals, the environment, and future generations, manufacturers, processors, and producers must take care. However, if there is a larger likelihood that the use would be useful or beneficial, some risk or potential for harm may be tolerated (beneficence to "do good"). It might undergo few more decades to shift nanotechnology from laboratory to field conditions.

## 9 Conclusion and Future Prospective

Considering huge raise in world population there is a high necessity to reach global food security by integrating nanotechnology with biotechnology which could improve the standard of living farmers, especially in countries like India [115]. Many scientific communities have been strongly believed in the field of nano science and reported that the nano based pesticides are potential delivery systems to maintain sustainability in the agriculture. According to the detailed analysis of recent literatures, the comparative data either qualitative or quantitative in comparison of nano pesticides with conventional pesticides is insufficient to support efficiency of nano formulations. Amalgamation of nanotechnology into a formulation helps in development of more number of plant protection products with different mode of action in concern with environmental sustainability and global food security. Moreover, most of the researches has been done on pharmaceutical drugs towards the development of nano-delivery carrying vehicles. So, there is a high necessity in developing a proper nano particle delivery channels which could provide a safer and greener pesticides. Despite of having several advantages nano-formulations have few drawbacks like less selective toxicity, low biodegradability, development of pesticide resistance towards pest and beneficial organisms due to injudicious application of pesticides.

By considering above factors, the upcoming prospective on nano-pesticides should be focused on (1) Improvement of nano-pesticide formulations through smart technology approach to overcome the issues faced due to persistent agro-chemicals (2) Modulation of ecological balanced nano solutions with the help of green chemistry (3) To develop the cost of effective nano-formulations. (4) Environmental toxicity indication test with nano-pesticides, and (6) Bio safety measurement of nano-pesticides in various agro ecosystems.

## References

1. Abd El-Wahab AS, Abd El-Fattah AY, El-Shafei WK, El Helaly AA (2020) Efficacy of aggregation nano gel pheromone traps on the catchability of *Rhynchophorus ferrugineus* (Olivier) in Egypt. Braz J Biol 81:452–460
2. Abdallah NA, Prakash CS, McHughen AG (2015) Genome editing for crop improvement: challenges and opportunities. GM Crops and Food 6:183–205
3. Abo-Arab RB, Amal MH, Hashem AS (2014) Comparative bioactivity of Aluminum Oxide ($Al_2O_3$), Titanium Dioxide ($TiO_2$) nanoparticles and malathion on Sitophilus oryzae L. and Sitophilus zeamais (Motsch.). Glob J Agric Food Saf Sci 1(2):25–37
4. Abou El-Ela AS, Ntiri ES, Munawar A, Shi XX, Zhang C, Pilianto J, Zhang Y, Chen M, Zhou W, Zhu ZR (2022) Silver and copper-oxide nanoparticles prepared with GA3 induced defense in rice plants and caused mortalities to the brown planthopper, Nilaparvata lugens (Stål). NanoImpact 1(28):100428
5. Adak T, Barik N, Patil NB, Gadratagi BG, Annamalai M, Mukherjee AK, Rath PC (2020) Nanoemulsion of eucalyptus oil: an alternative to synthetic pesticides against two major storage insects (*Sitophilus oryzae* (L.) and *Tribolium castaneum* (Herbst)) of rice. Ind Crops Prod 143:111–849
6. Adak T, Kumar J, Shakil NA, Walia S (2012) Development of controlled release formulations of imidacloprid employing novel nano-ranged amphiphilic polymers. J Environ Sci Health Part B 47:217–25
7. Akbar S, Tauseef I, Subhan F, Sultana N, Khan I, Ahmed U, Haleem KS (2020) An overview of the plant-mediated synthesis of zinc oxide nanoparticles and their antimicrobial potential. Inorg Nano Met Chem 50(4):257–271
8. Alimohamadian M, Aramideh S, Mirfakhraie S, Frozan M (2022) Silica nanoparticle: a potential of non-invasive and as a natural insecticide application for beet armyworm, *Spodoptera exigua* Hubner (Lepidoptera: Noctuidae) control. Agric Eng Int 24:248–257
9. Anton N, Vandamme TF (2011) Nano-emulsions and micro-emulsions: clarifications of the critical differences. Pharm Res 28:978–985
10. Athanassiou CG, Kavallieratos NG, Benelli G, Losic D, Usha Rani P, Desneux N (2018) Nanoparticles for pest control: current status and future perspectives. J Pest Sci 91:1–5
11. Athanassiou CK, Kavallieratos NG, Vayias BJ, Vassiliki KS (2008) Evaluation of a new enhanced diatomaceous earth formulation for use against the stored products pest Rhyzopertha dominica (Coleoptera: Bostrychidae). Int J Pest Manag 54(1):43–49
12. Banerjee I, Tripathi SK, Roy AS, Sengupta P (2014) Pesticide use pattern among farmers in a rural district of West Bengal. India J Nat Sci Biol Med 5:313
13. Barik TK, Sahu B, Swain V (2008) Nanosilica—from medicine to pest control. Parasitol Res 103(2):253–258
14. Behera L, Chandra R, Lenka S, Mahanty A, Kumar S, Rath PC (2023) Bacterial synthesized silver nanoparticle inhibits Rhizoctonia solani Kuhn, the causal organism for sheath blight disease of rice, association of rice research workers. Oryza 60(1): 166–174
15. Belhamel C, Boulekbache-Makhlouf L, Bedini S, Tani C, Lombardi T, Giannotti P, Conti B (2020) Nanostructured alumina as seed protectant against three stored product insect pests. J Stored Prod Res 87:101607

16. Bhagat D, Samanta SK, Bhattacharya S (2013) Efficient management of fruit pests by pheromone nanogels. Sci Rep 3:1294
17. Bin Hussein MZ, Yahaya AH, Zainal Z, Kian LH (2005) Nanocomposite-based controlled release formulation of an herbicide, 2, 4-dichlorophenoxyacetate incapsulated in zinc–aluminium-layered double hydroxide. Sci Technol Adv Mater 6(8):956–962
18. BirdLife (2008) Critically endangered birds: a global audit. BirdLife International, Cambridge, UK. http://www.birdlife.org/news/news/2008/09/Complete_Critical%20Birds_superlowres.pdf. Accessed 20 Jan 2009
19. Borei HA, El-Samahy MF, Galal OA, Thabet AF (2014) The efficiency of silica nanoparticles in control cotton leafworm, *Spodoptera littoralis* Boisd. (Lepidoptera: Noctuidae) in soybean under laboratory conditions. Glob J Agric Food Saf Sci 1:161–168
20. Brunel FE (2013) Complexation of copper (II) with chitosan gels: toward control of microbial growth. Carbohydr Polym 92:1348–1356
21. Carvalho FP (2006) Agriculture, pesticides, food security and food safety. Environ Sci Policy 9:685–692
22. Chin CP, Wu HS, Wang SS (2011) New approach to pesticide delivery using nanosuspensions: research and applications. Ind Eng Chem Res 50:7637–7643
23. Chouhan PN, Azimov A, Jabborova D, Singh S (2023) Review on the role of indigenous plants and plant derivatives of Ayurveda in bone healing. Plant Sci Today 10(sp2):143–151
24. Debnath N, Das S, Seth D, Chandra R, Bhattacharya SC, Goswami A (2011) Entomotoxic effect of silica nanoparticles against *Sitophilus oryzae* (L.). J Pest Sci 84:99–105
25. Debnath ND (2011) Entomotoxic effect of silica nanoparticles against Sitophilus oryzae (L). J Pest Sci 84:99–105
26. Dhaliwal GS, Jindal V, Dhawan AK (2010) Insect pest problems and crop losses: changing trends. Indian J Ecol 37(1):1–7
27. Dhawan AK, Peshin R (2009) Integrated pest management: concept, opportunities and challenges. In: Peshin R, Dhawan AK (eds) Integrated Pest Management: Innovation Development Process. Springer, Dordrecht, pp 51–81
28. Djiwanti SR, Noveriza R, Nurhayati H, Pasaribu G (2022) Application of bio-silica and citronella oil nanoemulsion, neem oil, and endophytic bacteria formula for the java tea root-knot nematode population suppression. IOP Conf Ser Earth Environ Sci 974:012072
29. Du J, Liu B, Zhao T, Xu X, Lin H, Ji Y, Li Y, Li Z, Lu C, Li P, Zhao H (2022) Silica nanoparticles protect rice against biotic and abiotic stresses. J Nanobiotechnology 20:1–8
30. Duan L, Ouyang K, Xu X, Xu L, Wen C, Zhou X, Qin Z, Xu Z, Sun W, Liang Y (2021) Nanoparticle delivery of CRISPR/Cas9 for genome editing. Front Genet 12:673286
31. El-Shetehy M, Moradi A, Maceroni M, Reinhardt D, Petri-Fink A, Rothen-Rutishauser B, Mauch F, Schwab F (2021) Silica nanoparticles enhance disease resistance in *Arabidopsis* plants. Nat Nanotechnol 16:344–353
32. FAO STAT (2020). http://www.fao.org/faostat/en/#data/QC/visualize
33. Gangwar P, Johri P, Datta R, Singh S, Trivedi M (2023) Overview on 1 phytopharmaceuticals and biotechnology of herbal plants. In: Phytopharmaceuticals and biotechnology of herbal plants. CRC Press, pp 1–17
34. Gao Y, Li D, Li D, Xu P, Mao K, Zhang Y, He S (2020) Efficacy of an adhesive nanopesticide on insect pests of rice in field trials. J Asia Pac Entomol 23(4):1222–1227
35. Giannousi K, Avramidis I, Dendrinou-Samara C (2013) Synthesis, characterization and evaluation of copper based nanoparticles as agrochemicals against *Phytophthora infestans*. RSC Adv 3:21743–21752
36. Goncalves C, Pereira P, Gama M (2010) Self-assembled hydrogel nanoparticles for drug delivery applications. Materials 3(2):1420–1460
37. Goswami A, Roy I, Sengupta S, Debnath N (2010) Novel applications of solid and liquid formulations of nanoparticles against insect pests and pathogens. Thin Solid Films 519:1252–1257
38. Goulson D, Nicholls E, Botías C, Rotheray EL (2015) Bee declines driven by combined stress from parasites, pesticides, and lack of flowers. Science 347:1255957. https://doi.org/10.1126/science.1255957

39. Goyal SK, Singh JP (2002) Demand versus supply of foodgrains in India: implications to food security. In: 13th international farm management congress. Wageningen, The Netherlands, p 20
40. Green JM, Beestman GB (2007) Recently patented and commercialized formulation and adjuvant technology. Crop Prot 26(3):320–327
41. Gupta G, Paul S, Singh S, Pietramellara G, Pathan SI, Danish S, Jha PN (2022) Exploring functional diversity and community structure of diazotrophic endophytic bacteria associated with Pennisetum glaucum growing under field in a semi-arid region. Land 11(7):991
42. Haider Z, Ayub AR, Tahir MU, Sajid SA, Khalid M (2020) Efficacy and characterization of synthesized zinc oxide nanoparticles against *Tribolium Castaneum* and *Trogoderma granarium*. Int J Sci Res 10:9912
43. Hajek A (2004) Natural enemies: an introduction to biological control. Cambridge University Press, Cambridge, UK
44. Hayles J, Johnson L, Worthley C, Losic D (2017) Nanopesticides: a review of current research and perspectives. In: Grumezescu AM (ed) New pesticides and soil sensors. Academic Press, Cambridge, pp 193–225
45. Hussain I, Singh NB, Singh A, Singh H, Singh SC (2016) Green synthesis of nanoparticles and its potential application. Biotechnol Lett 38:545–560
46. Ibrahim SS, Sahu U, Karthik P, Vendan SE (2023) Eugenol nanoemulsion as bio-fumigant: enhanced insecticidal activity against the rice weevil, *Sitophilus oryzae* adults. J Food Sci Technol 60:1435–1445
47. Jabborova D, Davranov K, Jabbarov Z, Bhowmik SN, Ercisli S, Danish S, Datta R (2022) Dual inoculation of plant growth-promoting Bacillus endophyticus and Funneliformis mosseae improves plant growth and soil properties in ginger. ACS Omega 7(39):34779–34788
48. Jasrotia P, Nagpal M, Mishra CN, Sharma AK, Kumar S, Kamble U, Bhardwaj AK, Kashyap PL, Kumar S, Singh GP (2022) Nanomaterials for postharvest management of insect pests: current state and future perspectives. Front Nanotechnol 3:811056
49. Joshi H, Choudhary P, Mundra SL (2019) Future prospects of nanotechnology in agriculture. Int J Chem Stud 7(2):957–963
50. Kalboush ZA, Hassan AA, Gabr WE (2016) Control of rice blast and brown spot diseases by synthesized zinc oxide nanoparticles. Egypt J Biol Pest Control 26(4)
51. Kaman PK, Dutta P (2019) Synthesis, characterization and antifungal activity of biosynthesized silver nanoparticle. Indian Phytopathol 72:79–88. https://doi.org/10.1007/s42360-018-0081-4
52. Kar S, Nayak RN, Sahoo NR, Bakhara CK, Panda MK, Pal US, Bal LM (2021) Rice weevil management through application of silica nano particle and physico-chemical and cooking characterization of the treated rice. J Stored Prod Res 94:101892
53. Kashyap PL, Kumar S, Jasrotia P, Singh DP, Singh GP (2020) Nanotechnology in wheat production and protection. In: Dasgupta N, Ranjan S, Lichtfouse E (eds) Environmental nanotechnology, vol 4. Springer, Cham, pp 165–194
54. Keck CM, Müller RH (2013) Nanotoxicological classification system (NCS)—a guide for the risk-benefit assessment of nanoparticulate drug delivery systems. Eur J Pharm Biopharm 84:445–448
55. Khan MR, Rizvi TF, Ahamad F (2019) Application of nanomaterials in plant disease diagnosis and management. In: Nanobiotechnology applications in plant protection, vol 2, pp 19-33
56. Khoobdel M, Ahsaei SM, Farzaneh M (2013) Insecticidal activity of polycaprolactone nanocapsules loaded with Rosmarinus officinalis essential oil in *Tribolium castaneum* (Herbst). Entomol Res 2017:175–184
57. Kim S, Kim K, Lamsal K, Kim Y, Kim S, Jung M, Sim S, Kim H, Chang S, Kim J, Lee Y (2009) An in vitro study of the antifungal effect of silver nanoparticles on oak wilt pathogen Raffaelea sp. J Microbiol Biotechnol 19(8):760–764
58. Kodandaram MH, Saha S, Rai AB, Prakash NS (2013) Compendium on pesticide use in vegetables. In: Extension Bulletin No. 50. ICAR-IIVR. Varanasi, U.P., India

59. Kohler HR, Triebskorn R (2013) Wildlife ecotoxicology of pesticides: can we track effects to the population level and beyond? Science 341:759–765
60. Kora AJ, Mounika J, Jagadeeshwar R (2020) Rice leaf extract synthesized silver nanoparticles: an in vitro fungicidal evaluation against *Rhizoctonia solani*, the causative agent of sheath blight disease in rice. Fungal Biol 124(7):671–681
61. Kumar A, Dixit CK (2017) Methods for characterization of nanoparticles. In: Advances in nanomedicine for the delivery of therapeutic nucleic acids. Woodhead Publishing, pp 43–58
62. Kumar N, Kumar R, Shakil NA, Sarkar DJ, Chander S (2019) Evaluation of fipronil nanoformulations for effective management of brown plant hopper (*Nilaparvata lugens*) in rice. Int J Pest Manag 65(1):86–93
63. Kumar S, Nehra M, Dilbaghi N, Marrazza G, Hassan AA, Kim KH (2019) Nano-based smart pesticide formulations: emerging opportunities for agriculture. J Control Release 294:131–153
64. Kumar S, Nehra M, Kedia D, Dilbaghi N, Tankeshwar K, Kim KH (2018) Carbon nanotubes: a potential material for energy conversion and storage. Prog Energy Combust Sci 64:219–253
65. Laborde A (2008) Pesticides. Children's health and environment: training package. World Health Organization, Geneva. https://www.who.int/ceh/capacity/Pesticides.pdf
66. Maddala VKS, Singh S (2023) Essential oils from plants and their role in nanomaterial synthesis characterization and applications. In: Secondary metabolites based green synthesis of nanomaterials and their applications. Singapore: Springer Nature Singapore, pp 191–207
67. Maddala VKS, Singh S, Bandi J (2024) Soil properties influencing nutrient signaling in plant soil systems. In: Essential minerals in plant-soil systems. Elsevier, pp 373–393
68. Madhavi V, Reddy A, Madhavi G, Reddy NB (2020) Nanoencapsulation of pesticides: Sustainable perspective in agriculture. In: AIP conference proceedings, vol 2208. AIP Publishing, p 1
69. Manikandan A, Sathiyabama M (2016) Preparation of chitosan nanoparticles and its effect on detached rice leaves infected with *Pyricularia grisea*. Int J Biol Macromol 84:58–61
70. Meddya S, Meshram S, Sarkar D, Datta R, Singh S, Avinash G, Thulasinathan T (2023) Plant stomata: an unrealized possibility in plant defense against invading pathogens and stress tolerance. Plants 12(19):3380
71. Muhlen AZ, Muhlen EZ, Niehus H, Mehnert W (1996) Atomic force microscopy studies of solid lipid nanoparticles. Pharm Res 13:1411–1416
72. Naeini AT, Adeli M, Vossoughi M (2010) Poly(citric acid)-block-poly(ethylene glycol) copolymers—new biocompatible hybrid materials for nanomedicine. Nanomedicine NBM 6(4):556–562
73. Nanopesticides (n.d.) Market Size, Growth, Trends, Report 2023–2032 (precedenceresearch.com)
74. Nuruzzaman MD, Rahman MM, Liu Y, Naidu R (2016) Nanoencapsulation, nano-guard for pesticides: a new window for safe application. J Agric Food Chem 64:1447–1483
75. Parveen R, Khare N, Singh S, Johri P (2023) An In Silico outlook for the detection and surveillance of evolving and persistent plant pathogens. In: Detection, diagnosis and management of soil-borne phytopathogens. Singapore: Springer Nature Singapore, pp 17–40
76. Patani A, Patel A, Prajapati D, Khare N, Singh S (2023) Various agriculture crop plant-based bioactive compounds and their use in nanomaterial synthesis and applications. In: Nanomaterials from agricultural and horticultural products. Singapore: Springer Nature, Singapore, pp 223–241
77. Patani A, Prajapati D, Shukla K, Patel M, Patani P, Patel A, Singh S (2024) Environmental stress–induced alterations in the micro-and macronutrients status of plant. In: Essential minerals in plant-soil systems. Elsevier, pp 181–195
78. Ponarulselvam S, Panneerselvam C, Murugan K, Aarthi N, Kalimuthu K, Thangamani S (2012) Synthesis of silver nanoparticles using leaves of *Catharanthus roseus* Linn. G. Don and their antiplasmodial activities. Asian Pac J Trop Biomed 2:574–580
79. Popp J, Pető K, Nagy J (2013) Pesticide productivity and food security: a review. Agron Sustain Dev 33:243–255

80. Pradhan S, Roy I, Lodh G, Patra P, Choudhury SR, Samanta A, Goswami A (2013) Entomotoxicity and biosafety assessment of PEGylated acephate nanoparticles: a biologically safe alternative to neurotoxic pesticides. J Environ Sci Health 48:559–569
81. Rahwanudin I, Susanto A, Panatarani C, Zainuddin A, Setiawati W (2022) Study of spinetoram nano suspension for environmentally friendly control of *Plutella xylostella* L. (Lepidoptera: Plutellidae). Biocatalysis and Agricultural Biotechnology, vol 44, p 102456
82. Raj SN, Anooj ES, Rajendran K, Vallinayagam S (2021) A comprehensive review on regulatory invention of nano pesticides in agricultural nano formulation and food system. J Mol Struct 1239:130517
83. Rajashekara H, Mishra KK, Aditya JP, Pattanayak A, Kant L (2023) Race distribution pattern of Magnaporthe oryzae causing rice blast in mid and high altitudes of North-Western Himalayan region of India. Indian Phytopathol. https://doi.org/10.1007/s42360-023-00665-2
84. Rajeswari E, Vidya Sagar B, Savani AK, Kannan C, Maheshwari TU, Devi GU, Ramanjineyulu P (2023) Unveiling the potential of rice rhizospheric microbes and indigenous organic sources for the management of rice blast. J Phytopathol 171(4–5):165–179
85. Reddy BS (2013) Non-pesticidal management of pests: status, issues and prospects—a review. Working Paper No. 130, RULNR Working Paper No. 22. Research Unit for Livelihoods and Natural Resources (Supported by Jamsetji Tata Trust). Centre for Economic and Social Studies Begumpet, Hyderabad-500016
86. Rizzati V, Briand O, Guillou H, Gamet-Payrastre L (2016) Effects of pesticide mixtures in human and animal models: an update of the recent literature. Chem Biol Interact 254:231–246
87. Rouhani M, Samih MA, Kalantari S (2013) Insecticidal effect of silica and silver nanoparticles on the cowpea seed beetle, *Callosobruchus maculatus* F.(Col.: Bruchidae), pp 297–305
88. Sabry AK, Salem HA, Metwally HM (2021) Development of imidacloprid and indoxacarb formulations to nanoformulations and their efficacy against *Spodoptera littoralis* (Boisd). Bull Natl Res Cent 45:1–7
89. Sao P, Chand Y, Kumar A, Singh S (2021) Potential drug target identification in porphyromonas gingivalis using in-silico subtractive metabolic pathway analysis. Bangladesh J Med Sci 20(4):887–896
90. Sao P, Parveen R, Khattri A, Sharma S, Tiwari N, Singh S (2022) Understanding the metabolomics of medicinal plants under environmental pollution: challenges and opportunities. In: Environmental pollution and medicinal plants, pp 193–205
91. Saranya S, Selvi A, Babujanarthanam R, Rajasekar A, Madhavan J (2020) Insecticidal activity of nanoparticles and mechanism of action. In: Siddhardha DB et al (eds) Model organisms to study biological activities and toxicity of nanoparticles, pp 243–66
92. Sasson Y, Levy-Ruso G, Toledano O, Ishaaya I (2007) Nanosuspensions: emerging novel agrochemical formulations. In: Ishaaya I, Horowitz AR, Nauen R (eds) Insecticides Design Using Advanced Technologies. Berlin, Springer, Heidelberg, pp 1–39
93. Scott-Fordsmand JJ, Fraceto LF, Amorim MJ (2022) Nano-pesticides: the lunch-box principle-deadly goodies (semio-chemical functionalised nanoparticles that deliver pesticide only to target species). J Nanobiotechnology 20:1–9
94. Sharma S, Kooner R, Arora R (2017) Insect pests and crop losses. In: Arora R, Sandhu S (eds) Breeding insect resistant crops for sustainable agriculture. Springer Nature, Singapore, pp 45–66. https://doi.org/10.1007/978-981-10-6056-4_2
95. Siddhartha VA, Bashyal BM, Gogoi R, Kumar R (2022) New nano-fungicides for the management of sheath blight disease (Rhizoctonia solani) in rice. Int J Pest Manag 68(3):217–226
96. Sigfridsson K, Nordmark A, Theilig S, Lindahl A (2011) A formulation comparison between micro-and nanosuspensions: the importance of particle size for absorption of a model compound, following repeated oral administration to rats during early development. Drug Dev Ind Pharm 37:185–192
97. Singh A, Sengar RS, Singh AK, Singh S, Kumar A, Ahmad K (2019) Impact of genetic engineering on agriculture food crops. Biotech Today Int J Biol Sci 9(1):17–24

98. Sioutas C, Delfino RJ, Singh M (2005) Exposure assessment for atmospheric ultrafine particles (UFPs) and implications in epidemiologic research. Environ Health Perspect 113:947–955
99. Soltani Nejad M, Bonjar GH, Khatami M, Amini A, Aghighi S (2017) In vitro and in vivo antifungal properties of silver nanoparticles against Rhizoctonia solani, a common agent of rice sheath blight disease. IET Nanobiotechnol 11(3):236–240
100. Song J, Soytong K, Kanokmedhakul S, Kanokmedhkul K, Poeaim S (2020) Natural product of nano-particles constructed from Chaetomium spp. to control rice blast disease caused by Magnaporthe oryzae. Int J Agric Biol 23(5):1013–20
101. Stackelberg PE, Kauffman LJ, Ayers MA, Baehr AL (2001) Frequently co-occurring pesticides and volatile organic compounds in public supply and monitoring wells, Southern New Jersey, USA. Environ Toxicol Chem Int J 20:853–865
102. Thabet AF, Boraei HA, Galal OA, El-Samahy MF, Mousa KM, Zhang YZ, Tuda M, Helmy EA, Wen J, Nozaki T (2021) Silica nanoparticles as pesticide against insects of different feeding types and their non-target attraction of predators. Sci Rep 11:14484
103. Thiruvengadam V, Bansod AV (2020) Characterization of silver nanoparticles synthesized using chemical method and its antibacterial property. Biointerface Res Appl Chem 10:7257–7264
104. Unsworth JB, Corsi C, Van Emon JM, Farenhorst A, Hamilton DJ, Howard CJ, Hunter R, Jenkins JJ, Kleter GA, Kookana RS, Lalah JO, Leggett M, Miglioranza KSB, Miyagawa H, Peranginangin N, Rubin B, Saha B, Shakil NA (2016) Developing global leaders for research, regulation, and stewardship of crop protection chemistry in the 21st century. J Agric Food Chem 64:52–60
105. Vani C, Brindhaa U (2013) Silica nanoparticles as nanocides against Corcyra cephalonica (S.), the stored grain pest. Int J Pharma Bio Sci 4(3)
106. Vedpriya A (2010) Living systems: eco-friendly nanofactories. Dig J Nanomater Bios 5(1):9–21
107. Verma N, Sao P, Srivastava A, Singh S (2021) Physiological and molecular responses to drought, submergence and excessive watering in plants. In: Harsh environment and plant resilience: molecular and functional aspects, pp 305–321
108. Vishwakarma SK, Ilyas T, Shahid M, Malviya D, Kumar S, Singh S, Singh HV (2024) Bacillus spp.: nature's gift to agriculture and humankind. In: Applications of bacillus and bacillus derived genera in agriculture, biotechnology and beyond. Singapore: Springer Nature, Singapore, pp 1–36
109. Vora Z, Pandya J, Vaikuntapu PR, Singh S, Asha S, Purama RK (2023) Genome-wide association of defense hormone crosstalk in plants. In: Hormonal cross-talk, plant defense and development. Academic Press, pp 353–371
110. Walker GW, Kookana RS, Smith NE, Kah M, Doolette CL, Reeves PT, Navarro DA (2017) Ecological risk assessment of nano-enabled pesticides: a perspective on problem formulation. J Agric Food Chem 66(26):6480–6486
111. Wang K, Peng Y, Chen J, Peng Y, Wang X, Shen Z, Han Z (2020) Comparison of efficacy of RNAi mediated by various nanoparticles in the rice striped stem borer (*Chilo suppressalis*). Pestic Biochem Physiol 165:104467
112. Wang L, Li X, Zhang G, Dong J, Eastoe J (2007) Oil-in-water nanoemulsions for pesticide formulations. J Colloid Interface Sci 314:230–235
113. Wang D, Saleh NB, Byro A, Zepp R, Demessie ES, Luxton TP, Ho TK, Burgess MR, Flury M, White JC, Su C(2022) Nano-enabled pesticides for sustainable agriculture and global food security. Nano Technol 17:347–360
114. Wani TA, Masoodi FA, Baba WN, Ahmad M, Rahmanian N, Jafari SM (2019) Nanoencapsulation of agrochemicals, fertilizers, and pesticides for improved plant production. In Advances in phytonanotechnology. Academic Press, pp 279–298
115. Watson SB, Gergely A, Janus ER (2011) Where is agronanotechnolgoy heading in the United States and European Union. Nat Resour Environ 26:8–12
116. Whitehouse P, Rannard S (2010) The application of nanodispersions to agriculture. Outlooks Pest Manag 21:190–192

117. Worrall EA, Hamid A, Mody KT, Mitter N, Pappu,HR (2018) Nanotechnology for plant disease management. Agronomy 8(12):285
118. Yadav J, Jasroti P, Kashyap PL, Bhardwaj AK, Kumar S, Singh M, Singh GP (2020) Nanopesticides: current status and scope for their application in agriculture. Plant Prot Sci 58:1–17
119. Yan S, Ren BY, Shen J (2021) Nanoparticle-mediated double-stranded RNA delivery system: a promising approach for sustainable pest management. Insect Sci 28:21–34
120. Zannat R, Rahman MM, Afroz M (2021) Application of nanotechnology in insect pest management: a review. SAARC J Agric 19:1–11
121. Zhi H, Zhou S, Pan W, Shang Y, Zeng Z, Zhang H (2022) The promising nanovectors for gene delivery in plant genome engineering. Int J Mol Sci 23:8501
122. Ziental D, Czarczynska-Goslinska B, Mlynarczyk DT, Glowacka-Sobotta A, Stanisz B, Goslinski T, Sobotta L (2020) Titanium dioxide nanoparticles: prospects and applications in medicine. Nanomaterials 10(2):387

# Silver Nanoparticles for Managing Fungal Diseases of Cocoa Crops

**Pranjal Kr Kaman, Vithanala Shiva Sai Swaroop, and Ajit Kumar Savani**

**Abstract** Nanotechnology is the design, character, creation and use of structures, materials and systems by controlling their shape and size at the nanometer scale. The main focus of this research is nanoscale materials and how they are used for various purposes in agriculture. Nanotechnology will become a new branch of science covering disciplines such as physics, chemistry, biology, information science and medicine in the coming years. In these systems, various metal nanoparticles such as silver, gold, zinc and iron are used in the prevention and treatment of plant diseases. Among various metal nanoparticles, silver nanoparticles are the most widely used. Silver nanoparticles exhibit unique physical and chemical properties compared to their macroscopic counterparts. Biosynthesized silver nanoparticles are more important than chemical synthesis because they are safe and do not produce toxic byproducts. More than 30 fungal diseases are known to cause disease in cocoa cultivation, of which *Phytophthora* spp., *Moniliophthora perniciosa* and *Moniliophthora roreri* are the most serious, and can cause commercial losses in crop cultivation. To date, there are no effective controls to control fungal diseases in cocoa. Therefore, it is possible to use biosynthesized silver nanoparticles for the management of major fungal diseases in cocoa.

**Keywords** Cocoa · Fungal · Nanoparticles · Silver nanoparticles

## 1 Introduction

The Olmec, Mayan, and Aztec civilizations were the first to cultivate cocoa (*Theobroma cacao*), or chocolate, in Central America. Its global spread can be attributed to pre-Columbian cultures. Chocolate is made from cocoa beans, which are the seeds

P. K. Kaman (✉) · V. Shiva Sai Swaroop
Department of Plant Pathology, Assam Agricultural University, Jorhat, Assam, India
e-mail: pranjal.k.kaman@aau.ac.in

A. K. Savani
ICAR-National Academy of Agricultural Research Management, Hyderabad, Telangana, India

 
D. Jabborova et al. (eds.), *Nanomaterials in Agroforestry Systems*, Smart Nanomaterials Technology, https://doi.org/10.1007/978-981-96-1337-3_12

of this fruit. The cocoa tree is native to the upper Amazon basin in Brazil, Ecuador, Peru and Colombia. Good farming techniques determine how cocoa is grown. Under normal circumstances, seedlings are planted after seeds are sown in nurseries. It is sometimes rare to see buried cocoa beans directly in the ground in some countries. Planting is usually done at the beginning of the rainy season to maintain soil moisture levels while the roots take hold. The cocoa tree needs high and consistent levels of humidity and shade to grow healthy and stay safe. For this purpose, cocoa is sometimes planted with other species such as banana or coconut trees. It takes three to four years for a cocoa tree to bear its first fruit, depending on the variety, and six to seven years for maximum harvest. Although the fruits grow throughout the year, there are usually four harvests: two small harvests at the beginning of the rainy season and a larger harvest at the end of the rainy season. Each fruit (called a pod) produced by the cocoa tree contains 25–40 seeds or beans, as well as soft flesh and immature beans [4]. In order to harvest coffee beans, the outer bark of the tree must be cut. Once the pods are removed, the beans undergo two stages of fermentation and drying before being sent to further processing. These are the most important stages of the production process, as they bring important changes to cocoa, giving it its taste and aroma [12, 101].

Around the world, cocoa is grown in several tropical and subtropical regions. Temperatures typically occur between 15 to 32 °C at elevations less than 300 mean above sea level, while they can occasionally reach 1100 mean above sea level in certain habitats. For the crop to grow well, the amount of rainfall should be distributed equally throughout the year, between 1500 and 3000 mm. Ivory Coast, Ghana, Indonesia, Ecuador, Nigeria, Cameroon, and Brazil are the top producers International Cocoa Organization [44]. As per the International Cocoa Organization, the output of cocoa reached 4697 thousand tonnes globally in 2019/2020, and it is expected to continue growing International Cocoa Organization [44]. In 2019, the market saw trade in raw cocoa and cocoa products valued at over 50,300 million dollars [5].

Like other crops, and cocoa plants are exposed to various diseases caused by plant pathogens at all stages of production (collection, harvest, fermentation, drying and storage). The climate and agriculture in all cocoa-growing countries encourage fungus growth, which reduces the quality of the final product. The quality of cocoa production is affected by many factors, including cosmetics, regional conditions where facilities and management are located and post-harvest processes such as fermentation, drying and storage. In particular, filamentous fungi can infect several stages of the cocoa processing chain, while poor agricultural practices can affect the quality characteristics of cocoa [15]. Many important fungal diseases have attracted attention in the past 20 years and pose a serious threat to sugarcane. Black spot disease, witch's broom disease, and frost bark rot are three diseases that can be very serious and cause significant damage [22, 26, 97] (Table 1).

**Table 1** Estimated annual reduction in potential cocoa production by major diseases. *Source* Taylor [97]

| Diseases | Pathogen | Region | Reduced production | |
|---|---|---|---|---|
| | | | (tons × 1000) | ($ million) |
| Black pod | *Phytophthora* spp. | Africa/Brazil/Asia | 450 | 423 |
| Witches' broom | *Crinipellis perniciosa* | Latin America | 250 | 235 |
| Frosty pod rot | *Moniliophthora roreri* | Latin America | 30 | 47 |
| Swollen shoot | CSSV | Africa | 50 | 28 |
| Vascular-streak dieback | *Oncobasidium theobromae* | Asia | 30 | 28 |

## 2 Major Fungal Diseases in Cocoa

One of the most important fungal diseases is witches' broom, caused by the basidiomycete fungus *Crinipellis perniciosa* (Stahel) Singer. The disease, first discovered in the Amazon in the eighteenth century [91], prevented the spread of cocoa grown in its region until recently. Over the last 10 years, Brazil's cocoa bean production has fallen from 400,000 metric tons to 100,000 metric tons, mainly due to the fungal disease *Crinipellis perniciosa.* In addition to Brazil, the disease has also spread to Panama, Peru, Ecuador, Venezuela in Central America and Colombia in South America. Trinidad and Tobago in the Caribbean also hosts this unique species [71, 75].

Frost pod rot is another serious disease caused by a fungus called *Moniliophthora roreri* that attacks cocoa beans in pods [21]. Although the fungus has not yet been reported in Brazil, it has spread from Panama to Costa Rica and Nicaragua in Central America. This disease can spread to other cocoa growing areas as the fungus can produce many spores in the air that give the pods a frosted appearance [23]. In Ecuador, Rorer [81] described *T. bicolor* (cacao blanco) and *Herrania balaoensis* (cacao de monte) as wild "cacao" affected by the disease. The current distribution of frost bark rot is limited to southern Central America (Nicaragua, Costa Rica, and Panama) and western South America (Ecuador, Peru, and Colombia). However, Brazil, one of the cocoa-growing regions of South America, is now under threat, if phytosanitary measures are not taken frequently (7–10 day schedule), yield loss predicted to be decrease by 25% or even below expectations [94].

Black pod, a disease that affects multiple species of the fungus-like bacterium known as *Phytophthora* and manifests itself in various ways, is one of the most frequently occurring fungi that destroy cacao around the world [32]. The most common species, which cause sporadic losses, are present in across the globe where cacao is produced. In West Africa, the world's top cacao-growing region is affected by the species *P. megakarya*, which is expanding and causing significant losses [31]. Black pods can cause annual crop losses that might vary from 30 to 90%. West and

Central Africa, which produce 60–70% of cocoa beans worldwide, is more prone to this disease. *Phytophthora* isolates from cocoa were previously categorized as *P. palmivora* (Butl.) Butler [11]. Cacao, rubber, papaya, pineapple, coconut, black pepper, citrus, avocado, and various decorative plants, have all been known to be targets of this species, which has been identified as one of the most significant infections in the tropics. Earlier research found some heterogeneity in the form and sorts of lesions that are isolated from other nations caused on cacao pods. *P. palmivora* isolates from cocoa were divided into four morphological categories in 1976 (MF1, MF2, MF3, and MF4). The morphological groupings were redefined by subsequent research. The MF1 form of *P. palmivora* was regarded as the species' normal form, and the MF2 form was a variation of the species [11]. *P. megakarya* Brasier and Gryphon, a new species, characterized the MF3 form, whereas *P. capsici* Leonian, a known species, was thought to represent the MF4 form [108]. *P. palmivora, P. capsici*, and *P. citrophthora* (Smith and Smith) Leonian have all been linked to the main cacao-growing region of Bahia, Brazil [49]. The prevalent and most significant species infecting cacao in Brazil appears to be *Phytophthora capsici*, which has also been found in other Central and South American nations, the West Indies, Indonesia, and India [20]. The least frequent species in Brazil is *Phytophthora citrophthora*, but it is also the most dangerous [49].

## 3 Nanoscience and Nanotechnology

The field of agricultural nanotechnology is still in its early phases of growth, despite its large range of applications in research and other areas of medical science. According to Rai et al. [78], the word "Nano" is derived from a Greek word that means "extremely small" or "dwarves". The physicist Richard Feynman presented the fundamental ideas of nanoscience and nanotechnology on December 29, 1959, at the California Institute of Technology (Cal Tech), under the title "There's a Plenty of Room at the Bottom" [25]. Professor Norio Taniguchi eventually came up with the name "Nanotechnology" by drawing on Feynman's investigations into ultra-precise machining. Nori Taniguchi invented the term "nanotechnology" in 1974 during a discussion about production engineering at the Tokyo International Conference. According to Rai et al. [78] and Huang et al. [38], the study of nanoscience and nanotechnology enables the well-developed application of exceptionally small objects and is capable of invading all other scientific fields, including engineering, biology, chemistry, materials science, metallurgy, and biotechnology. Biotechnology and nanotechnology are coupled to generate bionanotechnology, which seeks to advance many biosynthetic and friendly to the environment for the production of various nanomaterials [95]. Due to their distinctive properties compared to macroscopic particles, several studies on the creation of nanoparticles have generated significant interest in the newly growing field of science [86]. The huge array of innovative synthesis protocol creation and a variety of characterization methodologies are proof of nanotechnology's enormous advancement [89].

## 4 Nanosilver

The most commonly utilized and researched nanoparticle for biosystems is nanosilver. Its antimicrobial properties have long been recognized. Compared to bulk silver, more surface area and surface atom fraction on silver nanoparticles results in greater antibacterial activity. Colloidal nanosilver is a solution of well-dispersed, stabilized silver nanoparticles that is more effective than fungicide at adhering to bacteria and fungi. Silver is recognized to have antibacterial qualities and the ability to serve as a disinfectant. Because silver's ionic form has a higher antimicrobial activity than its non-ionic form, it inhibits the growth of unicellular microbes by interfering with the metabolism of enzymes through oligodynamic action [98]. The extreme reactivity of ionic silver and its easy reduction or oxidation into a metal depending on the medium it is present in make it unstable.

## 5 Creation of Silver Nanoparticle

Researchers within the discipline of material science are working to create new materials that outperform existing ones in terms of cost, utility, and characteristics. Various methods of physical, chemical, and biological production have been created to improve the functionality of nanoparticles, exhibiting superior capabilities, giving researchers more control over the particle size, dispersion, and appearance [30, 87, 90]. The creation of nanoparticles with improved authority over their composition, amount, purity, form, distribution, size, and quality through economical, ecologically friendly methods has never been easy for researchers [106].

### *5.1 Eco-Friendly Nanoparticle Synthesis*

Eco-Friendly synthesis is the creation of nanoparticles using living things or biologically derived materials. Plant extracts, live bacteria, or fungi can be used to make nanoparticles. Due to their low energy requirements, ability to operate at room temperature or below, and environmental friendliness, these techniques have advantages over more conventional methods of creating nanoparticles. These techniques use organisms that can typically be simply left to carry out their functions, are easily cultivated on straightforward organic media, and are renewable resources. Numerous creatures have been found to produce chalk and silica, two well-known examples of inorganic particles. More types of bacteria can convert metal ions to metal. By reducing iron compounds, several bacteria can create magnetic materials. These bacteria then incorporate magnetic nanoparticles into structures called magnetosomes within their cells. Certain species of bacteria have been successfully used in the production of nanoparticles. Both intracellularly and extracellularly, this is possible. The nitrate anion ($NO^3$), which is assumed to be used by the bacteria as a source of nitrogen, is left behind as metallic silver. In experiments, flowering plants and fungi have been utilized to create nanoparticles.

## 5.2 *Need for Green Synthesis*

Nanotechnology and biotechnology are connected through the green chemistry method known as the biological production of nanoparticles. It has been documented that phototrophic eukaryotes like plants can biosynthesize nanoparticles made of Au, Ag, Au-Ag alloy, Urannite ($UO_2$, a radioactive chemical), Tellurium, Selenium, Platinum, Palladium, Silica, Titania, Zirconia, Quantum dots, and Magnetite. Although biological nanoparticles are durable, their synthesis proceeds slowly and they are not monodispersed. The polydispersity of nanoparticles and consequent decline in synthesis rate are caused by variations in the concentration of artificially produced macromolecules or elements involved in the nucleation of particles throughout time. A combination of approaches, including photobiological technologies, may be utilized to solve these issues, including the optimization of various methods for microbial cultivation and extraction. To accelerate synthesis and enhance the properties of nanoparticles, a thorough understanding of the cellular, biochemical, and molecular mechanisms underlying the production of biological nanoparticles is essential. The potential of bacteria and plants as biological sources for the creation of nanoparticles has not yet been extensively investigated because of their enormous biodiversity. The major reaction that takes place during the biosynthesis of nanoparticles is reduction/oxidation. Nanoparticle biosynthesis was required because physical and chemical processes were too expensive. Chemical synthesis processes sometimes lead to the surface absorption of some hazardous compounds that may have unfavourable consequences in medical applications [66]. This is not an issue for biosynthesized nanoparticles made with a green synthesis technique [9]. Scientists therefore exploited plant extracts (phytochemicals) and microbial enzymes in their hunt for less expensive paths for the manufacture of nanoparticles. Because of their reducing or antioxidant properties, they frequently contribute to the reduction of metal compounds into their corresponding nanoparticles. Green synthesis is superior to physical and chemical processes because it is easier to scale up for large-scale synthesis, less expensive, and more ecologically adaptable. It also eliminates the need for harmful chemicals, high pressure, energy, and temperature.

### 5.2.1 Creation of Silver Nanoparticles from Fungi

Because fungi can release more proteins, they can produce more nanoparticles [58]. More proteins directly translate to more productive nanoparticles. Silver nanoparticle manufacturing by fungi is thought to involve two stages: the first is the $Ag^+$ ions being trapped at the fungal cells' surface, and the second is the enzymes within

**Table 2** Some examples of fungus for the creation of silver nanoparticles

| Sl No | Name of the fungus | References |
|---|---|---|
| 1 | *Phaenerochaete chrysosporium* | Vigneshwaran et al. [102] |
| 2 | *Aspergillus ustus* | Nayak and Anitha [62] |
| 3 | *Trichoderma viride* | Fayaz et al. [24] |
| 4 | *Trichoderma harzianum* | Singh and Raja [93] |
| 5 | *Pleurotus ostreatus* | Devika et al. [17] |
| 6 | *Penicilium* spp | Hemath et al. [36] |
| 7 | *Fusarium oxysporum* | Duran et al. [19] |
| 8 | *Aspergillus niger* | Gade et al. [27] |
| 9 | *Fusarium acuminatum* | Ingle et al. [42] |
| 10 | *Trichoderma asperellum* | Mukherjee et al. [61] |
| 11 | *Penicillium sp.* | Sadowski et al. [83] |
| 12 | *Phoma glomerata* | Birla et al. [10] |
| 13 | *Fusarium solani* | Ingle et al. [43] |
| 14 | *Fusarium semitectum* | Basavaraja et al. [8] |
| 15 | *Phoma* sp. 3.2883 | Chen et al. [13] |

those cells reducing the silver ions [60]. Extracellular enzymes like anthraquinones and naphthoquinones are said to aid in the reduction. Ahmad et al. [2] state that a shuttle quinine extracellular mechanism and NADPH-dependent nitrate reductase are believed to be responsible for the creation of nanoparticles.Although the precise mechanism underlying the synthesis of silver nanoparticles by fungus is still not entirely understood, it is thought that the aforementioned phenomenon is to blame. The extremely slow technique of creating silver nanoparticles using microorganisms is a significant disadvantage (Table 2).

### 5.2.2 Synthesis of Silver Nanoparticles from Bacteria

The *Pseudomonas stutzeri* AG259 strain, isolated from a silver mine, provided the first indication that bacteria may manufacture silver nanoparticles [35].

High concentrations of metal ions can support the growth and survival of certain bacteria. The microbes' resistance to the metal is what causes this phenomena. Husseiny et al. [39] list the following mechanisms as the root causes of resistance: efflux systems, changed toxicity and solubility as a result of biosorption, bioaccumulation, reduction or oxidation, formation of extracellular complexes or metal precipitation, and lack of particular metal transport mechanisms. Another factor is that even while these organisms can thrive in lower quantities of metal ions, exposing them to larger concentrations can make them hazardous. The nitrate reductase enzyme is the most generally acknowledged component of Ag production. Nitrate is changed

Table 3 Some examples of bacteria for the synthesis of silver nanoparticles

| Sl No | Name of the fungus | References |
|---|---|---|
| 1 | *Bacillus licheniformis* | Kalimuthu et al. [47] |
| 2 | *Escherichia coli* | Gurunathan et al. [34] |
| 3 | *Bacillus cereus* | Babu and Gunasekaran [6] |
| 4 | *Bacillus koriensis* | Sharma et al. [88] |
| 5 | *Klebsiella planticola* | Paulkumar et al. [69] |

into nitrite by the enzyme. In the presence of alpha-nicotinamide adenine dinucleotide phosphate reduced form (NADPH)-dependent nitrate reductase, the downstream processing step necessary in other circumstances for the in vitro cultivation of Ag-utilizing bacteria would be avoided [100] (Table 3).

### 5.2.3 Synthesis of Silver Nanoparticles from Plant Extracts

The main benefit of using plant extracts rather than microbes to produce silver nanoparticles is that the former are more readily available, typically safe and nontoxic, and have a variety of metabolites that can aid in the reduction of Ag ions. The basic mechanism of the method is phytochemical-induced plant-assisted reduction; the main phytochemicals involved are terpenoids, flavones, ketones, aldehydes, amides, and carboxylic acids; the ions are immediately reduced due to the action of water-soluble phytochemicals such as flavones, organic acids, and quinones [50, 51]. Studies have shown that xerophytes contain emodin, an anthraquinone that passes through tautomerization to produce silver nanoparticles. It was found that mesophytes contain three different kinds of benzoquinones: hydroquinone, dietchequinone, and remirin. Jha et al. [46] suggest that phytochemicals might be directly involved in the reduction of ions and the resulting silver nanoparticle formation (Fig. 1 and Table 4).

## 6 Management of Fungal Diseases of Cocoa Through Silver Nanoparticles

The fact that Phytophthora can live for years in soil and debris as zoospores makes controlling black pod difficult [20]. According to Evans and Prior [21], the disease may also be present in the canopy year-round, ready to spread rapidly when the climate is right for sporulation and dissemination. This is because susceptible pods may remain on the trees for much of the year. For chemical management, fungicides with metalaxyl- and copper-based active ingredients are used. These, however, are not successful, are expensive for small farmers, and are not practical from an economic standpoint [26, 70]. Chemicals are heavily used in tropical rainforests raises environmental issues, and there may be issues with side effects that aren't intended by the

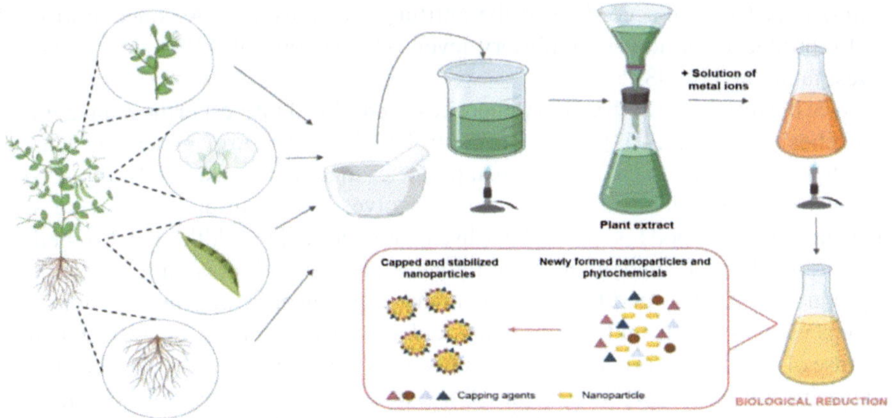


**Fig. 1** General steps of green synthesis of inorganic nanoparticles using plant extracts [80]

**Table 4** Some plant extracts for the creation of silver nanoparticles

| Sl No | Name of the fungus | References |
|---|---|---|
| 1 | *Acalypha indica* | Krishnaraj et al. [54] |
| 2 | *Allium sativum* | Ahmad et al. [1] |
| 3 | *Azadirachta indica* | Prathana et al. [74] |
| 4 | *Citrus sinensis* | Kaviya et al. [48] |
| 5 | *Cynodon dactylon* | Sahu et al. [84] |
| 6 | *Mangifera indica* | Philip [72] |
| 7 | *Medicago sativa* | Lukman et al. [56] |
| 8 | *Morinda pubescens* | Inbathamizh et al. [41] |
| 9 | *Piper betle L* | Usha and Rajasekharreddy [99] |
| 10 | *Terminalia chebula* | Jebakumar and Sethuraman [45] |

chemical and pathogen resistance. At the moment, cacao lacks the genetic resistance needed to control black pods [67, 104]. In such a situation the use of silver nanoparticles comes into play thereby inhibiting the zoospore creaion, zoospore germination, germ tube lengthening, and mycelial development. It was discovered that the fungus *Phytophthora palmivora*, which is responsible for several plant diseases, could be stopped in its tracks by bacterial silver nanoparticles. *Bacillus subtilis* extracellular nanoparticles have demonstrated substantial antifungal activity against *Phytophthora palmivora.* Silver nanoparticles produced extracellularly and derived from *Bacillus subtilis* (Mt3b) displayed a radial inhibition percentage of 81.81% against *Phytophthora palmivora* [105]. Titanium dioxide –silver ($TiO_2$-Ag) composites have been created using the Ultrasonic Batch Cleaning process and employed as an antifungal candidate against the pod rot fungus that affects cacao plants and is brought on by *Phytophthora palmivora.* $TiO_2$-Ag exhibits a good antifungal effect against *P. palmivora*, according to the antifungal activity test. A concentration of 2.50% produced the lowest inhibitory level, whereas one of 4.88% produced the lowest fatal rate [14, 33].

Since the turn of the 20th century, there has been a lot of interest in the management of witches' broom [21, 103]. Chemical control, biological control, genetic resistance, and phytosanitation are the four main approaches that may be used [53]. It has been demonstrated that phytosanitation, which involves removing and destroying sick plant parts, reduces pod loss and delays disease epidemics [82]. Although this method is laborious, it has been demonstrated in one study that 95% clearance is necessary to produce a 50% less pod loss [82]. Systematic chemical management of witches' brooms with protectant and systemic fungicides is not a practice in cocoa production because of the high costs and risks associated with contamination of cocoa beans and environmental health [21]. In such situations, utilizations of biologically synthesized silver nanoparticles are found to be promising because silver nanoparticles prevent fungi from producing defense mechanisms like spores. Silver nanoparticles cause the inactivation of the sulfhydryl group in the fungal cell membrane. They also create a number of hazardous chemicals, disrupt and change the structure of lipids and proteins connected to the membrane, and eventually kill the fungus. As a result, silver nanoparticles have antifungal potential [68].

In Peru, Panama, and Costa Rica, efforts are being made to manage frosty pod rot using alternate management methods, such as biological control, due to the difficulty in developing a viable and affordable fungicidal treatment [53]. This entails using mycoparasites, which are naturally existing fungi, to parasitize the pathogen and stop the spread of fungi spores. Trials in the field are being conducted with saprophytic fungi from the genera *Trichoderma* that were chosen for their ability to parasitize [73]. These microorganisms can be used to produce silver nanoparticles, which can be used to treat frosty pod rot [57].

## 7 Antifungal Mechanisms of Silver Nanoparticles

Silver nanoparticles' physical and chemical properties, including their size, shape, dispersion, and pH, affect their antifungal efficacy [37]. Pathogens can have their cell walls penetrated by silver nanoparticles that have a diameter of less than 12 nm, allowing them to enter their cytoplasm [65, 79]. Furthermore, Kim et al. [52] and Akther and Hemalatha [3] found that spherical AgNPs may effectively prevent the development of fungus at low concentrations. The smaller size of the silver particles that help in quick deposition on the fungal mycelium and then penetration inside it, as discovered by [96], may be the cause of the antifungal action. According to earlier research, silver particles smaller than a nanometer have unique features that may result from morphological, structural, and physiological alterations [63]. According to Hwang et al. [40], silver nanoparticles disrupt the metabolic process and respiration when they penetrate the fungal mycelium by reacting with cellular components. According to Morones et al. [59], metallic silver is generally unreactive but silver nanoparticles are extremely reactive because they produce $Ag^+$ ions. The ability of the nanoparticles to effectively enter microbial cells was also demonstrated [85], implying that sufficient microbial control might be achieved with lower concentrations of nano-sized silvers. According to a prior study [59], silver nanoparticles interfere with many transport mechanisms, including ion efflux. Silver ions can interfere with metabolic and respiratory processes in cells at low concentrations by interacting with molecules when they accumulate fast as a result of ion efflux malfunction. Reactive oxygen species (ROS), which harm cells by damaging proteins, lipids, and nucleic acids, are also known to be produced by silver ions as a result of their reactivity with oxygen [40, 96].

Previous cytological studies supported the findings that silver nanoparticles severely harmed the cellular components of pathogenic fungi's cell walls, damaged the integrity and structure of cell membranes, and resulted in wrinkled and depressed spores and mycelia. Then, mycelial respiration consumed less oxygen, the respiratory chain was damaged by the inactivation of important enzymes, and bound lipids and enzymes induced cell lysis. According to several studies [28, 107], eventually, the cells grew and twisted until they wilted and perished.

The molecular mechanism of silver nanoparticles has been gradually explained over the past two years by transcriptome analysis, which has given rise to a thorough understanding of potential differentially expressed genes involved in many biological processes [55, 77]. Silver nanoparticles, for instance, have a well-studied molecular mechanism against Fusarium sp. They may influence cellular energy utilisation, signal transduction pathways, cell structure, energy and substance metabolism, and the expression of the azole-related ATP-binding cassette (ABC) transporter.

In addition to serving as an energy source, carbohydrates are crucial parts of cell membranes and skeletons [18]. Given that the membranes and cell wall are made of highly cross-linked carbohydrates and glycoproteins, and silver nanoparticles work best against them [7, 29]. Plants utilise the carbon fixation pathway (CFPP) during photosynthesis to transform solar energy into biomass, bioproducts, and biofuel. Remarkably, there exist functional relationships between CFPP and the enzymes of many heterotrophic fungus [64]. The pathway that absorbed and transmitted light energy to the photosynthetic reaction centre may be significantly impacted by silver nanoparticles, as evidenced by the down-regulation of differentially expressed genes for "oxidative phosphorylation," "carbon fixation in photosynthetic organisms," and "methane metabolism" in fungal pathogens. Furthermore, fungi dramatically reduce oxidative phosphorylation, which is essential for aerobic cellular respiration. These results demonstrated that energy metabolic pathways were significantly blocked by silver nanoparticles [92].

Fungal infections used a range of cellular responses to silver nanoparticle stress in order to undo the alterations caused by the particles. For example, detoxification mechanisms for xenobiotics can be extracted from the environment or from complex mixtures formed during metabolic processes. Cytochrome P450 is engaged in over 90% of these oxidation processes and is responsible for the metabolism of a wide range of xenobiotics and endogenous compounds [109, 110].

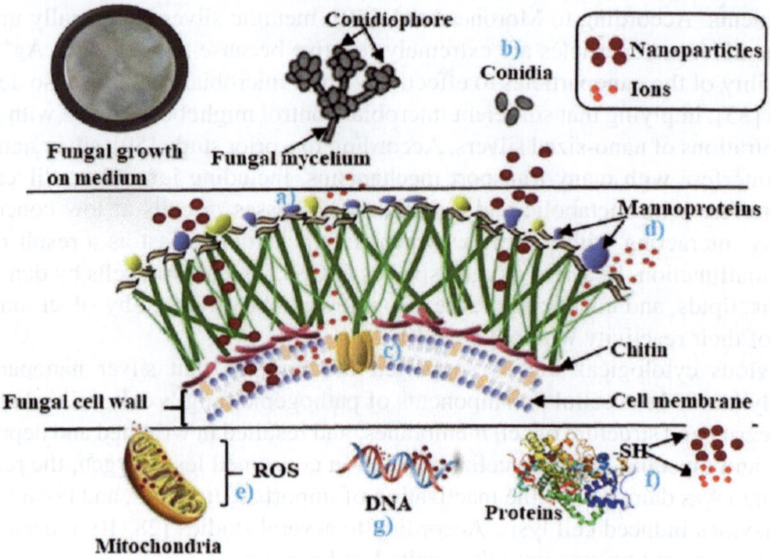


**Fig. 2** Possible mechanisms of action of metal nanoparticles on phytopathogenic fungi [16]

Silver nanoparticles have been linked to a significant amount of DNA breakage, cell death, and cell cycle arrest [76]. Genes that were differentially expressed for cellular senescence, cell growth and death, signalling pathways controlling stem cell pluripotency, and cellular community-eukaryotes became more expressed after a 24 h period (Fig. 2).

(a) When ions are released from nanoparticles, they attach themselves to specific protein groups, interfering with the permeability of cells and influencing the function of vital membrane proteins. (b) The conidia's growth and germination are suppressed by the nanoparticles. (c) Membrane potential is changed, electron transport is disrupted, and protein oxidation is caused by nanoparticles and released ions. (d) They also Hinder the oxidative electron transport of proteins. (e) In reaction to oxidative stress, they increase gene transcription, which affects the mitochondrial membrane's potential. (f) When different metallic nanoparticles catalyse oxidation processes, reactive oxygen species (ROS) are created. These activities seriously harm proteins, membranes, and deoxyribonucleic acid (DNA), as well as impair nutrient absorption. (g) The ions from the nanoparticles have a genotoxic effect that breaks down DNA and kills cells.

## 8 Conclusion

In conclusion, we can state that, at lower concentrations, nanoparticles are helpful in controlling fungal diseases in cocoa cultivations as compared to fungicides. By lowering environmental risks brought on by the non judicious use of pesticides, the use of nanoparticles as fungicides, bactericides, or viricides as plant protection materials will stop fungal infections in cocoa cultivations. However, research must be done on ecological concerns, other hazardous conditions, and the impact on the environment before it is used commercially. Prospects for future research involve investigating the application of organic nanocomposites or silver nanoparticles produced biotechnologically, whose surface biological ligands likely increase their fungicidal action.

## References

1. Ahamed M, Khan MM, Siddiqui MKJ, AlSalhi MS, Alrokayan SA (2011) Green synthesis, characterization and evaluation of biocompatibility of silver nanoparticles. Physica E Low Dimensio Sys Nanostruc 43(6):1266–1271
2. Ahmad A, Mukherjee P, Senapati S, Mandal D, Khan MI, Kumar R, Sastry M (2003) Extracellular biosynthesis of silver nanoparticles using the fungus Fusarium oxysporum. Colloids Surf B Bio 28(4):313–318
3. Akther T, Hemalatha S (2019) Mycosilver nanoparticles: synthesis, characterization and its efficacy against plant pathogenic fungi. Bionanoscien 9:296–301
4. Almeida AAFD, Valle RR (2007) Ecophysiology of the cacao tree. Braz J Plant Physiol 19:425–448
5. Anonymous (2019) International trade centre trade map—list of exporters for the selected product in 2019 product: 18 cocoa and cocoa preparations
6. Babu MMG, Gunasekaran P (2009) Production and structural characterization of crystalline silver nanoparticles from Bacillus cereus isolate. Colloids Surf B Bio 74:191–195
7. Barros D, Pradhan A, Pascoal C, Cássio F (2021) Transcriptomics reveals the action mechanisms and cellular targets of citrate-coated silver nanoparticles in a ubiquitous aquatic fungus. Environ Pollut 268:115913
8. Basavaraja S, Balaji SD, Lagashetty A, Rajasab AH, Venkataraman A (2008) Extracellular biosynthesis of silver nanoparticles using the fungus Fusarium semitectum. Mater Res Bull 43(5):1164–1170
9. Begum NA, Mondal S, Basu S, Laskar RA, Mandal D (2009) Biogenic synthesis of Au and Ag nanoparticles using aqueous solutions of black tea leaf extracts. Colloids Surf B Bio 71(1):113–118
10. Birla SS, Tiwari VV, Gade AK, Ingle AP, Yadav AP, Rai MK (2009) Fabrication of silver nanoparticles by Phoma glomerata and its combined effect against Escherichia coli, Pseudomonas aeruginosa and Staphylococcus aureus. Lett Appl Microbiol 48(2):173–179
11. Brasier CM, Griffin MJ (1979) Taxonomy of Phytophthora palmivora of cocoa. Trans Br Mycol Soc 72:111–143
12. Chaves-López C, Serio A, Grande-Tovar CD, Cuervo-Mulet R, Delgado-Ospina J, Paparella A (2014) Traditional fermented foods and beverages from a microbiological and nutritional perspective: the Colombian heritage. Compr Rev Food Sci Food Saf 13(5):1031–1048
13. Chen JC, Lin ZH, Ma XX (2003) Evidence of the production of silver nanoparticles via pretreatment of Phoma sp. 3.2883 with silver nitrate. Lett Appl Microbiol 37(2):105–108

14. Chouhan PN, Azimov A, Jabborova D, Singh S (2023) Review on the role of indigenous plants and plant derivatives of ayurveda in bone healing. Plant Sci Today 10(sp2):143–151
15. Copetti MV, Iamanaka BT, Pitt JI, Tanoak MH (2014) Fungi and mycotoxins in cocoa: from farm to chocolate. Int J Food Microbiol 178:13–20
16. Cruz-Luna AR, Cruz-Martínez H, Vásquez-López A, Medina DI (2021) Metal nanoparticles as novel antifungal agents for sustainable agriculture: current advances and future directions. J Fungi 7(12):1033
17. Devika R, Elumalai S, Manikandan E, Eswaramoorthy D (2012) Biosynthesis of silver nanoparticles using the fungus Pleurotus ostreatus and their antibacterial activity. Sci Rep 1(12):557
18. Diao FW, Dang ZH, Cui X, Xu J, Jia BB, Ding SL (2020) Transcriptomic analysis revealed distinctive modulations of arbuscular mycorrhizal fungi inoculation in halophyte Suaeda salsa under moderate salt conditions. Environ Exp Bot 183:104337
19. Durán N, Marcato PD, Alves OL, De Souza GI, Esposito E (2005) Mechanistic aspects of biosynthesis of silver nanoparticles by several Fusarium oxysporum strains. J Nanobiotech 3:1–7
20. Erwin DC, Bartnicki-Garcia S, Tsao PH (eds) (1983) Phytophthora: its biology, taxonomy, ecology, and pathology. American Phytopathological Society, St. Paul, MN
21. Evans HC (1981) Pod rot of cacao caused by Moniliophthora (Monilia) roreri, vol 24. Commonwealth Mycological Institute
22. Evans HC (2001) Risk assessment of fungal biocontrol agents of weeds and plant diseases. In: BMS international symposium on bioactive fungal metabolites. University of Swansea, pp 22–27
23. Evans HC, Stalpers JA, Sampson RA, Benny GL (1978) On the taxonomy of Monilia roreri, an important pathogen of Theobroma cacao in South America. Can J Bot 56:2528–2532
24. Fayaz AM, Balaji K, Girilal M, Yadav R, Kalaichelvan PT, Venketesan R (2010) Biogenic synthesis of silver nanoparticles and their synergistic effect with antibiotics: a study against gram-positive and gram-negative bacteria. Nanomed Nanotech Biol Med 6(1):103–109
25. Feynman R (1959) Lecture at the California institute of technology
26. Fulton RH (1989) The cacao disease trilogy: black pod, monilia pod rot, and witches'-broom. Plant Dis 73:601–603
27. Gade AK, Bonde PP, Ingle AP, Marcato PD, Duran N, Rai MK (2008) Exploitation of Aspergillus niger for synthesis of silver nanoparticles. J Mater Bioener 2(3):243–247
28. Gordienko MG, Palchikova VV, Kalenov SV, Belov AA, Lyasnikova VN, Poberezhniy DY (2019) Antimicrobial activity of silver salt and silver nanoparticles in different forms against microorganisms of different taxonomic groups. J Hazard Mater 378:120754
29. Gow NAR, Latge JP, Munro CA (2017) The fungal cell wall: structure, biosynthesis, and function. Microbiol Spectr 5:1–25
30. Granqvist GC, Bhurman AR (1976) Ultrafine metal particles. J Appl Phys 47:2200–2205
31. Gregory, P. H., and Maddison, A. C., eds. (1981). Epidemiology of Phytophthora on cocoa in Nigeria. Commonw Mycol Inst Kew Phytopathol 25
32. Gregory PH (ed) (1974) Phytophthora diseases of cocoa. Longman, London
33. Gupta G, Paul S, Singh S, Pietramellara G, Pathan SI, Danish S, Jha PN (2022) Exploring functional diversity and community structure of diazotrophic endophytic bacteria associated with Pennisetum glaucum growing under field in a semi-arid region. Land 11(7):991
34. Gurunathan S, Kalishwaralal K, Vaidyanathan R, Venkataraman D, Pandian SRK, Muniyandi J, Eom SH (2009) Biosynthesis, purification and characterization of silver nanoparticles using Escherichia coli. Colloids Surf B Bio 74(1):328–335
35. Haefeli C, Franklin C, Hardy K (1984) Plasmid-determined silver resistance in Pseudomonas stutzeri isolated from a silver mine. J Bacteriol 158(1):389–392
36. Hemath KS, Kumar G, Karthik L, Bhaskara Rao KV (2010) Extracellular biosynthesis of silver nanoparticles using the filamentous fungus Penicillium sp. Arch Appl Sci Res 2(6):161–167
37. Hong XS, Wen JJ, Xiong XH, Hu YY (2016) Shape effect on the antibacterial activity of silver nanoparticles synthesized via a microwave-assisted method. Environ Sci Pollut 23:4489–4497

38. Huang J, Chen C, He N, Hong J, Lu Y, Qingbiao L, Shao W, Sun D, Wang XH, Wang Y, Yiang X (2007) Biosynthesis of silver and gold nanoparticles by novel sundried Cinnamomum camphora leaf. Nanotech 18:105–106
39. Husseiny M, Aziz MAEBY, Mahmoud MA (2006) Biosynthesis of gold nanoparticles using Pseudomonas aeruginosa. Spectrochi Acta 67:1003–1006
40. Hwang ET, Lee JH, Chae YJ, Kim YS, Kim BC, Sang BI, Gu MB (2008) Analysis of the toxic mode of action of silver nanoparticles using stress-specific bioluminescent bacteria. Small 4(6):746–750
41. Inbathamizh L, Ponnu TM, Mary EJ (2013) In vitro evaluation of antioxidant and anticancer potential of Morinda pubescens synthesized silver nanoparticles. J Pharma Res 6(1):32–38
42. Ingle A, Gade A, Pierrat S, Sonnichsen C, Rai M (2008) Mycosynthesis of silver nanoparticles using the fungus Fusarium acuminatum and its activity against some human pathogenic bacteria. Cur Nanoscien 4:141–144
43. Ingle A, Rai M, Gade A, Bawaskar M (2009) Fusarium solani: a novel biological agent for the extracellular synthesis of silver nanoparticles. J Nanopart Res 11(8):2079–2085
44. International Cocoa Organization (1974) Quarterly bulletin of cocoa statistics, vol 1. International Cocoa Organization
45. Jebakumar IET, Sethuraman MG (2012) Instant green synthesis of silver nanoparticles using Terminalia chebula fruit extract and evaluation of their catalytic activity on reduction of methylene blue. Proc Biochem 47:1351–1357
46. Jha AK, Prasad K, Prasad K, Kulkarni AR (2009) Plant system: nature's nanofactory. Colloids Surf B Bio 73(2):219–223
47. Kalimuthu K, Babu RS, Venkataraman D, Bilal M, Gurunathan S (2008) Biosynthesis of silver nanocrystals by Bacillus licheniformis. Colloids Surf B Bio 65(1):150–153
48. Kaviya S, Santhanalakshmi J, Viswanathan B, Muthumary J, Srinivasan K (2011) Biosynthesis of silver nanoparticles using Citrus sinensis peel extract and its antibacterial activity. Spectrochim Acta Part A Mol Biomolec Spectrosco79(3):594–598
49. Kellam MK, Zentmyer GA (1986) Morphological, physiological, ecological, and pathological comparisons of Phytophthora species isolated from Theobroma cacao. Phytopath 76:159–164
50. Khare P, Kishore K, Sharma DK (2017) A study on the standardization parameters of Cassia angustifolia. Asian J Pharm Clin Res 10(7):329–332
51. Khare P, Kishore K, Sharma DK, Khare N (2024) Investigation of memory enhancing activity of combination extracts of Bauhinia variegata and Madhuca longifolia leaves against Colchicine: an experimental study and biochemical alterations in mice. Ind J Pharm Edu Res 58(1s):s282–s288
52. Kim SW, Jung JH, Lamsal K, Kim YS, Min JS, Lee YS (2012) Antifungal effects of silver nanoparticles (AgNPs) against various plant pathogenic fungi. Mycobiol 40:53–58
53. Krauss U, Hebbar P (1999) Research methodology in biocontrol of plant diseases. In: Workshop manual. CATIE, Turrialba, Costa Rica
54. Krishnaraj C, Ramachandran R, Mohan K, Kalaichelvan PT (2012) Optimization for rapid synthesis of silver nanoparticles and its effect on phytopathogenic fungi. Spectrochim. Acta Part A Mol Biomolec Spectrosco 93:95–99
55. Lu T, Qu Q, Lavoie M, Pan XJ, Peijnenburg WJGM, Zhou ZG (2020) Insights into the transcriptional responses of a microbial community to silver nanoparticles in a freshwater microorganism. Environ Pollut 258:113727
56. Lukman AI, Gong B, Marjo CE, Roessner U, Harris AT (2011) Facile synthesis, stabilization, and anti-bacterial performance of discrete Ag nanoparticles using Medicago sativa seed exudates. J Coll Inte Scien 353(2):433–444
57. Maddala VKS, Singh S (2023) Essential oils from plants and their role in nanomaterial synthesis characterization and applications. In: Secondary metabolites based green synthesis of nanomaterials and their applications. Singapore: Springer Nature, Singapore, pp 191–207
58. Mohanpuria P, Rana NK, Yadav SK (2008) Biosynthesis of nanoparticles: technological concepts and future applications. J Nanopart Res 10:507–517

59. Morones JR, Elechiguerra JL, Camacho A, Holt K, Kouri JB, Ramírez JT, Yacaman MJ (2005) The bactericidal effect of silver nanoparticles. Nanotech 16(10):2346
60. Mukherjee P, Ahmad A, Mandal D, Senapati S, Sainkar SR, Khan MI, Ramani R, Parischa R, Ajayakumar PV, Alam M, Sastry M, Kumar R (2001) Bioreduction of $AuCl^{4-}$ ions by the fungus, Verticillium sp. and surface trapping of the gold nanoparticles formed. Appl Chem 40(19):3585–3588
61. Mukherjee P, Roy M, Mandal BP, Dey GK, Mukherjee PK, Ghatak J, Tyagi AK, Kale SP (2008) Green synthesis of highly stabilized nanocrystalline silver particles by a non-pathogenic and agriculturally important fungus T. asperellum. Nanotechn 19(7):075103
62. Nayak BK, Anitha K (2014) Combined effects of antibiotics and AgNPs biosynthesized from Aspergillus ustus studied against few pathogenic bacteria. Int Pharm Tech Res 6(7):1976–1980
63. Nel A, Xia T, Madler L, Li N (2003) Toxic potential of materials at the nano level. Science 311:622–627
64. Nelson N, Ben-Shem A (2004) The complex architecture of oxygenic photosynthesis. Nat Rev Mol Cell Bio 5:971–982
65. Noori A, White JC, Newman LAJ (2017) Mycorrhizal fungi influence on silver uptake and membrane protein gene expression following silver nanoparticle exposure. J Nanopart Res 19:66
66. Parasharu K, Saxena A, Srivastava A (2009) Bioinspired synthesis of silver nanoparticles. Digest J Nanomater Biostruct 4(1):159–166
67. Parveen R, Khare N, Singh S, Johri P (2023) An in silico outlook for the detection and surveillance of evolving and persistent plant pathogens. In: Detection, diagnosis and management of soil-borne phytopathogens. Singapore: Springer Nature, Singapore, pp 17–40
68. Patani A, Patel A, Prajapati D, Khare N, Singh S (2023) Various agriculture crop plant-based bioactive compounds and their use in nanomaterial synthesis and applications. In: Nanomaterials from agricultural and horticultural products. Singapore: Springer Nature, Singapore, pp 223–241
69. Paulkumar K, Rajeshkumar S, Gnanajobitha G, Vanaja M, Malarkodi C, Annadurai G (2013) Eco-friendly synthesis of silver chloride nanoparticles using Klebsiella planticola (MTCC 2277). Int J Green Chem Bioproc 3(1):12–16
70. Pereira JL (1985) Chemical control of Phytophthora pod rot of cacao in Brazil. Cocoa Grow Bull 36:23–38
71. Pereira JL (1996) Management of witches' broom disease of cocoa: a contemporary retrospective. Cocoa Producers' Alliance, 8/10 Broad Street, P.O. Box 1718, Lagos, Nigeria
72. Philip D (2011) Mangifera indica leaf-assisted biosynthesis of well-dispersed silver nanoparticles. Spectrochim Acta Part A Mol Biomol Spectro 78:327–331
73. Piper S, Martínez A, Hidalgo E, Krauss U (2000) Effect of formulation on population dynamics of mycoparasites on the surface of cocoa pods. In: INCOPED 3rd international seminar on cocoa pest and diseases. Kota Kinabalu, Sabah, Malaysia
74. Prathna TC, Chandrasekaran N, Raichur AM, Mukherjee A (2011) Biomimetic synthesis of silver nanoparticles by Citrus limon (lemon) aqueous extract and theoretical prediction of particle size. Colloids Surf B Bio 82(1):152–159
75. Purdy LH, Schmidt RA (1996) Status of cacao witches'broom: biology, epidemiology, and management. Ann Rev Phytopath 34(1):573–594
76. Quevedo AC, Iseult L, Valsami-Jones E (2021) Cellular repair mechanisms triggered by exposure to silver nanoparticles and ionic silver in embryonic zebrafish cells. Environ Sci Nano 8:2507–2522
77. Rahman AH, Behera SK, Mishra A, Lundborg CS, Tripathy SK (2022) Transcriptomic regulation of Salmonella typhimurium during sonophotocatalysis and the effect of stress adaptation on the antibiotic resistance and tolerance post-treatment. Chem Engineer J 446:137442
78. Rai M, Yadav A, Gade A (2008) Current trends in phytosynthesis of metal nanoparticles. Cri Rev Biotechn 28(4):277–284
79. Raza MA, Kanwal Z, Rauf A, Sabri AN, Riaz S, Naseem S (2017) Size- and shape-dependent antibacterial studies of silver nanoparticles synthesized by wet chemical routes. NANO 6:1–15

80. Rónavári A, Igaz N, Adamecz DI, Szerencsés B, Molnar C, Kónya Z, Pfeiffer I, Kiricsi M (2021) Green silver and gold nanoparticles: biological synthesis approaches and potentials for biomedical applications. Molecules 26(4):844
81. Rorer JB (1918) Diseases and pests of cocoa in ecuador, and modern methods appropriate to the cultivation of cocoa. Report presented to the agricultural society of ecuador, Guayaquil
82. Rudgard SA, Butler DR (1987) Witches' broom disease in Rondonia, Brazil: pod infection in relation to pod susceptibility, wetness, inoculum, and phytosanitation. Plant Path 36:515–522
83. Sadowski Z, Maliszewska IH, Grochowalska B, Polowczyk I, Kozlecki T (2008) Synthesis of silver nanoparticles using microorganisms. Mater Scien Poland 26(2):419–424
84. Sahu N, Soni D, Chandrashekhar B, Sarangi BK, Satpute D, Pandey RA (2013) Synthesis and characterization of silver nanoparticles using Cynodon dactylon leaves and assessment of their antibacterial activity. Bioproc Biosys Eng 36:999–1004
85. Samuel U, Guggenbichler JP (2004) Prevention of catheter related infections: the potential of a new nano-silver impregnated catheter. Internat J Antimicro Agents 2(31):75–78
86. Sau TK, Rogach AL (2010) Non spherical noble metal nanoparticles: colloid-chemical synthesis and morphology control. Adv Mater 22(16):1781–1804
87. Shankar SS, Rai A, Ahmad A, Sastry M (2004) Biosynthesis of silver and gold nanoparticles from extracts of different parts of the geranium plant. Appl Nano Sci 1:69–77
88. Sharma S, Ahmad N, Prakash A, Singh VN, Ghosh AK, Mehta BR (2010) Synthesis of crystalline Ag nanoparticles (AgNPs) from microorganisms. Mater Scien Appl 1(01):1
89. Sharma VK, Yngard RA, Lin Y (2009) Silver nanoparticles: green synthesis and their antimicrobial activities. Adv Coll Interface Sci 14583–14596
90. Shibata S, Aoki K, Yano T, Yamane M (1998) Preparation of silica microspheres containing Ag nanoparticles. J Sci Tech 11:279–287
91. Silva P (1987) Cocoa and lizard or witch's broom. In: Technical bulletin (CEPLAC, Itabuna), vol 146
92. Singh A, Sengar RS, Singh AK, Singh S, Kumar A, Ahmad K (2019) Impact of genetic engineering on agriculture food crops. Biotech Today Int J Biol Sci 9(1):17–24
93. Singh P, Raja BR (2011) Biological synthesis and characterization of silver nanoparticles using the fungus Trichoderma harzianum. Asian J Exper Bio Sci 2(4):600–605
94. Soberanis W, Rıos R, Arévalo E, Zuniga L, Cabezas O, Krauss U (1999) Increased frequency of phytosanitary pod removal in cacao (Theobroma cacao) increases yield economically in eastern Peru. Crop Protec 18(10):677–685
95. Sobha K, Surendranath K, Meena V (2010) Emerging trends in nanobiotechnology. Biotechn Mol Biol Rev 5:1–12
96. Storz G, Imlay JA (1999) Oxidative stress. Cur Opin Microbiol 2:188–194
97. Taylor M (1998) The world cocoa situation. In: International forum in cocoa, Lima, Peru, 28–29th October 1998. LMC International, Ltd., London, UK
98. Thomas S, Mc Cubbin P (2003) A comparison of the antimicrobial effects of four silver-containing dressings on three organisms. J Wound Care 12(3):101–107
99. Usha RP, Rajasekharreddy P (2010) Green synthesis of silver-protein (core–shell) nanoparticles using Piper betle L. leaf extract and its ecotoxicological studies on Daphnia magna. Col Sur A Physicochem Engineer Aspects 389:188–194
100. Vaidyanathan R, Gopalram S, Kalishwaralal K, Deepak V, Pandian SRK, Gurunathan S (2010) Enhanced silver nanoparticle synthesis by optimization of nitrate reductase activity. Coll Surf B Bioint 75(1):335–341
101. Veiga Moreira IM, Miguel MGDCP, Duarte WF, Dias DR, Schwan RF (2013) Microbial succession and the dynamics of metabolites and sugars during the fermentation of three different cocoa (Theobroma cacao L.) hybrids. Food Res Int 54(1):9–17
102. Vigneshwaran N, Kathe AA, Varadarajan PV, Nachane RP, Balasubramanya RH (2006) Biomimetics of silver nanoparticles by white rot fungus, Phaenerochaete chrysosporium. Coll Surf B Biointerfaces 53(1):55–59
103. Vishwakarma SK, Ilyas T, Shahid M, Malviya D, Kumar S, Singh S, Singh HV (2024) Bacillus spp.: nature's gift to agriculture and humankind. In: Applications of Bacillus and

Bacillus derived genera in agriculture, biotechnology and beyond. Singapore: Springer Nature, Singapore, pp 1–36
104. Vora Z, Pandya J, Vaikuntapu PR, Singh S, Asha S, Purama RK (2023) Genome-wide association of defense hormone crosstalk in plants. In: Hormonal cross-talk, plant defense and development. Academic Press, pp 353–371
105. Wagi S, Ahmed A (2020) Bacterial nanobiotic potential. Green Proc Syn 9(1):203–211
106. Winterer M, Hahn H (2003) Nanoceramics by chemical vapour synthesis. J Metal 94(10):1084–1090
107. Xia ZK, Ma QH, Li SY, Zhang DQ, Cong L, Tian YL (2016) The antifungal effffect of silver nanoparticles on Trichosporon asahii. J Microbiol Immunol 49:182–188
108. Zentmyer GA, Kaosiri T, Idosu GO, Kellam MK (1981) Morphological forms of Phytophthora palmivora. In: Proceedings of 7th international cocoa research conference, 4–12 Nov 1979. Douala, Cameroon, pp 291–295
109. Zhu HH, Ai HL, Cao LW, Sui R, Ye HP, Du DY (2018) Transcriptome analysis providing novel insights for Cd-resistant tall fescue responses to Cd stress. Ecotoxicol Environ Saf 160:349–356
110. Zhuo R, Fan FF (2021) A comprehensive insight into the application of white rot fungi and their lignocellulolytic enzymes in the removal of organic pollutants. Sci Total Environ 778:146132

# Stress Management

# Application of Iron Oxide Nanoparticles for Promoting *Eucalyptus* Growth Under Salt Stress

**Karolina Waszkowska and Anna Lesiak**

**Abstract** Salt stress is a prominent environmental factor that profoundly influences the growth and evolution pathways of plants. Given their fixed position, plants require the evolution of robust mechanisms to acclimate to high-saline environments. The surge in intracellular osmotic pressure caused by salt stress can trigger the accumulation of sodium ions to levels that exert toxicity. The realm of nanotechnology, particularly featuring iron nanoparticles, presents a promising avenue to mitigate the adverse impacts of salt stress on plants. Within this discourse, we delve into a comprehensive exploration encompassing salt stress, its ramifications on ecosystems, intricate morphophysiological investigations involving *Eucalyptus* plants cultivated under saline conditions, and the transformative potential of iron oxide nanoparticles in alleviating salt stress, consequently enhancing the growth milieu for *Eucalyptus* vegetation.

**Keywords** Eucalyptus · Iron oxide nanoparticles · Salinity · Morpho-physiological studies · Biocompatibility

## 1 Introduction

With the shifts, in conditions, nowadays it has become crucial to comprehend how different plant species react both ecologically and physiologically to various stress factors. A particular stressor that poses a barrier for the growth and evolution of plants in regions, with poor soil quality and limited water availability, is salt stress [2, 82, 118, 124]. *Eucalyptus* is a known and valued type of tree and plant, due to its characteristics from both ecological and economic perspectives. It finds applications in fields, including wood and cellulose production, medicine, and essential

K. Waszkowska
LPHIA, SFR MATRIX, University of Angers, Angers, France

A. Lesiak (✉)
Institut de Chimie de Nice (ICN) UMR CNRS 7272, Parc Valrose, Université Côte d'Azur, Nice 06108, France
e-mail: anna.lesiak@univ-cotedazur.fr

 
D. Jabborova et al. (eds.), *Nanomaterials in Agroforestry Systems*, Smart Nanomaterials Technology, https://doi.org/10.1007/978-981-96-1337-3_13

oil extraction. Its reputation has spread across countries worldwide. However, the growth capacity of *Eucalyptus* has been significantly limited due to increasing soil salinity, which has consequences for these plants [11, 24]. The presence of salt stress disrupts the water and ion balance in *Eucalyptus* species negatively impacting their growth, photosynthesis, and overall health. By studying and analysing the underlying morphological processes that govern the response of *Eucalyptus* plants to salinity stress, we can gain insights for developing strategies that mitigate these harmful effects. Given the growing prevalence of salinity stress as a problem, understanding its impact on *Eucalyptus* becomes vital, for establishing land management practices and ensuring the survival of this unique tree species.

The application of iron oxide nanoparticles (IONPs) as fertilisers is very promising [53, 117]. These nanoparticles have distinctive properties that make them capable of transporting the essential nutrients required for optimal plant development [1]. The operation of nanoscale gives them an advantage in terms of surface area and reactivity, enabling targeted and precise dosing of nutrients. Incorporating iron oxide nanoparticles into fertilisation strategies can improve nutrient uptake by plants (even under difficult conditions such as salt stress), leading to improved growth, development, and overall health [92].

The aim of this comprehensive chapter is to analyse the multifaceted impact of high salinity on *Eucalyptus* plants by analysing morphological, biochemical and molecular studies available in the literature. By shedding light on how *Eucalyptus* trees cope with salt stress challenges, it may be possible to develop a way to increase their resilience and productivity in environments influenced by increased salt levels, through the use of Iron Oxide Nanoparticles, among other things. We have considered the problems of *Eucalyptus* plants in harsh conditions and how, using nanotechnology, this problem can be solved in the future.

## 2 Salt Stress and Their Impact on Ecosystems

### *2.1 Tolerance to Salt Stress*

When the level of soluble salts (mainly sodium chloride, NaCl) in the soil or in water (in aquatic or terrestrial ecosystems) is significantly elevated, this phenomenon is called salt stress, which has a significant impact on living organisms (flora and fauna) as well as ecological processes [59]. One example is plant growth and productivity are affected due to high soil salinity or salt stress [45, 94]. Elevated levels of NaCl cause disruption of the uptake of water and minerals through plant roots, which contributes to dehydration and nutrient deficiencies. This leads to inhibition of growth, reduced biomass production, and the risk of plant death. On the same token, salt stress is extremely harmful to organisms that live in freshwater ecosystems [72]. An example is fish and invertebrates that are adapted to life without high salinity and have specific mechanisms of osmoregulation that allow them to maintain an internal balance of salt and water. Moreover, salt stress contributes to the composition and distribution of plant species that are more sensitive to salt stress [13]. In this way, the structure of the ecosystem can be disturbed by the dominance of salt-tolerant species in ecosystems. Another factor contributing to the influence of salt stress on ecosystems is soil fertility [106]. Salinity alters soil fertility by negatively affecting the microbial activity and mineral and nutrient cycling processes. This reduced activity leads to reduced organic matter breakdown and the accessibility of minerals and nutrients that are essential for plants [103]. Besides, the primary productivity of ecosystems can be disrupted by salinity stress. Limited availability of minerals and nutrients, as well as reduced plant growth contribute to the limited flow of energy in the food chain, and thus affect the number and distribution of individual species of herbivores, carnivores, and decomposers [109]. Furthermore, high salinity has a very negative impact on water quality in aquatic ecosystems. This contributes to the increase in the density of water, which affects the mixing of layers and stratification of water, which has disastrous consequences for the availability of oxygen in deeper layers of water. Another important factor affected by salt stress is soil erosion. Elevated levels of NaCl break down soil aggregates, making the soil more sensitive to erosion by water and wind. Moreover, the distribution of wetland species as well as the functions of these ecosystems (such as mineral and nutrient cycling) can be affected by high salt concentrations. Wetlands and coastal areas are particularly vulnerable to salinity due to their proximity to the ocean [73]. In addition to the abovementioned factors, human activity is also important, which can be disturbed by high salinity [44]. In regions where inadequate irrigation methods or inefficient drainage are used, salinity levels can increase significantly, contributing to soil degradation and negatively impacting agricultural productivity. All these factors that are affected by salt stress can be mitigated through appropriate management strategies, such as adequate irrigation, planting salt-tolerant vegetation, and restoring already degraded habitats [81]. Understanding this dynamic and its consequences is very important for sustainable management of ecosystems and, above all, their protection.

## 2.2 Plant Response to Stress Condition

Habitually, living organisms evolve all the time to adapt to current conditions. Among other things, plants have developed various mechanisms that enable them to react and adjust to various stress conditions like drought, extreme temperatures, pathogens, deficiencies, and what is important from the perspective of this chapter: salt stress. These reactions are often very complex, and their changes are at the molecular, cellular and physiological level [34], which are schematically displayed in Fig. 1. One such reaction to stress conditions is the closure of the stomata [119]. During drought and extremely high temperatures, plants close their stomata, which minimizes water loss due to transpiration. On the other hand, it may limit $CO_2$ uptake for photosynthesis. Moreover, under the influence of stress, plants have developed the ability to change photosynthetic apparatuses [105], thanks to which it is possible to optimize energy uptake and minimize photodamage. Another reaction is the activation of stress-responsive genes, which activate under stressful conditions [75]. These genes are responsible for encoding proteins that protect plants from particular damage as well as help the plant cope with stress. Moreover, another mechanism is the accumulation of adaptable solutes, like proline or sugars, acting as osmoprotectants [4]. Thanks to these dissolved substances, plants have possibility to maintain the cellular osmotic balance as well as protect the cellular structure against destruction caused by stress. Another response that plants have developed to adapt to life under stress is the synthesis of stress proteins [112], such as heat shock proteins, or chaperones, which are designed to stabilize and repair already damaged proteins during stress. Furthermore, to prevent the production of reactive oxygen species (ROS) under stress conditions [47], plants have the ability to increase the synthesis of antioxidants, including superoxide dismutase, catalase and peroxidase, which contribute to the neutralization of ROS and thus prevent oxidative damage. Likewise, plants have developed the ability to accelerate root growth [35] as well as the development of root hairs [104], which during mineral and nutrient deficiencies caused by stress conditions, can increase their uptake from the soil. Moreover, under stress conditions, the levels of plant hormones [10, 28, 89, 121] can be disrupted, however they play crucial roles in stabilizing numerous stress responses. Therefore, plants have developed a change in hormonal balance that prevents such situations. Another way to deal with stress is to shed leaves, which prevents dehydration and deficiencies in minerals and nutrients that are necessary for the growth of more important components of the plant [86]. In addition, during severe stress, plants can enter a state of rest, which means that their growth is suspended until favourable conditions arise. Moreover, symbiosis is very important for plants under stress phenomenon [54, 67, 83]. Plants have created the possibility of living in symbiosis with certain microorganisms, such as mycorrhizae fungi, thanks to which better absorption of minerals, nutrients and water is possible, which enhances tolerance during stress. To sum up, depending on the plant varieties and the type, intensity and period of stress, the mechanisms leading to coping with stress can be varied and very dynamic. Understanding these reactions is very important, which allows the development of appropriate strategies that are responsible for protecting ecosystems, increasing the survival or productivity of plants in difficult conditions and the resilience of crops in agriculture.

## 2.3 Environmental Impact

The phenomenon of salt stress has disastrous consequences in ecosystems where significantly elevated salt levels occur naturally or as an outcome of human activity. An overview of literature shows that key impacts of salt stress affect both terrestrial and aquatic ecosystems [3, 27, 98, 113, 116]. One of the consequences of salinity is the degradation and reduction of soil fertility, because the excess of salt leads to disruption of its structure, which damages the filtration and drainage of water. This has serious consequences of water soaking as well as reduced availability of minerals

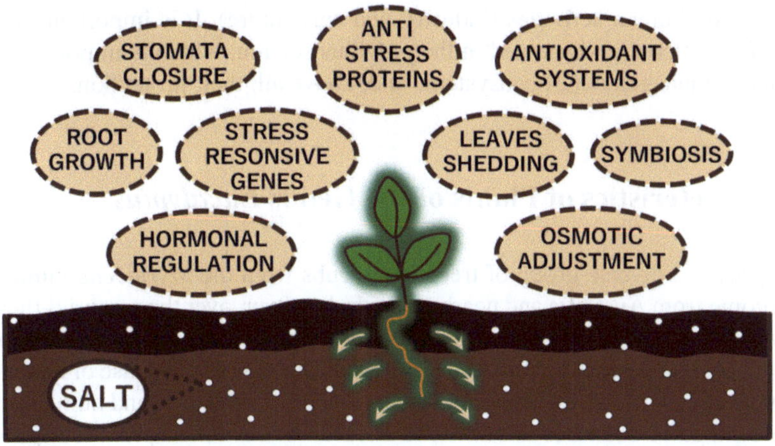


**Fig. 1** Schematically presented key plant reactions to salt stress

and nutrients for plants. Moreover, plant biodiversity decreases because of salinity. Salt stress in the environment changes the composition of plant communities, particularly favouring salt-tolerant plant species. This contributes to drastic changes in the ecosystem. Moreover as we have previously discussed wetlands and estuaries are particularly susceptible, to the impacts of salt stress due to their proximity to seas and oceans. This salt stress results in changes in the functioning of these ecosystems. It is important to highlight that one of the consequences of salt levels is the contamination of freshwater sources. The salts present in the soil get washed into groundwater posing threats to drinking water quality and the overall health of ecosystems. As mentioned earlier salt stress also has effects on soil stability contributing to erosion and subsequent sedimentation, in water bodies. These factors further compromise water and disrupt the aquatic ecosystem. Freshwater ecosystems are also vulnerable to disruption of osmoregulation in aquatic organisms, resulting in dehydration, impaired reproduction and, in the worst cases, even death. Moreover, the productivity of such ecosystems can be affected by salinity stress. Limited plant growth as well as reduced availability of minerals and nutrients adversely affect the flow of energy in the food chain, which affects the distribution of herbivores, carnivores and decomposers. By the same token, salinity has a negative effect on soil microbes, and this leads to reduced nutrient mineralization with consequent poor nutrient and mineral availability to plants. What is more, as a result of inadequate irrigation of economic habitats by humans, it can lead to the accumulation of salts in the soil. This results in lower availability of water for human consumption as well as for industry and agriculture. In the worst cases, the accumulation of salt in the soil contributes to desertification, a process in which fertile soil turns into an arid desert through limited plant growth. Salt stress negatively effects on the aquatic and terrestrial environment as well as on human activities (industry and agriculture). It is important to implement the practices we discussed in the previous section, which is important for the sustainable management of ecosystems and, above all, their protection.

## 3 Characteristics of Plants of the Genus *Eucalyptus*

*Eucalyptus* is a diverse group of trees and shrubs from the *Myrtaceae* family [40], which come from Australia and nearby islands, however, over the centuries they have been widely planted in many other regions of the world due to their unique properties and valuable wood, essential oils and pulpwood. Nonetheless because of factors such as climate change, soil conditions and the influence of salt stress and human activity, the percentage of countries and the size of areas where *Eucalyptus* trees grow can change dynamically. *Eucalyptus* has many unique properties,the most important uses of *Eucalyptus* are graphically presented in Fig. 2. Among other things, due to the presence of oils, the leaves of the *Eucalyptus* tree have a very strong aromatic (mint or camphor) smell. Furthermore, essential oils secreted by the glands of *Eucalyptus* leaves are widely used mainly in medicine as well as in the production of essential and aromatic oils [26]. For this reason, several species of *Eucalyptus* are used to treat respiratory problems as well as herbal remedies and in aromatherapy. Moreover, *Eucalyptus* oil is often used as a natural insect repellent for skin application. In addition, *Eucalyptus* trees have the ability to produce fruit called "gumnuts", the seeds of which play a key role in the dispersal of *Eucalyptus* species. In addition to medical importance, *Eucalyptus* trees have important commercial importance, where they are used in the production of wood, paper and construction or furniture, as this plant is also characterized by a rapid growth rate, making them popular in the production of wood or cellulose [96]. Most species of this tree can quickly regrow from the trunk after cutting it down. Furthermore, *Eucalyptus* trees are known from a source of biofuel and source of renewable energy. Moreover, the vast majority of *Eucalyptus* species are "evergreen" plants, so they can retain their leaves all year round, making them aesthetically appealing and, more importantly, contributing to their ability to photosynthesize throughout the year. However, in many places *Eucalyptus* is planted as protection against strong winds. What's more, most *Eucalyptus* species are drought tolerant and fire resistant. Over the years, many species have adapted to survive in arid regions that have low water availability. In environments particularly exposed to fire, they have developed the ability to regrow from buds protected under a unique bark after fire events. This bark has a characteristic pattern and is differentiated by *Eucalyptus* species. Furthermore, one of the most important characteristics of this plant is its attraction to wildlife, that is, *Eucalyptus* forests very often provide habitats and food sources for many wild animals such as mammals (for example, koalas [20], birds and insects). *Eucalyptus* flowers are very rich in nectar, which attracts pollinating insects (butterflies and bees, among others). This nectar is used to make flavourful *Eucalyptus* honey, which has unique taste and health benefits [80].

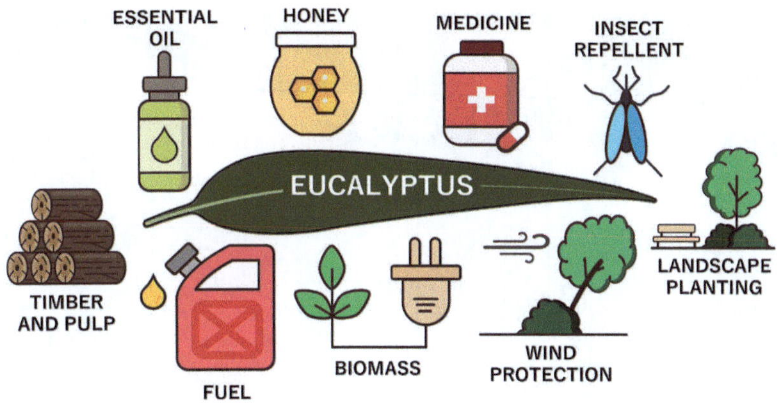


**Fig. 2** Common uses and applications of *Eucalyptus*

*Eucalyptus* dominates Australia and covers a large part of the country, occurring in a variety of ecosystems—from dry inland areas to coastal regions. *Eucalyptus* forests are characteristic of the Australian landscape. Figure 3 displays a simplified map of the world with marked countries where *Eucalyptus* cultivation can be found. Mainly, *Eucalyptus* is cultivated for commercial purposes. *Eucalyptus* trees have been strategically nurtured in regions, around the globe due to their remarkable growth rate and versatility in multiple industries. These industries include timber, paper and pulp production, as their effectiveness in preventing erosion and enhancing the aesthetic appeal of landscapes. For instance countries like China, Vietnam, India, Pakistan, Sri Lanka, Philippines, Thailand, Indonesia and Java, in Asia proudly host flourishing *Eucalyptus* plantations [100, 123]. It is often cultivated to produce paper or pulp, also used as firewood or as windbreaks. In addition, they are widely used in production of essential oils. In Europe [17, 21, 55], *Eucalyptus* is mainly grown in Portugal for its wood as well as paper and essential oils, however, due to the same uses, it can be found in smaller amounts in Spain. Moreover, in Great Britain, *Eucalyptus* was planted in coastal areas as protection from the wind. In addition, due to their ornamental properties, eucalyptus trees were planted in France, Italy, Greece and Cyprus. Generally, *Eucalyptus* is widely used in Middle Eastern countries. For example, in Israel and the United Arab Emirates, is planted for protection from the wind and is valued for its ornamental and shade-providing qualities. In addition, to Jordan, Saudi Arabia and Oman, *Eucalyptus* has been imported for reforestation purposes, as well as for development in arid and agricultural conditions. In Iran, *Eucalyptus* is valued for its wood. On the other hand, in African countries [25, 49, 50, 69] (such as Ethiopia, Tanzania, Uganda, Zambia, Zimbabwe, Malawi, Mozambique, Kenya or South Africa), *Eucalyptus* is used primarily as a fuel and building material, as well as protection against the wind, by reason of their rapid growth and capability to adapt to local conditions. What is more, Brazil [78] is one of the largest producers of *Eucalyptus* in the world next to Australia. In this country and in other South American [15, 42, 78] countries (such as Colombia, Uruguay, Venezuela, Argentina

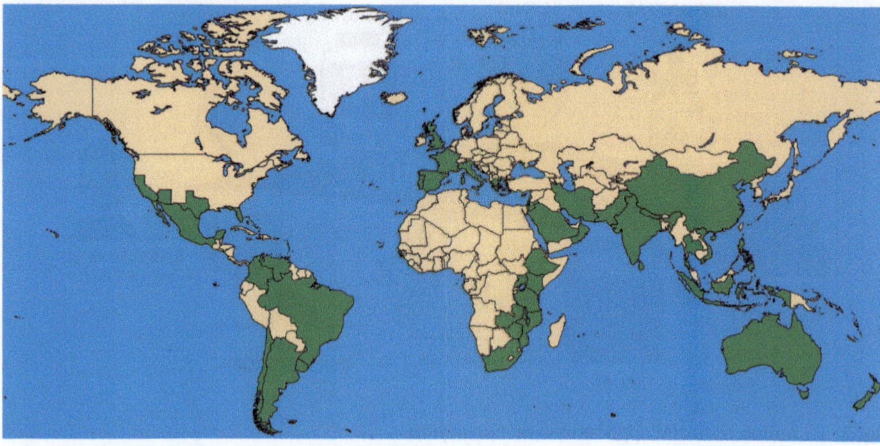

**Fig. 3** Simplified map of *Eucalyptus* cultivation (green colour)

or Chile), *Eucalyptus* trees and shrubs are widely used in the manufacturing of wood, fibre and paper, as well as for reforestation of areas. Furthermore, in Mexico [37] and some North American states [66, 87, 120] (such as Arizona, California, Florida), *Eucalyptus* has been planted for wind protection, shade and ornamental purposes, and has been introduced to Texas to control soil erosion. Summarizing, *Eucalyptus*, due to its unique properties, adaptability and rapid growth, has been brought too many parts of the world mainly for commercial and afforestation purposes. Notwithstanding, due to the topography and salt stress, many of these regions become invasive, leading to ecological problems. Careful management is important when bringing *Eucalyptus* species to new areas.

## 4 Morpho-Physiological Studies of *Eucalyptus* Grown Under Saline Condition

Studies of the effect of high salinity in soil or water, which affect the morphological and physiological characteristics of the growth of *Eucalyptus* plant growth, are primarily aimed at understanding how individual species can react and adapt to high levels of salt stress. Such studies are presented in Fig. 4. Moreover, the aim is to understand how the presence of high magnitude of salt can affect the growth and functioning of these species. One such aspect is research on growth and biomass, where, among other things, growth parameters of Eucalyptus species under salt stress are measured, such as height, stem diameter, or biomass accumulation [45, 102]. This makes it possible to determine the impact of salinity on the overall development of Eucalyptus plants. First, scientists focus on studying the characteristics of the root system, such as its length, volume, or branching system. These morphological changes determine how *Eucalyptus* species adapt to salt stress in uptake of nutrients, minerals and water. Furthermore, other studies focus on morphological changes in *Eucalyptus* leaves, such as their size, shape, and colour, among others, which are a response to salt stress [85]. Specific leaf surfaces as well as leaf thickness are also studied to understand the response to increased salinity. Other studies focus on gas exchange in leaves, where parameters such as photosynthesis rate, stomatal conductivity, and transpiration rate are measured [19]. They provide information such as the ability of *Eucalyptus* to carry out photosynthesis and regulate water loss under salt stress. Moreover, the evaluation of the efficiency of *Eucalyptus* photosynthesis under salt stress conditions and the efficiency of photosystem II is determined by studying the fluorescence of chlorophyll in *Eucalyptus* [36]. Other studies focus on water use efficiency, which is a key physiological feature that allows plants (not just *Eucalyptus*) to weather in high salinity conditions. It is calculated by comparing the amount of carbon associated with photosynthesis and the amount of water lost through transpiration [33]. Furthermore, gene expression patterns related to salt stress responses in *Eucalyptus* species are being analysed. These studies can reveal molecular processes related to the adaptation of the plant to saline circumstances [23]. Studies focussing on the analysis of the accumulation and distribution of ions (e.g., Na, Cl, K) under salinity conditions allow us to understand the dynamics of ions in identifying transport mechanisms in response to salt stress [11]. Furthermore, enzymes such as superoxide dismutase, catalase, and peroxidase are being tested to assess the ability of *Eucalyptus* to activate antioxidant defence systems under salinity-induced oxidative stress [48]. Another key solution is osmotic regulation studies, which help to determine the plant's ability to maintain cellular water balance, as *Eucalyptus* plants have the capability to accumulate solutes (e.g., proline, sugars) to cope with salt stress [18]. In conclusion, the above morpho-physiological studies of *Eucalyptus* species grown at elevated salt levels help to comprehend the mechanisms of tolerance and selection of salt-tolerant varieties and contribute to the development of practices that assist in the management of *Eucalyptus* plantations in areas affected by salinity.

## 5 Iron Oxide Nanoparticles

Nanomaterials have become an attractive group of materials due to their unique properties and low costs, including sensor technologies [16, 62] or as appropriate tools for balanced agricultural applications [39, 97]. Nanoparticles (NPs) can be obtained by conventional (chemical, physical) and biological methods. The last one, called also *green synthesis* of nanoparticles is a quite new research trend in nanotechnology. The choice of method for synthesizing iron oxide nanoparticles (IONPs) can affect their size, shape and crystalline structure, which has implications for their properties and subsequent applications [115]. The most important properties

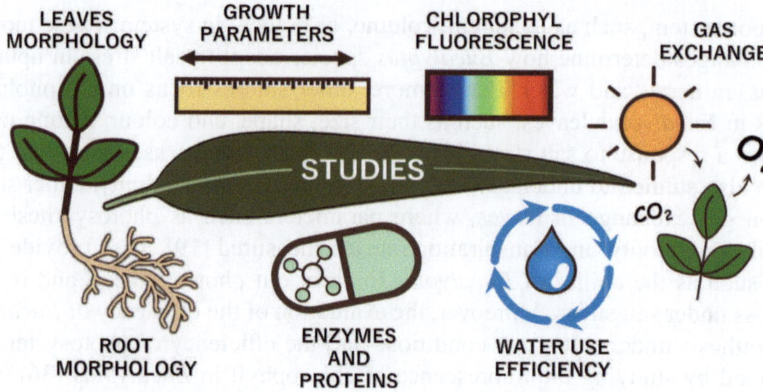


**Fig. 4** Common morpho-physiological studies of *Eucalyptus* grown under salt stress

of IONPs synthesis methods such as resource availability, particle size and shape control, biocompatibility and environmental impact are summarized in Table 1.

Conventional methods (like e.g. co-precipitation [7], thermal decomposition [52], hydrothermal/solvothermal [84] or sol-gel method [56]) allow precise control of reaction parameters such as temperature, reaction time or precursor concentration [76]. Moreover, experimental protocols are generally quite simple, have been extensively studied and optimized over the years, and can be performed with relatively basic equipment. Regardless of the number of advantages, these methods may also have

**Table 1** Comparison of the quality and properties of iron oxide nanoparticles based on the type of their synthesis

| | Conventional methods | Green synthesis | References |
|---|---|---|---|
| Resource availability | Typically based on synthetic reagents that may not be readily available or renewable | Use natural resources, such as plant extracts or microorganisms, which are often widely available and renewable | [8, 57] |
| Particle size and shape control | Due to precise conditions of reaction, offer better control over the size and shape of nanoparticles | Slightly less control over particle size and shape | [6, 60] |
| Biocompatibility | Usually require additional surface modifications to increase their biocompatibility for bioapplication | Due to the presence of natural compounds or biopolymers, often show good biocompatibility | [12, 125] |
| Environmental impact | Significantly negative impact on the environment; may generate toxic byproducts and/or waste that may be harmful to the human health and environment | More environmentally friendly and sustainable | [46, 114] |

some limitations, such as limited control over the monodispersity of the nanoparticles and the potential use of hazardous chemicals [61].

Meanwhile, by definition, green synthesis of IONPs is a method using sustainable methods, therefore is less toxic, more environmentally friendly, efficient and economical [41]. In addition, green synthesis uses natural or biological materials as reducing and stabilizing agents [90]. Thus, this approach uses, among other things, various plant extracts containing natural compounds with reducing properties (e.g. polyphenols, flavonoids, terpenoids),enzymes or metabolites derived from bacteria, fungi, and algae,or biopolymers (e.g., chitosan, starch, cellulose and proteins) which have functional groups that can reduce iron ions and stabilize the resulting nanoparticles [77, 91].

In general, the choice between conventional and biological methods for synthesizing IONPs depends on factors such as the intended application, environmental concerns and desired biocompatibility [93]. While conventional methods offer precise control over nanoparticle properties, biological methods provide a more environmentally friendly and sustainable approach, especially for bioapplications.

As mentioned earlier, the properties of IONPs depend on the type of synthesis and what is on their surface (among other things, after NPs surface functionalization) [95]. This makes it possible to obtain IONPs with a wide range of properties (Fig. 5). One of the main features of IONPs is their highly magnetic property, and their magnetic behaviour strongly depends on their size and crystal structure [70]. As with other types of nanoscale materials, IONPs have a high surface-to-volume ratio, which allows for increased reactivity and interaction with other materials, which can be crucial in catalytic applications [5]. Colloidal solutions of IONPs usually have a brownish colour, but their optical properties can also be observed and examined [22, 31, 110]. Formed by iron oxide NPs also can be used in conjunction with other substances or as photothermal agents on their own, because IONPs can generate heat after irradiation with infrared light [30]. The stability of IONPs is critical to their long-term activity. Stable nanoparticles are less susceptible to agglomeration or degradation over time, ensuring their effectiveness in a variety of applications [71, 111]. In addition, when appropriate coatings or surface modifications are applied to IONPs, they gain biocompatibility [65].

On this basis, research is being conducted on IONPs antibacterial activity [43], to use them as contrast agents [14], or as drug carriers [51]. However, it should be noted that while IONPs offer numerous advantages, their potential toxicity and biocompatibility must be carefully studied and considered for biomedical and environmental applications. Proper surface functionalization and careful design are crucial to ensure their safe and effective use in various fields [68].

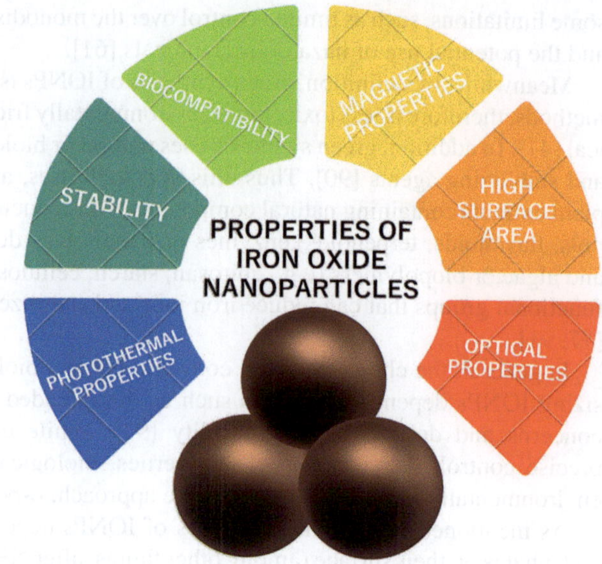


**Fig. 5** Schematic of the main properties of iron oxide nanoparticles (IONPs)

# 6 Application of Iron Oxide Nanoparticles on Plant Cultivation

Suitably obtained modified iron oxide nanoparticles are being considered as potential agents for agricultural development (as fertilizers and growth promoters). However, their spectrum of effects on plants depends on a wide range of factors. The development and stimulation of plant growth can be influenced by the physical properties of IONPs (e.g., size, shape), chemical properties (e.g., concentration and surface coverage), but also biological properties (e.g., biocompatibility, toxicity). As IONPs are definitely smaller than a typical iron oxide or iron molecule, it is possible for them to form complexes with different molecules to make iron more available to plant organs [32].

Studies conducted on various plant species have shown that interaction with IONPs can shape plant growth and biomass gain [9, 32, 63]. The results of these interactions are inherently dependent on the previously mentioned factors, such as nanoparticle concentration and dimensions, as well as exposure time. The observed effects represent a spectrum of responses, ranging from beneficial to inhibitory [58]. Iron is a micronutrient for plants, playing a key role in their metabolic functions. By acting as a channel for iron delivery, IONPs can potentially serve as a source of this important element [64]. In addition, optimum iron content in plants improves photosynthesis, so a fundamental process integrally linked to increased plant growth and overall productivity [29, 53, 88] Moreover, IONPs can interact with root surfaces and affect root morphology, affecting nutrient and water uptake. Furthermore, exposure to nanoparticles can induce changes in gene expression patterns in plants, leading to changes in various physiological processes [99].

When all the knowledge to date on the impact of IONPs on plant cultivation is collected, it can be stated that the application of IONPs for promoting *Eucalyptus* growth under salt stress holds several promising prospects (Fig. 6). As a cutting-edge area of research, the use of IONPs in agriculture and forestry shows potential benefits in mitigating the negative impacts of salt stress and enhancing plant growth [101] reported a detailed study on the subject, focusing the effect of various concentrations of IONPs on shoot cultures of *E. tereticornis* (commonly known as forest red gum) and to predict its potential as a nanosupplement for promoting the growth of *E. tereticornis* under extreme saline stress conditions. IONPs were synthesised by a chemical method and introduced into medium with cultures of *E. tereticornis.* In this study, visible plant growth was observed in terms of shoot growth, shoot biomass, root growth and chlorophyll content after supplementation with iron oxide nanoparticles, regardless of conditions (normal/salt stress). An optimum dose of IONPs (25 ppm) has been identified that promotes the growth of the shoot with a resistant defence system, although this growth was inhibited by reducing the dose due to the production of species of excessive reactive oxygen under abiotic stress conditions.

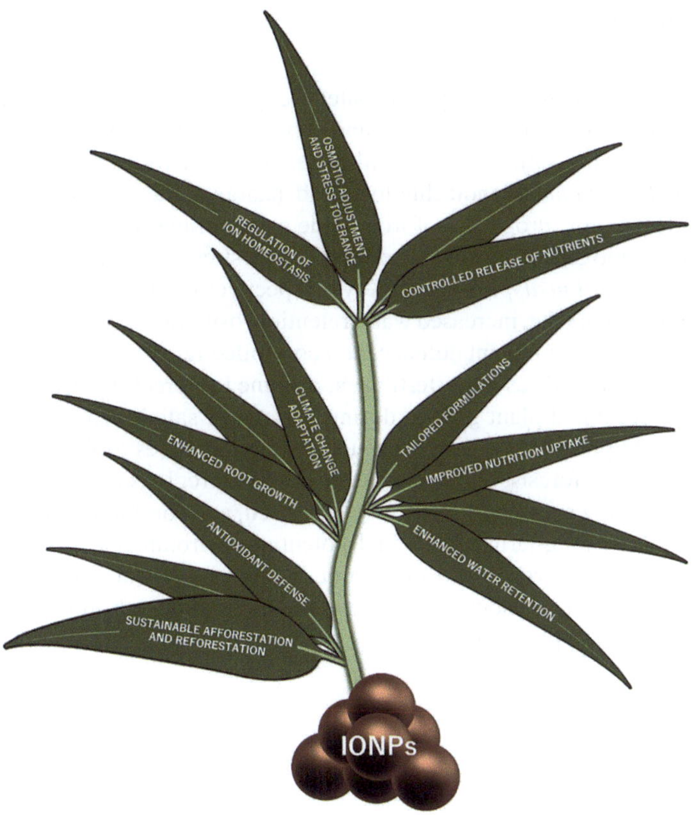


**Fig. 6** Prospects of using IONPs for promoting *Eucalyptus* growth under salt stress

By employing synthesis and functionalization techniques it is possible for IONPs to transport nutrients, such, as iron directly to the root area of plants. This specific delivery mechanism holds the potential to enhance the efficiency of absorption in soil environments with elevated salt levels that impede nutrient accessibility. Furthermore IONPs have the ability to alter soil characteristics leading to water retention and reduced water related stress, in plants [107]. IONPs can act as osmoprotectants, maintaining the water balance of cells and protecting plant tissues from damage [74, 108]. Thus, the use of IONPs in *Eucalyptus* cultivation may help these plants adapt to osmotic stress caused by high salt levels. Because IONPs can act as antioxidants [38, 122], removing reactive oxygen species (ROS) generated during salt stress, IONPs can enhance the antioxidant defences of *Eucalyptus plants*. This can be particularly beneficial in arid and semi-arid regions, where salt stress and water scarcity often co-exist. All the possibilities described can contribute to increasing the growth of *Eucalyptus* and thus to sustainable afforestation and reforestation in degraded or salinity-affected areas, helping to restore ecosystems and combat desertification.

## 7 Conclusion

*Eucalyptus* stands out as a widely distributed tree and plant variety, cherished for its distinct attributes from both ecological and economic standpoints. In contemporary times, the increasing salinity of the soil poses a greater restriction on the growth potential of *Eucalyptus*. Nanotechnology and nanomaterials can help solve these problems. The unique properties of iron oxide nanoparticles offer a range of potential benefits in mitigating the adverse effects of salt stress and enhancing the growth and productivity of *Eucalyptus* plants. Key perspectives for the use of IONPs include improved nutrient uptake, increased water retention, osmotic regulation, regulation of ionic homeostasis, antioxidant defence, and controlled release of nutrients. Furthermore, the use of IONPs as nano-fertilisers, designed to precisely release nutrients, can enhance sustained plant growth during periods of salinity stress. These applications hold the promise of supporting sustainable initiatives to foster new forests, rejuvenate existing forests, and restore ecosystems in regions affected by degradation or salinity. However, caution must be exercised, and careful research conducted to understand the long-term effects and potential environmental consequences of IONPs on *Eucalyptus* growth and soil health. Safety assessments, cost-effectiveness analyses, and careful consideration of potential environmental impacts are needed before widespread implementation.

## 8 Recommendations and Way Forward

Optimisation of the IONPs' physical and chemical properties, such as their shape and size, can help achieve their desired effect on the *Eucalyptus* growth. Additionally, research on the determination of the optimal dose to stimulate the growth of *Eucalyptus* without causing damage associated with excessive IONPs concentration, is crucial. Moreover, assessing the potential environmental impact of IONPs, in aspects such as persistence in soil and potential unintended effects on ecosystems, is a key to sustainable use of IONPs in *Eucalyptus* growth. The associated long-term effects should be investigated by scientists, taking into account factors such as sustained growth and resistance to IONPs, to provide information on sustainability when using IONPs in agriculture. Furthermore, focussing on functional techniques to deliver effective IONPs to the roots of *Eucalyptus* plants, is of great importance. This may increase the absorption of nutrients, especially in environments with high salinity. This research should also involve the interactions of IONPs with soil conditions, especially in saline environments. That may increase water retention, reduce stress, and improve the availability of nutrients. Given the potential benefits of IONPs in arid regions, comprehensive research can contribute to applications in water-stressed environments.

## References


1. Abdulwahid FS, Haider AJ, Al-Musawi S (2022) Iron oxide nanoparticles (IONPs): synthesis, surface functionalization, and targeting drug delivery strategies: mini-review. NANO 17(11):2230007
2. Acosta-Motos J, Ortuño M, Bernal-Vicente A, Diaz-Vivancos P, Sanchez-Blanco M, Hernandez J (2017) Plant responses to salt stress: adaptive mechanisms. Agronomy 7:18
3. Ahmad Z (2022) Impact of salt stress on morphology and physiology of maize plants. Plant Bull 1(1):31–53
4. Ahmed S, Heo T-Y, Roy Choudhury A, Walitang DI, Choi J, Sa T (2021) Accumulation of compatible solutes in rice (Oryza sativa L.) cultivars by inoculation of endophytic plant growth promoting bacteria to alleviate salt stress. Appl Biol Chem 64:1–14
5. Ajinkya N, Yu X, Kaithal P, Luo H, Somani P, Ramakrishna S (2020) Magnetic iron oxide nanoparticle (IONP) synthesis to applications: present and future. Mater (Basel) 13:4644
6. Akintelu SA, Oyebamiji AK, Olugbeko SC, Folorunso AS (2021) Green synthesis of iron oxide nanoparticles for biomedical application and environmental remediation: a review. Eclet Quim J 46:17–37
7. Al-Alawy AF, Al-Abodi EE, Kadhim RM (2018) Synthesis and characterization of magnetic iron oxide nanoparticles by co-precipitation method at different conditions. J Eng 24:60–72
8. Ali A, Zafar H, Zia M, ul Haq I, Phull AR, Ali JS, Hussain A (2016) Synthesis, characterization, applications, and challenges of iron oxide nanoparticles. Nanotechnol Sci Appl 9:49–67
9. Alkhatib R, Alkhatib B, Abdo N, Al-Eitan L, Creamer R (2019) Physio-biochemical and ultrastructural impact of ($Fe_3O_4$) nanoparticles on tobacco. BMC Plant Biol 19:1–12
10. Amir R, Munir F, Khan M, Iqbal T (2019) Use of plant hormones for the improvement of plant growth and production under salt stress. In: Salt stress, microbes, and plant interactions: causes and solution. Singapore: Springer, Singapore, pp 59–90

11. de Andrade JR, de Oliveira Maia Júnior S, da Silva JRR, da Silva VM, dos Santos CM, dos Santos Silva LK, Endres L, Ferreira VM (2022) Ion accumulation, antioxidant activity, growth and tolerance indices of Eucalyptus clones under salt stress. Acta Physiol Plant 44(5):52
12. Annu, Ali A, Ahmed S (2018) Green synthesis of metal, metal oxide nanoparticles, and their various applications. In: Handbook of ecomaterials. Cham: Springer International Publishing, pp 1–45
13. Assaf M, Korkmaz A, Karaman Ş, Kulak M (2022) Effect of plant growth regulators and salt stress on secondary metabolite composition in Lamiaceae species. South African J Bot 144:480–493
14. Avasthi A, Caro C, Pozo-Torres E, Leal MP, García-Martín ML (2020) Magnetic nanoparticles as MRI contrast agents. In: Page topics in current chemistry. Springer International Publishing, pp 1–43
15. Aylward J, Havenga M, Dreyer LL, Roets F, Wingfield BD, Pérez CA, Ramírez-Berrutti N, Carnegie AJ, Wingfield MJ (2021) Genetic diversity of Teratosphaeria pseudoeucalypti in Eucalyptus plantations in Australia and Uruguay. Australas Plant Pathol 50:639–649
16. Baluta S, Lesiak A, Cabaj J (2018) Graphene quantum dots-based electrochemical biosensor for catecholamine neurotransmitters detection. Electroanalysis 30:1781–1790
17. Bouvet A, Nguyen-The N, Melun F (2013) Nutrient concentration and allometric models for hybrid Eucalyptus planted in France. Ann For Sci 70:251–260
18. Cha-um S, Kirdmanee C (2010) Effects of water stress induced by sodium chloride and mannitol on proline accumulation, photosynthetic abilities and growth characters of eucalyptus (Eucalyptus camaldulensis Dehnh.). New For 40:349–360
19. Cha-um S, Somsueb S, Samphumphuang T, Kirdmanee C (2013) Salt tolerant screening in eucalypt genotypes (Eucalyptus spp.) using photosynthetic abilities, proline accumulation, and growth characteristics as effective indices. Vitr Cell Dev Biol - Plant 49:611–619
20. Charlton BD, Reby D, Ellis WAH, Brumm J, Fitch WT (2012) Estimating the active space of male koala bellows: propagation of cues to size and identity in a Eucalyptus forest. PLoS ONE 7:e45420
21. Costa J, Silva JS, Deus E, Pinho S, Pinto JF, Borralho N (2022) The genetics and ecology of post-fire Eucalyptus globulus recruitment in an isolated stand in Central Portugal. Forests 13:680
22. Dadashi S, Poursalehi R, Delavari H (2015) Structural and optical properties of pure iron and iron oxide nanoparticles prepared via pulsed Nd:YAG laser ablation in liquid. Procedia Mater Sci 11:722–726
23. Dai J-H, Hu A-Q, Zhang J-S, Liao W-H, Ma H-Y, Wu J-Z, Yu Y, Cao S-J (2021) NF-YB Mediated Active Responses of Plant Growth under Salt and Temperature Stress in Eucalyptus grandis. Plants 10:1107
24. Derbali F, Elouz F, Hanif MA, Hamrouni L (2021) In vitro evaluation of Eucalyptus urophylla behavior under salt stress. Glob J Bot Sci 9:51–58
25. Dessie AB, Abtew AA, Koye AD (2019) Determinants of the production and commercial values of Eucalyptus woodlot products in Wogera district. North Ethiopia Environ Syst Res 8:4
26. Dhakad AK, Pandey VV, Beg S, Rawat JM, Singh A (2018) Biological, medicinal and toxicological significance of Eucalyptus leaf essential oil: a review. J Sci Food Agric 98:833–848
27. Dmuchowski W, Baczewska-Dąbrowska A, Gozdowski D, Brągoszewska P, Gworek B, Suwara I, Chojnacki T, Jóźwiak A, Swiezewska E (2021) Effect of salt stress in urban conditions on two acer species with different sensitivity. Peer J 9:e10577
28. Egamberdieva D, Wirth S, Abd_Allah EF (2018) Plant hormones as key regulators in plant-microbe interactions under salt stress. In: Microorganisms for sustainability (MICRO), vol 5, pp 165–182
29. Elemike EE, Uzoh IM, Onwudiwe DC, Babalola OO (2019) The role of nanotechnology in the fortification of plant nutrients and improvement of crop production. Appl Sci 9:1–32

30. Estelrich J, Busquets M (2018) Iron oxide nanoparticles in photothermal therapy. Molecules 23:1567
31. Fazio E, Santoro M, Lentini G, Franco D, Guglielmino SPP, Neri F (2016) Iron oxide nanoparticles prepared by laser ablation: synthesis, structural properties and antimicrobial activity. Colloids Surf PhysChem Eng Asp 490:98–103
32. Feng Y, Kreslavski VD, Shmarev AN, Ivanov AA, Zharmukhamedov SK, Kosobryukhov A, Yu M, Allakhverdiev SI, Shabala S (2022) Effects of iron oxide nanoparticles ($Fe_3O_4$) on growth, photosynthesis, antioxidant activity and distribution of mineral elements in wheat (Triticum aestivum). Plants 11
33. Fricke W (2020) Energy costs of salinity tolerance in crop plants: night-time transpiration and growth. New Phytol 225:1152–1165
34. Fu C, Khan MN, Yan J, Hong X, Zhao F, Chen L, Ma H, Li Y, Li J, Wu H (2023) Mechanisms of nanomaterials for improving plant salt tolerance. Crop Environ 2:92–99
35. Fu Y, Yang Y, Chen S, Ning N, Hu H (2019) Arabidopsis IAR4 modulates primary root growth under salt stress through ros-mediated modulation of auxin distribution. Front Plant Sci 10
36. Fujii Y, Suyama K, Hayashi K, Tanabe T, Kawaoka A (2016) Evaluation of Salt Tolerance in Candidate Elite Eucalyptus globulus Conal Plants and Field Test. JAPAN TAPPI J 70:1301–1309
37. García C, Montero G, Coronado MA, Valdez B, Stoytcheva M, Rosas N, Torres R, Sagaste CA (2017) Valorization of Eucalyptus leaves by essential oil extraction as an added value product in Mexico. Waste Biomass Valorization 8:1187–1197
38. Ge X, Cao Z, Chu L (2022) The antioxidant effect of the metal and metal-oxide nanoparticles. Antioxidants 11:791
39. Giri VP, Shukla P, Tripathi A, Verma P, Kumar N, Pandey S, Dimkpa CO, Mishra A (2023) A review of sustainable use of biogenic nanoscale agro-materials to enhance stress tolerance and nutritional value of plants. Plants 12:815
40. Goetz P, Ghedira K (2012) Eucalyptus globulus Labill. (Myrtaceae): Eucalyptus. In: Phytothérapie anti-infectieuse, pp 271–279
41. Goutam SP, Saxena G, Roy D, Yadav AK, Bharagava RN (2020) Green synthesis of nanoparticles and their applications in water and wastewater treatment. In: Bioremediation of industrial waste for environmental safety. Singapore: Springer, Singapore, pp 349–379
42. Grover ZS, Cook RL, Zapata M, Byron Urrego J, Albaugh TJ, Zelaya A, Ozyhar T, Rubilar R, Carter DR, Campoe OC (2021) Eucalyptus grandis response to calcium fertilization in Colombia. For Sci 67:701–710
43. Gudkov SV, Burmistrov DE, Serov DA, Rebezov MB, Semenova AA, Lisitsyn AB (2021) Do iron oxide nanoparticles have significant antibacterial properties? Antibiotics 10:1–23
44. Gupta A, Mishra R, Rai S, Bano A, Pathak N, Fujita M, Kumar M, Hasanuzzaman M (2022) Mechanistic insights of plant growth promoting bacteria mediated drought and salt stress tolerance in plants for sustainable agriculture. Int J Mol Sci 23:3741
45. Ha-Tran DM, Nguyen TTM, Hung S-H, Huang E, Huang C-C (2021) Roles of plant growth-promoting rhizobacteria (PGPR) in stimulating salinity stress defense in plants: a review. Int J Mol Sci 22:3154
46. Hammad EN, Salem SS, Mohamed AA, El-Dougdoug W (2022) Environmental impacts of ecofriendly iron oxide nanoparticles on dyes removal and antibacterial activity. Appl Biochem Biotechnol 194:6053–6067
47. Hao S, Wang Y, Yan Y, Liu Y, Wang J, Chen S (2021) A review on plant responses to salt stress and their mechanisms of salt resistance. Horticulturae 7:132
48. Hasanuzzaman M, Nahar K, Fujit M (2013) Extreme Temperature Responses, Oxidative Stress and Antioxidant Defense in Plants. In: Abiotic Stress - Plant Responses and Applications in Agriculture. IntechOpen. DOI: 10.5772/54833
49. Hirsch H, Allsopp MH, Canavan S, Cheek M, Geerts S, Geldenhuys CJ, Harding G, Hurley BP, Jones W, Keet J-H, Klein H, Ruwanza S, van Wilgen BW, Wingfield MJ, Richardson DM (2020) Eucalyptus camaldulensis in South Africa—past, present, future. Trans R Soc South Africa 75:1–22

50. Hohenthal J, Räsänen M, Minoia P (2018) Political ecology of asymmetric ecological knowledges: diverging views on the Eucalyptus-water nexus in the Taita Hills, Kenya. J Polit Ecol 25
51. Hola K, Markova Z, Zoppellaro G, Tucek J, Zboril R (2015) Tailored functionalization of iron oxide nanoparticles for MRI, drug delivery, magnetic separation and immobilization of biosubstances. Biotechnol Adv 33:1162–1176
52. Hufschmid R, Arami H, Ferguson RM, Gonzales M, Teeman E, Brush LN, Browning ND, Krishnan KM (2015) Synthesis of phase-pure and monodisperse iron oxide nanoparticles by thermal decomposition. Nanoscale 7:11142–11154
53. Hyder S, Ul-Nisa M, Shahzadi, Shahid H, Gohar F, Gondal AS, Riaz N, Younas A, de Los Santos-Villalobos S, Montoya-Martínez AC, Sehar A, Latif F, Rizvi ZF, Iqbal R (2023) Recent trends and perspectives in the application of metal and metal oxide nanomaterials for sustainable agriculture. Plant Physiol Biochem 202:107960
54. Irshad A, Rehman RNU, Abrar MM, Saeed Q, Sharif R, Hu T (2021) Contribution of rhizobium-legume symbiosis in salt stress tolerance in medicago truncatula evaluated through photosynthesis, antioxidant enzymes, and compatible solutes accumulation. Sustainability 13:3369
55. Jiménez E, Vega JA, Fernández C, Pérez-Gorostiaga P, Cuiñas P, Fonturbel T, Alonso M, Rozados MJ, Bará S (2012) Changes in Eucalyptus globulus Labill. saplings growth and physiological parameters following fire-induced stem and crown damage in a plantation in north-western Spain. Eur J For Res 131:1967–1978
56. Kayani ZN, Arshad S, Riaz S, Naseem S (2014) Synthesis of iron oxide nanoparticles by Sol-Gel technique and their characterization. IEEE Trans Magn 50:1–4
57. Kiwumulo HF, Muwonge H, Ibingira C, Lubwama M, Kirabira JB, Ssekitoleko RT (2022) Green synthesis and characterization of iron-oxide nanoparticles using Moringa oleifera: a potential protocol for use in low and middle income countries. BMC Res Notes 15:149
58. Konate A, Wang Y, He X, Adeel M, Zhang P, Ma Y, Ding Y, Zhang J, Yang J, Kizito S, Rui Y, Zhang Z (2018) Comparative effects of nano and bulk-$Fe_3O_4$ on the growth of cucumber (Cucumis sativus). Ecotoxicol Environ Saf 165:547–554
59. Kumar S, Li G, Yang J, Huang X, Ji Q, Liu Z, Ke W, Hou H (2021) Effect of salt stress on growth, physiological parameters, and ionic concentration of water dropwort (Oenanthe javanica) cultivars. Front Plant Sci 12
60. Lassoued A, Dkhil B, Gadri A, Ammar S (2017) Control of the shape and size of iron oxide ($\alpha$-$Fe_2O_3$) nanoparticles synthesized through the chemical precipitation method. Results Phys 7:3007–3015
61. Laurent S, Forge D, Port M, Roch A, Robic C, Vander Elst L, Muller RN (2008) Magnetic iron oxide nanoparticles: synthesis, stabilization, vectorization, physicochemical characterizations, and biological applications. Chem Rev 108:2064–2110
62. Lesiak A, Drzozga K, Cabaj J, Bański M, Malecha K, Podhorodecki A (2019) Optical sensors based on II-VI quantum dots. Nanomaterials 9:192
63. Li J, Chang PR, Huang J, Wang Y, Yuan H, Ren H (2013) Physiological effects of magnetic iron oxide nanoparticles towards watermelon. J Nanosci Nanotechnol 13:5561–5567
64. Li M, Watanabe S, Gao F, Dubos C (2023) Iron nutrition in plants: towards a new paradigm? Plants 12:1–15
65. Ling D, Hyeon T (2013) Chemical design of biocompatible iron oxide nanoparticles for medical applications. Small 9:1450–1466
66. Lorentz KA, Minogue PJ (2015) Potential invasiveness for Eucalyptus species in Florida. Invasive Plant Sci Manag 8:90–97
67. Ma Z, Zhao X, He A, Cao Y, Han Q, Lu Y, Yong JWH, Huang J (2022) Mycorrhizal symbiosis reprograms ion fluxes and fatty acid metabolism in wild jujube during salt stress. Plant Physiol 189:2481–2499
68. Malhotra N, Lee JS, Liman RAD, Ruallo JMS, Villaflore OB, Ger TR, Der HC (2020) Potential toxicity of iron oxide magnetic nanoparticles: a review. Molecules 25:1–26

69. Mangwende E, Truter M, Aveling TAS, Chirwa PW (2021) Anthracnose leaf spot pathogens, Colletotrichum fructicola and Colletotrichum cigarro, associated with Eucalyptus seed produced in South Africa. Australas Plant Pathol 50:533–543
70. de Montferrand C, Hu L, Milosevic I, Russier V, Bonnin D, Motte L, Brioude A, Lalatonne Y (2013) Iron oxide nanoparticles with sizes, shapes and compositions resulting in different magnetization signatures as potential labels for multiparametric detection. Acta Biomater 9:6150–6157
71. Montiel Schneider MG, Martín MJ, Otarola J, Vakarelska E, Simeonov V, Lassalle V, Nedyalkova M (2022) Biomedical applications of iron oxide nanoparticles: current insights progress and perspectives. Pharmaceutics 14:204
72. van Moorsel SJ (2022) The importance of ecotype diversity on duckweed growth with and without salt stress. J Plant Ecol 15:1065–1079
73. Najjar R, Walker H, Anderson P, Barron E, Bord R, Gibson J, Kennedy V, Knight C, Megonigal J, O'Connor R, Polsky C, Psuty N, Richards B, Sorenson L, Steele E, Swanson R (2000) The potential impacts of climate change on the mid-Atlantic coastal region. Clim Res 14:219–233
74. Ndou N, Rakgotho T, Nkuna M, Doumbia IZ, Mulaudzi T, Ajayi RF (2023) Green synthesis of iron oxide (Hematite) nanoparticles and their influence on sorghum bicolor growth under drought stress. Plants 12:1425
75. Nefissi Ouertani R, Arasappan D, Abid G, Ben Chikha M, Jardak R, Mahmoudi H, Mejri S, Ghorbel A, Ruhlman TA, Jansen RK (2021) Transcriptomic analysis of salt-stress-responsive genes in Barley roots and leaves. Int J Mol Sci 22:8155
76. Nikam AV, Prasad BLV, Kulkarni AA (2018) Wet chemical synthesis of metal oxide nanoparticles: a review. Cryst Eng Comm 20:5091–5107
77. Nitta S, Numata K (2013) Biopolymer-based nanoparticles for drug/gene delivery and tissue engineering. Int J Mol Sci 14:1629–1654
78. de Oliveira NC, Ribeiro MF, Ottati A, de Tavares WS, Serrão JE, Zanuncio JC, Zanetti R, Wilcken CF (2022) The survival, development, and reproduction of Gonipterus platensis (Coleoptera: Curculionidae) on the main Eucalyptus (Myrtaceae) genotypes planted in Brazil. Peer J 10:e13698
79. de Oliveira TWG, Rubilar R, Sanquetta CR, Corte APD, Bozo D, Medina A, Mardones O, Emhart V, Quiroga JJ, Valenzuela H (2022) Changes in leaf physiology for Eucalyptus genotypes with increase in integral water stress and its consequence for initial growth in central Chile. Sci For 50
80. Palmieri N, Stefanoni W, Latterini F, Pari L (2022) Italian consumer preferences for Eucalyptus honey: an exploratory study. Sustainability 14:7741
81. Parihar P, Singh S, Singh R, Singh VP, Prasad SM (2015) Effect of salinity stress on plants and its tolerance strategies: a review. Environ Sci Pollut Res 22:4056–4075
82. Parvaiz A, Satyawati S (2008) Salt stress and phyto-biochemical responses of plants—a review. Plant Soil Environ 54:89–99
83. Rabhi NEH, Cherif-Silini H, Silini A, Alenezi FN, Chenari Bouket A, Oszako T, Belbahri L (2022) Alleviation of salt stress via habitat-adapted symbiosis. Forests 13:586
84. Rajamathi M, Seshadri R (2002) Oxide and chalcogenide nanoparticles from hydrothermal/solvothermal reactions. Curr Opin Solid State Mater Sci 6:337–345
85. Rasheed F, Bakhsh R, Qadir I (2020) Trade-off between shoot and root dry weight along with a steady CO assimilation rate ensures the survival of Eucalyptus camaldulensis under salt stress. J For Sci 66:452–460
86. Ritonga F, Ngatia J, Song R, Farooq U, Somadona S, Lestari A, Chen S (2021) Abiotic stresses induced physiological, biochemical, and molecular changes in Betula platyphylla: a review. Silva Fenn 55
87. Rockwood DL, Winandy JE, Gribbins NR (2022) Processing and wood factors influence medium density fiberboard production from young Eucalyptus grandis, E. amplifolia, corymbia torelliana, and cottonwood grown in Florida USA. Forests 13:266
88. Rui M, Ma C, Hao Y, Guo J, Rui Y, Tang X, Zhao Q, Fan X, Zhang Z, Hou T, Zhu S (2016) Iron oxide nanoparticles as a potential iron fertilizer for peanut (Arachis hypogaea). Front Plant Sci 7:1–10

89. Ryu H, Cho Y-G (2015) Plant hormones in salt stress tolerance. J Plant Biol 58:147–155
90. Sadiq MU, Shah A, Haleem A, Shah SM, Shah I (2023) Eucalyptus globulus mediated green synthesis of environmentally benign metal based nanostructures: a review. Nanomaterials 13:2019
91. Saif S, Tahir A, Chen Y (2016) Green synthesis of iron nanoparticles and their environmental applications and implications. Nanomaterials 6:209
92. Saleem S, Khan MS (2023) Phyto-interactive impact of green synthesized iron oxide nanoparticles and Rhizobium pusense on morpho-physiological and yield components of greengram. Plant Physiol Biochem 194:146–160
93. Samrot AV, Sahithya CS, Selvarani AJ, Purayil SK, Ponnaiah P (2021) A review on synthesis, characterization and potential biological applications of superparamagnetic iron oxide nanoparticles. Curr Res Green Sustain Chem 4:100042
94. Sarkar D, Singh S, Parihar M, Rakshit A (2021) Seed bio-priming with microbial inoculants: a tailored approach towards improved crop performance, nutritional security, and agricultural sustainability for smallholder farmers. Curr Res Environ Sustain 3:100093
95. Selvaraj R, Pai S, Vinayagam R, Varadavenkatesan T, Kumar PS, Duc PA, Rangasamy G (2022) A recent update on green synthesized iron and iron oxide nanoparticles for environmental applications. Chemosphere 308:136331
96. Seng Hua L, Wei Chen L, Antov P, Kristak L, Md Tahir P (2022) Engineering wood products from Eucalyptus spp. Adv Mater Sci Eng 2022:1–14
97. Shah IH, Sabir IA, Rehman A, Hameed MK, Albashar G, Manzoor MA, Shakoor A (2023) Co-application of copper oxide nanoparticles and Trichoderma harzianum with physiological, enzymatic and ultrastructural responses for the mitigation of salt stress. Chemosphere 336:139230
98. Sharma A, Devi YB, Meetei TT (2022) A review on impact of salt stress in soil health and its suitable control measure. Environ Conserv J 23:412–424
99. Siddiqi KS, Husen A (2017) Plant response to engineered metal oxide nanoparticles. Nanoscale Res Lett 12:92
100. Singh A, Singh P, Dhillon GPS, Sharma S, Singh B, Gill RIS (2023) Differential impacts of soil salinity and water logging on Eucalyptus growth and carbon sequestration under mulched versus unmulched soils in south-western Punjab. India Plant Soil 482:401–425
101. Singh D, Sillu D, Kumar A, Agnihotri S (2021) Dual nanozyme characteristics of iron oxide nanoparticles alleviate salinity stress and promote the growth of an agroforestry tree, Eucalyptus tereticornis Sm. Environ Sci Nano 8:1308–1325
102. Sixto H, González-González BD, Molina-Rueda JJ, Garrido-Aranda A, Sanchez MM, López G, Gallardo F, Cañellas I, Mounet F, Grima-Pettenati J, Cantón F (2016) Eucalyptus spp. and Populus spp. coping with salinity stress: an approach on growth, physiological and molecular features in the context of short rotation coppice (SRC). Trees 30:1873–1891
103. Sogoni A, Jimoh M, Kambizi L, Laubscher C (2021) The impact of salt stress on plant growth, mineral composition, and antioxidant activity in Tetragonia decumbens mill.: An underutilized edible halophyte in South Africa. Horticulturae 7:140
104. Song Y, Li S, Sui Y, Zheng H, Han G, Sun X, Yang W, Wang H, Zhuang K, Kong F, Meng Q, Sui N (2022) SbbHLH85, a bHLH member, modulates resilience to salt stress by regulating root hair growth in sorghum. Theor Appl Genet 135:201–216
105. Stefanov MA, Rashkov GD, Apostolova EL (2022) Assessment of the photosynthetic apparatus functions by chlorophyll fluorescence and P700 absorbance in C3 and C4 plants under physiological conditions and under salt stress. Int J Mol Sci 23:3768
106. Suddarth SRP, Ferreira JFS, Cavalcante LF, Fraga VS, Anderson RG, Halvorson JJ, Bezerra FTC, Medeiros SAS, Costa CRG, Dias NS (2019) Can humic substances improve soil fertility under salt stress and drought conditions? J Environ Qual 48:1605–1613
107. Tao Z, Zhou Q, Zheng T, Mo F, Ouyang S (2023) Iron oxide nanoparticles in the soil environment: adsorption, transformation, and environmental risk. J Hazard Mater 459:132107
108. Tawfik MM, Mohamed MH, Sadak MS, Thalooth AT (2021) Iron oxide nanoparticles effect on growth, physiological traits and nutritional contents of Moringa oleifera grown in saline environment. Bull Natl Res Cent 45:177

109. Thies J, Grossman J (2006) The soil habitat and soil ecology, pp 59–78
110. Tokoro H, Nakabayashi K, Nagashima S, Song Q, Yoshikiyo M, Ohkoshi S (2022) Optical properties of epsilon iron oxide nanoparticles in the millimeter- and terahertz- wave regions. Bull Chem Soc Jpn 95:538–552
111. Turrina C, Klassen A, Milani D, Rojas-González DM, Ledinski G, Auer D, Sartori B, Cvirn G, Mela P, Berensmeier S, Schwaminger SP (2023) Superparamagnetic iron oxide nanoparticles for their application in the human body: influence of the surface. Heliyon 9:e16487
112. Uma S (1995) Genetic variability in recovery growth and synthesis of stress proteins in response to polyethylene glycol and salt stress in finger millet. Ann Bot 76:43–49
113. Verma SS, Verma RS, Verma SK, Yadav AL, Verma AK (2018) Impact of salt stress on plant establishment, chlorophyll and total free amino acid content of ber (Zizyphus mauritiana Lamk.). J Pharmacogn Phytochem 7:556–559
114. Wang Y, Ding L, Yao C, Li C, Xing X, Huang Y, Gu T, Wu M (2017) Toxic effects of metal oxide nanoparticles and their underlying mechanisms. Sci China Mater 60:93–108
115. Xie W, Guo Z, Gao F, Gao Q, Wang D, Liaw B, Cai Q, Sun X, Wang X, Zhao L (2018) Shape-, size- and structure-controlled synthesis and biocompatibility of iron oxide nanoparticles for magnetic theranostics. Theranostics 8:3284–3307
116. Yadav SP, Bharadwaj R, Nayak H, Mahto R, Singh RK, Prasad SK (2019) Impact of salt stress on growth, productivity and physicochemical properties of plants: a review. Int J Chem Stud 7:1793–1798
117. Yadav VK, Ali D, Khan SH, Gnanamoorthy G, Choudhary N, Yadav KK, Thai VN, Hussain SA, Manhrdas S (2020) Synthesis and characterization of amorphous iron oxide nanoparticles by the sonochemical method and their application for the remediation of heavy metals from wastewater. Nanomaterials 10:1–17
118. Yang Y, Guo Y (2018) Unraveling salt stress signaling in plants. J Integr Plant Biol 60:796–804
119. Yastreb TO, Kolupaev YE, Shkliarevskyi MA, Dyachenko AI, Dmitriev AP (2020) Involvement of jasmonate signaling components in salt stress-induced stomatal closure in Arabidopsis thaliana. Cytol Genet 54:318–323
120. Yost JM, Wise SL, Love NLR, Steane DA, Jones RC, Ritter MK, Potts BM (2021) Origins, diversity and naturalization of Eucalyptus globulus (Myrtaceae) in California. Forests 12:1129
121. Yu Z, Duan X, Luo L, Dai S, Ding Z, Xia G (2020) How plant hormones mediate salt stress responses. Trends Plant Sci 25:1117–1130
122. Zakariya NA, Majeed S, Jusof WHW (2022) Investigation of antioxidant and antibacterial activity of iron oxide nanoparticles (IONPS) synthesized from the aqueous extract of Penicillium spp. Sensors Int 3:100164
123. Zhang Y, Wang X (2021) Geographical spatial distribution and productivity dynamic change of Eucalyptus plantations in China. Sci Rep 11:19764
124. Zhao S, Zhang Q, Liu M, Zhou H, Ma C, Wang P (2021) Regulation of plant responses to salt stress. Int J Mol Sci 22:4609
125. Zhu N, Ji H, Yu P, Niu J, Farooq M, Akram M, Udego I, Li H, Niu X (2018) Surface modification of magnetic iron oxide nanoparticles. Nanomaterials 8:810

# Applications of Nanobiostimulants and Nanofertilizers in Arid Zone Agroforestry Systems

**Marcelino Cabrera-De la Fuente, Paola Fincheira, Rocío Maricela Peralta-Manjarrez, Gonzalo Tortella, and Adalberto Benavides-Mendoza**

**Abstract** The chapter explores the integration of nanotechnology in agroforestry, particularly in arid regions where conventional farming methods fail to optimize productivity. The Introduction sets the stage by elucidating the pressing need for sustainable and efficient agriculture in arid zones. The Benefits of Agroforestry section delineates how the different multi-layered agroforestry systems enhance biodiversity and social benefits and optimize land and water use. The following section, Nanobiostimulants and Nanofertilizers in Agroforestry Plant Production, provides a list of the effectiveness of nanomaterials in nutrient uptake, water retention, and resistance against pests and diseases in different agroforest plant species. Furthermore, the section Nanobiostimulants and Nanofertilizers that could be used in Agroforestry Systems to Mitigate Environmental Challenges underscores the role that a series of nanomaterials can play in ameliorating the productivity of agroforestry systems. The chapter aims to guide researchers, policymakers, and technicians interested in sustainable agroforestry solutions via nanotechnology.

**Keywords** Nanotechnology · Biostimulation · Biostimulants · Nanomaterials · Nanoparticles · Fertilizers · Plant nutrition · Plant stress

M. Cabrera-De la Fuente · R. M. Peralta-Manjarrez · A. Benavides-Mendoza (✉)
Departmento de Horticultura, Universidad Autónoma Agraria Antonio Narro, Saltillo, Mexico
e-mail: adalberto.benavides@uaaan.edu.mx

P. Fincheira · G. Tortella
Centro de Excelencia en Investigación Biotecnológica Aplicada Al Medio Ambiente (CIBAMA), Universidad de La Frontera, Temuco, CP, Chile

G. Tortella
Departamento de Ingeniería Química, Facultad de Ingeniería y Ciencias, Universidad de La Frontera, Temuco, Chile



D. Jabborova et al. (eds.), *Nanomaterials in Agroforestry Systems*, Smart Nanomaterials Technology, https://doi.org/10.1007/978-981-96-1337-3_14

## 1 Introduction

The escalating climate crisis and burgeoning global population have put enormous strain on our agricultural systems, necessitating immediate attention and action from all stakeholders, including governing bodies. The challenge of securing food for humanity has never been as formidable as in the present twenty-first century, which has witnessed unparalleled technological progress in all fields. These advancements, while putting pressure on the environment, can also be harnessed to confront food scarcity and safety issues.

A reasonable approach would entail enhancing our capacity to grow adequate food for all sustainably in the near future, providing not only essential calories and nutrients for good health but also ensuring it is produced in an ecologically sustainable way.

One critical frontier lies in the arid zones, constituting approximately 41% of the Earth's terrestrial surface and housing over 2.5 billion people, many of whom are engaged in agriculture-based livelihoods. Water and atmospheric humidity scarcity and extreme temperatures majorly hinder agricultural productivity in arid zones [43].

Agroforestry is an integrated farming approach that emphasizes the diversification of different components in an agroecosystem, including woody perennials, palms, crops, livestock, and forages; it is a transformative solution to the intensifying environmental and socio-economic challenges in arid zones. Globally, a coverage of $307 \times 10^6$ ha of agroforestry production and $823 \times 10^6$ ha of production in the silvopastoral system is estimated [87]. Agroforestry, due to its ecological principles and approaches that underpin its design and management, is often deemed a practical application of agroecology. However, agroforestry in arid zones has been historically marginalized due to those mentioned above formidable environmental constraints of water availability and temperature extremes [71]. Nevertheless, agroforestry holds significant potential for combatting desertification and biodiversity loss and ensuring soil health and food security for many communities, given the application of the proper sustainable management practices and technological innovations [33], as is the case of nanobiostimulants and nanofertilizers.

Biostimulants and fertilizers (and biofertilizers) are chemical or biological materials widely used in agriculture. The biostimulants increase stress tolerance and crop adaptation to adverse conditions, and fertilizers ensure crop productivity, quality, and yield. The biostimulants and fertilizers taken to the nanoscale can be engineered and tailored to enhance nutrient uptake, improve soil fertility, and increase plant resistance to environmental stresses, thereby improving crop yield and sustainability in harsh environments; indeed, in different experimental settings and plant species, nanobiostimulants (NBs) and nanofertilizers (NFs) have shown greater efficiency than their conventional counterparts [76]. Nanotechnology is emerging as a promising tool in revolutionizing agriculture and the food production systems [58]. The use of NBs and NFs stands at the intersection of nanotechnology and agriculture, offering promising strategies to enhance productivity in general for agriculture, particularly for arid zone agroforestry systems [15, 49].

NBs, primarily comprising nanoparticles derived from beneficial elements (e.g., silicon and selenium), zeolites, biological polymers (e.g., chitosan and alginate), or nanoparticles (NPs) complexed with bioactive compounds, aim to stimulate plant growth and development without necessarily providing nutrients. They function through various mechanisms, such as enhancing metabolic processes, promoting nutrient absorption, and mitigating stress responses. The nano size offers significant advantages like increased surface area-to-volume ratio and distinctive physicochemical properties, allowing these NBs to interact efficiently with plant cells, facilitating their absorption and distribution, and reducing the losses of the products applied on soil and crops by leaching or weathering [15].

Conversely, NFs, obtained from essential or beneficial macro and micronutrient ions or minerals, are intended to offer efficient nutrient delivery systems. The NPs formulation enables slow and targeted release of nutrients, mitigating wastage from leaching, volatilization, or immobilization and reducing the risk of environmental contamination. This characteristic is particularly beneficial in arid environments where poor soil structure and low water availability limit traditional fertilizer effectiveness [76].

However, applying NBs and NFs in arid zone agroforestry remains a largely untapped field, necessitating further research and fieldwork. Despite the promise of nanotechnology, challenges persist in its application to extensive agriculture, specifically in arid regions. Technical hurdles must be addressed, such as optimizing particle size, shape, and composition for maximal effect, ensuring stability under extreme field conditions, and addressing potential ecotoxicological concerns. Moreover, understanding the social, economic, and ethical implications of nanotechnology applications in agriculture is vital for ensuring their successful integration into complex systems [15].

This manuscript intends to review the actual or potential applications of NBs and NFs in agroforestry systems. It aims to highlight their potential benefits and challenges in arid regions, presenting a comprehensive outlook on the transformative potential of nanotechnology in lessening the impacts of conventional biostimulants and fertilizers.

## 2 The Benefits of Agroforestry

In the context of the obtention of high and sustainable productivity in arid zones, agroforestry assumes tremendous significance and vast scope, encompassing many benefits spanning ecological, agricultural, and socio-economic domains. The benefits are listed below.

## 2.1 Ecological Benefits

Agroforestry practices are crucial in preserving and enhancing ecological balance in arid zones. Incorporating trees into farming systems can combat desertification by improving soil structure, reducing soil erosion, and strengthening the capacity of soil to retain moisture. The extensive root systems of trees help in water infiltration, reducing surface runoff and enabling more effective use of scant rainfall. Moreover, trees can sequester carbon and lessen the impacts of climate change while also enhancing biodiversity by providing habitat for plants and other organisms [33, 78].

## 2.2 Agricultural and Socio-Economic Benefits

Including trees within agricultural systems can significantly enhance crop productivity and resilience in arid zones [97]. Trees can provide a protective microclimate, reducing the impact of extreme temperatures on crops. Some trees, particularly nitrogen-fixing species, can enhance soil fertility by improving nutrient cycling. Trees can also serve as windbreaks, protecting crops from wind damage and reducing evaporation, conserving soil moisture. Furthermore, the diversified farming system reduces the hazard of crop failure in the face of pest outbreaks or extreme weather events [9, 93].

The socio-economic benefits of agroforestry in arid zones cannot be overemphasized. By increasing agricultural productivity and diversifying farm output, agroforestry enhances food security and income stability for rural households [102]. Farmers can benefit from various products like timber, firewood, fruits, nuts, and fodder, providing multiple income sources throughout the year. In addition, agroforestry can create jobs related to tree product harvesting, processing, and marketing, stimulating local economies [9].

Agroforestry recognizes the interactions between crops and trees and is acknowledged as a potential strategy for sustainably intensifying agriculture. Based on integrating the various components of the agroforestry complex, agroforestry systems used in arid zones are annotated in Table 1.

While each of the above agroforestry systems has unique advantages and challenges, all offer potential strategies for soil health, sustainable agriculture, and food production in arid zones. The system choice depends on the specific environmental conditions, socio-economic context, and the available resources and capacities of the farmers. The following section will discuss how nanobiostimulants and nanofertilizers can improve the response of crops and trees used in agroforestry in arid regions where environmental stress is prevalent.

**Table 1** Examples of agroforestry systems that are used in arid zones

| System | Description | References |
|---|---|---|
| Agro-silvo-pastoral system | Integrates crops, livestock, and trees. The species *Acacia senegal* is an example. Advantages include diversified income and enhanced sustainability. However, it requires complex management, and competition for resources among the different components can be an issue | [74] |
| Alley cropping | This practice involves the cultivation of crops between rows of trees. Drought-resistant trees like *Leucaena leucocephala* are often used in arid regions. It improves soil fertility and reduces soil erosion, but the competition for nutrients and water between trees and crops can impact crop yield | [96] |
| Forest farming | Involves the cultivation of shade-loving crops under a forest canopy. Species like Moringa oleifera are cultivated in arid zones. The system ensures efficient utilization of resources but requires careful management to balance light levels and minimize competition | [21] |
| Homegardens | This practice involves growing a diverse range of trees, shrubs, and crops around households. Fruit trees like date palm (*Phoenix dactylifera*) and fig (*Ficus carica*) are commonly grown. Homegardens offer food diversity and additional income but require considerable labor and can face challenges from pests | [74] |
| Multi-storey cropping | It involves growing crops of different heights together. In arid regions, overstorey trees like *Acacia* spp. may be combined with understory crops like groundnuts. This system maximizes land use and provides diverse products but can be complex to manage due to the interactions between various components | [18] |
| Parkland system | Characterized by scattered trees across crop fields, with species like Faidherbia albida common in arid regions. The system can improve soil fertility and microclimate, but the irregular distribution of trees can make mechanized farming difficult | [74] |
| Silvopastoral system | This system integrates trees with pasture and livestock. In arid zones, species such as *Acacia tortilis* and *Prosopis cineraria* are often used, providing shade and fodder for animals. Advantages include improved animal welfare, reduced feed costs, and enhanced biodiversity. However, water competition between trees and grass and potential overgrazing can be challenges | [74] |

(continued)

**Table 1** (continued)

| System | Description | References |
|---|---|---|
| Taungya system | Involves the growing of annual crops in the understory during the early stages of a tree crop. Trees like *Azadirachta indica* are often used. This system allows for efficient land use and additional income, but managing crop-tree interactions can be challenging | [74] |
| Windbreaks or shelterbelts | These are rows of trees or shrubs planted to protect crops from wind and dehydration damage. Species like *Casuarina equisetifolia* and *Eucalyptus spp.* are used in arid zones. While they protect soil from erosion and conserve moisture, they can compete with crops for resources | [59] |

# 3 Nanobiostimulants and Nanofertilizers in Agroforestry Plant Production

Agriculture and food production in arid zones present a formidable array of challenges and inconveniences due to the inherent climatic and edaphic conditions of these regions. Arid regions, characterized by less than 250 mm annual rainfall, low soil and atmospheric humidity, and high temperatures, create a harsh environment for agricultural activities, impacting both the viability and productivity of crops [62].

One of the most significant restrictions is water scarcity. Prolonged periods of drought and elevated evaporation rates lead to chronic water shortages, thus constraining the scope of farming activities. Moreover, this scarcity often leads to over-reliance on underground water sources, which can result in their over-exploitation, causing subsequent environmental and sustainability issues [81].

Soil fertility is another challenge. The topography of arid zones is frequently marked by poor soils that lack organic matter and essential nutrients and have poor water retention capabilities [27].

The extreme temperatures that characterize arid zones can also directly affect crop health. High temperatures can cause plant heat stress, reducing the stomatal gas exchange and photosynthesis rates, augmenting photorespiration and oxidative stress, and negatively impacting overall crop productivity. The low availability of photosynthates, the protein denaturation and dysfunction, the unfavorable changes in the membrane fluidity, and the higher energy expenditure (respiration + photorespiration) due to the plant's metabolic modulation against high temperatures decrease the energy budget of plants, with the concomitant reduction in the tolerance to pest and diseases, favoring the proliferation of harmful species that can devastate agricultural yields [28].

Regarding human aspects, farmers in arid zones often face economic challenges. The uncertainty of crop yields due to water scarcity, limited crop biodiversity, intrinsic low agricultural productivity, and variable climatic conditions, coupled with the high cost of irrigation technologies and soil amelioration methods, combined with inadequate access to credits and markets, put a significant financial strain on farmers. The volatile nature of farming in these areas can also deter investment in agriculture and limit access to farming resources and new technologies [39, 109].

How the use of nanobiostimulants and nanofertilizers can improve agricultural productivity in arid zones? Biostimulants are defined as a substance, microorganism, or physical stimulus that, when applied to plants or the surrounding water and soil, enhances the plant's growth, health, and tolerance to abiotic stresses by stimulating natural processes of metabolic modulation, adaptation, and defense. Biostimulants constitute a diverse group of beneficial elements and minerals, metabolites, polymers, microorganisms, and physical stimulus (e.g., UV light) that can enhance agricultural productivity in arid zones by directly improving plant metabolism and physiology and indirectly ameliorating soil health by improving soil structure, enhancing nutrient availability, and boosting beneficial soil microbial activity. The above leads to a more growth-promoting soil environment for plants. For example, some biostimulants stimulate the activity of beneficial soil microorganisms, which in turn increase organic matter decomposition, nutrient cycling, and soil structure [31]. By incorporating biostimulants into agroforestry practices, farmers in arid zones can improve their yields, making farming more resilient and sustainable in these harsh environments. In this sense, the use of nanobiostimulants, which have shown greater efficacy compared to conventional biostimulants (e.g., nanochitosan versus chitosan), can bring advantages to agroforestry producers in arid areas since they would allow a substantial improvement in the response of the plants in which they are applied [82].

Regarding fertilizers, they can significantly boost agricultural productivity in arid zones by enriching soil nutrient content. Arid soils often lack essential macronutrients such as N, P, K, Fe, Zn, Mn, and Cu. Adding fertilizers can replenish these essential nutrients, facilitating better plant growth and development [63]. However, the efficacy and efficiency of fertilizers in arid zones is not merely about their application but also their management. Some of the limitations for efficiently using nutrients in arid lands are water scarcity, soil salinity, high soil pH and soil alkalinity, low organic matter, and low nutrient and water holding capacity. The above limitations for the efficient use of nutrients cause the efficiency in using fertilizers to be very low, giving rise to low productivity and economic losses [67]. Additionally, the overuse or improper use of fertilizers can lead to issues like nutrient run-off, soil degradation, and groundwater contamination. Therefore, better farming techniques should be implemented to ensure nutrients are delivered when and where plants need them most. In this sense, using nanofertilizers can increase the efficiency of the applications of plant´s essential elements, reducing economic and ecological costs and improving plant productivity. An additional advantage of nanofertilizers is that they provide essential nutrients for crops and work as biostimulant agents. This dual action capacity makes them potentially valuable tools for agroforestry in arid zones [76].

Returning to the question, how can using nanobiostimulants and nanofertilizers improve agricultural productivity in arid zones? An explanation of the properties and mechanisms through which nanobiostimulants and nanofertilizers manage to

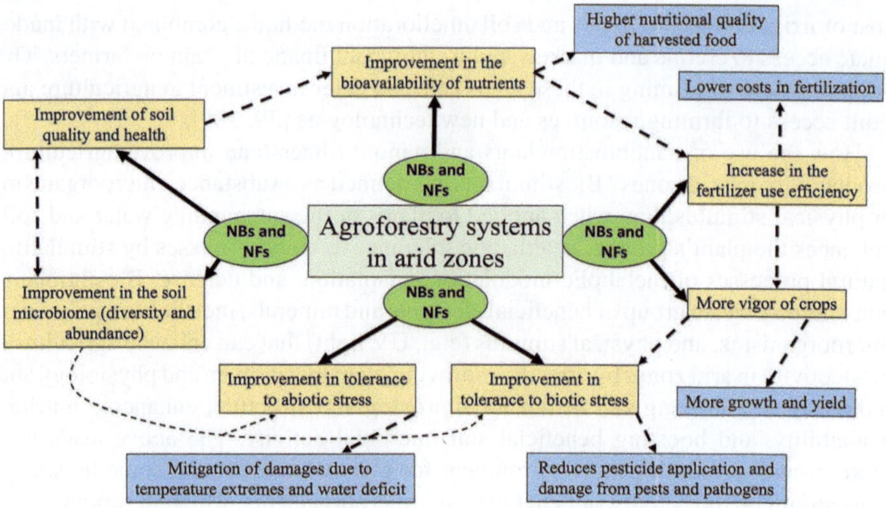


**Fig. 1** Mechanisms through which nanobiostimulants (NBs) and nanofertilizers (NFs) can improve the productivity of agroforestry systems in arid regions. The direct effects are noted in the orange boxes and the indirect effects in the blue boxes. The solid arrows indicate the direction of the direct impact of NBs and NFs, and the discontinuous ones are that of the indirect effects

improve performance compared to their conventional counterparts is noted in Fig. 1 and the following lines.

Nanobiostimulants are nano-sized materials that promote natural plant metabolic processes to improve nutrient efficiency, stress tolerance, and crop quality [79, 80]. Table 2 includes some of the properties and mechanisms of action of nanobiostimulants reported in the literature:

On the other hand, nanofertilizers represent an innovative approach to nutrition in agroforestry systems, with unique properties and mechanisms of action attributed to their nanoscale size and large surface area-to-volume ratio. Nanofertilizers are chemical agents with a dual biological impact [79, 80]. On the one hand, nanofertilizers efficiently deliver the necessary nutrients for the crops; on the other hand, due to their nanometric nature, they function as biostimulant agents, inducing defensive responses in plants, which translates into improved acclimatization [76]. Table 3 includes some key properties and mechanisms of action of nanofertilizers as reported in the literature.

Despite all the advantages reported in studies conducted, using nanobiostimulants and nanofertilizers in agroforestry systems is not widespread. Apart from using organic matter and compost, the application of conventional biostimulants and fertilizers is also not very extensive. Tables 4 and 5 were constructed by mentioning plant species (crops and trees) commonly used in agroforestry systems and linking them with existing (or non-existing) reports in Scopus searching to *Species name* AND

**Table 2** Mechanisms of action of nanobiostimulants reported in the literature that improve the growth, yield, or quality of crops

| Mechanism | Explanation | Reference |
|---|---|---|
| Improved absorption and mobility in the plant | In comparison with conventional biostimulants, nanobiostimulants can easily penetrate plant cell walls and membranes, leading to better absorption and mobility within the plant. Example nanoselenium versus selenium | [41] |
| Controlled release of nutrients or active metabolites | Nanobiostimulants can be designed to release inorganic or bioactive compounds in a controlled manner, reducing losses and enhancing the efficacy of the applications. Example nanolignin versus lignin | [60] |
| Enhanced root growth and nutrient uptake | As a result of better absorption and controlled release, nanobiostimulants can enhance root growth biomass and substrate exploration, leading to an increased volume for nutrient and water absorption. Some nanobiostimulants have also been reported to increase the expression of nutrient transporters in the plant, enhancing nutrient uptake. Example nanosilicon versus silicon | [26] |
| Modulation of plant metabolism | Nanobiostimulants can modulate plant metabolism, leading to increased production of growth-promoting hormones, enhanced photosynthetic efficiency, and improved stress tolerance. Example nanozinc versus zinc | [5] |
| Induction of systemic resistance | Some nanobiostimulants can induce systemic resistance in plants, making them more tolerant to pests and diseases. This is often achieved by triggering the plant's own defense mechanisms. Example iron nanomaterials | [77] |
| Antioxidant activity | Certain nanobiostimulants (e.g., humic substances and carbon nanomaterials) have antioxidant properties, helping plants to mitigate oxidative stress, which can be particularly beneficial under stress conditions such as drought, salinity, and extreme temperatures | [44] |
| Improved plant and soil microbiome | Some nanobiostimulants can promote beneficial plant–microbe interactions, enhancing plant growth and health. Example nanozeolites | [12] |

agroforestry AND nanobiostimulant OR nanofertilizer/*Species name* AND agroforestry AND nano biostimulant OR nano fertilizer/*Species name* AND nanobiostimulant OR nanofertilizer/*Species name* AND nano biostimulant OR nano fertilizer. Therefore, Table 4 indicates whether the information available in the Scopus database is directly related to using nanobiostimulants and nanofertilizers in species in agroforestry systems. For several species, such as *Moringa*, and especially for annual species, such as wheat and maize, there are many reports of the use and application of nanobiostimulants and nanofertilizers; however, Table 4 includes only those related to agroforestry systems or with potential agroforestry context.

On the other hand, Table 5 lists those species used in agroforestry systems, but no report related to the application of nanobiostimulants or nanofertilizers was found. It should be highlighted in the information presented in Table 5 that the absence of

**Table 3** Some of the action mechanisms through which nanofertilizers increase crop growth, yield, and stress tolerance

| Mechanism | Explanation | Reference |
|---|---|---|
| Increased nutrient use efficiency | Nanofertilizers improve nutrient use efficiency due to their high surface area, enhancing interaction with plant roots and the small particle size, facilitating penetration and movement within plant tissues. This ensures a more efficient uptake and use of nutrients, reducing environmental losses | [17] |
| Controlled release of nutrients | Nanofertilizers can encapsulate nutrients in a matrix that allows a slow and controlled release in response to environmental triggers or plant demand. This reduces the frequency of fertilizer application, decreases nutrient leaching, and ensures nutrient availability over a longer period | [86] |
| Enhanced root growth and nutrient uptake | Nanofertilizers can stimulate root growth and development, increasing the root surface area for nutrient and water absorption. They may also enhance the expression of nutrient transporters, facilitating nutrient uptake | [17] |
| Improved soil fertility | Nanofertilizers can improve soil fertility by altering soil pH, enhancing soil structure, increasing water-holding capacity, and promoting beneficial soil microorganisms | [50] |
| Induction of systemic resistance | Nanofertilizers can induce systemic tolerance in plants, enhancing their ability to withstand abiotic stresses such as drought, salinity, and extreme temperatures. Nanofertilizers can promote the production of stress-related proteins and antioxidants, helping plants to mitigate stress-related damage | [16] |
| Modulation of plant metabolism | Nanofertilizers can modulate plant metabolism to increase photosynthetic efficiency, enhance the synthesis of growth-promoting hormones, ameliorating overall plant growth and productivity | [103] |
| Pest and disease resistance | Nanofertilizers can play a role in enhancing plant resistance to pests and diseases, either through direct antimicrobial effects or by inducing the plant's own defense mechanisms | [110] |
| Improved seed germination and seedling vigor | Nanofertilizers can enhance seed germination and seedling vigor, improving crop establishment and yield | [1] |

information about the use of nanobiostimulants or nanofertilizers does not imply that their use is not advisable. Instead, it indicates the need for laboratory, greenhouse, or field research to determine the concentrations or quantities of specific nanobiostimulants or nanofertilizers to achieve a favorable metabolic or productive impact on that particular species.

**Table 4** Plant species used in agroforestry systems in different arid zones, and the reports on nanobiostimulants or nanofertilizers impact in the context of agroforestry production or research. The results come from a search in Scopus. The list of species was obtained using the Google search engine

| Plant species | Nanobiostimulants or nanofertilizer reported | References |
|---|---|---|
| *Adansonia digitata*. The fruit, leaves, and seeds of the baobab are edible, and the tree is also important for its role in maintaining biodiversity | Baobab plants sprayed with hydroxyapatite nanoparticles showed higher fresh weight (133.3% more than the control) and great improvement in the concentration of chlorophyll, carotenoids, and ascorbic acid, in comparison with control, DAP, and MAP | [99] |
| *Amaranthus* spp. Amaranth is grown both for its edible seeds and for its leaves, which can be consumed as a leafy vegetable | Nanohydroxyapatite combined with wollastonite can be used to decrease Cd uptake. An increase in biomass of 643–865% and a 74.8–75-1% decrease in Cd uptake was observed | [47] |
| *Chenopodium quinoa*. Quinoa is native to the Andean region and can withstand a range of environmental conditions | Chelate micronutrients (Fe, Zn, Mn, B) increased the absorption of N, P, and K in grains by 12.86, 127.27, and 98.64%, respectively, compared with control. In addition, 17.01% more protein, ash 4.56%, and fiber 2.23% were recorded | [53] |
| *Gossypium hirsutum*. Cotton can be grown in dryland systems primarily for its fiber | Applying ZnO NPs decreased the uptake of heavy metals (Cd and Pb) in seedlings. Therefore, a significant improvement was found in the seedlings' growth and the content of metabolites and protein | [84] |

(continued)

**Table 4** (continued)

| Plant species | Nanobiostimulants or nanofertilizer reported | References |
|---|---|---|
| *Helianthus annuus.* Sunflowers are grown in dryland systems for their seeds and oil | Different reports show favorable effects of NMs (nano-sulfur, nano-Se, NZnO) on growth, yield, quality, and tolerance to biotic and abiotic stress | [11, 100, 101] |
| *Hordeum vulgare.* Barley is a hardy cereal crop that is often used in dryland farming | Combining a biostimulant (mycorrhizal inoculation) and nano-Zn increases growth, yield, and quality under field conditions | [51, 72] |
| *Moringa* spp. The leaves of Moringa tree are used as a nutrient-rich and nutraceutical vegetable, and the seeds can be pressed for oil | Uso de nanofertilizantes (ZnO and $Fe_3O_4$ NPs) para reducir el estrés por salinidad | [98] |
| *Olea europaea.* The olive tree is a significant species in Mediterranean and Middle East agroforestry for its fruit and oil | Different studies indicate that the applications of nanofertilizers allow an increase in the efficiency of using fertilizers and the improvement of the yield and quality of the oil | [104, 105, 106] |
| *Phaseolus* spp. Beans are commonly grown in dryland systems as an important source of protein and minerals | Various studies have shown that bean plants and green beans respond favorably to NFs applications, improving growth, yield, quality, and physiological and biochemical characteristics | [10, 38, 66, 68, 73, 88, 90, 91] |

(continued)

**Table 4** (continued)

| Plant species | Nanobiostimulants or nanofertilizer reported | References |
|---|---|---|
| *Phoenix dactylifera.* Date palms are cultivated in many parts of the Middle East for their fruit | A nanobiostimulant (seaweed nanopowder, 50–100 mg $L^{-1}$) applied as a foliar spray determined significant improvements in chlorophyll concentration, antioxidants, and antioxidant enzyme activity. On the other hand, using NFs increased the weight of the fruits by 9.4% compared to conventional fertilizers | [8, 70, 95] |
| *Punica granatum.* Pomegranates are grown for their nutritious fruits | Different studies indicate that NFs show greater effectiveness than conventional fertilizers (for example, 1.8 kg of nano-N produces the same impact on yield as 16.3 kg N as urea). In the same way, it was found that the quality, the concentration of bioactive compounds, and the tolerance to stress are increased with the use of NFs | [23, 24, 25] |
| *Quercus* spp. Oaks are grown for their drought resistance and for the production of acorns, timber, and habitat provision for wildlife<br>*Quercus ilex*<br>*Quercus suber* | In *Quercus robur*, the application of Fe NPs improves mycorrhization with *Tuber borchii*, a fungus associated with truffle production | [61] |

(continued)

**Table 4** (continued)

| Plant species | Nanobiostimulants or nanofertilizer reported | References |
|---|---|---|
| *Sorghum bicolor*. Sorghum is a reliable source of grain in dry conditions and is also used for animal fodder | Using Fe and Zn, nanofertilizers demonstrated greater efficiency and effectiveness than conventional fertilizers. The yield improvement obtained with the NFs was 19.5%. In another study, no difference was found between fertilizers and NFs under conditions of absence of stress. Still, in stressful environments, NFs improved grain yield and quality | [7, 57] |
| *Triticum* spp. and *Triticum durum*. Wheat and Durum wheat are used in pasta and couscous production, wheat is a staple crop in many dryland agroforestry systems | There are a large number of studies about the favorable impact of NBs and NFs on wheat plants. However, the studies do not indicate a context of agroforestry production | [5, 6, 40, 46, 83] |
| *Vicia faba*. Faba beans are leguminous that can survive in low-water conditions and improve soil health | Several studies have shown the favorable impact of NBs and NFs on barley plants. However, the studies do not specifically refer to the context of agroforestry production | [4, 65, 75, 108] |

(continued)

**Table 4** (continued)

| Plant species | Nanobiostimulants or nanofertilizer reported | References |
|---|---|---|
| *Vigna unguiculata.* Cowpea is a key legume in many dryland farming systems due to its resilience to hot and dry conditions and its nitrogen-fixing capability | Foliar application of $TiO_2$ NPs doped with N, Fe, and Cu increased plant growth, productivity, soluble sugars, amino acids, soluble protein, photosynthetic pigments, and growth-stimulating hormones; decreased lipid peroxidation and hydrogen peroxide content. On the other hand, combining K and Fe nanochelates with biological biostimulants increased growth, yield, quality, osmotic regulation, chlorophyll, and photosynthesis. Favorable effects of soil and foliar-applied $MnO_2$ NPs on growth, yield, chlorophylls, and antioxidants were also observed | [54, 92, 69] |

(continued)

**Table 4** (continued)

| Plant species | Nanobiostimulants or nanofertilizer reported | References |
|---|---|---|
| *Vitis vinifera*. In dry regions, grapes are grown for wine production | In one study, it was found that nano-Ca was a more effective fertilizer than conventional Ca. Similarly, Zn nanofertilizers showed greater effectiveness than conventional fertilizers. On the other hand, a better crop response (yield and quality of the berries) was found when using a chelated NZn compared to NZnO | [29, 64] |
| *Zea mays*. Maize can be grown in a variety of conditions, including dryland agroforestry systems | Multiple studies have demonstrated the beneficial effects of NBs and NFs on maize plants. Nonetheless, the studies make no specific reference to agroforestry production | [2, 3, 14, 19, 22, 30, 35, 36, 45, 48, 56, 85] |

The examples in Table 4 about the favorable impact of nanobiostimulants or nanofertilizers on some species used in agroforestry systems indicate the technical feasibility of using these inputs. Table 5, on the other hand, suggests the need to research many species for which there is still a lack of information about using nanobiostimulants or nanofertilizers.

However, despite the technical feasibility of using nanobiostimulants and nanofertilizers, agroforestry in arid zones faces a series of technical, ecological, and economic challenges. The following can be mentioned among these challenges, which could be seen as factors with a dual impact, on the one hand as the factors that make the use of NBs and NFs recommendable or even obligatory to try to reduce the impact on the productivity of the agroforestry systems, but on the other hand, factors capable of slowing down the adoption of production techniques are based on NBs and NFs.

- Water scarcity. This represents a significant challenge for agroforestry growers, as both tree and crop growth and productivity are harshly affected by water shortage. Moreover, traditional irrigation methods may not be economically viable due to shortage of water resources.

**Table 5** Plant species used in agroforestry systems in arid zones do not have any report in Scopus (until August 2023) concerning nanomaterials or nanofertilizers used in agroforestry production or research. The list of species was obtained using the Google search engine

| Plant species |
|---|
| *Acacia* spp. Acacia trees are drought-tolerant and beneficial for soil enhancement because of their nitrogen-fixing capabilities |
| *Anacardium occidentale.* Known as Marañon or Cashew trees are grown for their fruits and nuts |
| *Arachis hypogaea.* Peanuts are grown for their nutritious seeds and are used in rotation with other crops to improve soil health |
| *Argania spinosa.* The Argan tree is native to North Africa and is mainly grown for its oil-rich seeds |
| *Bertholletia excelsa.* Brazil Nut Tree is cultivated for its edible nuts and is also important for timber |
| *Brassica napus.* Canola is grown for its oil-rich seeds |
| *Caesalpinia echinata.* Caatinga trees are native to South America and used for timber due to their hard and durable wood |
| *Callistemon* spp. Bottlebrush is used in agroforestry systems for its ornamental value and because it attracts pollinators |
| *Casuarina equisetifolia.* and *Casuarina* spp. and *Allocasuarina* spp. Casuarina species are used for timber, windbreaks, and soil improvement |
| *Ceratonia siliqua.* The carob tree is highly adapted to the Mediterranean climate and is valued for its pods that can be used as a chocolate substitute |
| *Cicer arietinum.* Chickpeas are a drought-tolerant legume crop that is widely used in Mediterranean cuisine |
| *Eragrostis tef.* Teff is a staple grain crop in North Africa, adaptable to different environmental conditions |
| *Eucalyptus* spp. Eucalyptus trees are native to Australia and are globally used for timber, oil, and honey production |
| *Ficus carica.* Figs trees are well-suited to dry climates and produce highly nutritious fruits |
| *Juniperus* spp. Junipers are drought-tolerant and used for their wood, berries, and for soil conservation |
| *Lens culinaris.* Lentils are leguminous crops that can cope with drought conditions and contribute to soil fertility by fixing nitrogen |
| *Manihot esculenta.* Yuca or Cassava is a major source of carbohydrates and can tolerate drought conditions |
| *Melaleuca* spp. These species are used for essential oil extraction and honey production |
| *Morus* spp. Mulberries are grown for their fruit, as well as for their leaves which are used in sericulture (silk production) |
| *Oryza sativa.* Rice dryland varieties are grown in parts of India and China |
| *Panicum miliaceum, Pennisetum glaucum.* Millets are often grown in dry conditions and can be used for both human consumption and livestock feed |

(continued)

**Table 5** (continued)

| Plant species |
|---|
| *Pinus cembroides* y *Pinus edulis*. Pinyon Pine are grown in agroforestry systems for their edible nuts and timber |
| *Pinus halepensis*. Aleppo pine tree is adapted to Mediterranean climates with dry summers and cool, wet winters. Its pine nuts can be harvested for human consumption |
| *Pistacia vera*. Pistachio trees are grown for their edible nuts |
| *Populus* spp. Poplar trees are fast-growing trees used for timber and are common in Asia and America |
| *Prosopis* spp. The Mesquite or Algarrobo, it's a drought-tolerant tree with edible seeds and pods. Its wood is used for fuel and construction |
| *Prunus dulcis*. Almonds are a major dryland crop in Mediterranean and Middle East regions. While they require a significant amount of water, they can still be grown in certain dryland conditions and provide high economic yield |
| *Robinia pseudoacacia*. The Black locusts are fast-growing, hardy trees that can enrich the soil with nitrogen |
| *Sclerocarya birrea*. Marula trees are native from Africa and known for their fruits that can be eaten fresh or fermented |
| *Tabebuia* spp. Guayacán trees are grown for timber and ornamental purposes |

- High temperatures. This factor can lead to increased evapotranspiration, aggravating the need for water to obtain productive agroforestry systems. Moreover, heat stress significantly reduces crop productivity.
- Poor soil fertility. High temperature and low rainfall conditions limit the accumulation of organic carbon in soils, which limits fertility, so the potential productivity of the agroforestry system is not obtained.
- Pest and disease challenges. The conditions in arid zones can make plants more susceptible to pests and diseases that may be more prevalent or destructive when plants do not produce enough photosynthates to maintain an adequate defense metabolism.
- Socio-economic challenges. Farmers in arid zones can face socio-economic challenges, lack of access to credit, and inadequate access to markets. These challenges can hinder their capacity to develop projects and benefit from agroforestry.
- Policy and institutional barriers. Policy and institutional barriers may arise that hinder the adoption and success of agroforestry in arid zones. These can include unclear land tenure and usage rights, lack of incentives for tree planting, and lack of integration of agroforestry into national agricultural and environmental strategies.
- Lack of knowledge and skills. Many farmers in arid zones lack the knowledge and skills needed to effectively implement improvements and new techniques that translate into greater quantity and sustainable quality of the products obtained from agroforestry systems. This can limit the adoption and success of agroforestry.

- Climate change. Changes in precipitation patterns, relative humidity, and temperatures are expected to exacerbate many of the challenges agroforestry growers face in arid zones, including increased water and heat stress.

The set of challenges mentioned above implies that, for the large-scale implementation of NBs and NFs in agroforestry systems, economic support, and guidance from extension agents from a long-term institutional effort is required, which considers the environmental, economic, and technological limitations, additionally to the sociocultural characteristics of the inhabitants of the arid regions.

Similarly, the above challenges underscore the need for innovative and context-specific solutions, such as the development and use of drought-tolerant and heat-tolerant tree and crop varieties, water-efficient irrigation technologies, and the use of nanobiostimulants and nanofertilizers to enhance plant growth and stress resistance. Furthermore, policy and institutional reforms, capacity building, and strengthening farmer support services are also critical.

## 4 Nanobiostimulants and Nanofertilizers That Could Be Used in Agroforestry Systems to Mitigate Environmental Challenges

The adverse environmental conditions prevailing in arid zones impose enormous challenges to obtaining (in a sustainable manner) high productivity and quality sufficient for the growing food and fiber needs of the human population. According to the experience of the authors of this chapter, with the appropriate use of NBs and NFs, it is possible to increase the efficiency of the use of inputs (e.g., efficiency in the use of water and fertilizers) at the same time as obtain improvements in yield and quality of crops (see Tables 2 and 3 for the description of mechanisms). As explained in Tables 4 and 5, examples of applications of nanobiostimulants and nanofertilizers in agroforestry systems are very scarce, but even so, the accumulated experience (in laboratory, greenhouses, and field) regarding the use of these materials indicates that their use is feasible and recommendable [13, 17]. Below are some specific examples of NBs and NFS whose use could be helpful in various arid environments, tree species, and annual crop species.

The order in which the NBs and NFs are listed indicates the perception of the authors regarding the feasibility of the application; that is, considering those above ecological, economic, and social limitations, the order in the list refers to the potential accessibility, cost, ease of storage, application, and use, and access to recommendations and advice regarding the use of each material for nanobiostimulation or nanofertilization. Some materials have a double impact since they are biostimulants and provide essential or beneficial nutrients for crops. This characteristic distinguishes some NBs as nanosilicon or nanoselenium and all the nanofertilizers: they are biostimulants and a source of nutrients [76]. Other nanobiostimulants, such as nanozeolites and carbon nanomaterials, induced biostimulation, and although they do not provide nutrients directly, they can improve soil health, fertility, and the efficient use of fertilizers [12].

## 4.1 Nano-Silicon

Some keyways nanosilicon can be advantageous for agroforestry production are: nanosilicon is an enhancer of plant stress resistance, including drought, heat, salinity, fungal pathogens, and pests. Nanosilicon can improve the photosynthetic efficiency of plants, thereby boosting their productivity and yield. Nanosilicon is also known to facilitate plant roots' uptake of nutrients and water and promote plant growth. This is particularly important in arid zones with low soil organic matter and nutrient content [26].

## 4.2 Nanozeolites

They are porous materials well-known for their absorption and ion exchange properties. Nanozeolites work as soil improvers due to their high cation exchange capacity (CEC) values. The CEC of natural zeolites can take values from 216 to 550 Cmol 100 $g^{-1}$, while nanozeolites can reach double these values [89]. Nanozeolites can improve soil fertility by holding onto nutrients that might otherwise be washed away or fixed by soil colloids. Once the nutrients are adsorbed on the nanozeolites, they are slowly released into the soil solution, providing a sustained supply of nutrients to the plants, and decreasing the frequency of fertilizer application. This property is particularly useful in arid zones where soil nutrient content can be low, and water scarcity makes nutrient conservation crucial.

On the other hand, nanozeolites can absorb and hold onto water and then release it slowly. This ability can help conserve water in arid zones by reducing water loss due to evaporation or runoff, ensuring that plants have a steady water supply. Due to their high surface area and absorption capacity, nanozeolites can help to remove contaminants from soil and water. They can absorb heavy metals, organic pollutants, and other harmful substances, thereby improving the quality of the environment for plant growth. Lastly, nanozeolites can be used directly as a pest control or delivery system for pesticides or other agrochemicals. They can slowly release these substances, improving their effectiveness and reducing the need for frequent applications [89].

## 4.3 Nanodusts or Nanopowders

The process of grinding different materials down to nanometric dimensions allows various biostimulant materials such as humic substances, composts, biochar, protein hydrolysates solids, and solids from other kinds of fermentates, plant materials, and algae lamina to function as nanometric materials; the above, adds an additional advantage to the biostimulant capacity of the conventional material [52]. Combining nanopowders of biostimulants with nanopowders of fertilizers containing essential or beneficial nutrients could provide a synergistic impact and increase their utility, reducing the costs of transportation, storage, and application to crops.

## 4.4 *Nanofertilizers*

A nanofertilizer or nanonutrient is a material engineered to the nanoscale, generally in the form of nanoparticles. The nanoparticle size typically ranges from 1 to 100 nm.

These nanoparticles' small size and high surface area allow for improved solubility, mobility, and nutrient uptake, leading to greater efficiency than traditional fertilizers. Moreover, nanofertilizers can be designed to release nutrients in a controlled manner in response to specific environmental triggers, reducing nutrient losses and environmental contamination [76].

While nanofertilizers offer several advantages in agriculture, especially in arid regions where efficient resource use is crucial, their widespread application has notable limitations and challenges. These constraints range from ecological and human health concerns to technical and economic factors and will be described in the next section of this chapter.

## 4.5 *Titanium Dioxide*

$TiO_2$ nanoparticles can be beneficial as biostimulants that enhance the ability of plants to tolerate stress. In an arid environment, plants often face heat stress, UV stress, and water scarcity. Nanotitanium can mitigate these stresses through improved metabolism and antioxidant production, thus improving photosynthesis efficiency, plant survival, and productivity. Similarly, nanotitanium might provide some resistance against certain pests and diseases [56, 94].

## 4.6 *Nanochitosan*

Chitosan is a linear polysaccharide derived from chitin. It can elicit plant defense responses, improve plant health and growth, and enhance stress tolerance, including drought resistance. Chitosan nanoparticles derived from chitosan have been shown to enhance plant growth, improve water use efficiency, and increase plant resistance to diseases and environmental stressors. Nanochitosan can positively impact soil health by improving its structure, nutrient content, and microbial activity, leading to better plant growth and productivity [89].

Nanochitosan can help improve water retention capacity in plants, thereby enhancing their drought resistance. It can help form a protective volume around plant roots and enhance their ability to absorb water and essential nutrients, even in low water availability conditions, such as arid regions. Nanochitosan can be used as a carrier of fertilizers, enhancing their efficiency by enabling slow release and targeted delivery. This method prevents the loss of nutrients and mitigates potential environmental damage. It can stimulate seed germination and root growth, promote photosynthesis, and enhance nutrient uptake. Some studies suggest that nanochitosan can enhance plant growth by modulating various biological pathways related to signaling and response to environmental stress.

Nanochitosan has significant antimicrobial, antifungal, and insecticidal properties, making it effective against various pests and diseases [89].

## 4.7 *Carbon Nanomaterials*

A large group of materials, including carbon nanotubes, carbon dots, graphene, and fullerenes. Carbon nanomaterials can improve plant growth by enhancing water and nutrient uptake, increasing photosynthesis, and boosting plant growth and development. Carbon nanomaterials can also enhance the stress tolerance of plants. In arid zones, they can help plants cope with water stress by improving water use efficiency and heat stress by enhancing thermotolerance. Carbon nanomaterials can help improve soil health by enhancing soil structure, nutrient content, and microbial activity. This can promote healthier and more productive agroforestry systems, especially in arid zones with poor soil quality [104]. On the other hand, due to their high surface area and reactivity, carbon nanomaterials can be used as carriers for pesticides and fertilizers, increasing their effectiveness and reducing the quantities needed. They can also reduce the environmental impact of these substances by limiting their leaching into the environment [34]. Maybe in the near future, carbon nanomaterials can be used to create biosensors that can monitor the agroforestry system's health, including pests, nutrient levels, and other factors. This can provide timely information for interventions and improve the overall productivity and system's sustainability [55].

## 4.8 *Nanoselenium*

Selenium is a beneficial and biofortifying nutrient for plants when present in small amounts, improving growth, nutritional quality, and productivity. Plants can absorb and utilize Se more efficiently in its nanometric form, potentially enhancing the above beneficial effects [41]. Nanoselenium can have a very high value as a nanobiostimulant nutrient in agroforestry production, particularly in arid zones. Nanoselenium can help increase the stress tolerance of plants, making them more resilient to harsh conditions, such as drought, temperature extremes, and salinity. Selenium and nanoselenium have the ability to reduce heavy metal and metalloid toxicity and reduce their bioavailability for plants, thus reducing their toxic effects on plants [41].

On the other hand, Se is an essential element for animal nutrition, including livestock and wildlife. Plants treated with low levels of nanoselenium can be biofortified and used as a source of Se, improving animal health and productivity [32].

## *4.9 Nanoencapsulated Biostimulants and Nutrients*

Using nanotechnological methods for encapsulating active compounds is regarded as an intelligent approach to enhance their controlled release and safeguard them from adverse environmental conditions. Nanoencapsulation involves enclosing biostimulants and nutrients in nanometer-scale capsules made of biodegradable materials such as polymers or lipids. This allows for controlled, slow release of the active compounds and prevents its degradation or leaching. The high surface area-to-volume ratio of the encapsulating nanomaterial enables better interaction with soil and plant roots and leaves [37].

Nanoencapsulated fertilizers release nutrients gradually, ensuring long-term availability and minimizing nutrient loss through leaching. Due to the above high efficiency of nutrient delivery, less fertilizer is needed, reducing environmental pollution and resource consumption. Some nanoencapsulated fertilizers (e.g., those based on biopolymers such as nanochitosan or glucans) can also improve the soil's physical and chemical properties, such as water retention and nutrient availability [20].

Combining biostimulants and fertilizers in the same nanoencapsulated material could offer synergistic benefits. For example, biostimulants can effectively enhance the plant's ability to utilize the nutrients released from nanoencapsulated fertilizers, or the biostimulants can prime plants to be more resilient to stresses like drought while nanoencapsulated fertilizers ensure a consistent nutrient supply. If applied together, NBs and NFs can reduce the overall requirements for water and conventional fertilizers, contributing to sustainable agriculture in arid regions [42].

## 5 Challenges and Opportunities for the Application of Nanomaterials in Agroforestry Systems

The future of agroforestry in arid zones will likely revolve around optimizing systems for these regions' unique environmental conditions and resource constraints. Technological advancements will play a critical role in determining the future of agroforestry in arid zones. Innovations such as precision agriculture, remote sensing, and advanced irrigation technologies can help improve the efficiency and effectiveness of agroforestry practices. Furthermore, developing and applying nanobiostimulants and nanofertilizers could offer promising strategies for enhancing nutrient uptake and improving plant stress resistance in arid environments.

NBs and NFs can offer a transformative approach to biostimulation and plant nutrition in agroforestry systems. However, as with any emerging technology, their application also brings challenges that must be addressed. For widespread and successful application of NBs and NFs in agroforestry, the following challenges must be resolved through concerted efforts in the political, social, economic, and ecological spheres and by the community of agricultural and forestry scientists and technicians. The challenges can guide various actions, including social, ecological, and technical research.

Policy support and institutional factors. The establishment and success of agroforestry systems largely depend on policy support and institutional backing. In addition to promoting incentives for tree planting and the integration of agroforestry into national agricultural and environmental strategies, the agricultural extension services need to provide education and training in agroforestry practices and using NBs and NFs tailored to arid regions.

Socio-Economic Factors. The economic viability of using NBs and NFs in agroforestry practices is crucial to their adoption.

Cost and accessibility. Currently, the production cost of NBs and NFS is relatively high compared to conventional biostimulants and fertilizers, making them less accessible for smallholder farmers. In addition, the technology needed to apply NBs and NFs may be out of reach for many farmers, especially in developing countries.

Regulation and standardization. The rapid development of nanotechnology in agriculture has outpaced the development of regulations and standards. One of the major challenges in the application of biostimulants is the lack of clear regulation and standardization. Clear regulatory guidelines are needed to ensure safe and effective use of NBs and NFs in agroforestry.

Cultural and community factors. The local knowledge, cultural practices, and preferences of communities in arid zones should be incorporated to design tailored management of NBs and NFs. Participatory approaches involving local communities in decision-making processes can lead to more appropriate and successful application of the new technologies.

Limited understanding of mechanisms. The mechanisms of action of many NBs and NFs are not fully understood. This lack of deep understanding can hinder their effective use and the development of more targeted and efficient products.

Potential environmental and health impacts. There are concerns about the potential environmental and health effects of NBs and NFs. While these products are generally considered safe in the short term, more research is needed to understand their long-term effects fully.

# 6 Conclusion

Applying NBs and NFs holds transformative potential for arid zone agroforestry systems, offering benefits ranging from improved nutrient use efficiency to enhanced plant stress tolerance. The mechanisms underlying these technologies exploit the unique attributes of nanomaterials, such as their inherent biostimulant capacity resulting from high surface area-to-volume ratio, tunable chemical properties, and the potential for targeted delivery. These characteristics are appropriate for resource-limited situations like agroforestry in arid zones, where conventional agronomic practices can fall short of sustaining productivity and environmental health.

Nanobiostimulants have shown efficacy in stimulating plant physiological processes, improving root architecture, nutrient absorption, and activating stress-responsive pathways. On the other hand, NFs offer advantages in terms of controlled nutrient release, reduced leaching, and enhanced nutrient absorption by plants. These materials offer an integrated and synergic approach to addressing biotic and abiotic stresses in arid agroforestry systems. In this chapter, plant species used in agroforestry systems were noted, and it was found that there are studies on the impact of NBs and NFs for a certain number of them. However, most studies do not refer to agroforestry production conditions. Additionally, many species used in agroforestry have not been studied regarding their response and feasibility of using NBs and NFs.

On the other hand, it is crucial to adopt a note of cautiousness. While the prospects are promising for the agroforestry systems, several limitations and uncertainties exist. Nanomaterials' environmental and human health implications remain active research and debate areas. Technical challenges in formulation stability, compatibility with existing agricultural practices, and the high cost of production are additional hurdles that require attention.

Future research directions should focus on the long-term ecological impacts of these nanomaterials, including potential bioaccumulation and effects on soil microbial communities. Furthermore, the socioeconomic and regulatory aspects must be carefully considered to ensure equitable access and safe utilization of these technologies. Detailed life cycle assessments, cost–benefit analyses, and field trials spanning diverse agroforestry systems and climatic conditions will be instrumental in guiding the responsible development and deployment of NBs and NFs in arid zones.

The authors of this chapter believe that integrating nanotechnology into agroforestry practices in arid regions offers a compelling pathway toward sustainable agriculture. While challenges exist, the potential benefits of yield and quality improvement, resource use efficiency, and environmental sustainability make this an area of research and development that is not only scientifically exciting but also critical for global long-term food security and ecosystem resilience.

## References


1. Abbasi Khalaki M, Moameri M, Asgari Lajayer B, Astatkie T (2021) Influence of nano-priming on seed germination and plant growth of forage and medicinal plants. Plant Growth Regul 93:13–28
2. Adhikari T, Kundu S, Biswas AK et al (2015) Characterization of zinc oxide nano particles and their effect on growth of Maize (Zea mays L.) Plant. J Plant Nutr 38:1505–1515
3. Adibah FSF, Jahan S, Fatihah HNN (2020) Betaine-rich Nano fertilizer improves growth parameters of Zea mays var. saccharata and Arabidopsis thaliana under salt stress. Bulgarian J Agr Sci 26:177–185
4. Alabade A, Al-Khashab Safwan, Kahlel A (2022) Response of three broad bean varieties ( Vicia faba L.) to boron, iron, and zinc nano fertilizers. RB 7:1–4
5. Ali AM, Ibrahim SM, Omer AM (2023) Foliar spraying of nano-silicate and nano-zinc on wheat (Triticum aestivum L.) under salt stress conditions enhances productivity and reduces the optimal nitrogen fertilizer rate. Commun Soil Sci Plant Anal 54:2731–2744
6. Alikhani M, Mirbolook A, Sadeghi J, Lakzian A (2023) Effect of a new slow-release zinc fertilizer based on carbon dots on the zinc concentration, growth indices, and yield in wheat (Triticum aestivum). Plant Physiol Biochem 200:107783
7. Al-Rubaie MAJ, Mohammed AR, Ali SH (2022) Nano fertilizer spraying affects the yield of Sorghum (Sorghum bicolor L.) varieties. Bionatura 7:1–15
8. Altemimy HMA, Altemimy IHH, Abed AM (2019) Evaluation the efficacy of nano-fertilization and Disper osmotic in treating salinity of irrigation water in quality and productivity properties of date palm Phoenix dactylifera L. IOP Conf Ser: Earth Environ Sci 388:012072
9. Altieri MA, Nicholls CI (2017) The adaptation and mitigation potential of traditional agriculture in a changing climate. Clim Change 140:33–45
10. Amaya-Olivas NI, Sánchez E, Hernández-Ochoa L et al (2023) Biofortification with magnesium nanofertilizer on bioactive compounds and antioxidant capacity in green beans. Notulae Botanicae Horti Agrobotanici Cluj-Napoca 51:12830–12830
11. Amin MA, Ismail MA, Badawy AA et al (2021) The potency of fungal-fabricated selenium nanoparticles to improve the growth performance of Helianthus annuus L. and control of cutworm Agrotis ipsilon. Catalysts 11:1551
12. Aminiyan MM, Hosseini H, Heydariyan A (2018) Microbial communities and their characteristics in a soil amended by nanozeolite and some plant residues: Short time in-situ incubation. EJSS 7:9–19
13. Andreotti C (2020) Management of abiotic stress in horticultural crops: Spotlight on biostimulants. Agronomy 10:1514
14. Aqaei P, Weisany W, Diyanat M et al (2020) Response of maize (Zea mays L.) to potassium nano-silica application under drought stress. J Plant Nutr 43:1205–1216
15. Arora S, Murmu G, Mukherjee K et al (2022) A comprehensive overview of nanotechnology in sustainable agriculture. J Biotechnol 355:21–41
16. Azameti MK, Imoro AWM (2023) Nanotechnology: A promising field in enhancing abiotic stress tolerance in plants. Crop Design 100037
17. Babu S, Singh R, Yadav D et al (2022) Nanofertilizers for agricultural and environmental sustainability. Chemosphere 292:133451
18. Bhandari DC, Meghwal PR, Lodha S (2014) Horticulture based production systems in Indian Arid Regions. In: Nandwani D (ed) Sustainable horticultural systems: Issues, technology and innovation. Springer International Publishing, Cham, pp 19–49

19. Bijanzadeh E, Barati V, Egan TP (2022) Foliar application of sodium silicate mitigates drought stressed leaf structure in corn (Zea mays L.). S Afr J Bot 147:8–17
20. Biradar SP, Mehta MR, Mahajan HP et al (2022) Chapter 5—Biological activities of chitosan-based nanomaterials. In: Kumar DRS, Madihally SV (eds) Role of Chitosan and Chitosan-based nanomaterials in plant sciences. Academic Press, pp 119–142
21. Chamberlain JL, Darr D, Meinhold K (2020) Rediscovering the contributions of forests and trees to transition global food systems. Forests 11:1098
22. Chen X, Chu S, Chi Y et al (2023) Unraveling the role of multi-walled carbon nanotubes in a corn-soil system: Plant growth, oxidative stress and heavy metal(loid)s behavior. Plant Physiol Biochem 200:107802
23. Davarpanah S, Tehranifar A, Abadía J et al (2018) Foliar calcium fertilization reduces fruit cracking in pomegranate (Punica granatum cv. Ardestani). Sci Hortic 230:86–91
24. Davarpanah S, Tehranifar A, Davarynejad G et al (2016) Effects of foliar applications of zinc and boron nano-fertilizers on pomegranate (Punica granatum cv. Ardestani) fruit yield and quality. Sci Hortic 210:57–64
25. Davarpanah S, Tehranifar A, Davarynejad G et al (2017) Effects of foliar nano-nitrogen and urea fertilizers on the physical and chemical properties of pomegranate (Punica granatum cv. Ardestani) fruits. HortScience 52:288–294
26. de Moraes ACP, Lacava PT (2022) Chapter 5—Use of silicon and nano-silicon in agro-biotechnologies. In: Etesami H, Al Saeedi AH, El-Ramady H et al (eds) Silicon and nano-silicon in environmental stress management and crop quality improvement. Academic Press, pp 55–65
27. De Pauw E, Göbel W, Adam H (2000) Agrometeorological aspects of agriculture and forestry in the arid zones. Agric For Meteorol 103:43–58
28. Desaint H, Aoun N, Deslandes L et al (2021) Fight hard or die trying: when plants face pathogens under heat stress. New Phytol 229:712–734
29. El Masri IY, Al Akiki M, Jamal Eldin N et al (2021) Conventional versus Nano-Ca fertilizers effects on traditional table grape Tfiefihi. J Plant Nutr 44:3020–3033
30. El-Ganainy SM, Mosa MA, Ismail AM, Khalil AE (2023) Lignin-loaded carbon nanoparticles as a promising control agent against Fusarium verticillioides in maize: Physiological and biochemical analyses. Polymers 15:1193
31. El-Ramady H, Abdalla N, Sári D et al (2023) Nanofarming: Promising solutions for the future of the global agricultural industry. Agronomy 13:1600
32. El-Ramady H, Faizy SE-D, Abdalla N et al (2020) Selenium and nano-selenium biofortification for human health: Opportunities and challenges. Soil Systems 4:57
33. Fahad S, Chavan SB, Chichaghare AR et al (2022) Agroforestry systems for soil health improvement and maintenance. Sustainability 14:14877
34. Fallah Z, Zare EN, Ghomi M et al (2021) Toxicity and remediation of pharmaceuticals and pesticides using metal oxides and carbon nanomaterials. Chemosphere 275:130055
35. Fathi A, Zahedi M, Torabian S (2017) Effect of interaction between salinity and nanoparticles (Fe2O3 and ZnO) on physiological parameters of Zea mays L. J Plant Nutr 40:2745–2755
36. Fatima A, Safdar N, Ain N et al (2023) Abscisic acid-loaded ZnO nanoparticles as drought tolerance inducers in Zea mays L. with physiological and biochemical attributes. J Plant Growth Regul 42:7280–7293
37. Fincheira P, Hoffmann N, Tortella G et al (2023) Eco-efficient systems based on nanocarriers for the controlled release of fertilizers and pesticides: Toward smart agriculture. Nanomaterials 13:1978
38. Franco-Lagos CL, Sánchez E, Palacio-Márquez A et al (2023) Efficacy of the application of boron nanofertilizer on biomass, yield, nitrogen assimilation and photosynthetic activity in green beans. Notulae Botanicae Horti Agrobotanici Cluj-Napoca 51:12795–12795
39. Gangwar P, Johri P, Datta R, Singh S, Trivedi M (2023) Overview on 1 Phytopharmaceuticals and biotechnology of herbal plants. In: Phytopharmaceuticals and biotechnology of herbal plants. CRC Press, pp 1–17

40. Gao Y, Dong C, Chen S et al (2023) Effect of nano carbon and nano calcium carbonate application on soil nutrient dynamics in winter wheat (Triticum aestivum L.). Commun Soil Sci Plant Anal 54:2800–2812
41. García Márquez V, Morelos Moreno Á, Benavides Mendoza A, Medrano Macías J (2020) Ionic selenium and nanoselenium as biofortifiers and stimulators of plant metabolism. Agronomy 10:1399
42. García-García AL, García-Machado FJ, Borges AA et al (2020) Pure organic active compounds against abiotic stress: A biostimulant overview. Front Plant Sci 11:575829
43. Gaur MK, Squires VR (2018) Geographic extent and characteristics of the world's arid zones and their peoples. In: Gaur MK, Squires VR (eds) Climate variability impacts on land use and livelihoods in drylands. Springer International Publishing, Cham, pp 3–20
44. Halawani RF, AbdElgawad H, Aloufi FA et al (2023) Synergistic effect of carbon nanoparticles with mild salinity for improving chemical composition and antioxidant activities of radish sprouts. Front Plant Sci 14:1158031
45. Hasan M, Rafique S, Zafar A et al (2020) Physiological and anti-oxidative response of biologically and chemically synthesized iron oxide: Zea mays a case study. Heliyon 6(8):e04595
46. Haydar MS, Ali S, Mandal P et al (2023) Fe–Mn nanocomposites doped graphene quantum dots alleviate salt stress of Triticum aestivum through osmolyte accumulation and antioxidant defense. Sci Rep 13:11040
47. Huang R, Mao P, Xiong L et al (2023) Negatively charged nano-hydroxyapatite can be used as a phosphorus fertilizer to increase the efficacy of wollastonite for soil cadmium immobilization. J Hazard Mater 443:130291
48. Ilyas MZ, Park H, Baek YS et al (2023) Efficacy of Carbon Nanodots and Manganese Ferrite (MnFe2O4) Nanoparticles in stimulating growth and antioxidant activity in drought-stressed maize inbred lines. Plants 12:2922
49. Jain T, Srivastava K, Singh R, Ansari MJ, Singh S, Dutta PK (2022) Role of nanotechnology 18 in the field of phytopharmaceuticals for the delivery of herbal drugs
50. Jakhar AM, Aziz I, Kaleri AR et al (2022) Nano-fertilizers: A sustainable technology for improving crop nutrition and food security. NanoImpact 27:100411
51. Jośko I, Kusiak M, Różyło K et al (2023) The life cycle study revealed distinct impact of foliar-applied nano-Cu on antioxidant traits of barley grain comparing with conventional agents. Food Res Int 164:112303
52. Juárez-Maldonado A, Ortega-Ortíz H, Morales-Díaz AB et al (2019) Nanoparticles and nanomaterials as plant biostimulants. Int J Mol Sci 20:162
53. Hasan KB, Leiby HR, Al Ghasheem N (2022) Effects of nano-chelated micronutrients and seaweed on nutrients uptake and chemical traits of quinoa (Chenopodium quinoa Willd.). Casp J Environ Sci 20:985–989
54. Kamal R, Mogazy AM (2023) Effect of doping on TiO2 nanoparticles characteristics: studying of fertilizing effect on cowpea plant growth and yield. J Soil Sci Plant Nutr 23:325–337
55. Karimi-Maleh H, Darabi R, Baghayeri M et al (2023) Recent developments in carbon nanomaterials-based electrochemical sensors for methyl parathion detection. J Food Measure 17:5371–5389
56. Karvar M, Azari A, Rahimi A et al (2021) Titanium dioxide nanoparticles (TiO2-NPs) enhance drought tolerance and grain yield of sweet corn (Zea mays L.) under deficit irrigation regimes. Acta Physiol Plant 44:14
57. Kazemi E, Ganjali HR, Mehraban A, Ghasemi A (2022) Yield and biochemical properties of grain sorghum (Sorghum bicolor L. Moench) affected by nano-fertilizer under field drought stress. CeR Res Commun 50:397–405
58. Khare N, Bhardwaj M, Chawla S, Praveen R, Singh S (2023) Redox responsive smart nano-materials to tackle hypoxia associated oxidative damage and inflammatory mediators using phytocompounds. In: Smart nanomaterials targeting pathological hypoxia. Springer Nature Singapore, Singapore, pp 313–325

59. Korwar GR, Prasad JVNS, Rao GR et al (2014) Agroforestry as a strategy for livelihood security in the Rainfed areas: Experience and expectations. In: Dagar JC, Singh AK, Arunachalam A (eds) Agroforestry systems in India: Livelihood security & ecosystem services. Springer India, New Delhi, pp 117–154
60. Latha M, Subramanian KS, Sundara Sharmila DJ et al (2023) Urea–Lignin/Chitosan nanocomposite as slow-release nanofertilizer. ACS Agric Sci Technol 3(6):463–476
61. Leonardi P, Lugli F, Iotti M et al (2020) Effects of biogenerated ferric hydroxides nanoparticles on truffle mycorrhized plants. Mycorrhiza 30:211–219
62. Maddala VKS, Singh S (2023) Essential oils from plants and their role in nanomaterial synthesis characterization and applications. In: Secondary metabolites based green synthesis of nanomaterials and their applications. Springer Nature Singapore, Singapore, pp 191–207
63. Maddala VKS, Singh S, Bandi J (2024) Soil properties influencing nutrient signaling in plant soil systems. In: Essential minerals in plant-soil systems. Elsevier, pp 373–393
64. Mahdavi S, Karimi R, Valipouri Goudarzi A (2022) Effect of nano zinc oxide, nano zinc chelate and zinc sulfate on vineyard soil Zn- availability and grapevines (Vitis vinifera L.) yield and quality. J Plant Nutr 45:1961–1976
65. Mahmoud AWM, Ayad AA, Abdel-Aziz HSM et al (2022) Foliar application of different iron sources improves morpho-physiological traits and nutritional quality of broad bean grown in sandy soil. Plants 11:2599
66. Márquez-Prieto AK, Palacio-Márquez A, Sanchez E et al (2022) Impact of the foliar application of potassium nanofertilizer on biomass, yield, nitrogen assimilation and photosynthetic activity in green beans. Notulae Botanicae Horti Agrobotanici Cluj-Napoca 50:12569–12569
67. Meddya S, Meshram S, Sarkar D, Datta R, Singh S, Avinash G, Thulasinathan T (2023) Plant stomata: An unrealized possibility in plant defense against invading pathogens and stress tolerance. Plants 12(19):3380
68. Medina-Pérez G, Fernández-Luqueño F, Trejo-Téllez LI, López_Valdéz FI, Pampillón-González L (2018) Growth and development of common bean (Phaseolus vulgaris L.) var. Pinto Saltillo exposed to iron, titanium, and zinc oxide nanoparticles in an agricultural soil. Appl Ecol Env Res 16:1883–1897
69. Mirsardoo F, Aien A, Abad HHS, Korehpaz S, (2023) The effect of biological and nanofertilizers on cowpea (Vigna unguiculata L.) yield, quantitative and qualitative traits in the southern Iranian climate. Turk J Field Crop 28:111–120
70. Mohamed AA, Sameeh MY, El-Beltagi HS (2023) Preparation of seaweed nanopowder particles using planetary ball milling and their effects on some secondary metabolites in date palm (Phoenix dactylifera L.) Seedlings. Life 13:39
71. Mondal S, Palit D (2022) Chapter 2—Challenges in natural resource management for ecological sustainability. In: Jhariya MK, Meena RS, Banerjee A, Meena SN (eds) Natural Resources Conservation and Advances for Sustainability. Elsevier, pp 29–59
72. Moshfeghi N, Heidari M, Asghari HR et al (2020) Foliar application of nano-Zn and mycorrhizal inoculation enhanced Zn in grain and yield of two barley (Hordeum vulgare) cultivars under field conditions. Aust J Crop Sci 475–484
73. Muñoz-Márquez E, Soto-Parra JM, Noperi-Mosqueda LC, Sánchez E (2022) Application of molybdenum nanofertilizer on the nitrogen use efficiency, growth and yield in green beans. Agronomy 12:3163
74. Muthee K, Duguma L, Majale C et al (2022) A quantitative appraisal of selected agroforestry studies in the Sub-Saharan Africa. Heliyon 8(9):e10670
75. Nasrallah AK, Kheder AA, Kord MA et al (2022) Mitigation of salinity stress effects on broad bean productivity using calcium phosphate nanoparticles application. Horticulturae 8:75
76. Naz M, Benavides-Mendoza A (2021) Nanofertilizers as tools for plant nutrition and plant biostimulation under adverse environment. In: Husen A (ed) Plant performance under environmental stress : hormones, biostimulants and sustainable plant growth Management. Springer International Publishing, Cham, pp 387–415
77. Noman M, Ahmed T, Shahid M et al (2023) Salicylic acid-doped iron nano-biostimulants potentiate defense responses and suppress Fusarium wilt in watermelon. J Adv Res. https://doi.org/10.1016/j.jare.2023.06.011

78. Pantera A, Mosquera-Losada MR, Herzog F, den Herder M (2021) Agroforestry and the environment. Agroforest Syst 95:767–774
79. Parveen R, Jain T, Parveen R, Singh S (2023) Genome-wide transcriptome profiling of crop plants. In: Genomics, transcriptomics, proteomics and metabolomics of crop plants. Academic Press, pp 145–171
80. Parveen R, Khare N, Singh S, Johri P (2023) An in silico outlook for the detection and surveillance of evolving and persistent plant pathogens. In: Detection, diagnosis and management of soil-borne phytopathogens. Springer Nature Singapore, Singapore, pp 17–40
81. Patani A, Patel A, Prajapati D, Khare N, Singh S (2023) Various agriculture crop plant-based bioactive compounds and their use in nanomaterial synthesis and applications. In: Nanomaterials from agricultural and horticultural products. Springer Nature Singapore, Singapore, pp 223–241
82. Patani A, Prajapati D, Shukla K, Patel M, Patani P, Patel A, Singh S (2024) Environmental stress–induced alterations in the micro-and macronutrients status of plant. In: Essential minerals in plant-soil systems. Elsevier, pp 181–195
83. Perea-Vélez YS, Carrillo-González R, González-Chávez M del CA et al (2023) Citrate-coated cobalt ferrite nanoparticles for the nano-enabled biofortification of wheat. Food Funct 14:4017–4035
84. Priyanka N, Geetha N, Manish T et al (2021) Zinc oxide nanocatalyst mediates cadmium and lead toxicity tolerance mechanism by differential regulation of photosynthetic machinery and antioxidant enzymes level in cotton seedlings. Toxicol Rep 8:295–302
85. Răcuciu M, Tecucianu A, Oancea S (2022) Impact of magnetite nanoparticles coated with aspartic acid on the growth, antioxidant enzymes activity and chlorophyll content of maize. Antioxidants 11:1193
86. Rahman MdH, Haque KMS, Khan MdZH (2021) A review on application of controlled released fertilizers influencing the sustainable agricultural production: A Cleaner production process. Environ Technol Innov 23:101697
87. Raj A, Jhariya MK, Banerjee A, et al (2022) Chapter 13—Agroforestry a model for ecological sustainability. In: Jhariya MK, Meena RS, Banerjee A, Meena SN (eds) Natural Resources conservation and advances for sustainability. Elsevier, pp 289–307
88. Ramírez-Estrada CA, Sánchez E, Flores-Cordova MA et al (2022) Efficiency and assimilation of nitrogen in bean plants through foliar application of zinc and molybdenum nano fertilizer. Not Bot Horti Agrobot Cluj-Napoca 50:12719–12719
89. Robledo-Olivo A, Cabrera-De la Fuente M, Benavides-Mendoza A (2021) Application of nanosilicon and nanochitosan to diminish the use of pesticides and synthetic fertilizers in crop production. In: Kharissova OV, Martínez LMT, Kharisov BI (eds) Handbook of nanomaterials and nanocomposites for energy and environmental applications. Springer International Publishing, Cham, pp 1–27
90. Salama DM, Abd El-Aziz ME, Shaaban EA, et al (2022) The impact of nanofertilizer on agro-morphological criteria, yield, and genomic stability of common bean (Phaseolus vulgaris L.). Sci Rep 12:18552
91. Salcido-Martínez A, Sánchez E, Licón-Trillo LP et al (2020) Impact of the foliar application of magnesium nanofertilizer on physiological and biochemical parameters and yield in green beans. Notulae Botanicae Horti Agrobotanici Cluj-Napoca 48:2167–2181
92. Samsoon S, Azam M, Khan A et al (2022) Green-synthesized $MnO_2$ nanofertilizer impact on growth, photosynthetic pigment, and non-enzymatic antioxidant of Vigna unguiculata cultivar. Biomass Conv Bioref. https://doi.org/10.1007/s13399-022-03686-5
93. Sarkar D, Dubey PK, Chaurasiya R, Sankar A, Shikha CN, Ganguly S, Meena VS, Meena SK, Parewa HP, Rakshit A (2021) Organic interventions conferring stress tolerance and crop quality in agroecosystems during the UN Decade on Ecosystem Restoration. Land Degrad Dev 32:4797–4816
94. Satti SH, Raja NI, Javed B et al (2021) Titanium dioxide nanoparticles elicited agro-morphological and physicochemical modifications in wheat plants to control Bipolaris sorokiniana. PLoS ONE 16:e0246880

95. Shareef HJ, Hzaa AYL, Elsheery NI (2023) Foliar iron and zinc nano-fertilizers enhance growth, mineral uptake, and antioxidant defense in date palm (Phoenix dactylifera L.) seedlings. Folia Oecologica 50:185–195
96. Sileshi GW, Mafongoya PL, Nath AJ (2020) Agroforestry systems for improving nutrient recycling and soil fertility on degraded lands. In: Dagar JC, Gupta SR, Teketay D (eds) Agroforestry for degraded landscapes: Recent advances and emerging challenges, vol 1. Springer, Singapore, pp 225–253
97. Singh A, Sengar RS, Singh AK, Singh S, Kumar A, Ahmad K (2019) Impact of genetic engineering on agriculture food crops. Biotech Today: Int J Biol Sci 9(1):17–24
98. Soliman AS, El-feky SA, Darwish E (2015) Alleviation of salt stress on Moringa peregrina using foliar application of nanofertilizers. J Hort Forest 7:36–47
99. Soliman AS, Hassan M, Abou-Elella F et al (2016) Effect of nano and molecular phosphorus fertilizers on growth and chemical composition of baobab (Adansonia digitata L.). J Plant Sci 11:52–60
100. Subramanian KS, Rajeswari R, Yuvaraj M et al (2022) Synthesis and characterization of nano-sulfur and its impact on growth, yield, and quality of sunflower (Helianthus annuus L.). Commun Soil Sci Plant Anal 53:2700–2709
101. Torabian S, Zahedi M, Khoshgoftar AH (2016) Effects of foliar spray of two kinds of zinc oxide on the growth and ion concentration of sunflower cultivars under salt stress. J Plant Nutr 39:172–180
102. Tungare K, Shahu R, Zambare V, Agarwal P, Jobby R, Nisar N, Jha P (2022) Toxicity mitigation of textile dye reactive blue 4 by hairy roots of Helianthus annuus and testing its effect in in vivo model systems. Biomed Res Int
103. Verma KK, Song X-P, Joshi A et al (2022) Recent trends in nano-fertilizers for sustainable agriculture under climate change for global food security. Nanomaterials 12:173
104. Verma SK, Das AK, Gantait S et al (2019) Applications of carbon nanomaterials in the plant system: A perspective view on the pros and cons. Sci Total Environ 667:485–499
105. Vishekaii ZR, Soleimani A, Fallahi E et al (2019a) The impact of foliar application of boron nano-chelated fertilizer and boric acid on fruit yield, oil content, and quality attributes in olive (Olea europaea L.). Sci Hortic 257:108689
106. Vishekaii ZR, Soleimani A, Ghasemnezhad M, Hasani A (2019b) The feasibility for replacement of urea with nitrogen nano-chelated fertilizer in olive (Olea europaea L.) orchards. Iran J Plant Physiol 10:3047–3058
107. Vishekaii ZR, Soleimani A, Fallahi E et al (2023) Response of olive (Olea europaea L.) trees to foliar spray of nano chelated and chemical potassium fertilizers. J Plant Nutr 46:1159–1171
108. Yang J, Yan Z, Xu D, Wang X (2021) Enhanced growth of broad beans (Vicia faba L.) through separating antagonistic nutrients using nitrogen-doped carbon nanotubes. ACS Sustainable Chem Eng 9:16437–16449
109. Zerssa G, Feyssa D, Kim D-G, Eichler-Löbermann B (2021) Challenges of smallholder farming in Ethiopia and opportunities by adopting climate-smart agriculture. Agriculture 11:192
110. Zhao L, Bai T, Wei H et al (2022) Nanobiotechnology-based strategies for enhanced crop stress resilience. Nat Food 3:829–836

# Scope of Nanomaterials in Phytoremediation Actions of Agricultural Crops

**Magín González-Moscoso, Yolanda González-García, Hermes Pérez-Hernández, and Antonio Juárez-Maldonado**

**Abstract** Currently, agriculture must focus on managing sustainable agricultural systems in the long term. However, soil contamination by a variety of contaminants has made it increasingly difficult to obtain safe and quality food to meet population demand. Paradoxically, human activity itself is responsible for the contamination of soils through different materials such as heavy metals, hydrocarbons, organic and inorganic solvents, and plastics, among others. They can cause damage to plants, reduce growth and yield, and ultimately affect the availability and quality of food. To deal with the problem of soil contamination, phytoremediation has been studied, a strategy that has given good results. Within phytoremediation different routes can be followed, such as phytoextraction, phytostabilization, phytovolatilization, and phytodegradation, which provide different solutions to the problem of soil contamination. The *Brassica* genus stands out, since some species have great phytoremediation and heavy metal hyperaccumulation potential because they synthesize substances that help in the translocation of heavy metal ions. It has been shown that at least 10 genotypes of *B. juncea* have the potential to decontaminate agricultural soils, while *B. napus* can accumulate more than 1000 mg Pb $kg^{-1}$ of dry matter, which demonstrates its ability to extract heavy metals from the soil. In addition to this, better results have been achieved through the use of nanomaterials that have unique properties, in conjunction with phytoremediation. This strategy, called nanophytoremediation, seems to be an important tool, which will surely have a positive impact in the near future on agricultural soil contamination problems. Nanophytoremediation consists of the nanomaterials that adsorb pollutants and degrade them, and so are accumulated by plants. The great advantage of this technology is that it is less expensive and has

M. González-Moscoso
Department of Nanotechnology, Polytechnic University of Chiapas, Suchiapa, Mexico

Y. González-García
National Institute of Forestry, Agricultural and Livestock Research, Northwest Regional Research Center, Todos Santos Experimental Field, La Paz, Mexico

H. Pérez-Hernández · A. Juárez-Maldonado (✉)
Department of Botany, Autonomous Agrarian University Antonio Narro, Saltillo, Mexico
e-mail: antonio.juarez@uaaan.edu.mx

 
D. Jabborova et al. (eds.), *Nanomaterials in Agroforestry Systems*, Smart Nanomaterials Technology, https://doi.org/10.1007/978-981-96-1337-3_15

less negative impact on the environment than any physical and chemical remediation technology. However, nanomaterials can also play an additional role in dealing with heavy metal contamination problems in the soil, since it has been observed in certain species such as *Solanum lycopersicum*, which can significantly reduce their absorption. This can potentially decrease the accumulation of heavy metals in foods, decreasing the risk to human health.

**Keywords** Heavy metals · Nanotechnology · Pollutants · Pollutant removal · Stabilization of pollutants · Volatilization of pollutants

## 1 Introduction

Currently, agriculture faces several important challenges that must be faced to ensure that agricultural production systems are sustainable in the long term [132]. Furthermore, if we consider that climate change is influencing different environmental factors that can induce stress in plants, the management of agricultural systems becomes even more complex [50]. In agriculture, the soil is essential, since most agricultural production systems are currently developed on it. In addition to the fact that soil is important since it is the basis of all terrestrial life, it provides ecosystem services and has a great diversity of beneficial microorganisms for plants [124].

One of the great challenges for agriculture derives from soil contamination, since due to human activity, soils have been contaminated with different materials or molecules such as heavy metals (HM), hydrocarbons, organic and inorganic solvents, and plastics, among others [120, 127]. This has generated a global problem with different levels of severity for agriculture [140].

Although HM are found naturally in the environment [54], the main origin is human activities among which are mining, industrial activities, waste leaks, sewage sludge, and agricultural fertilization [21, 24, 42, 113]. Hydrocarbons are a clear example of how human activity has generated problems, since due to the processes of exploration, production, transportation, storage, leaks in pipelines, accidental spills, and supply, oil has contaminated vast areas of soil [80, 90]. Moreover, the oil itself is a source of HM such as copper (Cu), iron (Fe), vanadium (V), cadmium (Cd), and lead (Pb), which will contaminate the soil [39]. As if this were not enough, there is evidence that plants can absorb hydrocarbons, which apart from the negative effects they can have on the plants themselves, can reach higher trophic levels, and generate adverse effects on other species [46].

Another soil contamination problem, although less common, is radiation contamination, which comes mainly from nuclear accidents that release radioactivity [141]. This problem can be severe, since it is persistent and can accumulate in organisms for a prolonged time [109]. Additionally, recently the contamination of terrestrial environments by micro and nano plastics has been studied, which has increased due to the use of plastic materials, and their poor handling and disposal [48, 73]. Particularly in agriculture, the problem arises from the use of plastic mulches and waste applications, in addition to the application of compost that may also contain plastics [48, 73].

The impacts of soil contaminants on plants are diverse, they can induce damage to leaves and stomata, induce senescence, diminish photosynthesis, alter membrane permeability, and negatively impact the development of plant-sensitive species, among many others [101, 126].

Possibly, phytoremediation is the main strategy used to deal with soil contamination problems, that is, the use of an edible or non-edible plant to degrade, eliminate, absorb, and immobilize diverse contaminants from terrestrial and aquatic systems [5]. Among the most common phytoremediation strategies are phytoextraction, phytostabilization, phytovolatilization, and phytodegradation [66]. Phytoextraction is the absorption of contaminants from the soil or water through the roots and transfers them to the plant biomass [14, 94]. Phytostabilization is when plants accumulate pollutants in the root tissue due to root exudates and chelation with metal-binding molecules [103]. Phytovolatilization occurs when plants absorb pollutants and convert them into less dangerous volatile chemical compounds through transpiration [31]. Phytodegradation is the transformation of pollutants into simpler molecules through metabolic processes by the plant itself through enzymes produced by the roots or by the joint action of plants and endophytic and/or rhizospheric bacteria [86].

However, although this technique has given positive results and can be considered low cost, it also presents disadvantages such as the accumulation of contaminants in plant tissues that make it non-consumable, low production of plant biomass, and time necessary to achieve the objective of removing contaminants from the soil [29, 55].

For its part, nanotechnology, due to the unique characteristics that nanomaterials (NM) have such as size (<100 nm), large surface area, and greater adsorption capacity, is considered a promising technology to help remediate contaminated soils [121, 131]. Furthermore, unlike conventional materials, the physicochemical properties of NM are more effective in activating the defense systems of crops and strengthening the immunity and growth of plants, especially when they develop under stress conditions [67], which applied to plants useful for phytoremediation can increase their efficiency.

The union of phytoremediation with NM is a new field of knowledge, defined as nanophytoremediation, which includes nanoscale materials used for the adsorption of contaminants and their degradation, as well as the use of plants used to accumulate contaminants [122]. It is considered that this technology can be extremely important in the recovery of contaminated soils [106]. This is why the aim of this chapter is to address the issues related to the use of nanotechnology as another tool to improve the phytoremediation capacity, to deal with pollution problems in agricultural soils more efficiently [133].

## 2 Pollutants in the Soil

Soils are the basis of all terrestrial life and provide ecosystem services, in addition to having a great diversity of microorganisms that perform beneficial functions [124]. However, the soils have become contaminated, which has generated a global problem with different degrees of severity, with agricultural fields being the most affected [110, 140]. The most documented soil contaminants are HM, hydrocarbons, organic and inorganic solvents, and burning of garbage residues, and currently great attention has been generated by plastic pollution [127] (Fig. 1).

Contaminants in the soil have a transformation process that includes redox reactions, precipitation, adsorption, biodegradation, bioavailability, phytoavailability, and environmental toxicity [111]. Analyzing the impact of soil pollution at a global level is a challenge since there are different types of soils and climates that contribute considerably to contaminants [65]. Finally, existing soil remediation technologies generally require long treatment times [20]. Therefore, it is important to develop new strategies and options that are more efficient and environmentally friendly [112].

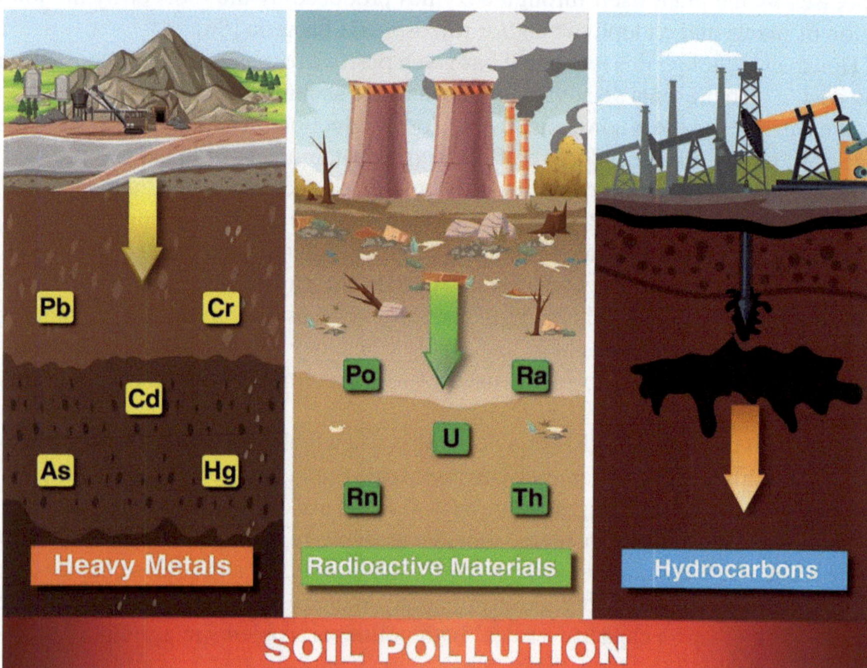


**Fig. 1** Main soil pollutants and their origin

## *2.1 Heavy Metals*

Heavy metals are metallic property elements with a comparatively high density (>5 g $cm^{-3}$) to water that can cause toxicity to various aspects and occur naturally in the environment, however, exceeding concentrations can be harmful [54]. This surplus originates mainly from human activities, for example, mining, industrial emissions, waste leakage, sewage sludge, and agricultural fertilization [21, 24, 42]. These anthropogenic activities are derived from population and industry growth.

HM in the soil such as lead (Pb), mercury (Hg), chromium (Cr), cadmium (Cd), Thallium (Tl), and arsenic (As) in high concentrations are toxic for the development of plants and organisms [61, 100]. HM are considered contaminants because they have high resistance to degradation, their toxic effects on organisms, their ability to persist for a long time in soils, and their translocation [125]. Unlike organic pollutants, HM cannot be degraded by microorganisms, these elements can only be transformed from one chemical state to another [45, 52]. Furthermore, it has been reported that soils contaminated with HM negatively impact the structure and diversity of microorganisms [43].

Pb constitutes 0.0002% of the Earth's crust and is a high toxic metal (the second most); naturally, its concentration is very low [102]. However, activities of human beings such as coal-fired power plants, coal mines, smelting slag, and vehicle emissions contribute large amounts of Pb [2].

Cd is generally found naturally as the $Cd^{2+}$ ion, and it is very rare for it to occur alone; it is commonly found associated with other minerals [74]. Cd does not undergo microbial or chemical degradation, it is a chemically very stable element and is not essential for organisms [147]. It has great mobility in soils and can be absorbed quickly from the soil to crops [142].

Cr in the soil according to its oxidation state is mainly found in trivalent and hexavalent forms, the latter being the most toxic because it is more soluble [58]. Particularly trivalent chromium, its mobility and toxicity are low, and it is also easily absorbed into clay minerals in the form of different complexes [23].

Hg is the element that occupies number 66 in quantity on the Earth's crust and has no reported biological function [77]. Hg in soil may be present in three oxidation states, elemental mercury, mercurious and mercuric, each one has different properties which makes the evaluation of contaminated soils complex [87].

As is commonly found in two oxidation states: 1) arsenite (AsIII) and 2) arsenate (AsV) [146]. This element is very toxic, but AsIII is 60 times more toxic than AsV [137]. As can easily enter crops because it is similar to phosphorus and can be transported in its absorption channels [1]. Therefore, it is a risk to human health because it can easily enter the food chain.

## 2.2 Petroleum Hydrocarbons

Oil is one of the most dangerous pollutants due to the enormous quantities that are spilled in the processes of exploration, production, transportation, storage, pipeline leaks, accidental spills, and supply [80, 90]. Oil pollution is a global problem in aquatic and terrestrial systems. This contaminant is a viscous liquid mixture that mainly contains aliphatic, aromatic compounds, alkanes, and resins, among other toxic substances [139, 149]. Polycyclic aromatic hydrocarbons (composed of benzene rings) are part of the group of persistent organic pollutants, this specific characteristic means that they do not degrade rapidly [13]. On the other hand, oil has HM fractions such as copper, iron, vanadium, Cd, and Pb, which will be incorporated into the soil as part of the pollution [39].

Oil pollution causes an effect on the properties of the soil, both physically and chemically [135]. This contaminant significantly reduces the cation exchange capacity, phosphorus, calcium, and magnesium contents [35]. Furthermore, it has been reported that the higher the concentration of oil in the soil, the electrical conductivity and water retention capacity decrease considerably [97]. Regarding the biological aspect, it has been reported that oil concentrations above 20,000 mg $kg^{-1}$ in the soil decrease the diversity and structure of the microbial populations [30].

## 2.3 Radioactive Materials

Although it is less common than contamination by HM or hydrocarbons, nuclear accidents can release radioactivity into ecosystems and cause radiation contamination through the deposit of radioactive elements into the ground [141]. Contamination by radioactive elements is persistent and can accumulate in organisms for a long time [109]. Additionally, these radioactive elements can easily accumulate in agricultural products [129], where the translocation will be greater if the quantity of radioactive elements in the soil is high [84]. Among the main radioactive elements that can be found naturally are uranium (U), thorium (Th), polonium (Po), radon (Rn), xenon (Xe), and krypton (Kr) [89, 99]. These radionuclides are present in the environment in different isotopic forms, which is why living organisms can be exposed to ionizing radiation [4]. Regarding human health, exposure to natural radionuclides at high concentrations can cause cancer [49].

Radiation is found naturally in the environment and can release radionuclides such as uranium that will accumulate in the topsoil [70]. However, uranium is also released by anthropogenic activities such as the nuclear industry, agriculture, and mining causing pollution and a risk to living organisms [68].

Polonium is a radioactive element that is generated from the uranium decay chain and has an average life of approximately 138 days and a radiation energy of 5.3 MeV [108]. Polonium can be absorbed into soil particles as humic substances and mineral colloids [114].

Radon is a radioactive noble gas that is formed from uranium, it originates from the radioactive decay of uranium [12]. Interestingly, 40% of the natural radiation to which the human population is exposed comes from this element [62].

### 2.4 *Micro and Nano Plastics*

One of the most recently studied pollution problems in terrestrial environments is that caused by micro and nano plastics. This problem is generated by the increase in the use of plastic materials in several human activities, as well as their poor handling and disposal [48, 73].

In the area of agriculture, it has been reported that the problem arises from the use of plastic mulches and other waste applications, which represent the first source of contributions of micro and nano plastics to the soil [73]. However, also the application of compost is a source of these plastics [48].

## 3 Impacts of Pollutants in Agricultural Plants

Two types of direct damage that contaminants cause to plants have been reported, one occurs as a result of exposure to elevated concentrations of contaminants, which induces visible damage to the leaves such as necrotic lesions [95]. While the second type is more subtle, since it requires prolonged exposure to the contaminant, is observed as a growth and/or yield of the plants limited, and does not present clear visible symptoms [101]. Among the main soil pollutants are HMs, hydrocarbons, organic and inorganic solvents, and plastic pollution, which can present both types of damage [127]. Derived from this, the impact of contaminants on plants can induce a variety of negative effects on plants, they can cause damage to leaves and stomata, premature senescence, decreased photosynthesis, altered membrane permeability and growth, and yield reduction in sensitive plant species [69, 101].

### 3.1 *Impact of Heavy Metals on Agricultural Plants*

It is possible that HM are the main contamination problem in agricultural soils today, and therefore, one of those that will have the greatest impact on plants used in agriculture. It is well known that HM contamination negatively impacts agricultural crops by reducing their yields and decreasing nutritional quality [130]. However, the toxicity of HM in plants is dependent on factors including plant species, growth conditions and stage of development, toxicity of the specific elements, physical and chemical soil properties, bioavailability of HM ions in soil solution, and properties of soil rhizosphere [75, 104].

HM can alter the structure and therefore also the normal function of cellular components, in addition to directly interfering at physiological, metabolic, biochemical, and molecular levels of plants, generating oxidative stress, inhibiting photosynthetic phosphorylation, inactivate enzymes/proteins of both the plant and the soil, induce genotoxicity, generate genetic modifications (modulate gene expression), and hormonal deregulation, in addition, they indirectly affect plants due to the growth limitation, proliferation, and soil microbial diversity [100, 104, 105].

Particularly, when HM induce oxidative stress, i.e., hypergeneration of ROS, can cause significant damage to plant cellular structures, such as protein and lipid peroxidation, affectation of nucleic acids, inhibition of enzymatic activity, and ultimately can cause cell death [105].

For example, Pb, which is considered one of the most toxic HM, causes a variety of damages to plants throughout growth and development, alters the water and nutritional status in plants, and induces oxidative damage. Moreover, Pb alters enzymatic activities, induces membrane damage, and interferes with stomatal closure due to the induction of abscisic acid and the negative correlation with potassium. In addition, this HM alters the photosynthetic apparatus and the reduced biosynthesis of chlorophylls affecting carbon metabolism [154].

### 3.2 Impact of Hydrocarbons on Agricultural Plants

Petroleum hydrocarbons (PH) originating from crude oil distillates (diesel, gasoline, lubricating oil, and others) are very important pollutants globally because they are highly toxic, mutagenic, and carcinogenic [59].

When PH are absorbed/adsorbed by organisms, they can cause sublethal or lethal effects, e.g., alter the cell membrane, resulting in modifications in membrane fluidity, integrity, and function [59, 92]. Particularly, in plants, PH affect germination and nutrient uptake and translocation, at the cellular level inducing oxidative damage and alters the metabolism, therefore affecting plant physiology and morphology and reducing plant yield [38, 59].

### 3.3 Impact of Micro and Nano Plastics on Agricultural Plants

Microplastic contamination in soils has become very relevant in recent times due to potential influences on soil properties that can impact significantly plant development and soil fertility [73]. Their presence affects a variety of soil and plant characteristics, it has been documented that these pollutants seriously impact soil ecosystem functions that are fundamental, for example, microbial activity and nutrient cycles [48, 53].

Soil properties related to erosion risk, structural integrity, and water storage capacity are generally negatively affected by microplastic inputs to the soil. While the effects of soil microplastics on rhizosphere function are diverse, in some cases are positive impacts (improved associations between plants and symbiotic fungi), however, they generally induce at least some negative impact on plant development [73].

Interestingly, biodegradable plastics appear to present a greater risk to plant development in comparison to chemical plastic polymers [48]. Therefore, it is necessary to consider this information to make better decisions in the use of plastics in agriculture.

In this sense, Meng et al. [76] demonstrated that LDPE-MP (low-density polyethylene) did not show significant effects on root and shoot biomass of *Phaseolus vulgaris* L., while Bio-MP (polylactic acid mixed with polybutylene adipate-co-terephthalate) significantly inhibited it. Furthermore, both types of microplastics presented negative impacts on specific root nodules, suggesting that regardless of the origin of these materials, they may be a potential risk to soil–plant systems.

## 4 Phytoremediation of Contaminated Soils

To date, there is relevant information related to phytoremediation techniques to streamline the treatment process of soils contaminated with different types of compounds (organic and inorganic) and HM in an efficient, sustainable, and low-cost manner. Phytoremediation is the use of an edible or non-edible plant to degrade, eliminate, absorb, and immobilize diverse contaminants from terrestrial and aquatic systems [5]. Some plant species have potential mechanisms that allow the decontamination of heavy metals and a high capacity to survive contaminant stress. Studies suggest that tolerance to contaminants depends on the plant genotype, the speed of absorption, and the ability to bioconcentrate contaminating substances in the tissues. Additionally, in the plant–metal interaction, bioavailability of metal, environmental conditions, and the soil matrix are factors that allow the phytoremediation strategy, in which the molecular genetics in plants and soil-chemical mechanisms are involved. In genetic mechanisms, proteins are responsible for the homeostasis of HM, i.e., plants regulate the absorption of metals and maintain the survival plant [41, 83].

Additionally, plants must be tolerant to HM, have short life cycles, and have a bioconcentration factor (BCF) and translocation factor (TF) greater than 1. BCF indicates the root-to-soil ratio of HM, while TF is the shoot-to-root ratio of HM [17, 60]. According to the plant species, plant–metal interaction, accumulation, and absorption patterns, plants are classified into three groups: (a) excluders, (b) excretors, and (c) accumulators. The excluders are the ones that stand out for accumulating higher amounts of HM in the roots ($TF < 1$). Excretors release heavy metals through their glands or trichomes from the leaf biomass. Finally, accumulators have a metal bioaccumulation factor greater than 1 ($BCF > 1$) [17]. In general way, there is a list of plants with the potential capacity to accumulate contaminants on a large scale, to mention some species: *Brassica spp, Alyssum bertholonii, Thlaspi caerulescens, Arabidopsis halleri, Arundo donax, Typha spp, Atriplex lentiformis, Atriplex halimus* subsp. *Schweinfurthii, Berkheya coddii, Boehmeria nivea, Canna indica, Dalbergia sissoo, Helianthus annuus, Hydrocotyle ranunculoides, Lagerstroemia indica, Ludwigia peploides, Medicago sativa, Nicotiana tabacum, Noccaea caerulescens, Pistia stratiotes, Pteris vittata, Solanum nigrum, Suaeda fruticosa, Thlaspi caerulescens, Usnea amblyoclada, Sesbania exaltata, Sesuvium portulacastrum, Melilotus officinalis, Amaranthus retroflexus, Pennisetum purpureum,* among others [86, 98].

Among the most common phytoremediation strategies are phytoextraction, phytostabilization, phytovolatilization, and phytodegradation (Fig. 2). The accumulation of contaminants by plants is a complex system in which at least three steps are involved: (1) transport of membranes through the plasmalemma of the root cells, (2) loading and translocation of the xylem, and (3) detoxification and sequestration of metals throughout the plant and at the cellular level [66].

The phytoremediation strategy is a promising method based on the use of plants that can tolerate high concentrations of HM and pollutants present in the soil and environment. Unlike soil remediation techniques, e.g., precipitation and chemical leaching, thermal treatments, electroremediation, and soil replacement, phytoremediation is a method applicable to agricultural soils and less expensive than the rest. However, although there are advantages, there are also disadvantages that are listed below [55]. Advantages: (a) It is a low-cost technology with zero ecological impact, therefore, it is considered environmentally friendly,(b) It can be applied in situ and prevents the spread of contaminants; (c) Does not require sophisticated personnel and equipment; and (d) Technique without noise emission compared to the other methods. Disadvantages: (a) Many studies have been evaluated in the laboratory,

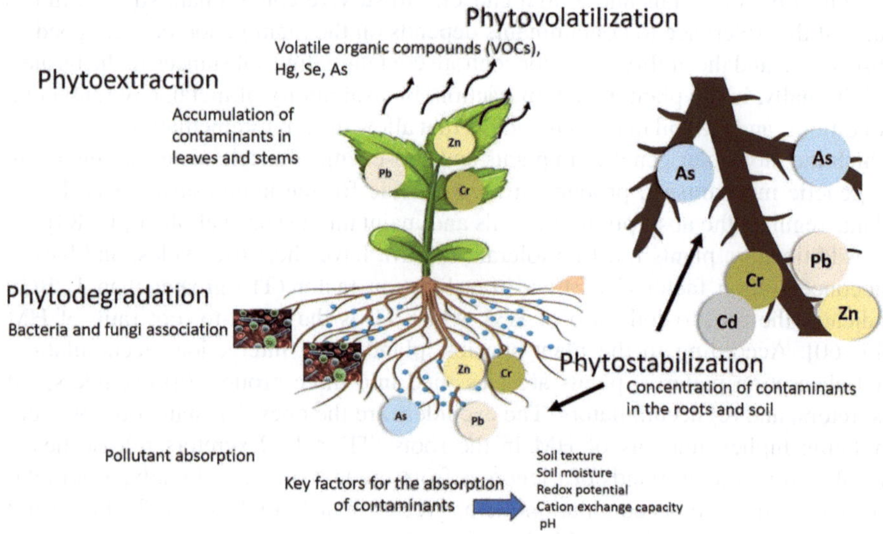


**Fig. 2** Most common phytoremediation strategies and plant–pollutants interactions

therefore, there are doubts about the effectiveness in the long term and real situations (field); (b) Contaminants can accumulate in leaves, stems, and fruits, making the products unfeasible to consume; (c) Not all the species studied adapt to climatic environments, in many cases, they are site-specific plant species; (d) Many plant species have low biomass production; (e) In some cases, plants are effective for a specific contaminant; and (f) Unlike physical and chemical treatments, their effectiveness is slow.

## 4.1 Phytoextraction Strategy

Phytoextraction is the absorption, of pollutants (from the soil or water) through the roots and transfers them to the plant biomass (stems, leaves, and fruits). A little more than 400 pollutant hyperaçcumulator plants are recognized. For this to be fulfilled, the plants must have a high biomass production and be fast growing. In this line, plants of the *Brassica* genus are considered hyperaccumulators of heavy metals, and therefore, can be used as potential phytoremediators [14]. The physiological and biochemical potential of these plants to tolerate the adverse effects of these pollutants is due to the efficient defense mechanism, which includes enzymatic and non-enzymatic compounds [93].

Within a variety of plants (80 genotypes), at least 10 genotypes of Indian mustard plants (*Brassica juncea*) were shown to have the potential to decontaminate agricultural soils, the plants concentrated Cd and Pb in they different organs (leaves, stems, and roots). In particular, the accumulation of both metals in the sprouts exceeded the permissible limit for human consumption (0.20 mg $kg^{-1}$). The researchers indicated that the uptake and transport of metals in mustard plants are related to the exposure time, soil pH (5.5), and the availability of the metal in plant roots through plasma membrane cation channels. Likewise, the authors suggest that soil exudates are a factor that modifies soil pH and consequently makes Cd and Pb more available [37]. Other studies reinforce these findings with other plant species, [153] suggested that the release of citric acid by parts of the roots of *Sedum plumbizincicola* L. decreased the soil pH, which led to higher dissolution of metals such as Cd and Zn, consequently, greater uptake by plants. When comparing plant species, the accumulation of HM was higher in *S. plumbizincicola* in comparison to the wheat crop.

Furthermore, the authors suggest that organic acids released by plants promote the conversion of metals to the available fraction in the soil, thus facilitating the remediation efficiency. Researchers have shown that the extraction of metals absorbed by plants varies depending on the rhizosphere of the plant species [119].

On the other hand, the Pb in soil has low solubility due to its sorption in the soil, thus making it difficult for plants to absorb it. However, it has been reported that in *B. napus*, they accumulate above 1000 mg $kg^{-1}$ of dry matter. As far as is known, Pb enters through the apoplastic pathway and calcium channels to the root cells. During translocation, Pb accumulates in root vacuoles. Furthermore, it has been reported that the accumulation and immobilization are given in the form of phosphates, reducing the adverse effects on plants and consequently increasing the phytoextraction of the HM through metal–ligand complexes [57]. Additionally, studies document that *Brassica* species synthesize substances that help in the translocation of HM. For example, low molecular weight phytochelatins are responsible for the transportation of metal ions from root tissues to the vacuoles of leaf and stem cells [79].

Since Cd has high mobility and solubility in water, absorption by roots is facilitated. During the process, the ZIP transporters (AtIRT1) are the main ones responsible for transporting heavy metals to the phloem of the plants. However, YSL (Yellow-Stripe 1-Like) proteins, calcium transport channel, and ATP-binding cassette transporter are involved in the absorption of this non-essential element for plants [18, 148, 150]. In detail, studies report that Cd, with the help of the proteins and channels involved, crosses through the symplast and is transported to the xylem. However, through the apoplastic route, Cd enters when the Casparin bands in the root are at the beginning of formation [93]. However, it is important to highlight that the bioavailability of toxic metals as well as their absorption by plants is regulated by the properties of the soil matrix, i.e., texture, humidity, redox potential, cation exchange capacity, and pH [93].

## 4.2 *Phytostabilization Strategy*

In phytostabilization, plants accumulate contaminants in the root tissue. In this strategy, the basic mechanism takes place in roots through exudates and chelation with metal-binding molecules [103]. Efficient phytostabilization depends on the plant species, which must be tolerant to contaminants and have an abundant root system since, for this technique, the roots play an important function in the immobilization of toxic compounds [152].

In addition, phytostabilization involves the participation of microorganisms and antioxidant compounds. The authors suggest that the presence of microorganisms, particularly solubilizing bacteria, is the main factor in the production of organic acids, chelating agents, and metabolites, substances that participate in the metal immobilization process [103, 115]. Phytostabilization depends on the solubility and mobility of metabolites exuded in roots, like sugars, polysaccharides, amino acids, peptides, and proteins. Studies have shown that rice plants (*Oryza sativa* L.) intercropped with *Thalia dealbata* decreased Cd concentrations. The decrease in Cd was achieved due to the fine roots of *T. dealbata* take Cd from the rice rhizosphere. Even the amounts of the metal in the rice grains were very low. In fact, the authors argued that the grains could be safely consumed [134].

Specifically, by root exudates, HM are stabilized without being absorbed by plants [123]. In the soil, the high concentrations of Cr (VI) affect the mobility and absorption of essential minerals like P, Ca, Mg, Zn, and Fe, among others, due to the masking of sorption sites and the formation of insoluble complexes, causing a nutrient imbalance in plants [117]. Cr is very soluble in the soil, so plants that accumulate metals have the advantage of extracting the element. When the soil has high levels of organic matter and a pH between 5.0 and 5.5, Cr forms complexes with organic acids, increasing the solubility and mobility through the roots [138]. Studies affirm that Cr (III), considered less harmful, enters through the apoplastic route while Cr (VI), the most toxic state, enters through the symplastic route. The translocation and accumulation capacity of Cr in plant tissues depends on the plant species and factors associated with the soil and the environment [88]. Regarding the direct mediators that influence the absorption of Cr into plant tissue, through calcium transporters and phosphate proteins, both Cr (III) and Cr (VI) are directed mainly to the cytosol and, in lesser quantities, to the vacuoles [93].

For all of the above, phytostabilization is used to immobilize highly toxic contaminants. In general, the roots or rhizosphere of plants abruptly stop the contaminant's movement. According to the literature, it can be said that phytostabilization is an effective strategy for soil decontamination and the conservation of both groundwater and surface water [3].

### 4.3 *Phytovolatilization Strategy*

In phytovolatilization, plants absorb pollutants and convert them into less dangerous volatile chemical compounds through transpiration. The plants most studied in these strategies are *B. juncea* and *A. thaliana*, which absorb pollutants and convert them into volatile organic compounds (VOCs) inside the plant, which are then released into the environment [31]. For example, it was shown that *B. juncea* volatilizes large amounts of Se into the atmosphere through the chemical forms dimethylselenide (DMSe) and dimethyldiselenide (DMDSe). Also, it has been shown that *B. juncea* plants volatilize more Se when the plants absorb Se-methionine (SeMet) since it is the most available form. In this process, plants absorb Se through sulfate transport proteins [118].

Moreover, the microorganisms in the soil facilitate the volatilization of As. [36] demonstrated that *A. donax* plants, in combination with plant growth-promoting bacteria (PGPR), managed to volatilize more than 70% of the initial content of As in the soil. The results were interesting since the As in the plant biomass was less than 0.20%.

Mercury is another element that has been phytoremediated with the phytovolatilization method. However, the effectiveness depends on the physical state and availability of the pollutant in the plant rhizosphere [81].

### 4.4 *Phytodegradation Strategy*

Phytodegradation is the transformation of pollutants in simpler molecules through metabolic processes by the plant itself through enzymes produced by the roots or by the joint action of plants and endophytic and rhizospheric bacteria. Organisms associated with plants have genes linked to the degradation of pollutants. In addition, they improve plant development and induce tolerance to toxic compounds [28, 86].

To degrade Benzo(a)pyrene (BaP), a compound that is part of the polycyclic aromatic hydrocarbons (PAH), Kotoky and Pandey [56] revealed that the *Melia azedarach* L. plant in the presence of rhizospheric bacteria managed to degrade up to 85% of the BaP in the soil. The results demonstrated the capacity of bacteria to produce biosurfactants and solubilize the contaminant. The authors verify the effectiveness of the plant–microbe association to degrade PAH of soil. It has been shown that *Bacillus subtilis* (endophytic bacteria) isolated from the roots of *Ficus benghalensis* L. has the ability to secrete biosurfactants and contribute to the degradation and recovery of oil by 40% [96].

Nebeská et al. [85] reported that *Miscanthus* × *giganteus* (Mxg) grew in sites contaminated with aliphatic hydrocarbons and PAH, and its association with soil microorganisms becomes effective for oil degradation. Even the diversity of microorganisms was greater in contaminated soils than in controls. In detail, the results revealed that the increase in biomass was related to soil degradation and that the consortium with microbes makes a novel and ecological technique.

## 5 Phytoremediation Assisted with Nanomaterials

Nanomaterials (NM) have small size (<100 nm) which gives them unique and tunable physicochemical properties; they are considered to have immense potential due to the variety of reported applications in multiple sectors such as medicine, healthcare, food sector, environment, agriculture, electronics, and pharmacy [121]. In agricultural systems, the use of NM has a variety of advantages over conventional materials, such as increased effectiveness, reduced input needs, and reduced environmental toxicity, which is why nanotechnology applied to agriculture has become relevant in the last decade [27]. NM is increasingly used in agroecosystems in order to alleviate abiotic/biotic stress and remediate soil, this is because NM applied in adequate quantities induces positive functions in defense and alleviation of various types of stress in agricultural plants [67]. In addition, they have been used for various purposes in agriculture, since they function as growth regulators and can be used as nanopesticides, nanofertilizers, nanoantimicrobial agents, and specific transporters in plants, in addition to reducing the risks of abiotic stress [27, 121].

Due to their unique characteristics such as size, large surface area, and high adsorption capacity, nanomaterials are considered a promising technology to remediate polluted soils [121, 131]. With the great advantage that unlike conventional materials, NM activates the defense systems of stressed plants more effectively and therefore strengthen the immunity and growth [67]. Furthermore, all the advances that have been made in materials science have allowed to understand many more aspects of the molecular complexity and their functions of NMs in plants, which has allowed us to obtain various positive results [27].

Particularly, in the area of phytoremediation, it is considered that NM can be used in conjunction with plants to remediate HM and emerging organic pollutants in the soil more efficiently through increasing the immobilization of contaminants, as well as accelerating degradation and regulating the physiology of agricultural plants and the microbial populations of the soil rhizosphere to improve plant immune responses [67, 121].

## 5.1 *Nanophytoremediation*

The union of phytoremediation with NM is a new field of knowledge, in this sense, [122] defined nanophytoremediation as an environmentally friendly technology that uses NM for the adsorption of contaminants and their degradation, as well as the use of some species of plants to accumulate pollutants. The integration of NM as agents that improve the solubility of the contaminant and phytoremediation can be a relevant strategy in the remediation of polluted soils [106].

Nanophytoremediation consists of two main steps: (1) Nanomaterials adsorb pollutants and degrade them and (2) Degraded materials are accumulated by plants [82]. Additionally, this new technology is typically cheaper and with fewer negative impacts on the environment in comparison with any physical and chemical remediation technologies [11].

NM can stimulate plant development and can improve the absorption of HM by plants, improving the phytoremediation capacity of contaminated soils [91]. However, it must be taken into account that the success of the remediation of pollutants in the soil not only is dependent on the plant species, type of nanomaterial, and quantities but also on the treatment time [151].

Regarding the nanoremediation strategy, it has been reported that iron nanoparticles (Fe NPs) show the ability to immobilize up to 20% of Pb in the soil; however, after 120 days, the immobilization efficiency decreases [26]. Furthermore, the capacity to immobilize metals in soil with the use of nanomaterials may depend on soil properties, nanomaterial concentrations, metal characteristics, and the presence of other elements in the soil [32]. Interestingly, the NPs size increases the capacity to react with the contaminant and to be absorbed in susceptible sites, which can result in improved degradation, and they can also migrate to deeper sites in the soil to react with the contaminants [72].

Currently, there is a series of research that showed positive effects of the use of NM on the development of agricultural crops under conditions of soil contamination, either in sites with the real problem or in conditions simulated in experiments. However, it is important to consider the objective of using NM, since in some cases, it increases the ability of plants to absorb HM, while in other cases, it decreases it (Table 1). It can then be considered that in plants that are commonly used for phytoremediation, their capacity to absorb HM can be increased through the use of NM.

**Table 1** Application of different nanomaterials as agents to improve the phytoremediation of polluted soils

| Type of nanomaterial | Pollutant | Plant | Effects | References |
|---|---|---|---|---|
| Silicon nanoparticles | As | *Solanum lycopersicum* L. | Reduced arsenic translocation | González-Moscoso et al. [34] |
| Nanoscale zerovalent iron (nZVI) | Pb | *Lolium perenne* L. | Greater accumulation of Pb with a concentration of 100 mg $kg^{-1}$ nZVI | Huang et al. [44] |
| $TiO_2$ nanoparticles | Sb | *Sorghum bicolor* (L.) Moench | Greater concentration capacity of *S. bicolor* for Sb, reaching an accumulation of 1624.1 μg | Zand et al. [143] |
| $TiO_2$ nanoparticles | Cd | *Trifolium repens* L. | Greater capacity to absorb cadmium | Zand et al. [144] |
| Nanoscale zerovalent iron (nZVI) | As, Hg | *Medicago sativa* L. | It immobilized As in the soil and increased the uptake of Hg by the plant | Baragaño et al. [10] |
| Silicon dioxide nanoparticles | As, Cd | *Oryza sativa* L. | Translocation decreased 29 and 68% respectively | Wang et al. [136] |
| Selenium nanoparticles | Cd | *Coriandrum sativum* L. | Cadmium absorption decreased | Babashpour-Asl et al. [7] |
| $TiO_2$ nanoparticles | Pb | *Sorghum bicolor* (L.) Moench | Increased in the accumulation ability of *S. bicolor* for Pb | Daryabeigi Zand et al. [19] |
| $TiO_2$ nanoparticles | Cd | *Brassica juncea* L. | Eliminated Cd from the soil by up to 55.11% | Bakshi and Kumar [8] |
| Nanoscale zerovalent iron (nZVI) | Cd | *Trifolium repens* L. | Increased in Cd accumulation capacity of *T. repens* | Zand et al. [145] |
| Hydroxyapatite nanoparticles | Ni, Cu, Pb | *Arachis hypogaea* L. | Stabilized the HM on the soil | El-Nagar and Abdel-Halim [22] |
| FeO nanoparticles | As | *Triticum aestivum* L. | Restriction of translocation in roots and shoots | Manzoor et al. [71] |

(continued)

**Table 1** (continued)

| Type of nanomaterial | Pollutant | Plant | Effects | References |
|---|---|---|---|---|
| Copper nanoparticles functionalized with aspartic acid | Pb | *Zea mays* L. | Reduced lead absorption by roots | Ullah et al. [128] |
| Nanobiocarbon | Cd | *Brassica chinensis* L. | Stabilized cadmium ions in the soil | Liu et al. [64] |
| Nano-$SiO_2$ Nano-$CeO_2$ | Polycyclic aromatic hydrocarbons | *Sedum spectabile* (Boreau) H.Ohba | Elimination of polycyclic aromatic hydrocarbons | Liu et al. [63] |
| Iron-doped Zinc oxide nanoparticles | Chromite | *Triticum aestivum* L. | Restriction on translocation | Jehan et al. [51] |
| Nanosilica | Pb, Cd | *Secale montanum* Guss | It stabilized the HM in the soil and accumulated in the roots | Moameri and Abbasi Khalaki [78] |
| Magnesium oxide nanoparticles | Pb | *Daucus carota* L. | Reduction in the absorption and translocation of Pb | Faiz et al. [25] |
| $TiO_2$ nanoparticles | Petroleum | *Eleusine indica* (L.) Gaertn | Remediation efficiency of 65% | Ikhajiagbe and Osayamen [47] |
| Multi-walled carbon nanotubes | Pb, Cd | *Calendula officinalis* L. | The absorption of Pb and Cd in their tissues increased | Sharifi et al. [116] |
| Nanoscale zerovalent iron | Lindane | *Brassica napus* L. | Reduction in the accumulation of lindane in the soil | Hidalgo et al. [40] |
| Silver nanoparticles | Fipronil | *Plantago major* L. | Increased degradation of fipronil and greater accumulation in tissues | Romeh [107] |
| Silver nanoparticles | Pb, Cd, As, Hg, Cr | *Abelmoschus esculentus* (L.) Moench | Soil contamination was reduced by up to 60% | Azeez et al. [6] |
| Goethite nanospheres | As | *Nasturtium officinale* W.T.Aiton | Immobilization of As in the soil, reducing its availability | Baragaño et al. [9] |
| Nanoscale zerovalent iron | Cd | *Sorghum bicolor* (L.) Moench | Reduction in Cd accumulation in the root | Cheng et al. [16] |

(continued)

**Table 1** (continued)

| Type of nanomaterial | Pollutant | Plant | Effects | References |
|---|---|---|---|---|
| Multi-walled carbon nanotubes | Cd | *Boehmeria nivea* (L.) Gaudich | Increased uptake and translocation of Cd in the leaves and stem of ramie | Gong et al. [33] |
| Multi-walled carbon nanotubes | Cd, As | *Solanum nigrum* L. | Less uptake and accumulation of As by the plant. Decrease in Cd concentration in stem. Reduction of oxidative damage caused by Cd and As | Chen et al. [15] |

# 6 Conclusion

The problem of soil contamination, particularly in the agricultural area, is of utmost importance due to the implications it has not only on plants but also due to the potential risks it entails for human health. There are several types of pollutants in the soil, among which heavy metals, hydrocarbons, and more recently micro and nano plastics stand out, which negatively impact the growth and development of agricultural plants. To deal with the problem of soil contamination, phytoremediation has been studied, a strategy that has given good results. This strategy encompasses four categories, namely, phytoextraction, phytostabilization, phytovolatilization, and phytodegradation, each with different particular mechanisms of action. However, the scope of phytoremediation has not been sufficient to deal with the severe contamination problems of agricultural soils. Fortunately, with the development of nanotechnology, the application of nanomaterials has been combined with phytoremediation to achieve more promising results than those observed by phytoremediation alone. This strategy, called nanophytoremediation, seems to be an important tool, which will surely have a positive impact in the near future on agricultural soil contamination problems. Different studies demonstrate positive effects of using NM to assist phytoremediation, and thus achieve better results to address soil contamination. However, NM can increase the capacity of plants to absorb HM, but they can also decrease it. Hence, it is essential to take into account the plant species that are being used during phytoremediation, to establish if what is sought is for HM to enter the plants (aerial part or root), or only be degraded in the soil. Finally, the use of nanomaterials will make the strategy chosen more effective to reduce the negative impact of pollution on agricultural soils.

## References


1. Abbasi S, Lamb D, Rahman MA, Naidu R, Megharaj M (2021) Response of phosphorus sensitive plants to arsenate. Environ Technol Innov 24:102008. https://doi.org/10.1016/j.eti.2021.102008
2. Abbaszade G, Tserendorj D, Salazar-Yanez N, Zacháry D, Völgyesi P, Tóth E, Szabó C (2022) Lead and stable lead isotopes as tracers of soil pollution and human health risk assessment in former industrial cities of Hungary. Appl Geochem 145:105397. https://doi.org/10.1016/j.apgeochem.2022.105397
3. Ali S, Abbas Z, Rizwan M, Zaheer I, Yavaş İ, Ünay A, Abdel-DAIM M, Bin-Jumah M, Hasanuzzaman M, Kalderis D (2020) Application of floating aquatic plants in phytoremediation of heavy metals polluted water: a review. Sustainability 12(5):1927. https://doi.org/10.3390/su12051927
4. Asaduzzaman K, Mannan F, Khandaker MU, Farook MS, Elkezza A, Amin YBM, Sharma S, Kassim HBA (2015) Assessment of natural radioactivity levels and potential radiological risks of common building materials used in bangladeshi dwellings. PLoS One 10. https://doi.org/10.1371/journal.pone.0140667
5. Awa SH, Hadibarata T (2020) Removal of heavy metals in contaminated soil by phytoremediation mechanism: a review. Water Air Soil Pollut 231(2):47. https://doi.org/10.1007/s11270-020-4426-0
6. Azeez L, Adebisi SA, Adetoro RO, Oyedeji AO, Agbaje WB, Olabode OA (2022) Foliar application of silver nanoparticles differentially intervenes remediation statuses and oxidative stress indicators in *Abelmoschus esculentus* planted on gold-mined soil. Int J Phytoremediation 24:384–393. https://doi.org/10.1080/15226514.2021.1949578
7. Babashpour-Asl M, Farajzadeh-Memari-Tabrizi E, Yousefpour-Dokhanieh A (2022) Foliar-applied selenium nanoparticles alleviate cadmium stress through changes in physio-biochemical status and essential oil profile of coriander (*Coriandrum sativum* L.) leaves. Environ Sci Pollut Res 29:80021–80031. https://doi.org/10.1007/S11356-022-19941-1/METRICS
8. Bakshi M, Kumar A (2023) Co-application of $TiO_2$ nanoparticles and hyperaccumulator Brassica juncea L. for effective Cd removal from soil: assessing the feasibility of using nano-phytoremediation. J Environ Manage 341:118005. https://doi.org/10.1016/J.JENVMAN.2023.118005
9. Baragaño D, Alonso J, Gallego JR, Lobo MC, Gil-Díaz M (2020) Zero valent iron and goethite nanoparticles as new promising remediation techniques for as-polluted soils. Chemosphere 238. https://doi.org/10.1016/j.chemosphere.2019.124624
10. Baragaño D, Forján R, Álvarez N, Gallego JR, González A (2022) Zero valent iron nanoparticles and organic fertilizer assisted phytoremediation in a mining soil: arsenic and mercury accumulation and effects on the antioxidative system of Medicago sativa L. J Hazard Mater 433. https://doi.org/10.1016/j.jhazmat.2022.128748
11. Biswal T (2023) Nano-phytoremediation and its applications. In: Phytoremediation: management of environmental contaminants, vol 7, pp 335–364. https://doi.org/10.1007/978-3-031-17988-4_16/COVER
12. Celen YY, Gunay O, Oncul S, Narin B (2023) Measurement of soil radon concentration in Balikesir and examination of its effects on health. J Radiat Res Appl Sci 16:100718. https://doi.org/10.1016/j.jrras.2023.100718
13. Chaber P, Gworek B (2020) Surface horizons of forest soils for the diagnosis of soil environment contamination and toxicity caused by polycyclic aromatic hydrocarbons (PAHs). PLoS One 15. https://doi.org/10.1371/journal.pone.0231359
14. Chaudhry H, Nisar N, Mehmood S, Iqbal M, Nazir A, Yasir M (2020) Indian Mustard Brassica juncea efficiency for the accumulation, tolerance and translocation of zinc from metal contaminated soil. Biocatal Agric Biotechnol 23:101489. https://doi.org/10.1016/j.bcab.2019.101489

15. Chen X, Wang J, Hayat K, Zhang D, Zhou P (2021) Small structures with big impact: multi-walled carbon nanotubes enhanced remediation efficiency in hyperaccumulator Solanum nigrum L. under cadmium and arsenic stress. Chemosphere 276. https://doi.org/10.1016/j.chemosphere.2021.130130
16. Cheng P, Zhang S, Wang Q, Feng X, Zhang S, Sun Y, Wang F (2021) Contribution of nano-zero-valent iron and arbuscular mycorrhizal fungi to phytoremediation of heavy metal-contaminated soil. Nanomaterials 11. https://doi.org/10.3390/nano11051264
17. Dahmani-Muller H, Van Oort F, Gélie B, Balabane M (2000) Strategies of heavy metal uptake by three plant species growing near a metal smelter. Environ Pollut 109(2):231–238. https://doi.org/10.1016/S0269-7491(99)00262-6
18. Dar FA, Pirzadah TB, Malik B (2020) Accumulation of heavy metals in medicinal and aromatic plants. In: Aftab T, Hakeem KR (eds) Plant micronutrients. Springer International Publishing, pp 113–127. https://doi.org/10.1007/978-3-030-49856-6_6
19. Daryabeigi Zand A, Vaezi Heir A, Khodaei H (2021) Integrated remediation approach for metal polluted soils using plants, nanomaterials and root-associated bacteria. J Dispers Sci Technol 43:1674–1688. https://doi.org/10.1080/01932691.2021.1878900
20. Deng B, Carter RA, Cheng Y, Liu Y, Eddy L, Wyss KM, Ucak-Astarlioglu MG, Luong DX, Gao X, JeBailey K, Kittrell C, Xu S, Jana D, Torres MA, Braam J, Tour JM (2023) High-temperature electrothermal remediation of multi-pollutants in soil. Nat Commun 14https://doi.org/10.1038/s41467-023-41898-z
21. Dou C, Cui H, Zhang W, Yu W, Sheng X, Zheng X (2023) Copper and cadmium accumulation and phytoextraction potential of native and cultivated plants growing around a copper smelter. Agronomy 13:2874. https://doi.org/10.3390/agronomy13122874
22. El-Nagar DA, Abdel-Halim KY (2021) Remediation of heavy metals in contaminated soil by using nano-bentonite, nano-hydroxyapatite, and nano-composite. Land Degrad Dev 32:4562–4573. https://doi.org/10.1002/ldr.4052
23. Ertani A, Mietto A, Borin M, Nardi S (2017) Chromium in agricultural soils and crops: a review. Water Air Soil Pollut 228. https://doi.org/10.1007/s11270-017-3356-y
24. Etesami H (2018) Bacterial mediated alleviation of heavy metal stress and decreased accumulation of metals in plant tissues: mechanisms and future prospects. Ecotoxicol Environ Saf 147:175–191. https://doi.org/10.1016/j.ecoenv.2017.08.032
25. Faiz S, Yasin NA, Khan WU, Shah AA, Akram W, Ahmad A, Ali A, Naveed NH, Riaz L (2022) Role of magnesium oxide nanoparticles in the mitigation of lead-induced stress in *Daucus carota*: modulation in polyamines and antioxidant enzymes. Int J Phytoremediation 24:364–372. https://doi.org/10.1080/15226514.2021.1949263
26. Fajardo C, Sánchez-Fortún S, Costa G, Nande M, Botías P, García-Cantalejo J, Mengs G, Martín M (2020) Evaluation of nanoremediation strategy in a Pb, Zn and Cd contaminated soil. Sci Total Environ 706:136041. https://doi.org/10.1016/j.scitotenv.2019.136041
27. Farooq MA, Hannan F, Islam F, Ayyaz A, Zhang N, Chen W, Zhang K, Huang Q, Xu L, Zhou W (2022) The potential of nanomaterials for sustainable modern agriculture: present findings and future perspectives. Environ Sci Nano 9:1926–1951. https://doi.org/10.1039/D1EN01124C
28. Feng NX, Yu J, Zhao HM, Cheng YT, Mo CH, Cai QY, Li YW, Li H, Wong MH (2017) Efficient phytoremediation of organic contaminants in soils using plant–endophyte partnerships. Sci Total Environ 583:352–368. https://doi.org/10.1016/j.scitotenv.2017.01.075
29. Gangwar P, Johri P, Datta R, Singh S, Trivedi M (2023) Overview on 1 phytopharmaceuticals and Biotechnology of herbal plants. In: Phytopharmaceuticals and biotechnology of herbal plants. CRC Press, pp 1–17
30. Gao H, Wu M, Liu H, Xu Y, Liu Z (2022) Effect of petroleum hydrocarbon pollution levels on the soil microecosystem and ecological function. Environ Pollut 293:118511. https://doi.org/10.1016/J.ENVPOL.2021.118511
31. Ghosh M (2005) A review on phytoremediation of heavy metals and utilization of its byproducts. Appl Ecol Environ Res 3(1):1–18. https://doi.org/10.15666/aeer/0301_001018

32. Gil-Díaz M, Pinilla P, Alonso J, Lobo MC (2017) Viability of a nanoremediation process in single or multi-metal(loid) contaminated soils. J Hazard Mater 321:812–819. https://doi.org/10.1016/j.jhazmat.2016.09.071
33. Gong X, Huang D, Liu Y, Zeng G, Wang R, Xu P, Zhang C, Cheng M, Xue W, Chen S (2019) Roles of multiwall carbon nanotubes in phytoremediation: Cadmium uptake and oxidative burst in: *Boehmeria nivea* (L.) Gaudich. Environ Sci Nano 6:851–862. https://doi.org/10.1039/c8en00723c
34. González-Moscoso M, Juárez-Maldonado A, Cadenas-Pliego G, Meza-Figueroa D, SenGupta B, Martínez-Villegas N (2022) Silicon nanoparticles decrease arsenic translocation and mitigate phytotoxicity in tomato plants. Environ Sci Pollut Res. https://doi.org/10.1007/s11356-021-17665-2
35. Grifoni M, Rosellini I, Angelini P, Petruzzelli G, Pezzarossa B (2020) The effect of residual hydrocarbons in soil following oil spillages on the growth of *Zea mays* plants. Environ Pollut 265. https://doi.org/10.1016/j.envpol.2020.114950
36. Guarino F, Miranda A, Castiglione S, Cicatelli A (2020) Arsenic phytovolatilization and epigenetic modifications in *Arundo donax* L. assisted by a PGPR consortium. Chemosphere 251:126310. https://doi.org/10.1016/j.chemosphere.2020.126310
37. Gurajala HK, Cao X, Tang L, Ramesh TM, Lu M, Yang X (2019) Comparative assessment of Indian mustard (*Brassica juncea* L.) genotypes for phytoremediation of Cd and Pb contaminated soils. Environmental Pollution 254:113085. https://doi.org/10.1016/j.envpol.2019.113085
38. Haider FU, Ejaz M, Cheema SA, Khan MI, Zhao B, Liqun C, Salim MA, Naveed M, Khan N, Núñez-Delgado A, Mustafa A (2021) Phytotoxicity of petroleum hydrocarbons: sources, impacts and remediation strategies. Environ Res 197:111031. https://doi.org/10.1016/j.envres.2021.111031
39. Hegazy AK, Hussein ZS, Mohamed NH, Safwat G, El-Dessouky MA, Imbrea I, Imbrea F (2023) Assessment of *Vinca rosea* (Apocynaceae) potentiality for remediation of crude petroleum oil pollution of soil. Sustainability (Switzerland) 15. https://doi.org/10.3390/su151411046
40. Hidalgo J, Anza M, Epelde L, Becerril JM, Garbisu C (2022) Zero-valent iron nanoparticles and organic amendment assisted rhizoremediation of mixed contaminated soil using *Brassica napus*. Environ Technol Innov 28. https://doi.org/10.1016/j.eti.2022.102621
41. Hong-Bo S, Li-Ye C, Cheng-Jiang R, Hua L, Dong-Gang G, Wei-Xiang L (2010) Understanding molecular mechanisms for improving phytoremediation of heavy metal-contaminated soils. Crit Rev Biotechnol 30(1):23–30. https://doi.org/10.3109/07388550903208057
42. Hu Q, Li J, Wang Y, Huang P, He X (2023) Evaluation and source analysis of heavy metal pollution in grassland soils under different management modes in Altay, Xinjiang. Agronomy 13. https://doi.org/10.3390/agronomy13102621
43. Hu X, Wang J, Lv Y, Liu X, Zhong J, Cui X, Zhang M, Ma D, Yan X, Zhu X (2021) effects of heavy metals/metalloids and soil properties on microbial communities in farmland in the vicinity of a metals smelter. Front Microbiol 12. https://doi.org/10.3389/fmicb.2021.707786
44. Huang D, Qin X, Peng Z, Liu Y, Gong X, Zeng G, Huang C, Cheng M, Xue W, Wang X, Hu Z (2018) Nanoscale zero-valent iron assisted phytoremediation of Pb in sediment: impacts on metal accumulation and antioxidative system of *Lolium perenne*. Ecotoxicol Environ Saf 153:229–237. https://doi.org/10.1016/j.ecoenv.2018.01.060
45. Huang M, Zhu Y, Li Z, Huang B, Luo N, Liu C, Zeng G (2016) Compost as a soil amendment to remediate heavy metal-contaminated agricultural soil: mechanisms, efficacy, problems, and strategies. Water Air Soil Pollut 227
46. Hunt LJ, Duca D, Dan T, Knopper LD (2019) Petroleum hydrocarbon (PHC) uptake in plants: a literature review. Environ Pollut 245:472–484. https://doi.org/10.1016/j.envpol.2018.11.012
47. Ikhajiagbe B, Osayamen KI (2019) Application of silver nanoparticles during bioremediation of petroleum hydrocarbon-polluted soil by *Eleusine indica*—inhibition or improvement? Beckley. Res J Chem Sci 9:7–16

48. Iqbal S, Xu J, Allen SD, Khan S, Nadir S, Arif MS, Yasmeen T (2020) Unraveling consequences of soil micro- and nano-plastic pollution on soil-plant system: implications for nitrogen (N) cycling and soil microbial activity. Chemosphere 260:127578. https://doi.org/10.1016/j.chemosphere.2020.127578
49. Isinkaye MO, OlaOlorun OA, Chandasekaran A, Adekeye AS, Dada TE, Tamilarasi A, Sathish V, Khandaker MU, Almujally A, Tamam N, Sulieman A (2023) Quantification of radiological hazards associated with natural radionuclides in soil, granite and charnockite rocks at selected fields in Ekiti State, Nigeria. Heliyon, e22451. https://doi.org/10.1016/j.heliyon.2023.e22451
50. Jabborova D, Davranov K, Jabbarov Z, Bhowmik SN, Ercisli S, Danish S, Datta R (2022) Dual inoculation of plant growth-promoting *Bacillus endophyticus* and *Funneliformis mosseae* improves plant growth and soil properties in ginger. ACS Omega 7(39):34779–34788. https://doi.org/10.1021/acsomega.2c02353
51. Jehan S, Khattak SA, Khan S, Ali L, Waqas M, Kamran A (2023) Comparative efficacy of Parthenium hysterophorus (L.) derived biochar and iron doped zinc oxide nanoparticle on heavy metals (HMs) mobility and its uptake by *Triticum aestivum* (L.) in chromite mining contaminated soils. Int J Phytoremediation 25:1890–1900. https://doi.org/10.1080/15226514.2023.2204968
52. Khan AG (2020) Promises and potential of in situ nano-phytoremediation strategy to mycorrhizo-remediate heavy metal contaminated soils using non-food bioenergy crops (*Vetiver zizinoides* & *Cannabis sativa*). Int J Phytoremediation 22:900–915. https://doi.org/10.1080/15226514.2020.1774504
53. Khare P, Kishore K, Sharma DK (2017) A study on the standardization parameters of *Cassia angustifolia*. Asian J Pharm Clin Res 10(7):329–332
54. Klik B, Brtnicky M, Jaskulska I, Gusiatin MZ, Jaskulski D, Holatko J, Baltazar T, Liniauskiene E, Radziemska M (2023) Unlocking the saponite potential in aided phytostabilisation of multi-metal-contaminated soils. Minerals 13:1354. https://doi.org/10.3390/min13111354
55. Koptsik GN (2014) Problems and prospects concerning the phytoremediation of heavy metal polluted soils: a review. Eurasian Soil Sci 47(9):923–939. https://doi.org/10.1134/S1064229314090075
56. Kotoky R, Pandey P (2020) Rhizosphere mediated biodegradation of benzo(A)pyrene by surfactin producing soil bacilli applied through Melia azedarach rhizosphere. Int J Phytorem 22(4):363–372. https://doi.org/10.1080/15226514.2019.1663486
57. Kumar B, Smita K, Cumbal Flores L (2017) Plant mediated detoxification of mercury and lead. Arab J Chem 10:S2335–S2342. https://doi.org/10.1016/j.arabjc.2013.08.010
58. Kumar P, Tokas J, Singal HR (2019) Amelioration of Chromium VI Toxicity in Sorghum (*Sorghum bicolor* L.) using Glycine Betaine. Sci Rep 9. https://doi.org/10.1038/s41598-019-52479-w
59. Kuppusamy S, Maddela NR, Megharaj M, Venkateswarlu K (2020) Ecological impacts of total petroleum hydrocarbons. Total petroleum hydrocarbons. Springer International Publishing, Cham, pp 95–138
60. Li C, Yang G, Liu Z, Cai J (2022) Overview of phytoremediation technology for heavy metal contaminated soil. In: E3S web of conferences, vol 350, p 01006. https://doi.org/10.1051/e3sconf/202235001006
61. Li C, Zhou K, Qin W, Tian C, Qi M, Yan X, Han W (2019) A review on heavy metals contamination in soil: effects, sources, and remediation techniques. Soil Sediment Contam 28:380–394. https://doi.org/10.1080/15320383.2019.1592108
62. Liu H, Wang M, Chen G, Zhou H, Dong J, Yang L, Li T, Meng Z, Gu R, Gan H, Wu Z, Liu S, Sun Y, Yuan Y, Dou G (2023) Effects of radon exposure on gut microbiota and its metabolites short-chain fatty acids in mice. Toxicology 486. https://doi.org/10.1016/j.tox.2023.153449
63. Liu J, Wang Y, Wang M, Feng X, Liu R, Xue Z, Zhou Q (2023) Improving the uptake of PAHs by the ornamental plant *Sedum spectabile* using nano-$SiO_2$ and nano-$CeO_2$. Sci Total Environ 870:161808. https://doi.org/10.1016/J.SCITOTENV.2023.161808
64. Liu W, Li Y, Feng Y, Qiao J, Zhao H, Xie J, Fang Y, Shen S, Liang S (2020) The effectiveness of nanobiochar for reducing phytotoxicity and improving soil remediation in cadmium-contaminated soil. Sci Rep 10. https://doi.org/10.1038/s41598-020-57954-3

65. Liu YR, van der Heijden MGA, Riedo J, Sanz-Lazaro C, Eldridge DJ, Bastida F, Moreno-Jiménez E, Zhou XQ, Hu HW, He JZ, Moreno JL, Abades S, Alfaro F, Bamigboye AR, Berdugo M, Blanco-Pastor JL, de los Ríos A, Duran J, Grebenc T, Illán JG, Makhalanyane TP, Molina-Montenegro MA, Nahberger TU, Peñaloza-Bojacá GF, Plaza C, Rey A, Rodríguez A, Siebe C, Teixido AL, Casado-Coy N, Trivedi P, Torres-Díaz C, Verma JP, Mukherjee A, Zeng XM, Wang L, Wang J, Zaady E, Zhou X, Huang Q, Tan W, Zhu YG, Rillig MC, Delgado-Baquerizo M (2023) Soil contamination in nearby natural areas mirrors that in urban greenspaces worldwide. Nat Commun 14. https://doi.org/10.1038/s41467-023-37428-6
66. Lombi E, Tearall KL, Howarth JR, Zhao FJ, Hawkesford MJ, McGrath SP (2002) Influence of iron status on cadmium and zinc uptake by different ecotypes of the hyperaccumulator *Thlaspi caerulescens*. Plant Physiol 128(4):1359–1367. https://doi.org/10.1104/pp.010731
67. Ma C, Han L, Shang H, Hao Y, Xu X, White JC, Wang Z, Xing B (2023) Nanomaterials in agricultural soils: ecotoxicity and application. Curr Opin Environ Sci Health 31:100432. https://doi.org/10.1016/j.coesh.2022.100432
68. Ma M, Wang R, Xu L, Xu M, Liu S (2020) Emerging health risks and underlying toxicological mechanisms of uranium contamination: lessons from the past two decades. Environ Int 145:106107. https://doi.org/10.1016/j.envint.2020.106107
69. Maddala VKS, Singh S, Bandi J (2024) Soil properties influencing nutrient signaling in plant soil systems. In: Essential minerals in plant-soil systems. Elsevier, pp 373–393
70. Mandeng EPB, Bidjeck LMB, Bessa AZE, Ntomb YD, Wadjou JW, Doumo EPE, Dieudonné LB (2019) Contamination and risk assessment of heavy metals, and uranium of sediments in two watersheds in Abiete-Toko gold district, Southern Cameroon. Heliyon 5. https://doi.org/10.1016/j.heliyon.2019.e02591
71. Manzoor N, Ali L, AL-Huqail AA, Alghanem SMS, Al-Haithloul HAS, Abbas T, Chen G, Huan L, Liu Y, Wang G (2023) Comparative efficacy of silicon and iron oxide nanoparticles towards improving the plant growth and mitigating arsenic toxicity in wheat (*Triticum aestivum* L.). Ecotoxicol Environ Saf 264. https://doi.org/10.1016/j.ecoenv.2023.115382
72. Marcon L, Oliveras J, Puntes VF (2021) *In situ* nanoremediation of soils and groundwaters from the nanoparticle's standpoint: a review. Sci Total Environ 791:148324. https://doi.org/10.1016/j.scitotenv.2021.148324
73. Mbachu O, Jenkins G, Kaparaju P, Pratt C (2021) The rise of artificial soil carbon inputs: reviewing microplastic pollution effects in the soil environment. Sci Total Environ 780:146569. https://doi.org/10.1016/j.scitotenv.2021.146569
74. McLaughlin MJ, Smolders E, Zhao FJ, Grant C, Montalvo D (2021) Managing cadmium in agricultural systems. In: Advances in agronomy. Academic Press Inc., pp 1–129
75. Meddya S, Meshram S, Sarkar D, Datta R, Singh S, Avinash G, Thulasinathan T (2023) Plant stomata: an unrealized possibility in plant defense against invading pathogens and stress tolerance. Plants 12(19):3380. https://doi.org/10.3390/plants12193380
76. Meng F, Yang X, Riksen M, Xu M, Geissen V (2021) Response of common bean (*Phaseolus vulgaris* L.) growth to soil contaminated with microplastics. Sci Total Environ 755:142516. https://doi.org/10.1016/j.scitotenv.2020.142516
77. Meyer L, Guyot S, Chalot M, Capelli N (2023) The potential of microorganisms as biomonitoring and bioremediation tools for mercury-contaminated soils. Ecotoxicol Environ Saf 262:115185. https://doi.org/10.1016/j.ecoenv.2023.115185
78. Moameri M, Abbasi Khalaki M (2019) Capability of Secale montanum trusted for phytoremediation of lead and cadmium in soils amended with nano-silica and municipal solid waste compost. Environ Sci Pollut Res 26:24315–24322. https://doi.org/10.1007/s11356-017-0544-7
79. Mohamed AA, Castagna A, Ranieri A, Sanità Di Toppi L (2012) Cadmium tolerance in *Brassica juncea* roots and shoots is affected by antioxidant status and phytochelatin biosynthesis. Plant Physiol Biochem 57:15–22. https://doi.org/10.1016/j.plaphy.2012.05.002
80. Mohammed Suhail F, Adnan Hussein Z (2023) Rule of Rhizobia and Bacillus in phytoremediation of contaminated soil with diesel oil. J Saudi Soc Agric Sci. https://doi.org/10.1016/j.jssas.2023.08.003

81. Mudgal V, Raninga M, Patel D, Ankoliya D, Mudgal A (2023) A review on phytoremediation: sustainable method for removal of heavy metals. Mater Today: Proc 77:201–208. https://doi.org/10.1016/j.matpr.2022.11.261
82. Mustafa K, Shakeel I, Kanwal J, Farrukh S, Mussaddiq S, Saddiq N, Younas M (2022) Nano-phytoremediation technology in environmental remediation. In: Phytoremediation technology for the removal of heavy metals and other contaminants from soil and water, pp 433–459. https://doi.org/10.1016/B978-0-323-85763-5.00029-5
83. Navarro-León E, Oviedo-Silva J, Ruiz JM, Blasco B (2019) Possible role of HMA4a TILLING mutants of Brassica rapa in cadmium phytoremediation programs. Ecotoxicol Environ Saf 180:88–94. https://doi.org/10.1016/j.ecoenv.2019.04.081
84. Nduka JK, Umeh TC, Kelle HI, Ozoagu PC, Okafor PC (2022) Health risk assessment of radiation dose of background radionuclides in quarry soil and uptake by plants in Ezillo-Ishiagu in Ebonyi South-Eastern Nigeria. Case Stud Chem Environ Eng 6. https://doi.org/10.1016/j.cscee.2022.100269
85. Nebeská D, Trögl J, Ševců A, Špánek R, Marková K, Davis L, Burdová H, Pidlisnyuk V (2021) *Miscanthus x giganteus* role in phytodegradation and changes in bacterial community of soil contaminated by petroleum industry. Ecotoxicol Environ Saf 224:112630. https://doi.org/10.1016/j.ecoenv.2021.112630
86. Nedjimi B (2021) Phytoremediation: a sustainable environmental technology for heavy metals decontamination. SN Appl Sci 3(3):286. https://doi.org/10.1007/s42452-021-04301-4
87. O'Connor D, Hou D, Ok YS, Mulder J, Duan L, Wu Q, Wang S, Tack FMG, Rinklebe J (2019) Mercury speciation, transformation, and transportation in soils, atmospheric flux, and implications for risk management: a critical review. Environ Int 126:747–761. https://doi.org/10.1016/j.envint.2019.03.019
88. Oliveira H (2012) Chromium as an environmental pollutant: insights on induced plant toxicity. J Bot 2012:1–8. https://doi.org/10.1155/2012/375843
89. Orfano M, Perego J, Cova F, Bezuidenhout CX, Piva S, Dujardin C, Sabot B, Pierre S, Mai P, Daniel C, Bracco S, Vedda A, Comotti A, Monguzzi A (2023) Efficient radioactive gas detection by scintillating porous metal–organic frameworks. Nat Photonics 17:672–678. https://doi.org/10.1038/s41566-023-01211-2
90. Ossai IC, Ahmed A, Hassan A, Hamid FS (2020) Remediation of soil and water contaminated with petroleum hydrocarbon: a review. Environ Technol Innov 17:100526. https://doi.org/10.1016/j.eti.2019.100526
91. Pakash P, Chandran SS (2023) Nano-phytoremediation of heavy metals from soil: a critical review. Pollutants 3:360–380. https://doi.org/10.3390/pollutants3030025
92. Parveen R, Khare N, Singh S, Johri P (2023) An in silico outlook for the detection and surveillance of evolving and persistent plant pathogens. In: Detection, diagnosis and management of soil-borne phytopathogens. Springer Nature Singapore, Singapore, pp 17–40
93. Pasricha S, Mathur V, Garg A, Lenka S, Verma K, Agarwal S (2021) Molecular mechanisms underlying heavy metal uptake, translocation and tolerance in hyperaccumulators-an analysis. Environmental Challenges 4:100197. https://doi.org/10.1016/j.envc.2021.100197
94. Patani A, Patel A, Prajapati D, Khare N, Singh S (2023) Various agriculture crop plant-based bioactive compounds and their use in nanomaterial synthesis and applications. In: Nanomaterials from agricultural and horticultural products. Springer Nature Singapore, Singapore, pp 223–241
95. Patani A, Prajapati D, Shukla K, Patel M, Patani P, Patel A, Singh S (2024) Environmental stress–induced alterations in the micro-and macronutrients status of plant. In: Essential minerals in plant-soil systems. Elsevier, pp 181–195
96. Pathak KV, Keharia H (2014) Application of extracellular lipopeptide biosurfactant produced by endophytic *Bacillus subtilis* K1 isolated from aerial roots of banyan (*Ficus benghalensis*) in microbially enhanced oil recovery (MEOR). 3 Biotech 4(1):41–48. https://doi.org/10.1007/s13205-013-0119-3
97. Patowary R, Patowary K, Devi A, Kalita MC, Deka S (2017) Uptake of Total Petroleum Hydrocarbon (TPH) and Polycyclic Aromatic Hydrocarbons (PAHs) by *Oryza sativa* L. grown

in soil contaminated with crude oil. Bull Environ Contam Toxicol 98:120–126. https://doi.org/10.1007/s00128-016-1990-5
98. Patra DK, Pradhan C, Patra HK (2020) Toxic metal decontamination by phytoremediation approach: concept, challenges, opportunities and future perspectives. Environ Technol Innov 18:100672. https://doi.org/10.1016/j.eti.2020.100672
99. Prabhath RK, Sreejith SR, Nair MG, Rao DD, Pradeepkumar KS (2015) Determination of 210Po concentration in commercially available infant formulae and assessment of daily ingestion dose. J Radiat Res Appl Sci 8:470–476. https://doi.org/10.1016/j.jrras.2015.05.002
100. Qin G, Niu Z, Yu J, Li Z, Ma J, Xiang P (2021) Soil heavy metal pollution and food safety in China: effects, sources and removing technology. Chemosphere 267:129205. https://doi.org/10.1016/j.chemosphere.2020.129205
101. Rai PK (2016) Impacts of particulate matter pollution on plants: implications for environmental biomonitoring. Ecotoxicol Environ Saf 129:120–136. https://doi.org/10.1016/j.ecoenv.2016.03.012
102. Raj K, Das AP (2023) Lead pollution: impact on environment and human health and approach for a sustainable solution. Environ Chem Ecotoxicol 5:79–85. https://doi.org/10.1016/j.enceco.2023.02.001
103. Rane NR, Tapase S, Kanojia A, Watharkar A, Salama ES, Jang M, Kumar Yadav K, Amin MA, Cabral-Pinto MMS, Jadhav JP, Jeon BH (2022) Molecular insights into plant–microbe interactions for sustainable remediation of contaminated environment. Biores Technol 344:126246. https://doi.org/10.1016/j.biortech.2021.126246
104. Rashid A, Schutte BJ, Ulery A, Deyholos MK, Sanogo S, Lehnhoff EA, Beck L (2023) Heavy metal contamination in agricultural soil: environmental pollutants affecting crop health. Agronomy 13:1–30. https://doi.org/10.3390/agronomy13061521
105. Rizvi A, Zaidi A, Ameen F, Ahmed B, Alkahtani MDF, Khan MS (2020) Heavy metal induced stress on wheat: phytotoxicity and microbiological management. RSC Adv 10:38379–38403. https://doi.org/10.1039/d0ra05610c
106. Romeh AA, Ibrahim Saber RA (2020) Green nano-phytoremediation and solubility improving agents for the remediation of chlorfenapyr contaminated soil and water. J Environ Manag 260. https://doi.org/10.1016/j.jenvman.2020.110104
107. Romeh AAA (2018) Green silver nanoparticles for enhancing the phytoremediation of soil and water contaminated by fipronil and degradation products. Water Air Soil Pollut 229. https://doi.org/10.1007/s11270-018-3792-3
108. Rudnicki-Velasquez P, Boryło A, Kaczor M, Wieczorek J, Rutkowska J (2023) Study of Polonium (210Po) activity concentration in fruit wines derived from different locations in Poland. Molecules 28. https://doi.org/10.3390/molecules28010438
109. Saniewski M, Wietrzyk-Pełka P, Zalewska T, Węgrzyn MH (2022) Current radioactive fallout contamination along a trans-European gradient assessed using terricolous lichens. Chemosphere 304. https://doi.org/10.1016/j.chemosphere.2022.135281
110. Sao P, Parveen R, Khattri A, Sharma S, Tiwari N, Singh S (2022) Understanding the metabolomics of medicinal plants under environmental pollution: challenges and opportunities. In: Environmental pollution and medicinal plants, CRC Press, pp 193–205
111. Sarkar B, Mukhopadhyay R, Ramanayaka S, Bolan N, Ok YS (2021) The role of soils in the disposition, sequestration and decontamination of environmental contaminants. Philos Trans R Soc B: Biol Sci 376. https://doi.org/10.1098/rstb.2020.0177
112. Sarkar D, Rakshit A (2020) Safeguarding the fragile rice–wheat ecosystem of the Indo-Gangetic Plains through bio-priming and bioaugmentation interventions. FEMS Microbiol Ecol 96:fiaa221. https://doi.org/10.1093/femsec/fiaa221
113. Sarkar D, Shikha RS, Ganguly S, Rakshit A (2017) Management of increasing soil pollution in the ecosystem. Adv Res 12:1–9. https://doi.org/10.9734/AIR/2017/36622
114. Sethy NK, Sutar AK, Rath P, Jha VN, Ravi PM, Triphathi RM (2015) A review of radio chemical analysis and estimation of $^{210}$Po in soil matrices. J Radiat Res Appl Sci 590–596. https://doi.org/10.1016/j.jrras.2015.07.001

115. Shah AA, Nawaz A, Kanwal L, Hasan F, Khan S, Badshah M (2015) Degradation of poly(ε-caprolactone) by a thermophilic bacterium *Ralstonia* sp. Strain MRL-TL isolated from hot spring. Int Biodeterior Biodegradation 98:35–42. https://doi.org/10.1016/j.ibiod.2014.11.017
116. Sharifi P, Bidabadi SS, Zaid A, Abdel Latef AAH (2021) Efficacy of multi-walled carbon nanotubes in regulating growth performance, total glutathione and redox state of *Calendula officinalis* L. cultivated on Pb and Cd polluted soil. Ecotoxicol Environ Saf 213:112051. https://doi.org/10.1016/j.ecoenv.2021.112051
117. Sharma A, Kapoor D, Wang J, Shahzad B, Kumar V, Bali AS, Jasrotia S, Zheng B, Yuan H, Yan D (2020) Chromium bioaccumulation and its impacts on plants: an overview. Plants 9(1):100. https://doi.org/10.3390/plants9010100
118. Sharma S, Singh B, Manchanda VK (2015) Phytoremediation: role of terrestrial plants and aquatic macrophytes in the remediation of radionuclides and heavy metal contaminated soil and water. Environ Sci Pollut Res 22(2):946–962. https://doi.org/10.1007/s11356-014-3635-8
119. Shehzad J, Khan I, Zaheer S, Farooq A, Chaudhari SK, Mustafa G (2023) Insights into heavy metal tolerance mechanisms of Brassica species: physiological, biochemical, and molecular interventions. Environ Sci Pollut Res 30(50):108448–108476. https://doi.org/10.1007/s11356-023-29979-4
120. Singh A, Sengar RS, Singh AK, Singh S, Kumar A, Ahmad K (2019) Impact of genetic engineering on agriculture food crops. Biotech Today: Int J Biol Sci 9(1):17–24. https://doi.org/10.5958/2322-0996.2019.00002.4
121. Singh PM, Tiwari A, Maity D, Saha S (2022) Recent progress of nanomaterials in sustainable agricultural applications. J Mater Sci 57:10836–10862. https://doi.org/10.1007/s10853-022-07259-9
122. Srivastav A, Yadav KK, Yadav S, Gupta N, Singh JK, Katiyar R, Kumar V (2019) Nano-phytoremediation of pollutants from contaminated soil environment: current scenario and future prospects. In: Phytoremediation: management of environmental contaminants. Springer International Publishing, pp 383–401
123. Tahir M, Khan MB, Shahid M, Ahmad I, Khalid U, Akram M, Dawood A, Kamran M (2022) Metal-tolerant Pantoea sp. WP-5 and organic manures enhanced root exudation and phytostabilization of cadmium in the rhizosphere of maize. Environ Sci Pollut Res 29(4):6026–6039. https://doi.org/10.1007/s11356-021-16018-3
124. Thiele-Bruhn S (2021) The role of soils in provision of genetic, medicinal and biochemical resources. Philos Trans R Soc B: Biol Sci 376:20200183. https://doi.org/10.1098/rstb.2020.0183
125. Tomczyk P, Wdowczyk A, Wiatkowska B, Szymańska-Pulikowska A (2023) Assessment of heavy metal contamination of agricultural soils in Poland using contamination indicators. Ecol Indic 156. https://doi.org/10.1016/j.ecolind.2023.111161
126. Tungare K, Shahu R, Zambare V, Agarwal P, Jobby R, Nisar N, Jha P (2022) Toxicity mitigation of textile dye reactive blue 4 by hairy roots of *Helianthus annuus* and testing its effect in in vivo model systems. Biomed Res Int 958939. https://doi.org/10.1155/2022/1958939
127. Ukaogo PO, Ewuzie U, Onwuka CV (2020) Environmental pollution: causes, effects, and the remedies. In: Microorganisms for sustainable environment and health. Elsevier, pp 419–429
128. Ullah R, Ullah Z, Iqbal J, Chalgham W, Ahmad A (2023) Aspartic acid-based nano-copper induces resilience in Zea mays to applied lead stress via conserving photosynthetic pigments and triggering the antioxidant biosystem. Sustainability (Switzerland) 15. https://doi.org/10.3390/su151612186
129. Urushadze TF, Manakhov DV (2017) Radioactive contamination of the soils of Georgia. Ann Agrar Sci 15:375–379. https://doi.org/10.1016/j.aasci.2017.07.009
130. Vasilachi IC, Stoleru V, Gavrilescu M (2023) Analysis of heavy metal impacts on cereal crop growth and development in contaminated soils. Agriculture (Switzerland) 13(10):1983. https://doi.org/10.3390/agriculture13101983
131. Verma A, Roy A, Bharadvaja N (2021) Remediation of heavy metals using nanophytoremediation. In: Advanced oxidation processes for effluent treatment plants, pp 273–296. https://doi.org/10.1016/B978-0-12-821011-6.00013-X

132. Verma N, Sao P, Srivastava A, Singh S (2021) Physiological and molecular responses to drought, submergence and excessive watering in plants. In: Harsh environment and plant resilience. Springer, Cham. pp 305–321. https://doi.org/10.1007/978-3-030-65912-7_12
133. Vishwakarma SK, Ilyas T, Shahid M, Malviya D, Kumar S, Singh S, Singh HV (2024). Bacillus spp.: nature's gift to agriculture and humankind. In: Applications of bacillus and bacillus derived genera in agriculture, biotechnology and beyond. Springer Nature Singapore, Singapore, pp 1–36
134. Wang J, Lu X, Zhang J, Ouyang Y, Wei G, Xiong Y (2020) Rice intercropping with alligator flag (*Thalia dealbata*): a novel model to produce safe cereal grains while remediating cadmium contaminated paddy soil. J Hazard Mater 394:122505. https://doi.org/10.1016/j.jhazmat.2020.122505
135. Wang L, Cheng Y, Naidu R, Bowman M (2021) The key factors for the fate and transport of petroleum hydrocarbons in soil with related *in/ex situ* measurement methods: an overview. Front Environ Sci 9. https://doi.org/10.3389/fenvs.2021.756404
136. Wang X, Jiang J, Dou F, Sun W, Ma X (2021) Simultaneous mitigation of arsenic and cadmium accumulation in rice (*Oryza sativa* L.) seedlings by silicon oxide nanoparticles under different water management schemes. Paddy Water Environ 19:569–584. https://doi.org/10.1007/s10333-021-00855-6
137. Wang YY, Chai LY, Yang WC (2019) Arsenic distribution and pollution characteristics. In: Arsenic pollution control in nonferrous metallurgy. Springer Singapore, pp 1–15
138. Wani KI, Naeem M, Aftab T (2022) Chromium in plant-soil nexus: speciation, uptake, transport and sustainable remediation techniques. Environ Pollut 315:120350. https://doi.org/10.1016/j.envpol.2022.120350
139. Wu Y, Cheng Z, Wu C, Zhao H, Bao P, Cui X (2023) Water conditions and arbuscular mycorrhizal symbiosis affect the phytoremediation of petroleum-contaminated soil by Phragmites Australis. Environ Technol Innov 32:103437. https://doi.org/10.1016/j.eti.2023.103437
140. Xie X, Li D, Yan J, Pei J, Wu W, Liu Z, Ding X (2023) Complex resistivity spectrum of pollutant soils with low-concentration heavy metals. Heliyon 9. https://doi.org/10.1016/j.heliyon.2023.e20541
141. Xoubi N (2020) Assessment of environmental radioactive surface contamination from a hypothetical nuclear research reactor accident. Heliyon 6. https://doi.org/10.1016/j.heliyon.2020.e04968
142. Yang Y, Ge Y, Zeng H, Zhou X, Peng L, Zeng Q (2017) Phytoextraction of cadmium-contaminated soil and potential of regenerated tobacco biomass for recovery of cadmium. Sci Rep 7. https://doi.org/10.1038/s41598-017-05834-8
143. Zand A, Tabrizi AM, Heir AV (2020) Co-application of biochar and titanium dioxide nanoparticles to promote remediation of antimony from soil by Sorghum bicolor: metal uptake and plant response. Heliyon 6. https://doi.org/10.1016/j.heliyon.2020.e04669
144. Zand AD, Mikaeili Tabrizi A, Vaezi Heir A (2020) Application of titanium dioxide nanoparticles to promote phytoremediation of Cd-polluted soil: contribution of PGPR inoculation. Bioremediat J 24:171–189. https://doi.org/10.1080/10889868.2020.1799929
145. Zand AD, Tabrizi AM, Heir AV (2020) Incorporation of biochar and nanomaterials to assist remediation of heavy metals in soil using plant species. Environ Technol Innov 20. https://doi.org/10.1016/j.eti.2020.101134
146. Zeng D, Pu G, Chen X, Wang K, Mo L, Liao J (2023) Phytoremediation of arsenic contaminated soils by *Arundo donax* L. enhanced with Earth Total Support (ETS). Sustain Chem Environ 3:100036. https://doi.org/10.1016/j.scenv.2023.100036
147. Zeng X, Xu H, Lu J, Chen Q, Li W, Wu L, Tang J, Ma L (2020) The immobilization of soil cadmium by the combined amendment of bacteria and hydroxyapatite. Sci Rep 10. https://doi.org/10.1038/s41598-020-58259-1
148. Zhang L, Wen A, Wu X, Pan X, Wu N, Chen X, Chen Y, Mao D, Chen L, Luan S (2019) Molecular identification of the magnesium transport gene family in *Brassica napus*. Plant Physiol Biochem 136:204–214. https://doi.org/10.1016/j.plaphy.2019.01.017

149. Zhang T, Liu Y, Zhong S, Zhang L (2020) AOPs-based remediation of petroleum hydrocarbons-contaminated soils: efficiency, influencing factors and environmental impacts. Chemosphere 246. https://doi.org/10.1016/j.chemosphere.2019.125726
150. Zhang XD, Zhao KX, Yang ZM (2018) Identification of genomic ATP binding cassette (ABC) transporter genes and Cd-responsive ABCs in *Brassica napus*. Gene 664:139–151. https://doi.org/10.1016/j.gene.2018.04.060
151. Zhu Y, Xu F, Liu Q, Chen M, Liu X, Wang Y, Sun Y, Zhang L (2019) Nanomaterials and plants: positive effects, toxicity and the remediation of metal and metalloid pollution in soil. Sci Total Environ 662:414–421. https://doi.org/10.1016/j.scitotenv.2019.01.234
152. Zine H, Midhat L, Hakkou R, El Adnani M, Ouhammou A (2020) Guidelines for a phytomanagement plan by the phytostabilization of mining wastes. Scientific African 10:e00654. https://doi.org/10.1016/j.sciaf.2020.e00654
153. Zou J, Song F, Lu Y, Zhuge Y, Niu Y, Lou Y, Pan H, Zhang P, Pang L (2021) Phytoremediation potential of wheat intercropped with different densities of Sedum plumbizincicola in soil contaminated with cadmium and zinc. Chemosphere 276:130223. https://doi.org/10.1016/j.chemosphere.2021.130223
154. Zulfiqar U, Farooq M, Hussain S, Maqsood M, Hussain M, Ishfaq M, Ahmad M, Anjum MZ (2019) Lead toxicity in plants: impacts and remediation. J Environ Manag 250:109557. https://doi.org/10.1016/j.jenvman.2019.109557

# Energy Aspects

# Role of Nanocomposites in Bioenergy Production

**Zhihao Yu, Kai Yan, Jingfei Wang, Run Jing, and Xuebin Lu**

**Abstract** As one of the environmentally friendly and renewable carbon resources, biomass feedstocks can be further valorized into various high-end chemicals and liquid biofuels through chemical catalysis. To date, bioenergy is emerging as a promising candidate to replace the utilization of non-renewable fossil fuels. The development of biomass energy production technologies is seen as an important strategy for human society to alleviate its huge dependence on non-renewable resources and to avoid excessive emissions of greenhouse gases. Nanocomposites play an important role in biomass energy production owing to their modifiable catalyst nanostructures, versatile active sites and their controllable catalytic effects. In this chapter, we intend to demonstrate the key catalytic role of nanocomposites for the catalytic synthesis of levulinic acid esters derived from biomass feedstocks, valeric biofuels and furan-based biofuels, which are considered to be carbon-based bioenergy molecules with promising applications. The viewpoints offered herein this chapter might be conducive to the theoretical perception of the key role of multifunctional active sites of nanocomposites and the scientific design of novel nanocomposites for the next-generation bioenergy production.

**Keywords** Heterogeneous catalysis · Biomass · Nanocomposites · Bioenergy · Multifunctional catalysis

---

Z. Yu · K. Yan · J. Wang · R. Jing · X. Lu (✉)
School of Environmental Science and Engineering, Tianjin University, Tianjin, P.R. China
e-mail: xbltju@tju.edu.cn

X. Lu
School of Ecology and Environment, Tibet University, Lhasa, P.R. China



D. Jabborova et al. (eds.), *Nanomaterials in Agroforestry Systems*, Smart Nanomaterials Technology, https://doi.org/10.1007/978-981-96-1337-3_16

## 1 Introduction

With the growing exhaustion of non-renewable fossil resources as well as the worsening prominence of worldwide energy crisis, the development of alternative energy sources is of great practical importance. Biomass, the only renewable carbon resource, is the one that holds the most promise for replacing fossil resources, which can serve as a feedstock to manufacture high quality liquid fuels and a broad range of oxygenated chemical products for greener industrial production. Chemical catalysis is recognized as a promising approach for the upgrading of biomass feedstocks and their derived platform molecules towards value-added biofuels (including fuel additives). Rational design of novel multifunctional catalytic materials is pivotal for achieving a high productivity of bioenergy products from biomass-derived carbon-based molecules.

Nanocomposites constitute a multi-phase solid substance comprising two or more types of materials that have differing properties, both physically and chemically, at least one of which is at a nanoscale. The unique force, thermal, acoustic, optical, electrical and magnetic properties of nanocomposites allow them to show promising applications in research areas such as catalysis, environment and energy. The nanostructures of nanocomposites are highly tunable, which allows them to exhibit geometrical and electronic structures that can be flexibly modulated. Such features of nanocomposites enable them to respond precisely to specific catalytic needs through rational design and tailor-made engineering. Therefore, nanocomposites are considered promising for catalytic biomass conversion with complex catalytic purposes.

In this chapter, we present in detail the applications of nanocomposites in bioenergy production with three representative biofuel molecules, namely levulinic acid esters, valeric esters and furan-based biofuels, as typical cases. In particular, catalytic synthesis routes for aforementioned biofuel molecules from different biomass feedstocks are presented, and the catalytic effects of nanocomposite active sites and synergistic effects between multiple active sites are deciphered. The facilitating roles of acid sites (including multi-acid site synergy), metal sites (including multi-metal site synergy), metal–acid site synergy and metal-support synergy have been widely involved in this chapter. The viewpoints offered herein might be conducive to the theoretical perception of the key role of multifunctional active sites of nanocomposites and the scientific design of novel nanocomposites for the next-generation bioenergy production.

# 2 Nanocomposites-Promoted Catalytic Synthesis of Levulinate Ester Biofuels

## 2.1 Synthetic Mechanism of Levulinate Esters

It is practically feasible to obtain ethyl levulinate from biomass sugars (cellulose, glucose, fructose), furans (furfural and furfuryl alcohol), and levulinic acid, through complex tandem reactions. In general, biomass is first depolymerized into sugars and then dehydrated into furan compounds, and subsequently converted into ethyl levulinate through steps involving etherification, isomerization, dehydration and ring-opening steps (Fig. 1). Biomass polysaccharides like cellulose require catalysts with strong acid sites in their reactions, with some processes require Brønsted acid sites and others requiring synergistic interactions between different acid sites in response to a multi-step tandem reaction for the formation of ethyl levulinate, as detailed below. In addition, ethyl levulinate yields can be more easily obtained from biomass-derived levulinic acid. As shown in Fig. 2, Pasquale et al. [49] produced ethyl levulinate using biomass-derived levulinic acid as the initial feedstock. The esterification of levulinic acid can be referred to as a Fischer esterification reaction in simple terms. First, levulinic acid is adsorbed on the catalyst's Brønsted acid sites to form an intermediate. The carbonyl carbon of the levulinic acid's intermediate is highly electrophilic leading to easy reaction with the nucleophilic oxygen atom of ethanol to form the carbonyl ion. The carbonyl ion then forms a new carbonyl ion by proton transfer, followed immediately by dehydration and deprotonation of the previous carbonyl ion to give the ester [25, 47].

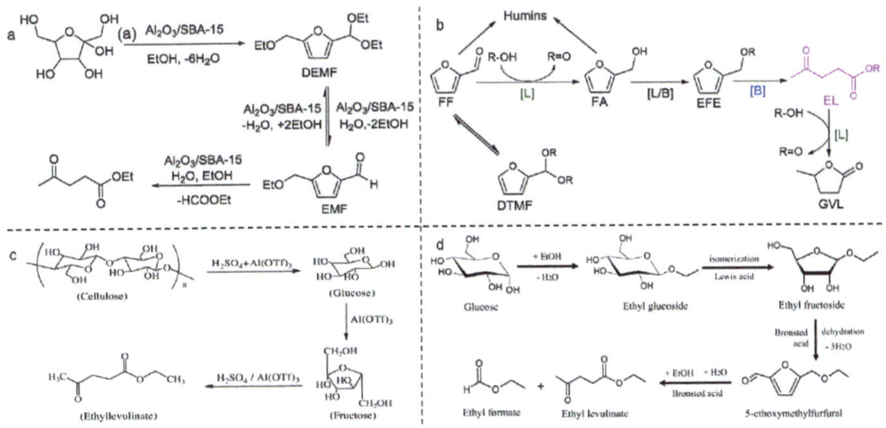


**Fig. 1** **a** The fructose conversion into ethyl levulinate [3]. **b** Proposed reaction pathway of conversion furfural into ethyl levulinate in ethanol [32]. **c** The cellulose conversion to ethyl levulinate [9]. **d** Plausible mechanism pathway of glucose conversion to ethyl levulinate [73]

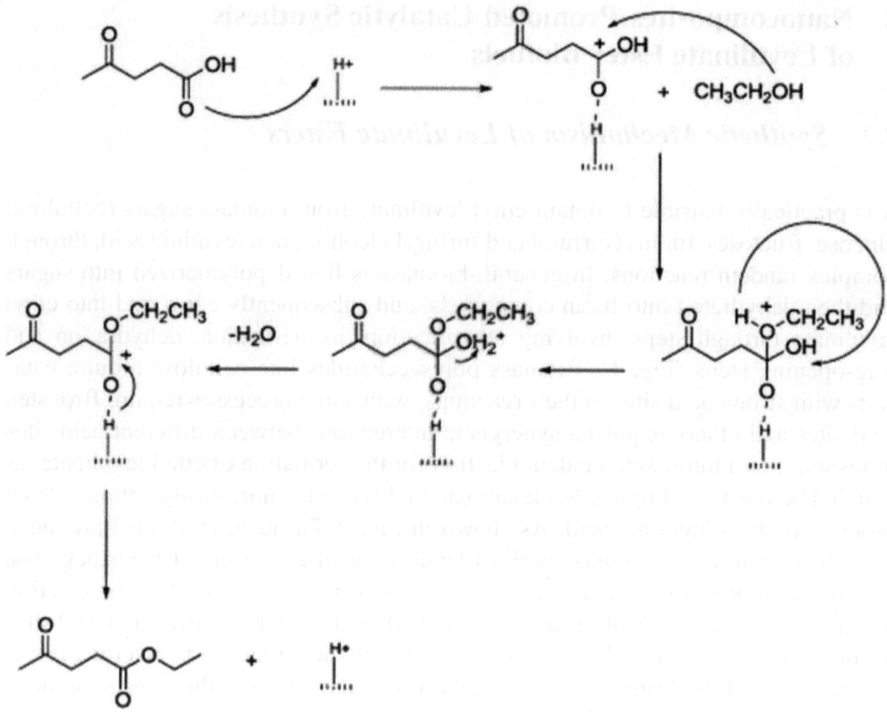

Fig. 2 Proposed mechanism for levulinic acid esterification [49]

## 2.2 Synthesis of Levulinic Acid Esters from Levulinic Acid

Ethyl levulinate can be easily synthesized via the esterification of levulinic acid. The conversion of levulinic acid can be effectively promoted by catalysts containing Brønsted acid sites [27, 45, 49, 52]. The catalytic results of various catalysts have been sorted out in Table 1. Nandiwale et al. [45] used the desilicated ZSM-5 loaded dodecyl phosphate catalyst for the esterification of levulinic acid. The conversion of levulinic acid was observed to increase from 28 to 94% when the loading of dodecyl phosphate was increased from 0 to 15% (Entry 1, Table 1). It was found that this could be ascribed to the remarkable increments in total acidity (43.14–84.31%). Pasquale et al. [49] prepared silica-containing Wells–Dawson heteropolysaccharide for the esterification reaction to ethyl levulinate (Fig. 3). It was found that the doping of phosphotungstic acid improved the acid strength, thus ensuring the efficient conversion of LA (Entry 2, Table 1). Kong et al. [27] also demonstrated that the use of commercially available silica spheres modified with silicotungstic acid can effectively facilitate the synthesis of ethyl levulinate. The experimental results showed that the increase in the dosage of silicotungstic acid increased the yield of ethyl levulinate (Entry 3–6, Table 1). Ramli et al. [52] prepared phosphotungstic acid/$ZrO_2$ (loading amounts = 15, 20, 25 wt.%) catalysts for the formation of levulinic acid esters. The 20 wt.% HPW/$ZrO_2$ exhibited

**Table 1** Ethyl levulinate synthesis from levulinic acid

| Entry | Feedstock | Catalyst | Product | Tem. (°C) | Time (h) | Conv. (%) | Sel. (%) | References |
|---|---|---|---|---|---|---|---|---|
| 1 | Levulinic acid | 15 wt.% DTPA/ DH-ZSM-597 | Ethyl levulinate | 78 | 4 | 94 | 100 | Nandiwale et al. [45] |
| 2 | Levulinic acid | WD HPA-$SiO_2$ | Ethyl levulinate | 78 | 10 | 100 | 79.0 | Pasquale et al. [49] |
| 3 | Levulinic acid | 10 wt.% STA/ SGS | Ethyl levulinate | 84 | 4 | 100 | 85.3 | Kong et al. [27] |
| 4 | Levulinic acid | 20 wt.% STA/ SGS | Ethyl levulinate | 84 | 4 | 100 | 96.5 | Kong et al. [27] |
| 5 | Levulinic acid | 30 wt.% STA/ SGS | Ethyl levulinate | 84 | 4 | 100 | 96.9 | Kong et al. [27] |
| 6 | Levulinic acid | 40 wt.% STA/ SGS | Ethyl levulinate | 84 | 4 | 100 | 97.0 | Kong et al. [27] |
| 7 | Levulinic acid | $ZrO_2$ | Ethyl levulinate | 150 | 3 | 54.7 | 64.2 | Ramli et al. [52] |
| 8 | Levulinic acid | HPW | Ethyl levulinate | 150 | 3 | 82.3 | 55.6 | Ramli et al. [52] |
| 9 | Levulinic acid | 15 wt.% HPW/ Zr | Ethyl levulinate | 150 | 3 | 90.1 | 87.5 | Ramli et al. [52] |
| 10 | Levulinic acid | 20 wt.% HPW/ Zr | Ethyl levulinate | 150 | 3 | 99.4 | 97.3 | Ramli et al. [52] |
| 11 | Levulinic acid | 25 wt.% HPW/ Zr | Ethyl levulinate | 150 | 3 | 97.2 | 62.3 | Ramli et al. [52] |

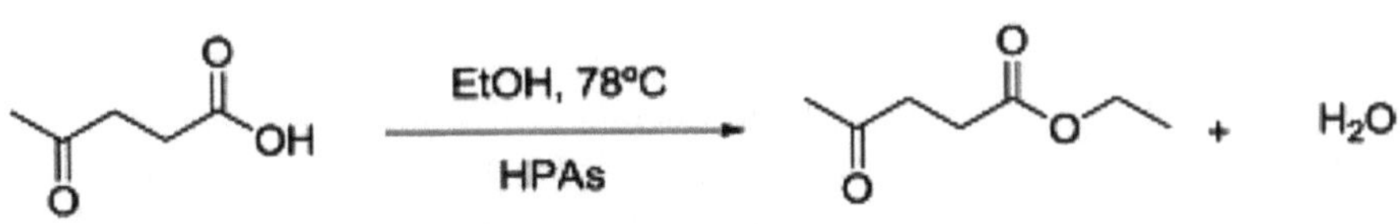


**Fig. 3** Reaction route for the synthesis of ethyl levulinate from levulinic acid [49]

the highest ethyl levulinate yield of 97.3% (Entry 7–11, Table 1). Characterization results indicated that this could be due to the high acidity and surface area of the 20 wt.% HPW/$ZrO_2$ catalyst.

## 2.3 Synthesis of Levulinic Acid Esters from Furfural and Furfuryl Alcohol

An increase of Brønsted acid sites has been shown to help promote the synthesis of furfural and furfuryl alcohol to ethyl levulinate [6, 37]. As shown in Fig. 4, Chhabra et al. [6] used activated carbon nanostructured catalysts loaded with phosphomolybdic acid (PMA/C) for the conversion of furfuryl alcohol to alkyl levulinates (Entries 1–5, Table 2). Catalytic tests revealed that the ethyl levulinate yield increased from 25 to 32% when the loading of phosphomolybdic acid was increased from 75 to 100 mg (Entries 3, 4 in Table 2). This was mainly ascribed to the increase of active acid sites, which facilitated the formation of ethyl levulinate. In addition, the effect of temperature on the ethyl levulinate yield was also investigated. The elevations in temperature are not conducive to the production of ethyl levulinate, as shown by entries 1, 3 and 5 in Table 2. It was found that this may be due to the polymerization of the reactants due to the high reaction temperature. In addition, the sulfonic acid group of the catalyst can serve as a strong Brønsted acid site. Liu and Li et al. [37] prepared MIL-101(Cr) catalysts for furfuryl alcohol transformation to ethyl levulinate. It was found that a comparatively favorable catalytic activity with 79.2% yield of ethyl levulinate and an almost complete conversion of furfuryl alcohol obtained mainly depended on the intensity of Brønsted acid sites (Entry 6, Table 2). In addition, various sulfonic acid-based catalysts were also summarized for application in furfuryl alcohol to ethyl levulinate conversion, and the specific performance results are shown in Entries 7–8 in Table 2.

Rational modulation of Brønsted and Lewis acid sites can improve the catalytic performance of furfural compounds conversion to ethyl levulinate [32, 38, 55, 63]. Li et al. [32] fabricated a bifunctional Zr-Al/SBA-15 catalyst for the formation of ethyl levulinate from furfural (Entry 9 in Table 2). It was observed that Lewis acid sites could have prompted the Meerwein–Ponndorf–Verley reduction of furfural into furfuryl alcohol, and Brønsted acid sites facilitated the further formation of ethyl levulinate. By optimally adjusting the ratio of $ZrO_2$ and $Al_2O_3$, the yield of ethyl levulinate could reach 67.2%. Liu and Pan et al. [38] synthesized mesoporous MIL-101(Cr)-$SO_3H$ (MMSs) catalysts for the formation of ethyl levulinate. At 150 °C and 2 h, 83.8% selectivity of ethyl levulinate and a complete conversion of furfuryl alcohol could be obtained. The characterization results confirmed that the synergistic

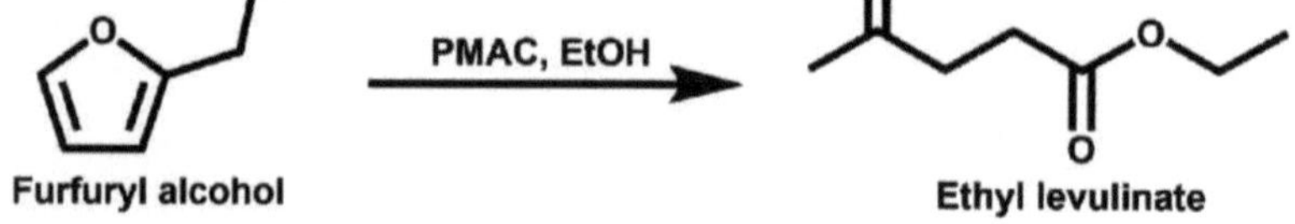


**Fig. 4** Ethyl levulinate synthesis from furfuryl alcohol [6]

**Table 2** Ethyl levulinate synthesis from furfuryl alcohol

| Entry | Feedstock | Catalyst | Product | Tem. (°C) | Time (h) | Conv. | Sel. (%) | References |
|---|---|---|---|---|---|---|---|---|
| 1 | Furfuryl alcohol | PMA/C (100 mg) | Ethyl levulinate | 140 | 2 | – | 42 | Chhabra et al. [6] |
| 2 | Furfuryl alcohol | PMA/C(100 mg) | Ethyl levulinate | 140 | 3 | – | 63 | Chhabra et al. [6] |
| 3 | Furfuryl alcohol | PMA/C (75 mg) | Ethyl levulinate | 160 | 2 | – | 25 | Chhabra et al. [6] |
| 4 | Furfuryl alcohol | PMA/C (100 mg) | Ethyl levulinate | 160 | 2 | – | 32 | Chhabra et al. [6] |
| 5 | Furfuryl alcohol | PMA/C (100 mg) | Ethyl levulinate | 180 | 2 | – | 25 | Chhabra et al. [6] |
| 6 | Furfuryl alcohol | MIL-101(Cr)–$SO_3H$ | Ethyl levulinate | 140 | 2 | 100% | 79.2 | Liu and Li et al. [37] |
| 7 | Furfuryl alcohol | UiO-66(Zr)–$SO_3H$ | Ethyl levulinate | 140 | 2 | 23.4% | 3.1 | Akiyama et al. [1] |
| 8 | Furfuryl alcohol | $Fe_3O_4$@$SiO_2$–$SO_3H$ | Ethyl levulinate | 140 | 2 | 99.5% | 61.6 | Prieto et al. [51] |
| 9 | Furfural | Zr-Al/SBA-15 | Ethyl levulinate | 150 | 5 | 92.8% | 71.4 | Li et al. [32] |
| 10 | Furfuryl alcohol | UCC-S-Fe-300 | Ethyl levulinate | 80 | 4 | 100% | 95.8 | Zainol et al. [74] |
| 11 | Furfuryl alcohol | $Zr_{0.25}$TPA/β-zeolite | Ethyl levulinate | 130 | 5 | 94% | 53 | Yogita et al. [72] |
| 12 | Furfuryl alcohol | $Zr_{0.5}$TPA/β-zeolite | Ethyl levulinate | 130 | 5 | 100% | 78 | Yogita et al. [72] |
| 13 | Furfuryl alcohol | $Zr_{0.75}$TPA/β-zeolite | Ethyl levulinate | 130 | 5 | 100% | 96 | Yogita et al. [72] |
| 14 | Furfuryl alcohol | Sn/Hmordenite | Ethyl levulinate | 180 | 2 | 100% | 95 | Sk et al. [55] |

physicochemical properties, proper acid density, mesopore size, and available—$SO_3H$ sites could contribute to the catalytic performance of MMS(0.3)-0.15 catalyst. Zainol et al. [74] used sulfonated and Fe doped carbon cryogels (UCC-S-Fe) for the formation of ethyl levulinate. A high product yield of 95.8% was obtained at 80 °C, 4 h (Entry 10, Table 2). The sulfonation treatment of UCC followed by the iron doping can improve catalytic activity. The introduction of iron enables UCC-S-Fe-300 to offer Lewis acid sites for the glucose isomerization, and the Brønsted acid sites favor the promotion of the further ethanolysis reaction, thus enhancing the final yield of ethyl levulinate.

Yogita et al. [72] prepared Zr-containing tungstophosphoric acid (TPA) loaded on β-zeolite catalysts for the formation of ethyl levulinate. Among these catalysts, $Zr_{0.75}$TPA/β-zeolite exhibited the highest activity with a 96% yield of ethyl levulinate, as shown in Entries 11–13 in Table 2. The addition of Zr produced Lewis acid sites, and TPA could offer abundant Brønsted acid sites. The FT-IR also confirmed the coexistence of both Brønsted and Lewis acid sites in the catalyst. The catalytic activity of furfuryl alcoholysis depends mainly on the intensity of acid sites. A series of H-mordenite catalysts loaded with Sn were synthesized by Sk et al. [55] to catalyze the furfuryl alcohol to ethyl levulinate. The catalytic tests revealed that the 10 wt.% Sn/H-mordenite catalyst had the most excellent catalytic performance, and 95% of ethyl levulinate could be obtained at 180 °C, 2 h reaction conditions (Entry 14 in Table 2). It was found that the total acidity and Sn dispersion of the H-mullite carrier had a significant effect on the reactivity.

## 2.4 Synthesis of Levulinic Acid Esters from Biomass Sugars

It has been demonstrated that the Brønsted acid site helps to promote the synthesis of fructose to ethyl acetylpropionate [2, 50, 62, 77]. Zhong et al. [77] prepared sulfonated mesoporous structured silica–carbon catalysts for the synthesis of fructose to ethyl levulinate in ethanol solvent in yields up to 80% (Entry 1, Table 3). The characterization revealed that the catalysts have a peculiar layered pore structure, where the mesopores facilitate the entry and fast transport of the substrate, but the presence of micropores facilitates the achievement of fast sugar catalysis. The rich Brønsted acid sites are key to the generation of ethyl levulinate from 5-hydroxymethylfurfural. And it was confirmed that alcohols such as ethanol can protect stabilize 5-hydroxymethylfurfural to form ethyl levulinate, while the presence of water tends to favor for the generation of humic acid from 5-HMF. Rode et al. synthesized a series of SBA-15 loaded phosphotungstic acid (PWA) catalysts for the fructose transformation to 5-hydroxymethylfurfural or 5-ethoxymethylfurfural. Reaction testing revealed that 95% conversion of fructose could be achieved on 20% PWA/SBA-15, while 5-hydroxymethylfurfural was further etherified, and the yields of 5-EMF and ethyl levulinate were 67% and 12%, respectively. The increase in PWA content caused an incremental acidity in the composite materials thereby increasing the reactivity.

Rational modulation of Brønsted acid and Lewis sites can also improve biomass sugar transformation to ethyl levulinate. Song et al. [56] designed sulfonic acid functionalized $ZrO_2$/organosilicon catalysts ($SO_4^{2-}/ZrO_2$-PMO-$SO_3H$) for the production of ethyl levulinate. The proportion of acid sites and porosity of $SO_4^{2-}/ZrO_2$-PMO-$SO_3H$ were optimized by adjusting the proportion of Si/Zr. Catalysts with an initial Si/Zr molar ratio of 1.0 showed the highest yields of ethyl levulinate (42.3%). Ce–Si pillared Montmorillonite (CeSiM)-loaded tungsten phosphate ($H_6P_2W_{18}O_{64}$) multifunctional catalysts were synthesized by Lai and Yan et al. [30] for the formation of ethyl levulinate. The glucose conversion was close to 100% and the ethyl levulinate yield was 56.2%. The doping of phosphotungstic acid and cerium imparted large specific surface area as well as strong acidity sites to the DPW-CeSiM catalyst, thus showing a high catalytic performance compared to other catalysts (Entries 2–9 in

**Table 3** Ethyl levulinate synthesis from biomass sugars

| Entry | Feedstock | Catalyst | Product | Tem. (°C) | Time | Conv. | Sel. | References |
|---|---|---|---|---|---|---|---|---|
| 1 | Fructose | $Si_{66}C_{33}$-550-$SO_3H$ | Ethyl levulinate | 140 | 24 h | – | 76% | Zhong et al. [77] |
| 2 | Fructose | PWA/SBA-15 | Ethyl levulinate | 100 | 24 h | 67% | 12% | [50] |
| 3 | Fructose | CMK-HPM-50 | Ethyl levulinate | 160 | 3 h | 98% | 72% | Ayashi et al. [2] |
| 4 | Fructose | $[C_3N][SO_3CF_3]$-HCSs-1 | Ethyl levulinate | 140 | 2 h | 100% | 89.7% | Sun and Zhang et al. [62] |
| 5 | Glucose | $SO_4^{2-}$/ $ZrO_2$-PMO-$SO_3H$ | Ethyl levulinate | 170 | 12 h | – | 42.3% | Song et al. [56] |
| 6 | Glucose | DPW-CeSiM | Ethyl levulinate | 170 | 4 h | 100% | 56.2% | Lai et al. [30] |
| 7 | Glucose | Sn/ZrP$SO_3H$ | Ethyl levulinate | 170 | 10 h | – | 49.3% | Tian et al. [64] |
| 8 | Glucose | AC-Fe-$SO_3H$ | Ethyl levulinate | 200 | 3 h | – | 19.1% | Zhang and Chen [76] |
| 9 | Glucose | 2ML-SZ-SBA-15 | Ethyl levulinate | 140 | 24 h | – | 24.2% | Morales et al. [43] |
| 10 | Sucrose | DPW-CeSiM | Ethyl levulinate | 170 | 4 h | – | 58.2% | Lai et al. [30] |
| 11 | Fructose | DPW-CeSiM | Ethyl levulinate | 170 | 4 | – | 64.7 | Lai et al. [30] |
| 12 | Cellulose | DPW-CeSiM | Ethyl levulinate | 170 | 4 | – | 36.7 | Lai et al. [30] |
| 13 | Glucose | UFCS-Zn | Ethyl levulinate | 180 | 6 | – | 27.4 | Zainol et al. [73] |
| 14 | Cellulose | Al-OCS-0.1 | Ethyl levulinate | 200 | 5 | – | 50.8 | Huang and Hao et al. [21] |

Table 3). In addition, the DPW-CeSiM catalyst showed high catalytic performance in the translation of sucrose, fructose and cellulose, to ethyl levulinate, as shown in Entries 10–12 in Table 3. Zinc-doped sulfonated urea-furaldehyde carbon freeze gels (UFCS-Zn) acid catalysts were synthesized for glucose alcoholysis reaction by Zainol et al. [73]. The UFCS-Zn catalyst for glucose alcoholysis reaction provided a maximum yield of 27.4% ethyl levulinate (Entry 13 in Table 3). It was found that the introduction of sulfonic acid groups and Zn provided the necessary Brønsted and Lewis acid sites for the multi-step conversion of glucose.

The formation of ethyl levulinate from cellulose is a more complex process than that from fructose and glucose. Typically, cellulose is hydrolyzed to glucose monomer under acid-catalyzed conditions. Glucose is then isomerized to produce fructose, which is then hydrolyzed to give 5-hydroxymethylfurfural. Finally, 5-hydroxymethyl furfural is dehydrated to form levulinic acid, and levulinic acid is esterified with ethanol to form ethyl levulinate. Huang and Hao et al. [21] synthesized a sulfonated oxidatively ordered mesoporous carbon (OOMC) catalyst loaded with $Al_2(SO_4)_3$. The nanocomposites exhibited an excellent activity in catalyzing the reaction of cellulose-to-ethyl levulinate at 200 °C for 5 h, with a satisfactory ethyl levulinate yield at 50.8% (entry 14 in Table 3).

# 3 Nanocomposites-Promoted Catalytic Synthesis of Valeric Biofuels

## *3.1 Synthetic Mechanism of Valeric Biofuels*

Valeric acid esters have been regarded as next-generation biofuels, which are more compatible in nature with existing fossil fuels than conventional biomass-based fuel molecules (γ-valerolactone, 2-methyltetrahydrofuran, ethanol, etc.). In addition, valeric acid ester molecules exhibit more superior properties both in terms of preparation process and fuel performance. The generation of valeric acid biofuel mainly involves four consecutive reaction steps, in the presence of acid: (1) hydrolysis of lignocellulose to produce levulinic acid; (2) levulinic acid hydrogenation to form γ-valerolactone; (3) conversion of γ-valerolactone to valeric acid; (4) valeric acid esterification to valeric acid esters. Besides, valeric biofuels can also be converted from furan compounds. The pathway for the conversion of various feedstocks into valeric biofuels is shown in Fig. 5. It's worth noting that the rate-determining step for the synthesis of expected product is ring-opening process of γ-valerolactone, which usually requires strong acid sites. For the widely reported valeric acid ester synthesis from levulinic acid or γ-valerolactone, bifunctional catalysts with metal and acid sites, such as Pd/MCM-41, Ru/H-ZSM-5, Pd/ZSM-5, Ru/SBA-$SO_3H$, Co@ZSM-5, Ni/K-ZSM-5, and Co/H-Y, provide better reaction results. The synthesis of valeric acid esters mainly requires coordination between the metal and acid sites.

## *3.2 Synthesis of Valeric Biofuels from Levulinic Acid and Its Esters*

Several metal-loaded zeolite bifunctional catalysts for levulinic acid conversion have been applied for the efficient manufacture of valeric acid biofuels. Weckhuysen et al. developed an efficient Ru/H-ZSM5 catalyst to obtain valeric acid with 91.3% yield under gentle conditions, and better control of the density of acid sites is the success to high productivity [40]. The highest yield of valeric acid (99%) was achieved with Pt/HMFI having an average nanocluster size at about 1.9 nm without solvent. The

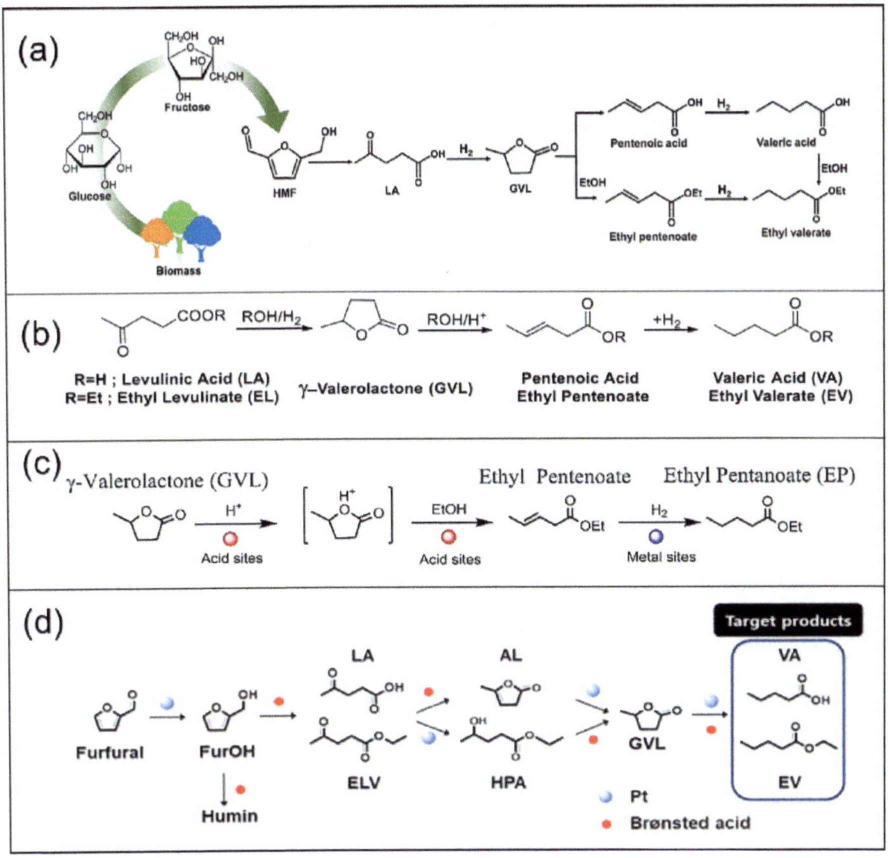

**Fig. 5** **a** The reaction pathway by which glucose is converted to valeric acid and valeric esters [24]. **b** Reaction pathway for levulinic acid/ethyl levulinate conversion to valeric acid/ethyl valerate [44]. **c** Reaction mechanism for the conversion of γ-valerolactone to ethyl valerate over metal–acid bifunctional catalysts [18]. **d** Reaction network in the conversion of furfural to valeric acid and ethyl valerate [7]

catalytic system was directed by the cooperative interaction between Brønsted acid sites on HMFI and Pt clusters [25]. The Pd/AlMCM-41 catalyst allowed a direct synthetic of valeric acid from levulinic acid with 45.1% yield. Mesoporous supports (such as MCM-41, ZrMCM-41 and AlMCM-41) can effectively resist the leaching and clustering of Pd nanoparticles [67].

In addition to the above precious metal loading, there are also non-precious metal loaded catalysts that can achieve satisfactory catalytic performance. Li et al. first reported a bifunctional Co/HZSM-5 catalyst, which can serve as a promising alternative to precious metal catalysts for the levulinic acid conversion to valeric biofuels (Table 4, Entry 1). Co nanoparticles encapsulated in HZSM-5 crystallography catalyzed the consecutive hydrogenation of ketone and alkene groups, while the

**Table 4** Valeric biofuels synthesis from levulinic acid and its esters

| Entry | Feedstock | Catalyst | Product | Tem. | Time (h) | Conv. (%) | Sel. (%) | References |
|---|---|---|---|---|---|---|---|---|
| 1 | Levulinic acid | Co/HZSM-5 | Valeric acid+ethyl valerate | 240 °C | 3 | 93 | 91 | Sun and Gao et al. [60] |
| 2 | Levulinic acid | ZSM-5@(Co/$SiO_2$) | Ethyl valerate | 250 °C | 2 | 92 | 62 | Wang and Wang etal. [69] |
| 3 | Levulinic acid | ZSM-5@(Co/$SiO_2$) | Ethyl valerate | 250 °C | 6 | 100 | 88 | Wang and Wang et al. [69] |
| 4 | Levulinic acid | W–Ni/$TiO_2$ | Valeric acid | 270 °C | 6[a] | 73.5 | 48.5 | Kumar et al. [28] |
| 5 | Levulinic acid | W–Ni/$TiO_2$ | Valeric acid | 270 °C | 12[a] | 72.9 | 48.7 | Kumar et al. [28] |
| 6 | Levulinic acid | W–Ni/$TiO_2$ | Valeric acid | 270 °C | 24[a] | 73.8 | 48.3 | Kumar et al. [28] |
| 7 | Levulinic acid | W–Ni/$TiO_2$ | Valeric acid | 270 °C | 48[a] | 73.4 | 48.5 | Kumar et al. [28] |
| 8 | Levulinic acid | W–Ni/$TiO_2$ | Valeric acid | 270 °C | 60[a] | 72.3 | 47.5 | Kumar et al. [28] |
| 9 | Levulinic acid | 4Nb-40Cu/ZPS | Valeric acid | 150 °C | 2 | 95.6 | 96.7 | Karanwal et al. [24] |
| 10 | Levulinic acid | 4Nb-40Cu/ZPS | Valeric acid | 150 °C | 2 | 96.1 | 97.3 | Karanwal et al. [24] |
| 11 | Levulinic acid | Ru/MnOx | Valeric acid+ethyl valerate | 523 K | 6 | 100 | 15 | Pan et al. [48] |
| 12 | Levulinic acid | Ru/MgO | Valeric acid+ethyl valerate | 523 K | 6 | 100 | 3 | Pan et al. [48] |
| 13 | Levulinic acid | Ru/CeOx | Valeric acid+ethyl valerate | 523 K | 6 | 100 | 6 | Pan et al. [48] |
| 14 | Levulinic acid | Ru/ZSM-5 | Valeric acid+ethyl valerate | 523 K | 6 | 100 | 29 | Pan et al. [48] |
| 15 | Levulinic acid | Ru/C | Valeric acid+ethyl valerate | 523 K | 6 | 100 | 1 | Pan et al. [48] |
| 16 | Levulinic acid | Ru/$ZrO_2$ | Valeric acid+ethyl valerate | 523 K | 6 | 100 | 4 | Pan et al. [48] |

(continued)

**Table 4** (continued)

| Entry | Feedstock | Catalyst | Product | Tem. | Time (h) | Conv. (%) | Sel. (%) | References |
|---|---|---|---|---|---|---|---|---|
| 17 | Levulinic acid | $Ru/TiO_2$ | Valeric acid+ethyl valerate | 523 K | 6 | 100 | 6 | Pan et al. [48] |
| 18 | Levulinic acid | $Ru/SiO_2$ | Valeric acid+ethyl valerate | 523 K | 6 | 100 | 10 | Pan et al. [48] |
| 19 | Levulinic acid | $Ru/Nb_2O_5$ | Valeric acid+ethyl valerate | 523 K | 6 | 99 | 3 | Pan et al. [48] |
| 20 | Levulinic acid | Ru-SBA-15 | Valeric acid+ethyl valerate | 523 K | 6 | 99 | 2 | Pan et al. [48] |
| 21 | Levulinic acid | Ru/ $SBA\text{-}SO_3H\text{-}4$ | Valeric acid+ethyl valerate | 523 K | 6 | 100 | 90 | Pan et al. [48] |

[a] Continuous operation conditions

zeolite catalyzed the ring-opening reaction of γ-valerolactone intermediates. Homogeneous embedding of Co nanoparticles in HZSM-5 crystallography could stabilize the Co nanoparticles. So that, under liquid phase conditions, burning and filtration did not occur even in the presence of water [60]. Wu et al. used ZSM-5@($Co/SiO_2$) as a bifunctional metal/acid catalyst in the ethyl levulinate hydrogenation with ethanol as the solvent (Table 4, Entries 2–3). First, the ethyl levulinate was hydrogenated at the metal site to produce ethyl 4-hydroxyvalerate. Then the ethyl 4-hydroxyvalerate was converted to γ-valerolactone via dehydration, and γ-valerolactone was cycloaditioned to valeric acid via the coordinated effect between acid and metal sites. It was found that ethyl 4-hydroxyvalerate or valeric acid is more easily converted to ethyl valerate over ZSM-5@($Co/SiO_2$) with tinier Co particle sizes, bigger total acid amounts, and greater Brønsted acid sites [68].

Liquid-phase dealumination and coke deposition of zeolite materials have been identified as major problems for catalyst deactivation in biomass-related liquid-phase reactions. Well-dispersed ultrasmall Ru nanoclusters (the particle size is approximately 1 nm) were confined in the micropores of Y zeolite, providing the desired site proximity, which greatly improved the hydrodeoxygenation of ethyl levulinate for the selective synthesis of valeric biofuels. The promoting of catalyst stability was due to the addition of La, which prevents zeolite lattice deconstruction by inhibiting the dealumination and desilylation of zeolites [19]. The acid-regulating effect of K addition on Ni/HZSM-5 catalyst could reduce the strong acidity of catalyst while modulating the ratio of Brønsted and Lewis acid. The coke analysis showed that the acidity of the coke could be adjusted by the addition of K to change the heavier coke fraction (alkylated polyaromatics) to a lighter coke fraction (alkylated monoaromatics), thus effectively extending the operating period in fixed-bed reactor of the Ni/HZSM-5 [61].

Venugopal et al. prepared highly efficient Ni/$TiO_2$ catalysts by simple maceration, where Lewis acid sites were engaged in the dehydration of levulinic acid, whereas Brønsted acid sites appeared to launch the ring-opening process of γ-valerolactone to valeric acid and hydrocarbons [29]. They also explored the effect of W on the reductive behavior of Ni/$TiO_2$ and Brønsted acidity during the tandem reaction of levulinic acid to valeric acid. W-modified Ni/$TiO_2$ was selected for the levulinic acid hydrogenation to produce γ-valerolactone, while the interplay of Ni with W was responsible for the production of valeric acid [28]. The enhancement of Brønsted acid sites on the W-modified Ni/$TiO_2$ prompted the generation of valeric acid via the intermediate ring-opening. W-modified Ni/$TiO_2$ also remained stable over 60 h under continuous operation condition (Table 4, Entries 4–8). The cooperation of Ni and Ni-W interactions is active for the tandem conversion of levulinic acid to valeric acid. Levulinic acid could also be converted to valeric acid via a one-pot conversion on Nb-Cu/ZPS. Under gentle conditions, levulinic acid was completely converted to valeric acid in aqueous medium with 99.8% conversion (Table 4, Entries 9–10). Among them, ZPS exhibited strong Lewis acid sites, which enhanced the adsorption of levulinic acid. Meanwhile, the synergistic effect of Lewis acid and Brønsted acid bound by $Nb_2O_5$ and the $Cu^0$ sites could stimulate the tandem hydrogenation, cyclization, ring-opening, and hydrogenation of levulinic acid to produce valeric acid (as shown in Fig. 6) [24].

On this basis, the direct reaction of levulinic acid to valerate without separating γ-valerolactone intermediates was expected to further simplify the reaction process. To achieve this goal, a deeper recognition of the influence of catalyst support was needed, especially the effect of carrier acidity on the selectivity of levulinic acid hydrogenation. Luo et al. investigated the levulinic acid hydrogenation over four Ru catalysts with catalyst supports of non-acidic ($Nb_2O_5$ and $TiO_2$) and strongly acidic (H-ZSM5 and H-β) [41]. The results showed that the zeolite catalysts could directly synthesize valeric acid from levulinic acid in one-pot without separating the intermediate γ-valerolactone. The loss of acid sites in the process of dealumination caused catalyst deactivation. H-ZSM5 was found to be more resistant to dealumination than H-β. Ru/SBA-$SO_3H$ bifunctional catalyst was fabricated by Pan et al. [48] (Table 4, Entries 11–21). The selectivity of ethyl valerate and valerate was improved by the enhancement of acid site on the support, and the yield of ethyl valerate and valerate could reach 94% (probable pathways are shown in Fig. 7). Mariscal et al. used amorphous $SiO_2$-$Al_2O_3$, beta zeolite and ZSM5 as supports, kinds of Pd-based catalysts were prepared by the primary wet impregnation method [44]. The best yield of 92% was obtained Pd/ZSM5 at 240 °C within 8 h. This could be attributed to the suitable acidity of the catalyst, both in terms of the intensity and amounts of acid sites.

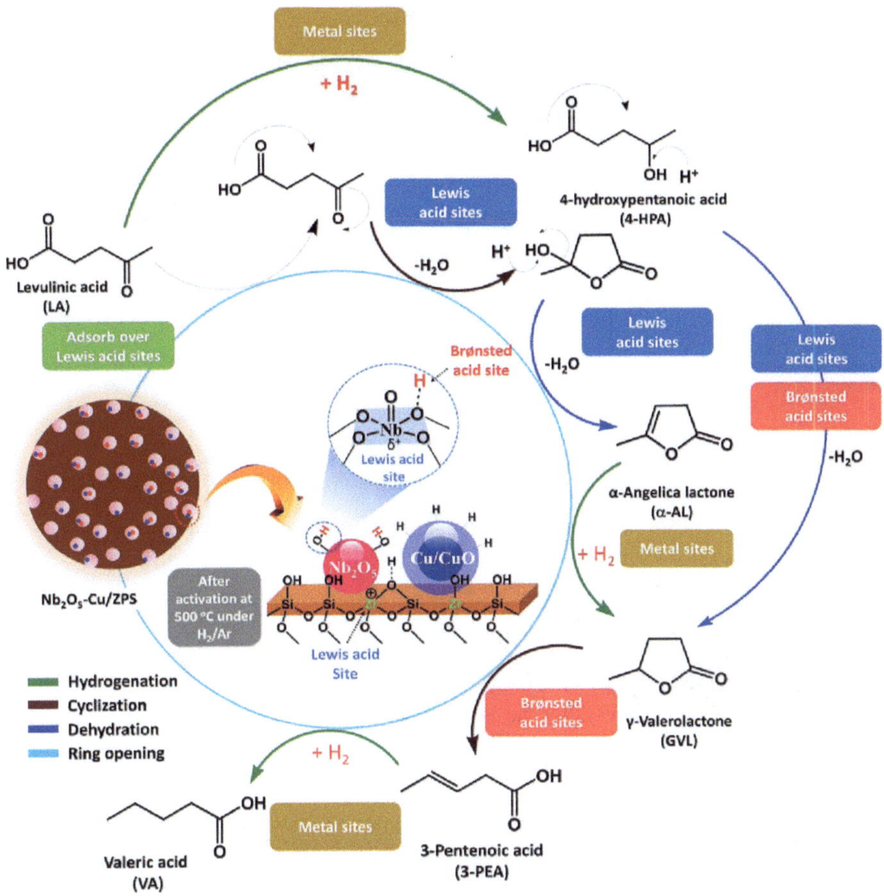


**Fig. 6** Plausible reaction pathway for the direct conversion of levulinic acid to valeric acid over bimetallic Nb-Cu/ZPS catalyst [24]

### 3.3 *Synthesis of Valeric Biofuels from γ-Valerolactone*

In the presence of zeolite-loaded metal catalysts containing metal centers and acid sites, γ-valerolactone hydrogenation produces valeric acid in good product yields. Proper adjustment of zeolite acidity can reduce the deposition of heavy carbonaceous substances during the catalytic process, thus effectively extending the catalyst lifetime. With 200 °C and 3 MPa $H_2$, the Ni/La-Y maintained 90% of the valeric acid esters yield even after 1000 h. While the Ni/H-Y was gradually deactivated within 200 h (Table 5, Entries 1–2). The combination of multiple characterization techniques revealed that the addition of levulinic acid not only modulated the acidity of zeolites and effectively inhibits coke generation, but also preserved the acid sites by avoiding the zeolite dealumination during the reaction [18]. In addition, Ni/ZSM-5 catalysts

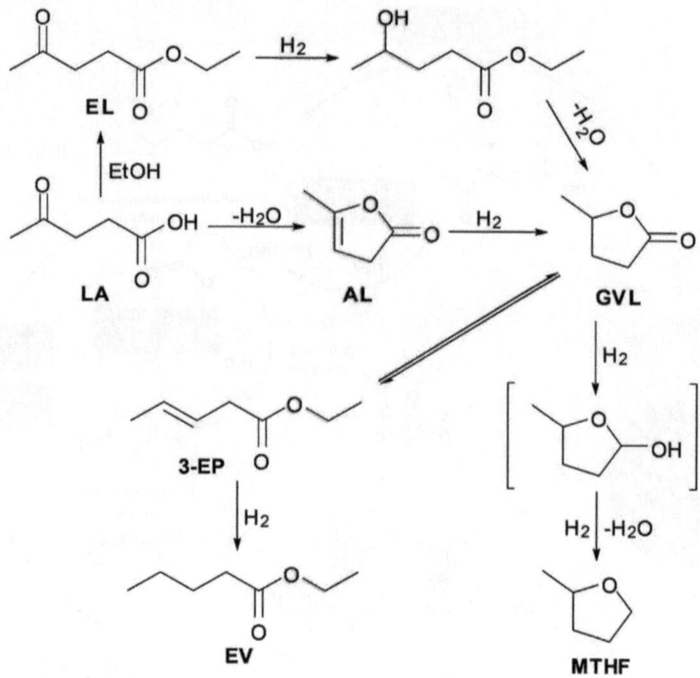


**Fig. 7** Probable reaction pathways for the conversion of levulinic acid to ethyl valerate over Ru/SBA-$SO_3H$ [48]

modified with promoters (Cr, Mo and W) were investigated for the gas-phase conversion of γ-valerolactone to ethyl valerate. Among the three different promoters, the Mo-modified catalyst was considered as the best candidate (Table 5, Entries 3–7). The C–O bond opening of γ-valerolactone on the methyl side led to the rapid hydrogenation and esterification of pentanoic acid as an intermediate, which favored for the selective transformation of γ-valerolactone to ethyl valerate (as shown in Fig. 8). (Velisoju and [66]).

In addition to zeolites, some other solid acids, such as $ZrO_2$, niobium pentoxide-cerium oxide (NbCe) and amorphous silica-zirconia (SiZr), are also used as the catalyst components for the synthesis of valeric biofuels. The Cu/$ZrO_2$ catalyst synthesized by Li et al. performed an excellent activity for the catalytic conversion of γ-valerolactone to pentyl valerate (85.4% γ-valerolactone conversion and 98.0% pentyl valerate selectivity) (Table 5, Entry 8), Liu and Fan et al. [36] which was mainly due to the interplay between $Cu^0$ and $Cu^+$, and the high dispersion of nanoparticles, which enhanced the adsorption and polarization of C=O bonds by γ-valerolactone and the dissociation of $H_2$ for the hydrogenation step. The Pd-NbCe/C showed excellent performance in the preparation of valeric acid esters from γ-valerolactone (Table 5, Entry 9) [4]. The γ-valerolactone ring-opening occurred at

**Table 5** Valeric biofuels synthesis from γ-valerolactone

| Entry | Feedstock | Catalyst | Product | Tem. | Time (h) | Conv. (%) | Sel. (%) | References |
|---|---|---|---|---|---|---|---|---|
| 1 | γ-valerolactone | Ni/La-Y | Ethyl valerate | 200 °C | 1000[a] | 91 | 98.9 | He et al. [18] |
| 2 | γ-valerolactone | Ni/H-Y | Ethyl valerate | 200 °C | 200[a] | 72 | 94.4 | He et al. [18] |
| 3 | γ-valerolactone | Ni/HZ5 | Ethyl valerate | 250 °C | 50 | 9.1 | 58.6 | Velisoju et al. [66] |
| 4 | γ-valerolactone | Cr-Ni/HZ5 | Ethyl valerate | 250 °C | 50 | 8.6 | 68.5 | Velisoju et al. [66] |
| 5 | γ-valerolactone | Mo-Ni/HZ5 | Ethyl valerate | 250 °C | 50 | 9.6 | 92 | Velisojua et al. [66] |
| 6 | γ-valerolactone | W–Ni/HZ5 | Ethyl valerate | 250 °C | 50 | 9.1 | 80.2 | Velisoju et al. [66] |
| 7 | γ-valerolactone | Mo-Ni/HZ5 | Ethyl valerate | 300 °C | 50 | 99.2 | 91.5 | Velisoju et al. [66] |
| 8 | γ-valerolactone | $Cu/ZrO_2$ | Pentyl valerate | 230 °C | 10 | 85.4 | 98.1 | Liu and Fan et al. [36] |
| 9 | γ-valerolactone | Pd–NbCe/C | Valeric acid | 538 K | 25 | 92 | 79 | Buitrago-Sierra et al. [4] |
| 10 | γ-valerolactone | $Cu/SiO_2$ | Pentyl valerate | 250 °C | 10 | 91 | 92 | Scotti et al. [54] |

[a] Continuous-flow system

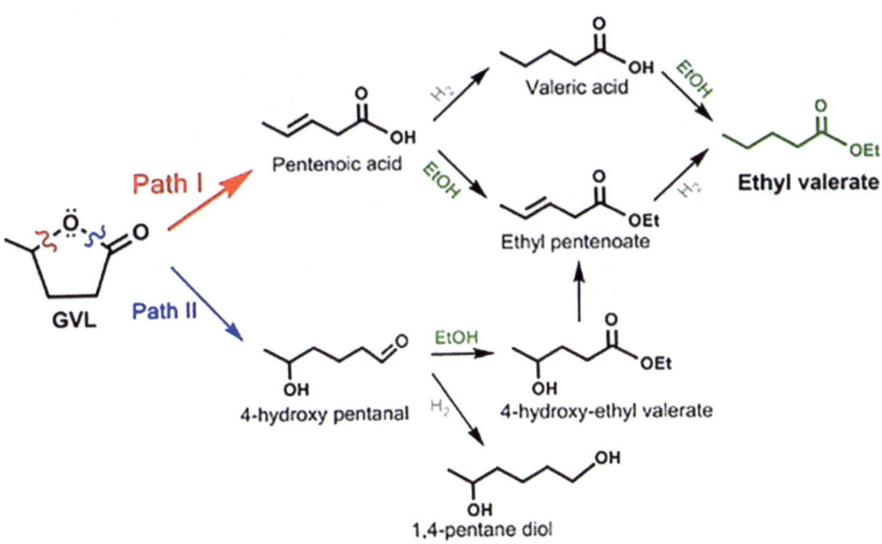


**Fig. 8** Proposed reaction pathways for γ-valerolactone conversion over metal-modified Ni/ZSM-5 catalysts [66]

the acid site of Nb, while the hydrogenation to produce valeric acid occurred at the Pb particles.

In addition to this, there are catalyst systems in which both acid and hydrogenation activity are attributed to the presence of metal particles without the need for acid sites. Ravasio et al. found that finely divided metal particles could perform Lewis acidity associated with catalysis. This property, coupled with the significant hydrogenation activity of metals, allowed the design of novel bifunctional catalysts, such as Cu/$SiO_2$, without an acid support. The Cu particles played a role not only in hydrogenation reactions but also, by virtue of its Lewis acidity, in the process of the reactant activation to nucleophilic addition. Such features facilitated the efficient and selective conversion of γ-valerolactone to pentyl valerate with 92% product selectivity (Table 5, Entry 10) [54].

## 3.4 Synthesis of Valeric Biofuels from Furan Compounds

The furfural conversion to valeric acid and its esters requires five consecutive steps alternating between metallic and acidic sites. The skeleton Al in Pt/H-ZSM-5 synthesized by Cho et al. selectively enriched around the sealed Pt nanoparticles, which was known as the halo effect [7]. Such a halo effect was able to prompt the multistep tandem reaction of furfural to valeric acid/ethyl valerate in one pot with 86% product yields (Table 6, Entry 1). The high product yield on Pt/H-ZSM-5 could be due to the close relationship between acid and metal sites, which effectively mediated the tandem reaction requiring alternating metal and acid sites, i.e., the halo effect reduced the distance between the intermediates to access the active site to inhibit catalyst deactivation. Further, the authors investigated a model for the tandem conversion of furfural with acetone and ethanol [8]. The two encapsulated catalysts, Pt/Na-ZSM-5, and Pt/H-ZSM-5, exhibited selective switching results (Table 6, Entries 2–3), which suggested that Pt/H-ZSM-5 could prompt the furfural hydrogenation preferentially rather than the aldol condensation (as shown in Fig. 9). It was demonstrated that the concentration of ethanol is a key parameter for the selectivity control. A moderate ethanol concentration facilitates the provision of valerate/ethyl valerate through catalytic transfer hydrogenation pathways in zeolite micropores and exposure of the intermediates to Brønsted acid sites prior to Pt nanoparticles.

**Table 6** Valeric biofuels synthesis from furan compounds

| Entry | Feedstock | Catalyst | Product | Tem. (°C) | Time (h) | Product yield (%) | References |
|---|---|---|---|---|---|---|---|
| 1 | Furfural | Pt@H-ZSM-5 | Valeric acid/ethyl valerate | 140 | 24 | 86 | Cho et al. [7] |
| 2 | Furfural | Pt@Na-ZSM-5 | 4-(2-furyl)butan-2-one/ 4-(2-furyl)butan-2-ol | 160 | 24 | 69 | Cho et al. [8] |
| 3 | Furfural | Pt@H-ZSM-5 | Valeric acid/ethyl valerate | 160 | 24 | 80 | Cho et al. [8] |

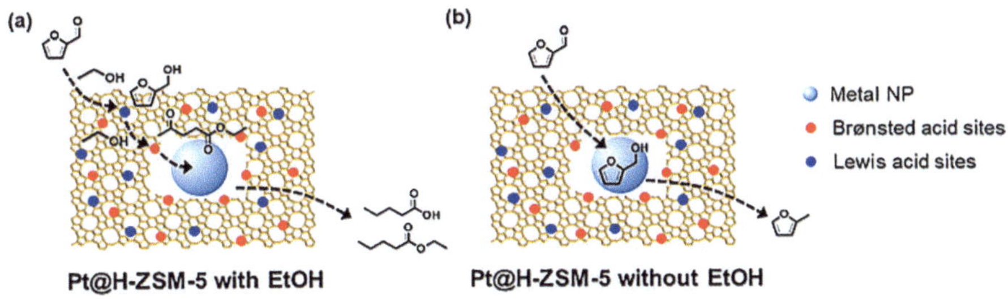


**Fig. 9** Schematic of the conversion of furfural over Pt@H-ZSM-5 **a** in the presence of ethanol and **b** in the absence of ethanol [8]

# 4 Nanocomposites-Promoted Catalytic Synthesis of Furan-Based Biofuels

## *4.1 Synthetic Mechanism of Furan-Based Biofuels*

Furan-based biofuels mainly include 2,5-dimethylfuran, 2-methylfuran, 2-methyltetrahydrofuran, etc. 2,5-Dimethylfuran is a highly promising biofuel that is typically obtained through the hydrogenation and dehydration of 5-hydroxymethylfurfural (Fig. 10a), which is characterized by its high energy density [5, 65]. 2-Methylfuran and 2-methyltetrahydrofuran are both important bio-gasoline fuels that exhibit excellent performance as additives in gasoline. Furthermore, 2-methylfuran can also be used as an additive for diesel or jet fuel. Both 2-methylfuran and 2-methyltetrahydrofuran can be derived from furfural [10, 12, 13, 22, 23, 31, 77], and 2-methyltetrahydrofuran can also be obtained from γ-valerolactone or levulinic acid (Fig. 10b). This section mainly summarizes the synthesis of these three furan-based biofuels on nanocomposite materials, with particular emphasis on the synergistic effects between the metal and acidic sites of nanocomposite materials.

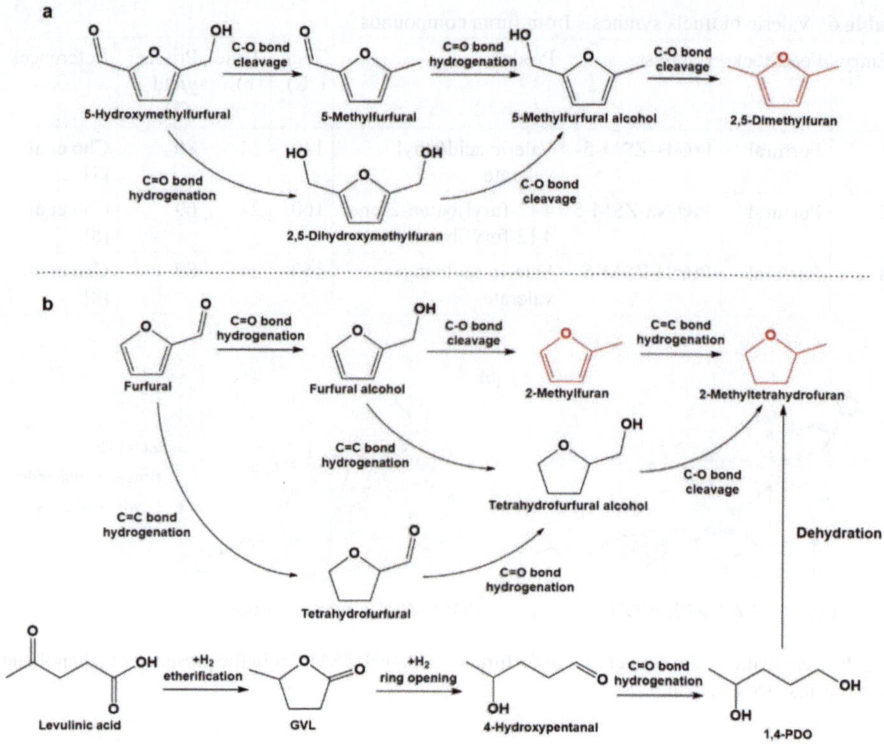


**Fig. 10** **a** The synthesis pathway of 2,5-dimethylfuran from 5-hydroxymethylfurfural [71]. **b** The synthesis pathway of 2-methylfuran and 2-methyltetrahydrofuran from furfural and γ-valerolactone [20, 70]

## 4.2 *Synthesis of 2,5-Dimethylfuran from 5-Hydroxymethylfurfural*

The transformation of 5-hydroxymethylfurfural to 2,5-dimethylfuran mainly involves hydrogenation and deoxygenation steps. Chitra Sarkar et al. developed Cu-Pd bimetallic nanoparticles encapsulated in a metal–organic framework (MOF), which showed high catalytic activity in this reaction, with a maximum yield of 96.5% for 2,5-dimethylfuran (Table 7, Entry 1–2) [53]. The enhanced catalytic performance was attributed to the geometric and electrical phenomena that transpire at the Cu-Pd interface, where Pd adjusted the local atomic structural environment by increasing the Pd–Pd bond distance and reducing the Cu–Cu bond length, thereby enhancing the catalytic activity. Similarly, for the Cu-Pd bimetallic system, Gunawan et al. calculated the total reaction barriers and the adsorption energies of reactants and products on three catalysts, namely, Pd(111), Cu(111), and $Cu_3Pd(111)$ [39]. The Pd(111) surface exhibited a greater total reaction barrier compared to the $Cu_3Pd(111)$ surface. Furthermore, the adsorption energy of 2,5-dimethylfuran on the Pd(111)

**Table 7** 2,5-dimethylfuran synthesis from 5-hydroxymethylfurfural

| Entry | Feedstock | Catalyst | Product | Tem. (°C) | Time (h) | Conv. (%) | Sel. (%) | References |
|---|---|---|---|---|---|---|---|---|
| 1 | 5-hydroxymethylfurfural | Cu-Pd@C-A | 2,5-dimethylfuran | 140 | 7 | 48.8 | 36.6 | Sarkar et al. [53] |
| 2 | 5-hydroxymethylfurfural | Cu-Pd@C-B | 2,5-dimethylfuran | 140 | 7 | 100 | 97 | Sarkar et al. [53] |
| 3 | 5-hydroxymethylfurfural | Ni-Mn(3:1)/AC | 2,5-dimethylfuran | 140 | 1 | 100 | 98.5 | Liu and Shi et al. [39] |
| 4 | 5-hydroxymethylfurfural | Ni-Mn(2:1)/AC | 2,5-dimethylfuran | 140 | 1 | 100 | 93.2 | Liu and Shi et al. [39] |
| 5 | 5-hydroxymethylfurfural | $Cu/Fe_2O_3-Al_2O_3$ | 2,5-dimethylfuran | 150 | 10 | 100 | 93.3 | Esteves et al. [11] |
| 6 | 5-hydroxymethylfurfural | $Cu/Al_2O_3$ | 2,5-dimethylfuran | 150 | 10 | 100 | 93.9 | Esteves et al. [11] |
| 7 | 5-hydroxymethylfurfural | $Cu/Fe_2O_3$ | 2,5-dimethylfuran | 150 | 10 | 32.7 | 14.37 | Esteves et al. [11] |
| 8 | 5-Hydroxymethylfurfural | 0.4Ni/ZSM-5 | 2,5-dimethylfuran | 180 | 7 | 91.2 | 96.2 | Guo et al. [17] |
| 9 | 5-hydroxymethylfurfural | Pd-Co9S8/S-CNT | 2,5-dimethylfuran | 120 | 13 | 96.0 | 83.7 | Liao et al. [34] |
| 10 | 5-hydroxymethylfurfural | Ni-OMD3 | 2,5-dimethylfuran | 200 | 6 | 99.9 | 98.7 | Goyal et al. [14] |
| 11 | 5-hydroxymethylfurfural | $Cu/ZrO_2$(CZ-90) | 2,5-dimethylfuran | 180 | 7 | 100 | 98.4 | Li and Yang et al. [33] |

surface exceeded that on the $Cu_3Pd(111)$ surface. 2,5-dimethylfuran was not easily desorbed from the Pd(111) surface and underwent excessive hydrogenation to form 2,5-dimethyltetrahydrofuran. Cu(111) had a higher energy barrier for dissociating $H_2$ adsorption and producing $H_2O$, which prevented the hydrodeoxygenation of 5-hydroxymethylfurfural even though its overall energy barrier was significantly lower than that of Pd(111) and Cu3Pd(111) surfaces. It was concluded that $Cu_3Pd(111)$ was the optimal catalyst for this reaction. A bifunctional Ni-Mn/AC catalyst was created by Liu et al. to produce 2,5-dimethylfuran from 5-hydroxymethylfurfural [16]. Excessively high temperature of 200 °C and extended reaction time were found to reduce the selectivity of the target product 2,5-dimethylfuran while enhancing the selectivity of an excessive hydrogenation byproduct 2,5-dimethyltetrahydrofuran (Table 7, Entry 3–4). The catalytic activity of Ni alone for the reaction were much lower compared to the Ni-Mn catalyst, where the introduction of $MnO_x$ provided moderate acid sites that facilitated the dissociation of C–O bonds. However, excessive addition of Mn also led to the production of ring-opening byproducts.

Typically, in hydrogenation and deoxygenation reactions, the characteristics of the catalyst supports have a direct bearing on the catalytic activity of bifunctional catalysts. Recently, Esteves et al. investigated how different catalyst supports impact the transformation of 5-hydroxymethylfurfural to 2,5-dimethylfuran employing Cu-based catalysts (Table 7, Entry 5–7) [11]. They investigated the behavior of Cu supported on $Al_2O_3$, $Fe_2O_3$, $Nb_2O_5$, and their combinations. $Cu/Al_2O_3$ and $Cu/Fe_2O_3$-$Al_2O_3$ yielded the highest 2,5-dimethylfuran productivity during the first hour and the entire reaction time, reaching 94% and 90% yields, respectively. $Cu/Fe_2O_3$ exhibited the lowest 5-hydroxymethylfurfural conversion throughout the reaction due to Cu nanoparticle agglomeration and low metal dispersion. For hydrogenation and deoxygenation reactions, the product yield was directly influenced by the characteristics of the metal and acid sites. The $Cu/Al_2O_3$ catalyst produced a high 2,5-dimethylfuran yield by facilitating better copper dispersion and providing moderate Lewis acid sites thanks to its high specific surface area alumina support.. Srivastava et al. also investigated the influence of supports, $CeO_2$, $ZrO_2$, and $Al_2O_3$, on the Cu–Co catalyst in the transformation of 5-hydroxymethylfurfural to 2,5-dimethylfuran [58]. Cu–Co/$CeO_2$ had larger Cu nanoparticles and lower acidity, resulting in weaker C–O activation. Cu–Co/$Al_2O_3$ exhibited a higher activity in the hydrogenation/dehydration reaction, which was assigned to a high metal dispersion, and suitable weak acid sites. However, Cu–Co/$ZrO_2$ showed relatively good activity but poor 2,5-dimethylfuran selectivity due to strong acid sites, leading to excessive hydrogenation byproducts.

In addition to metal–metal interactions, modulation of metal-support interactions is also critical for the synthesis of furan-based biofuels. Guo et al. prepared Ni/ZSM-5 catalyst for the transformation of 5-hydroxymethylfurfural to 2,5-dimethylfuran (Table 7, Entry 8) [35]. The Ni metal sites activated hydrogen molecules into hydrogen atoms, promoting the C=O hydrogenation. ZSM-5 had acid sites that could activate C–O bonds, followed by hydrogenolysis. Liao et al. used S-modified carbon nanotubes (SCNT) as the support to load Pd-Co bimetallic nanoparticles [34]. The highest selectivity for 2,5-dimethylfuran was 83.7% (Table 7, Entry 9), which could be attributed to the SCNT providing anchoring sites for metals, leading to a highly even distribution of Pd and Co nanoparticles and the cooperative effect of Pd-$Co_9S_8$ bimetallic centers. Similar to the S-modified support providing anchoring sites in Liao et al.'s work, Goyal et al. loaded Ni onto N-rich mesoporous carbon materials to convert 5-hydroxymethylfurfural to 2,5-dimethylfuran [14]. N atoms and Ni nanoparticles (<5 nm) exhibited a metal-support synergy, and the strong interaction between the two groups of atoms allowed the Ni nanoparticles to be steadily dispersed on the support, enhancing the total reduction of Ni and thus improving the hydrogenation activity of the catalyst (99.9% 5-hydroxymethylfurfural conversion, 98.7% 2,5-dimethylfuran selectivity, Table 7, Entry 10). Li et al. prepared Cu/$ZrO_2$ catalyst using isopropanol as a solvent (hydrogen donor) and synthesized controllable VO-CuO (oxygen vacancies near Cu metal) and VZr-$CuO^{\delta+}$dual-interface active sites for the transformation of 5-hydroxymethylfurfural to 2,5-dimethylfuran [30]. By offering distinct active sites for intermediate products and reactants, the dual-interface sites successfully prevented coupling reactions brought on by the competitive adsorption. (Table 7, Entry 11).

## 4.3 *Synthesis of 2-Methylfuran from Furfural*

2-Methylfuran is typically derived from furfural conversion that involves the hydrogenation of the C=O bond and the hydrogenolysis of the C–O bond. Golub et al. investigated the effects of pyrolysis temperature and Co/Cu ratio on the $Co_xCu_{1-x}MOF_{74}$ catalyst for furfural hydrogenation [13]. Cu exhibited strong adsorption for carbonyl oxygen during the hydrogenation but repelled the furan ring, thereby showing higher selectivity towards furfuryl alcohol. On the other hand, Co did not repel the furan ring and exhibited lower furfuryl alcohol selectivity, instead of favoring the hydrogenolysis to produce 2-methylfuran. The two metals formed a core–shell structure (Cu-shell, Co-core) after a $N_2$ pyrolysis treatment (400–900 °C). Based on characterization results, the outer layer of the catalyst tended to form a more complete Cu shell at high temperatures, resulting in a drop in furfuryl alcohol conversion but an increase in selectivity. At lower temperatures (below 600 °C), the incomplete Cu shell exposed more Co, resulting in higher selectivity towards 2-methylfuran. What's more, higher Co:Cu ratio has been shown to boost activity and change selectivity in favor of 2-methylfuran. Furfuryl alcohol selectivity of 66–89% and 2-methylfuran selectivity of 10–25% were obtained from the bimetallic catalysts' selective conversion of furfural. In addition, Dong et al. conducted an impressive study in which they utilized a two-stage packed Cu-Pd catalyst to achieve a direct conversion of furfural into 2-methyltetrahydrofuran at room temperature with a yield of 97.1% (Table 8, Entry 1–2) [10]. $Cu_2Si_2O_5(OH)_2$ located at the top of the reactor catalyzed the hydrogenation and deoxygenation of the C=O bond in furfural to synthesize 2-methylfuran. Meanwhile, the hydrogenation of 2-methylfuran's C=C bond was aided by Pd/$SiO_2$ which was located at the reactor's bottom.

**Table 8** 2-Methylfuran synthesis from furfural and xylose

| Entry | Feedstock | Catalyst | Product | Tem. (°C) | Time | Conv. (%) | Sel. (%) | References |
|---|---|---|---|---|---|---|---|---|
| 1 | Furfural | $Cu_2Si_2O_5(OH)_2$ | 2-methylfuran | 170 | / | 94.4 | 84.6 | Dong et al. [10] |
| 2 | Furfural | $Cu_2Si_2O_5(OH)_2$+Pd/$SiO_2$ | 2-methylfuran | 170 | / | 99.1 | 65.6 | Dong et al. [10] |
| 3 | Furfural | Pd^$SO_3$H@Y-5 | 2-methylfuran | 130 | 6 h | 99.5 | 99.3 | Jin et al. [23] |
| 4 | Furfural | Pd^$SO_3$H@Y-10 | 2-methylfuran | 130 | 6 h | 99.5 | 98.9 | Jin et al. [23] |
| 5 | Furfural | Cu-MCF-LT | 2-methylfuran | 190 | 5 h | 95 | 76 | Jiménez-Gómez et al. [22] |
| 6 | Furfural | Rh@H-BEA (Si/Al=12.5) | 2-methylfuran | 150 | 24 h | 87 | 98 | Zhang et al. [77] |
| 7 | Furfural | Rh@Na-BEA (Si:Al=68) | 2-methylfuran | 150 | 24 h | 75 | 0 | Zhang et al. [77] |

Bifunctional catalysts involving metal and acid sites have been widely used for the synthesis of 2-methylfuran from furfural. Jin et al. developed a method to incorporate sulfonic acid groups and Pd nanoparticles into zeolite crystals, creating synergistic active sites ($Pd^\wedge SO_3H@Y$) [23]. The sulfonic acid groups functioned as the acid sites, and Pd as the metal sites. The $Pd^\wedge SO_3H@Y$ catalyst exhibited a 2-methylfuran selectivity of 99.3% (Table 8, Entry 3–4), due to the near proximity of Pd nanoparticles and acid sites. Furthermore, the rigid zeolite structure stabilized the metal–acid interface, resulting in stable catalytic performance during continuous cycling experiments. Adsorbed Cu nanoparticles atop porous silica supports (Cu-MCF-LT) by Jiménez-Gómez et al. allowed furfural to be gas-phase converted to 2-methylfuran. (Table 8, Entry 5) [22]. The hydrogenation reaction was promoted by the presence of tiny Cu particles and weak acid sites on the supports. Zhang et al. prepared Rh@BEA catalysts by changing the Si/Al ratio and proton or sodium exchange in the zeolite support to modify its acid property [77]. Experimental results showed that Rh@H-BEA, which had the highest Al content (Si:Al=12.5) and a proton-exchanged silica-alumina zeolite support, provided both Lewis and Brønsted acid sites, resulting in a 2-methylfuran selectivity of 98% (Table 8, Entry 6–7). In contrast, Rh@Na-BEA, which had a low Al content (Si:Al=68) and a sodium-exchanged silica-alumina zeolite support lacking acid sites, primarily produced the hydrogenation product furfuryl alcohol.

## *4.4 Synthesis of 2-Methyltetrahydrofuran from Levulinic Acid and γ-Valerolactone*

The production of 2-methyltetrahydrofuran from levulinic acid and γ-valerolactone mainly involves the successive steps of hydrogenation, ring-opening and dehydration. The majority of current research focuses on the creation of bimetallic catalysts, with one metal providing hydrogenation active sites and another positively charged metal providing acid sites. Zhang et al. developed $NiMoO_x/Al_2O_3$ for the hydrogenolysis of γ-valerolactone to create 1,4-pentanediol and 2-methyltetrahydrofuran. The overall yield of these two products was 94.0% (Table 9, Entry 1) [75]. The Ni atoms served as active centers for the dissociation of hydrogen molecules, while the surface-defect $MoO_x$ species acted as acid sites with a medium-strength acidity. γ-valerolactone can also be converted to 1,4-pentanediol through ring-opening and hydrogenation, followed by dehydration to form 2-methyltetrahydrofuran. Levulinic acid was converted into 2-methyltetrahydrofuran by utilizing a silicon-supported Co catalyst [46]. Using a silicon-supported Co catalyst… At 200 °C in steady-state conditions, the major product was γ-valerolactone, with a yield of 98% (Table 9, Entry 2). Higher reaction temperatures (above 225 °C) could increase the hydrogenation activity and favour the ring-opening of γ-valerolactone, resulting in the formation of 2-methyltetrahydrofuran in 70% yield. The Co(0) metal sites and

**Table 9** 2-Methyltetrahydrofuran synthesis from levulinic acid and γ-valerolactone

| Entry | Feedstock | Catalyst | Product | Tem. (°C) | Time | Conv. (%) | Sel. (%) | References |
|---|---|---|---|---|---|---|---|---|
| 1 | γ-valerolactone | Ni-MoOx/$Al_2O_3$-600 | 2-Methyltetrahydrofuran, 1,4-pentanediol | 200 | 4 h | 95 | 31 | Zhang et al. [75] |
| 2 | Levulinic acid | Co/$SiO_2$ | 2-Methyltetrahydrofuran, γ-valerolactone | 200 | / | 100 | 70 | Novodárszki et al. [46] |
| 3 | γ-valerolactone | RhMo/$SiO_2$(0.25) | 2-Methyltetrahydrofuran | 120 | 6 h | 76 | 86 | Huang and Kudo et al. [20] |
| 4 | γ-valerolactone | Cu/$Al_2O_3$ | 2-Methyltetrahydrofuran, 1,4-pentanediol | 200 | 2 h | 91 | 81 | Liu and Zhao et al. [35] |
| 5 | γ-valerolactone | $Zn_{0.5}Cu/Al_2O_3$ | 2-Methyltetrahydrofuran, 1,4-pentanediol | 200 | 2 h | 92 | 25 | Liu and Zhao et al. [35] |
| 6 | γ-valerolactone | Cu/$Al_2O_3$ | 2-Methyltetrahydrofuran | 140 | 2.5 h | 98.5 | 98.9 | Sun and Saito et al. [59] |
| 7 | γ-valerolactone | 1 Ni-4%Co/$Al_2O_3$ | 2-Methyltetrahydrofuran | 230 | 5 h | 86 | 93.0 | Soszka et al. [57] |
| 8 | Levulinic acid | Pt–Mo/H-β | 2-Methyltetrahydrofuran | 130 | 24 h | >99 | 86 | Mizugaki et al. [42] |

CoOx Lewis acid sites in the catalyst enabled the hydrogenation and dehydrogenation processes. Huang et al. conducted further research on the transformation of γ-valerolactone to 2-methyltetrahydrofuran [20]. They achieved selective hydrogenation and deoxygenation to produce 2-methyltetrahydrofuran using RhRe and RhMo supported on silica catalysts, with the highest selectivity reaching 86% (Table 9, Entry 3). Using n-heptane as a solvent, Rh allowed for high reactivity at low temperatures. However, the selectivity over $Rh/SiO_2$ toward 2-methyltetrahydrofuran was rather low, resulting in a further production of 2-pentanol. The addition of Mo and Re provided an additional acidity and improved the selectivity of 2-methyltetrahydrofuran. Liu et al. investigated the use of $Cu/Al_2O_3$ and $ZnCu/Al_2O_3$ catalysts to convert γ-valerolactone to 1,4-pentanediol and 2-methyltetrahydrofuran [35]. The $Cu/Al_2O_3$ with 10 wt.% Cu produced roughly equal amounts of 1,4-pentanediol and 2-methyltetrahydrofuran (Table 9, Entry 4–5). Zn was added to create a Zn-Cu alloy, which inhibited Cu(0) oxidation while lowering surface Lewis acidity. This improved 1,4-pentanediol selectivity by preventing 1,4-pentanediol from dehydrating into 2-methyltetrahydrofuran.

More generally, acid sites can be provided by solid acid supports, which made metal-loaded solid acid catalysts extensively applied nanocomposites for the synthesis of 2-methyltetrahydrofuran. To capitalize on the complementary effects of metal and acid sites in the support, Sun et al. synthesized $Cu/Al_2O_3$ to facilitate the conversion of γ-valerolactone into 2-methyltetrahydrofuran [59]. The $Cu/Al_2O_3$ catalyst achieved the highest γ-valerolactone conversion of 98.5% with a 2-methyltetrahydrofuran selectivity of 98.9% (Table 9, Entry 6). It was concluded that the large particle size of copper and higher acid concentration were the determining factors for the high productivity and selectivity. A bimetallic Ni-Co/γ-$Al_2O_3$ catalyst with the right proportion of Ni demonstrated a high yield of 2-methyltetrahydrofuran, as reported by Soszka et al. (Table 9, Entry 7) [27]. The authors precisely controlled two steps of the reaction. Metal sites are required for the first step, which involves opening γ-valerolactone to generate 1,4-pentanediol, and the design of Ni-Co alloy enhances the availability of Ni, reducing its susceptibility to hydrogen poisoning. In the subsequent phase, a significant quantity of weak and moderate acid sites are needed for the dehydration of 1,4-pentanediol into the cyclic form, these sites are supplied by $Al_2O_3$. Mizugaki et al. focused on the dual role of the catalyst support in the conversion of levulinic acid to 2-methyltetrahydrofuran (Table 9, Entry 8) [42]. They prepared a Pt–Mo/H-β catalyst with H-β zeolite as the support. In addition to acting as an acid site during the dehydration of 1,4-pentanediol to produce 2-methyltetrahydrofuran, the H-β zeolite effectively supported the dispersion of Pt nanoparticles and MoOx, fostering their mutual enhancement during the hydrogenation reaction.

## 5 Concluding Remarks

Nanocomposites play an important role in biomass energy production owing to their modifiable catalyst nanostructures, versatile active sites and their controllable catalytic effects. In this chapter, we demonstrate the key catalytic role of nanocomposites as multifunctional catalysts for the manufacture of typical bioenergy chemicals, e.g., levulinic acid esters, valeric biofuels and furan-based biofuels, which have been intensively focused on by related studies in recent years. Particularly, catalytic synthesis routes for these chemicals are presented, and we further concentrate our attention on catalytic effects of nanocomposite active sites and synergistic effects between multiple active sites on the bioenergy synthesis processes. For the current study, the exploitation of the theoretical implications of the coordination of multiple sites of nanocomposites on surface reactions and the enrichment of nanocomposites synthesis methods for more precise nanoengineering are still considered to be the main technical challenges in this field.

For future research, many advanced technological approaches that have gradually been emerging recently are expected to be adopted to proactively cope with these challenges. For example, theoretical computational techniques (including density functional theory as well as molecular dynamics, etc.) can be applied to recognize the surface reaction processes of nanocomposites at a theoretical level. In-situ characterization techniques (including in-situ infrared spectroscopy, in-situ Raman spectroscopy, etc.) can be used to probe the catalytic effects of nanocomposites under realistic reaction conditions. The application of the above concepts will potentially contribute to the creation of novel multifunctional nanocomposites for more efficient valorization of biomass into liquid fuels.

**Acknowledgements** The authors wish to thank the project sponsorship from the Postdoctoral Science Foundation of China (No. 2023M732589), and the National Natural Science Foundation of China (No. 52066017, 22308253).

## References

1. Akiyama G, Matsuda R, Sato H, Takata M, Kitagawa S (2011) Cellulose hydrolysis by a new porous coordination polymer decorated with sulfonic acid functional groups. Adv Mater 23(29):3294–3297
2. Ayashi N, Najafi Chermahini A, Saraji M (2022) Biomass conversion to alkyl levulinates using heteropoly acid carbon mesoporous composites. Process Saf Environ Prot 160:988–1000
3. Babaei Z, Najafi Chermahini A, Dinari M (2018) Alumina-coated mesoporous silica SBA-15 as a solid catalyst for catalytic conversion of fructose into liquid biofuel candidate ethyl levulinate. Chem Eng J 352:45–52
4. Buitrago-Sierra R, Serrano-Ruiz JC, Rodríguez-Reinoso F, Sepúlveda-Escribano A, Dumesic JA (2012) Ce promoted Pd–Nb catalysts for γ-valerolactone ring-opening and hydrogenation. Green Chem 14(12)

5. Chen S, Wojcieszak R, Dumeignil F, Marceau E, Royer S (2018) How catalysts and experimental conditions determine the selective hydroconversion of furfural and 5-hydroxymethylfurfural. Chem Rev 118(22):11023–11117
6. Chhabra T, Rohilla J, Krishnan V (2022) Nanoarchitectonics of phosphomolybdic acid supported on activated charcoal for selective conversion of furfuryl alcohol and levulinic acid to alkyl levulinates. Mol Catal 519:112135
7. Cho HJ, Kim D, Li S, Su D, Ma D, Xu B (2019) Molecular-level proximity of metal and acid sites in zeolite-encapsulated Pt nanoparticles for selective multistep tandem catalysis. ACS Catal 10(5):3340–3348
8. Cho HJ, Kim D, Xu B (2020) Selectivity control in tandem catalytic furfural upgrading on zeolite-encapsulated Pt nanoparticles through site and solvent engineering. ACS Catal 10(8):4770–4779
9. Dai J, Peng L, Li H (2018) Intensified ethyl levulinate production from cellulose using a combination of low loading $H_2SO_4$ and $Al(OTf)_3$. Catal Commun 103:116–119
10. Dong F, Zhu Y, Ding G, Cui J, Li X, Li Y (2015) One-step conversion of furfural into 2-methyltetrahydrofuran under mild conditions. Chemsuschem 8(9):1534–1537
11. Esteves LM, Brijaldo MH, Oliveira EG, Martinez JJ, Rojas H, Caytuero A, Passos FB (2020) Effect of support on selective 5-hydroxymethylfurfural hydrogenation towards 2,5-dimethylfuran over copper catalysts. Fuel 270
12. Geng W, Li W, Liu L, Liu J, Liu L, Kong X (2020) Facile assembly of Cu-$Cu_2O$/N-reduced graphene oxide nanocomposites for efficient synthesis of 2-methylfuran. Fuel 259
13. Golub KW, Sulmonetti TP, Darunte LA, Shealy MS, Jones CW (2019) Metal–organic-framework-derived Co/Cu–carbon nanoparticle catalysts for furfural hydrogenation. ACS Appl Nano Mater 2(9):6040–6056
14. Goyal R, Sarkar B, Bag A, Siddiqui N, Dumbre D, Lucas N, Bhargava SK, Bordoloi A (2016) Studies of synergy between metal–support interfaces and selective hydrogenation of HMF to DMF in water. J Catal 340:248–260
15. Gu X-M, Zhang B, Liang H-J, Ge H-B, Yang H-M, Qin Y (2017) Pt/HZSM-5 catalyst synthesized by atomic layer deposition for aqueous-phase hydrogenation of levulinic acid to valeric acid. J Fuel Chem Technol 45(6):714–722
16. Gunawan R, Cahyadi HS, Insyani R, Kwak SK, Kim J (2021) Density functional theory investigation of the conversion of 5-(Hydroxymethyl)furfural into 2,5-dimethylfuran over the Pd(111), Cu(111), and Cu3Pd(111) surfaces. J Phys Chem C 125(19):10295–10317
17. Guo D, Liu X, Cheng F, Zhao W, Wen S, Xiang Y, Xu Q, Yu N, Yin D (2020) Selective hydrogenolysis of 5-hydroxymethylfurfural to produce biofuel 2, 5-dimethylfuran over Ni/ZSM-5 catalysts. Fuel 274
18. He J, Lin L, Liu M, Miao C, Wu Z, Chen R, Chen S, Chen T, Su Y, Zhang T, Luo W (2022) A durable Ni/La-Y catalyst for efficient hydrogenation of γ-valerolactone into pentanoic biofuels. J Energy Chem 70:347–355
19. He J, Wu Z, Gu Q, Liu Y, Chu S, Chen S, Zhang Y, Yang B, Chen T, Wang A, Weckhuysen BM, Zhang T, Luo W (2021) Zeolite-tailored active site proximity for the efficient production of pentanoic biofuels. Angew Chem Int Ed Engl 60(44):23713–23721
20. Huang X, Kudo S, Ashik UPM, Einaga H, Hayashi J-I (2020) Selective hydrodeoxygenation of γ-valerolactone over silica-supported Rh-based bimetallic catalysts. Energy Fuels 34(6):7190–7197
21. Huang Z, Hao S, Yuan H (2022) Synthesis of ethyl levulinate from cellulose over a double acid site catalyst. J Chem Technol Biotechnol 97(1):240–253
22. Jiménez-Gómez CP, Cecilia JA, Alba-Rubio AC, Cassidy A, Moreno-Tost R, García-Sancho C, Maireles-Torres P (2022) Tailoring the selectivity of Cu-based catalysts in the furfural hydrogenation reaction: influence of the morphology of the silica support. Fuel 319
23. Jin Z, Yi X, Wang L, Xu S, Wang C, Wu Q, Wang L, Zheng A, Xiao F-S (2019) Metal-acid interfaces enveloped in zeolite crystals for cascade biomass hydrodeoxygenation. Appl Catal B: Environ 254:560–568

24. Karanwal N, Verma D, Butolia P, Kim SM, Kim J (2020) One-pot direct conversion of levulinic acid into high-yield valeric acid over a highly stable bimetallic Nb-Cu/Zr-doped porous silica catalyst. Green Chem 22(3):766–787
25. Khder AS, El-Sharkawy EA, El-Hakam SA, Ahmed AI (2008) Surface characterization and catalytic activity of sulfated tin oxide catalyst. Catal Commun 9(5):769–777
26. Kon K, Onodera W, Shimizu K-I (2014) Selective hydrogenation of levulinic acid to valeric acid and valeric biofuels by a Pt/HMFI catalyst. Catal Sci Technol 4(9):3227–3234
27. Kong X, Wu S, Li X, Liu J (2016) Efficient conversion of levulinic acid to ethyl levulinate over a silicotungstic-acid-modified commercially silica-gel sphere catalyst. Energy Fuels 30(8):6500–6504
28. Kumar VV, Naresh G, Deepa S, Bhavani PG, Nagaraju M, Sudhakar M, Chary KVR, Tardio J, Bhargava SK, Venugopal A (2017) Influence of W on the reduction behaviour and Brønsted acidity of $Ni/TiO_2$ catalyst in the hydrogenation of levulinic acid to valeric acid: pyridine adsorbed DRIFTS study. Appl Catal A: Gen 531:169–176
29. Kumar VV, Naresh G, Sudhakar M, Tardio J, Bhargava SK, Venugopal A (2015) Role of Brønsted and Lewis acid sites on $Ni/TiO_2$ catalyst for vapour phase hydrogenation of levulinic acid: kinetic and mechanistic study. Appl Catal A: Gen 505:217–223
30. Lai F, Yan F, Wang P, Qu F, Shen X, Zhang Z (2021) Efficient one-pot synthesis of ethyl levulinate from carbohydrates catalyzed by Wells-Dawson heteropolyacid supported on Ce–Si pillared montmorillonite. J Clean Prod 324:129276
31. Li H, Liu H, Cai C, Wang H, Huang Y, Li S, Yang B, Wang C, Liao Y, Ma L (2023) Tandem conversion xylose to 2-methylfuran with NiCu/C catalyst. Catal Commun 175
32. Li M, Wei J, Yan G, Liu H, Tang X, Sun Y, Zeng X, Lei T, Lin L (2020) Cascade conversion of furfural to fuel bioadditive ethyl levulinate over bifunctional zirconium-based catalysts. Renew Energy 147:916–923
33. Li X, Yang P, Zhang X, Liu Y, Miao C, Feng J, Li D (2021) Insights into the role of dual-interfacial sites in Cu/ZrO(2) catalysts in 5-HMF hydrogenolysis with isopropanol. ACS Appl Mater Interfaces 13(19):22292–22303
34. Liao W, Zhu Z, Chen N, Su T, Deng C, Zhao Y, Ren W, Lü H (2020) Highly active bifunctional Pd-Co9S8/S-CNT catalysts for selective hydrogenolysis of 5-hydroxymethylfurfural to 2,5-dimethylfuran. Mol Catal 482
35. Liu Q, Zhao Z, Arai M, Zhang C, Liu K, Shi R, Wu P, Wang Z, Lin W, Cheng H, Zhao F (2020) Transformation of γ-valerolactone into 1,4-pentanediol and 2-methyltetrahydrofuran over Zn-promoted $Cu/Al_2O_3$ catalysts. Catal Sci Technol 10(13):4412–4423
36. Liu S, Fan G, Yang L, Li F (2017) Highly efficient transformation of γ-valerolactone to valerate esters over structure-controlled copper/zirconia catalysts prepared via a reduction-oxidation route. Appl Catal A: Gen 543:180–188
37. Liu X-F, Li H, Zhang H, Pan H, Huang S, Yang K-L, Yang S (2016) Efficient conversion of furfuryl alcohol to ethyl levulinate with sulfonic acid-functionalized MIL-101(Cr). RSC Adv 6(93):90232–90238
38. Liu X, Pan H, Zhang H, Li H, Yang S (2019) Efficient catalytic upgradation of bio-based furfuryl alcohol to ethyl levulinate using mesoporous acidic MIL-101(Cr). ACS Omega 4(5):8390–8399
39. Liu Y, Shi X, Hu J, Liu K, Zeng M, Hou Y, Wei Z (2022) Highly effective activated carbon-supported Ni-Mn bifunctional catalyst for selective hydrodeoxygenation of 5-hydroxymethylfurfural to 2,5-dimethylfuran. Chemsuschem 15(13):e202200193
40. Luo W, Bruijnincx PCA, Weckhuysen BM (2014) Selective, one-pot catalytic conversion of levulinic acid to pentanoic acid over Ru/H-ZSM5. J Catal 320:33–41
41. Luo W, Deka U, Beale AM, van Eck ERH, Bruijnincx PCA, Weckhuysen BM (2013) Ruthenium-catalyzed hydrogenation of levulinic acid: influence of the support and solvent on catalyst selectivity and stability. J Catal 301:175–186
42. Mizugaki T, Togo K, Maeno Z, Mitsudome T, Jitsukawa K, Kaneda K (2016) One-Pot transformation of levulinic acid to 2-methyltetrahydrofuran catalyzed by Pt–Mo/H-β in water. ACS Sustain Chem Eng 4(3):682–685

43. Morales G, Osatiashtiani A, Hernández B, Iglesias J, Melero JA, Paniagua M, Robert Brown D, Granollers M, Lee AF, Wilson K (2014) Conformal sulfated zirconia monolayer catalysts for the one-pot synthesis of ethyl levulinate from glucose. Chem Commun 50(79):11742–11745
44. Muñoz-Olasagasti M, Sañudo-Mena A, Cecilia JA, Granados ML, Maireles-Torres P, Mariscal R (2019) Direct conversion of levulinic acid into valeric biofuels using Pd supported over zeolites as catalysts. Top Catal 62(5–6):579–588
45. Nandiwale KY, Sonar SK, Niphadkar PS, Joshi PN, Deshpande SS, Patil VS, Bokade VV (2013) Catalytic upgrading of renewable levulinic acid to ethyl levulinate biodiesel using dodecatungstophosphoric acid supported on desilicated H-ZSM-5 as catalyst. Appl Catal A: Gen 460–461:90–98
46. Novodárszki G, Solt HE, Valyon J, Lónyi F, Hancsók J, Deka D, Tuba R, Mihályi MR (2019) Selective hydroconversion of levulinic acid to $\gamma$-valerolactone or 2-methyltetrahydrofuran over silica-supported cobalt catalysts. Catal Sci Technol 9(9):2291–2304
47. Osiglio L, Romanelli G, Blanco M (2010) Alcohol acetylation with acetic acid using borated zirconia as catalyst. J Mol Catal A: Chem 316(1):52–58
48. Pan T, Deng J, Xu Q, Xu Y, Guo Q-X, Fu Y (2013) Catalytic conversion of biomass-derived levulinic acid to valerate esters as oxygenated fuels using supported ruthenium catalysts. Green Chem 15(10)
49. Pasquale G, Vázquez P, Romanelli G, Baronetti G (2012) Catalytic upgrading of levulinic acid to ethyl levulinate using reusable silica-included Wells-Dawson heteropolyacid as catalyst. Catal Commun 18:115–120
50. Patil CR, Rode CV (2018) Synthesis of diesel additives from fructose over PWA/SBA-15 catalyst. Fuel 217:38–44
51. Prieto G, Tüysüz H, Duyckaerts N, Knossalla J, Wang G-H, Schüth F (2016) Hollow nano-and microstructures as catalysts. Chem Rev 116(22):14056–14119
52. Ramli NAS, Sivasubramaniam D, Amin NAS (2017) Esterification of levulinic acid using $ZrO_2$-supported phosphotungstic acid catalyst for ethyl levulinate production. BioEnergy Res 10(4):1105–1116
53. Sarkar C, Koley P, Shown I, Lee J, Liao Y-F, An K, Tardio J, Nakka L, Chen K-H, Mondal J (2019) Integration of interfacial and alloy effects to modulate catalytic performance of metal–organic-framework-derived Cu–Pd nanocrystals toward hydrogenolysis of 5-hydroxymethylfurfural. ACS Sustain Chem Eng 7(12):10349–10362
54. Scotti N, Dangate M, Gervasini A, Evangelisti C, Ravasio N, Zaccheria F (2014) Unraveling the role of low coordination sites in a Cu metal nanoparticle: a step toward the selective synthesis of second generation biofuels. ACS Catal 4(8):2818–2826
55. Sk H, Balla P, Ponnala B, Ginjupalli S, Nekkala N, Koppadi KS, Komandur VRC (2022) Efficient transformation of furfuryl alcohol into ethyl levulinates via alcoholysis reaction catalyzed by $SnO_2$/H-mordenite catalyst. Catal Surv Asia 26(2):104–114
56. Song D, Zhang Q, Sun Y, Zhang P, Guo Y-H, Hu J-L (2018) Design of ordered mesoporous sulfonic acid functionalized $ZrO_2$/organosilica bifunctional catalysts for direct catalytic conversion of glucose to ethyl levulinate. ChemCatChem 10(21):4953–4965
57. Soszka E, Jędrzejczyk M, Keller N, Ruppert AM (2023) High yield production of 2-methyltetrahydrofuran biofuel with reusable Ni-Co catalysts. Fuel 332
58. Srivastava S, Jadeja GC, Parikh J (2017) Influence of supports for selective production of 2,5-dimethylfuran via bimetallic copper-cobalt catalyzed 5-hydroxymethylfurfural hydrogenolysis. Chin J Catal 38(4):699–709
59. Sun D, Saito T, Otsuka S, Ozawa T, Yamada Y, Sato S (2020) Selective hydrogenation of $\gamma$-valerolactone to 2-methyltetrahydrofuran over $Cu/Al_2O_3$ catalyst. Appl Catal A: Gen 590
60. Sun P, Gao G, Zhao Z, Xia C, Li F (2014) Stabilization of cobalt catalysts by embedment for efficient production of valeric biofuel. ACS Catal 4(11):4136–4142
61. Sun P, Gao G, Zhao Z, Xia C, Li F (2016) Acidity-regulation for enhancing the stability of Ni/HZSM-5 catalyst for valeric biofuel production. Appl Catal B: Environ 189:19–25
62. Sun Y, Zhang Q, Zhang P, Song D, Guo Y (2018) Nitrogen-Doped carbon-based acidic ionic liquid hollow nanospheres for efficient and selective conversion of fructose to 5-ethoxymethylfurfural and ethyl levulinate. ACS Sustain Chem Eng 6(5):6771–6782

63. Tang K, Xie S, Cofield GR, Yang X, Tian E, Lin H (2018) Catalytic transfer hydrogenation of furfural for the production of ethyl levulinate: interplay of lewis and brønsted acidities. Energ Technol 6(9):1826–1831
64. Tian L, Zhang L, Liu Y, He Y, Zhu Y, Sun R, Yi S, Xiang J (2020) Clean production of ethyl levulinate from kitchen waste. J Clean Prod 268:122296
65. Tuan Hoang A, Viet Pham V (2021) 2-methylfuran (MF) as a potential biofuel: a thorough review on the production pathway from biomass, combustion progress, and application in engines. Renew Sustain Energy Rev 148
66. Velisoju VK, Jampaiah D, Gutta N, Bentrup U, Brückner A, Bhargava SK, Akula V (2020) Conversion of γ-valerolactone to ethyl valerate over metal promoted Ni/ZSM-5 catalysts: influence of $Ni^0/Ni^{2+}$ heterojunctions on activity and product selectivity. ChemCatChem 12(5):1341–1349
67. Wang A, Lu Y, Yi Z, Ejaz A, Hu K, Zhang L, Yan K (2018) Selective production of γ-valerolactone and valeric acid in one-pot bifunctional metal catalysts. ChemistrySelect 3(4):1097–1101
68. Wang D, Wang B, Ding Y, Yuan Q, Wu H, Guan Y, Wu P (2017) Robust synthesis of green fuels from biomass-derived ethyl esters over a hierarchically core/shell-structured ZSM-5@(Co/SiO(2)) catalyst. Chem Commun (Camb) 53(73):10172–10175
69. Wang S, Cheng A, Liu F, Zhang J, Xia T, Zeng X, Fan W, Zhang Y (2023) Catalytic conversion network for lignocellulosic biomass valorization: a panoramic view. Ind Chem Mater 1(2):188–206
70. Weng R, Lu X, Ji N, Fukuoka A, Shrotri A, Li X, Zhang R, Zhang M, Xiong J, Yu Z (2021) Taming the butterfly effect: modulating catalyst nanostructures for better selectivity control of the catalytic hydrogenation of biomass-derived furan platform chemicals. Catal Sci Technol 11(24):7785–7806
71. Yogita BS, Rao CS, Lingaiah N (2021) The selective conversion of furfuryl alcohol to ethyl levulinate over Zr-modified tungstophosphoric acid supported on β-zeolites. New J Chem 45(6):3224–3233
72. Zainol MM, Asmadi M, Amin NAS, Roslan MNF (2022) Glucose-derived bio-fuel additive via ethanolysis catalyzed by zinc modified sulfonated carbon. Mater Today: Proc 57:1008–1013
73. Zainol MM, Asmadi M, Iskandar P, Wan Ahmad WAN, Amin NAS, Hoe TT (2021) Ethyl levulinate synthesis from biomass derivative chemicals using iron doped sulfonated carbon cryogel catalyst. J Clean Prod 281:124686
74. Zhang G, Li W, Fan G, Yang L, Li F (2019) Controlling product selectivity by surface defects over MoO-decorated Ni-based nanocatalysts for γ-valerolactone hydrogenolysis. J Catal 379:100–111
75. Zhang J, Chen J (2016) Modified solid acids derived from biomass based cellulose for one-step conversion of carbohydrates into ethyl levulinate. J Energy Chem 25(5):747–753
76. Zhang Y, Li A, Kubů M, Shamzhy M, Čejka J (2022) Highly selective reduction of biomass-derived furfural by tailoring the microenvironment of Rh@BEA catalysts. Catal Today 390–391:295–305
77. Zhong R, Yu F, Schutyser W, Liao Y, de Clippel F, Peng L, Sels BF (2017) Acidic mesostructured silica-carbon nanocomposite catalysts for biofuels and chemicals synthesis from sugars in alcoholic solutions. Appl Catal B: Environ 206:74–88

# Translocation and Risk Assessment

# Nanomaterials Journey in Citrus Trees: A Pivotal Agroforestry Exploration

**Iqra Attique, Mubashra Inam, and Sumaira Anjum**

**Abstract** Phyto-nanotechnology, employing smart nanomaterials with precise target specificity, has revolutionized agroforestry by enhancing crop yield and quality. It offers applications in Citrus tree cultivation for disease detection, stress tolerance, and growth enhancement. Citrus plants contribute significantly to agro-economy in terms of provision of fruits and pharmaceutically and industrially important metabolites that can also be elicited using nanomaterials. While a substantial body of literature explores the nexus between nanomaterials and Citrus trees, the understanding of the intricate transport mechanisms underlying nanomaterials within plants and their consequential physiological responses remains relatively limited. The literature reviewed in this chapter is on the nanomaterial administration techniques, the routes of their uptake by the plant, the subsequent transport mechanisms and processes involved in nanoparticle delivery in plants and their physiological and environmental responses. It also sheds light on the potential risks of nanomaterials and the strategies and regulations established to cope with them. Conclusively, the future research aspects in the systematic study of nanomaterials in plants are also discussed.

**Keywords** Nanomaterials · Citrus trees · Phyto-nanotechnology · Agroforestry · Translocation · Risk assessment

## 1 Introduction

With a lack in evolutionary methods to cope with the increasing agricultural requirements of the developing world, scientists introduced Phyto-nanotechnology, a concept utilizing smart nanomaterials with peculiar physiochemical properties in complex agroforestry systems in order to optimize the quality and yield of the produce [94]. The principle characteristics of these smart nanodevices that make them

Iqra Attique and Mubashra Inam—Authors contributed equally.

I. Attique · M. Inam · S. Anjum (✉)
Department of Biotechnology, Kinnaird College for Women, Lahore, Pakistan
e-mail: sumaira.anjum@kinnaird.edu.pk

 
D. Jabborova et al. (eds.), *Nanomaterials in Agroforestry Systems*, Smart Nanomaterials Technology, https://doi.org/10.1007/978-981-96-1337-3_17

extraordinary, is their target specificity, mainly due to their size compatibility with nanoscopic cellular organelles, eliminating any form of hindrance in uptake, translocation and functionality [33]. Essentially, target-based systems allow for an automated, time-controlled, integrative and optimized network that carries and delivers foreign material directly to the desired component in the agricultural set-up, avoiding interruption with the surrounding biological systems [56, 81].

In terms of applicability, nanomaterials can be of pertinent use in the agroforestry of ubiquitous crop plants such as Citrus trees, aiding in the detection and treatment of diseases, monitoring of plant pathogens, inducing tolerance for environmental stress, and enhancing growth [17, 53]. These flowering trees, harbor common fruits such as oranges, limes, grapefruits, and lemons etc., and are considered immensely valuable in the industry of agri-food, cosmetics, bio-fuel synthesis, and packaging [120]. Moreover, since the COVID-19 pandemic, the pharmaceutical industry has widely sourced vitamin C from Citrus trees to manufacture immunity boosting medication thus creating a higher demand for their cultivation [1].

While integrating nanotechnology with Citrus tree agroforestry systems has a myriad of benefits, a range of potential risks can also arise, hindering their success. Contamination of the environment, including the aquatic ecosystem, the atmosphere and the soil medium, is one of the most concerning prospects. The process of engineering nanoparticles often produces wastewater, sludge or debris that accidentally ends up in landfills and sewage canals. Subsequently they reach their ultimate sink, the soil, constantly being absorbed by nearby plants and organisms [18]. Apart from the internal structural damage caused by the movement of the nanoparticles within the plant system, their accumulation above the threshold concentration can invariably result in irreversible disruption of their physiological and biochemical pathways, alteration in their morphology, and cause genotoxicity [131]. In terms of plant health, the resultant flora will suffer from a significant decrease in the rate of transpiration and photosynthesis, slower rate of seed germination, inevitably giving rise to plants lower in quality, yield and total biomass [34]. Moreover, once the plant dies off and is biodegraded, the accumulated nanoparticles are recycled back into the ecosystem continuing to pose threats [77].

Nevertheless, these repercussions are mainly caused by improper management of the areas treated with nanomaterials and can be avoided in a well maintained, closely regulated agroforest. In addition, the enzymatic and non-enzymatic innate defense mechanisms of plants against stress induction help protect them from the harms of nanomaterials [42, 87]. Yet the aggravating concerns revolving around the engineering of novel nanomaterials and their toxic impact on the environmental has prompted further research on their uptake, translocation and accumulation by plants [21].

The goals of this chapter involve exploring the interaction between nanomaterials and Citrus trees by discussing the various methods of nanoparticle administration into plants, elaborating some of the inherent plant barriers that must be overcome for the nanomaterials to be taken up, and explaining the transportation pathways involved in assimilating them into different parts of the plant. Furthermore, insights into the factors influencing the distinct processes and the potential risks associated with un-regulated phyto-nanotechnology are also discussed.

## 2 Administration of Nanomaterials

The uptake of nanoparticles by a specific plant is dependent on a number of determinants that vary with the nature of the nanoparticle, its interaction with environmental elements, and the morphology of the plant [93]. The three primary methods of administration include: (i) Foliar spray, (ii) Trunk injection, and (iii) Root exposure, all classified on the basis of the part of the plant that is targeted during the process. Figure 1 demonstrates the general pathway adopted by nanoparticles when travelling through the three prime regions of the plant [88].

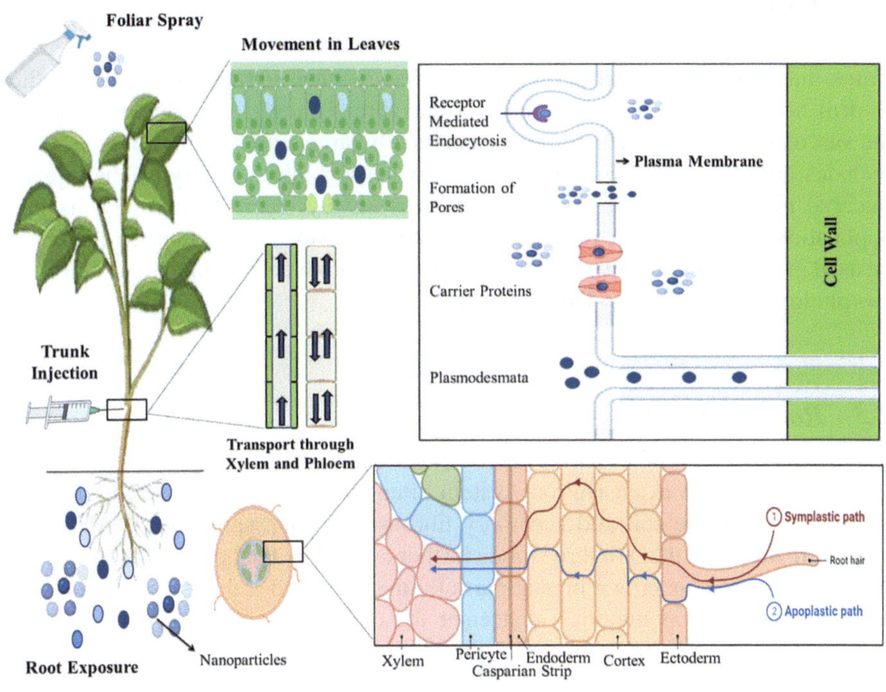


**Fig. 1** Schematic representation of the three principal routes of uptake of nanoparticles by plants: (i) Foliar spray (ii) Trunk Injection (iii) Root Exposure, The sub-cellular methods of invasion and the translocation pathways involved

### 2.1 Foliar Sprays

A preparation of nanoparticles, usually in the form of nano-powders, nano-aerosols, or nano-suspensions, is sprayed onto the leaves of the plant where they enter the system through the stomata and are transported to various parts of the plant via the symplastic and apoplastic pathways [46]. Despite the relatively small, ovulated leaf structure of citrus trees with an average leaf area of 5 $m^2$/fruit [36], foliar spray application has been widely used for the administration of fertilizers in the citrus industry. In Florida, Citrus nurseries are overcoming plant nutrient deficiencies by foliarly providing zinc, magnesium, manganese, copper, and boron to their crops reporting better efficiency, faster uptake of nutrients by the plant and a reduction in the loss of nanofertilizers as compared to traditional methods [41].

### 2.2 Trunk Injection

Trunk injection method utilizes injector devices, such as syringes or micro-needles to drill holes into the stem of the plant and directly insert the nanomaterial into the vascular tissue [14]. This process specifically targets the vascular bundle which includes both the xylem and phloem that are responsible for carrying the injected material to different plant organs. Being a relatively recent technology, its field application is limited and remains under study however, it has been reported to be used in the targeted delivery of plant protection products to Apple trees that show morphological similarity to Citrus tree trunks [133].

### 2.3 Root Exposure

Citrus trees have an extensive root system often comprising of a main tap root that grows deep into the soil and accessory fibrous roots that spread out horizontally absorbing nutrients that are three times further away than the height of the tree [15]. In agroforests, plants grown in nanoparticle supplemented soil uptake nutrients and subsequently the nanomaterials that enter the cell wall of the root, cross the cell membrane of the root epidermis, and ultimately invade the xylem vessel via several transport mechanisms [74].

# 3 Uptake of Nanomaterials in Citrus Trees

## *3.1 Mucilage and Exudates*

Plants release an amalgamation of polysaccharide rich secretions from different regions such as the root, stem, leaves, and seed that act as adhesives, protectants, aids plants retain water, and helps acquire nutrients [31]. In terrestrial plants such as Citrus trees, the mucilage and exudate released by the root hair and the cells lining the border of the root cap are primarily responsible for altering the biological, physical, and chemical composition of the soil around them which further interferes with nutrient/nanoparticle absorption by the plant [82]. The interaction between mucilage and nanoparticles is based on the solubility, size and surface charge of the latter which in turn determines their bioavailability to the plant [23, 69]. The involvement of mucilage and exudates from any plant part, other than the roots, in the uptake of nanoparticles is currently under investigation however, a research reporting the accumulation of Pb nanoparticles in necrotic leaves was hypothesized to be due to entrapment by the mucilage of lysed, damaged cells [90, 128].

Plant mucilage, often with the help of soil microorganisms, has the ability to decrease the pH of the surrounding rhizosphere which stimulates the dissolution of, otherwise insoluble nanoparticles present within that area [89, 111]. Research reveals that exudates, strong enough to oxidize gold nanoparticles (AuNPs) are released by plant roots that notably increase their dissolvability and subsequently their absorbability [122]. Furthermore, nanoparticles that are already soluble may often dissolve completely by being disintegrated into smaller units before being taken up by the roots and translocated to the shoot [68].

Since the surface of root hairs is negatively charged, nanoparticles bearing a positive charge often accumulate in the rhizosphere primarily due to electrostatic forces of attraction [141]. On the other hand, nanoparticles that are either neutral or charged negatively are absorbed and translocated at a relatively higher rate because of their minimal attachment to the identically charged root hair [145]. Nonetheless, occasional accumulation of these nanoparticles indicates the presence of additional, stronger forces that can override electrostatic repulsion [24]. The establishment of hydrogen bonds and covalent bonds may explain the stated accumulation and uptake of nanoparticles [109]. Precise size exclusion limit of nanoparticles through mucilage is difficult to determine as the acidic environment of the soil interrupts with the observation techniques employed in most experiments [68, 113]. Across a range of terrestrial plants and nanoparticles of varying sizes, plant mucilage and exudates exhibit a broad protective action against the uptake of nanoparticles, extending particularly against ones that are small, positively charged [143].

## 3.2 Cuticle

Plants are majorly covered by a layer of waxy cuticle that envelopes all parts exposed to air and some portions of the root rhizodermis. The cuticle of the leaves is composed of wax, cutin, and pectin and is responsible for the protection of the plant against excessive dehydration, attack by pathogens, and invasion of unwanted foreign particles [108, 137] While this hydrophobic layer acts as a natural primary barrier, repulsing the inward and outward movement of most polar and non-polar entities, its surface contains two channels: a hydrophilic channel and a lipophilic channel that allow the infiltration of certain components within the size range of 0.6–4.8 nm [3, 26]. Nonetheless, negatively charged mesoporous silica nanoparticles of 20 nm and neutrally charged lipid-based nanoparticles ranging from 150 to 300 nm have also been reported to be accumulated on the cuticle, lining the anticlinal cell wall, indicating variation in pore sizes [51, 79]. Yet another study revealed the ability of titanium dioxide nanoparticles (nano-$TiO_2$) to invade by introducing holes into the cuticle thus the need for in depth research and direct observation remains [61].

Hydrophilic nanoparticles opt for the polar pathways to infiltrate the plant through different leaf openings such as the stomata, trichomes, hydathodes, and surface wounds. The primary function of these apertures is to regulate the absorption and secretion of water molecules because of which they are inherently thin and pervious, allowing charged nanoparticles to enter or exit through them. However, plants' ability to absorb nanoparticles via the epidermis is constrained by the small size of the pore channels in the cuticle. Current research has thus far only supported the stomata to be the sole entry route for nanoparticles [66, 144]. Detailed studies have shown that water based nanoparticles must be smaller than 1.1 μm in order for plants to naturally absorb them through their stomata [26]. Additional investigation has revealed that only when leaves were treated with a surfactant were nanoparticles larger than 100 $\mu m^3$ discovered. Thus, it was established that the use of these wetting agents resulted in a greater absorption via the stomata [54].

## 3.3 Cell Wall Pores

The plant cell is confined within a dense web of biopolymers that are tightly intertwined to create a multilamellar matrix that surrounds the plant cell in a manner that prevents access to the plasma membrane (Albersheim P. 2011. Plant Cell Walls: From Chemistry to Biology. New York, USA: Garland Science). The structure is further fortified by the presence of suberin, papilla, lignin, callose, pectin, fibers and compounds such as $CaCO_3$, $SiO_2$, and $MgCO_3$ that also increase its impermeability to foreign materials [6]. Topographical EM studies, gas adsorption, and absorption of dye-labeled nanoscopic molecules are some of the techniques that have been employed to define the SEL of the nanoparticles that can pass through the pores of cell walls, the value of which is estimated to be 10 nm, though nanoparticles as large as 100 nm have also been detected [78]. Nonetheless, SEL varies with species of plant, thickness of cell wall, pore size, and nature of the nanoparticle [76]. Nanoparticles penetrate the cell wall by diffusion, receiving access to the cell membrane, however, nanoparticles exceeding the SEL are believed to access the symplast by injurious tissue infiltration or biotransformation, though evidence for it is limited [7].

As the cell wall functions as a detoxification and storage unit for the plant cell, nanoparticles may accumulate in it too [102]. Amorphous silicon, often conjugated with fibers of the cell wall to increase structural rigidity, has the ability to sequester heavy metal such as Al, Mn and Zn resulting in their immobilization as they remain adsorbed to Si surface [86]. A similar phenomenon is possible with absorbed nanoparticles.

Differences in the composition of the cell wall in monocots and dicots result in variations in their respective permeability to nanoparticles. The three main factors that account for a stronger, more impermeable cell wall in monocots are: (i) the cross linking between pectin polymers and cellulose in monocots is significantly stronger than that in dicots, (ii) monocots contain a higher concentration of Si in their cell wall and (iii) the parallel pattern of the veins in the leaves of monocots that provides 3.6–4.2 times extra resistance to damage and tears [13]. Consequently, dicots, including all Citrus trees are more susceptible to nanoparticle penetration.

## 3.4 Cell Membrane

Regions of the plant with thin walls, especially developing root hair and pollen tubes largely depend on the selective absorptivity of the cell membrane to mediate the uptake of foreign particles. Entities that are non-polar and smaller in size can easily enter the plant cell through different parts of the plasma membrane via the process of diffusion however, larger compounds, carrying a charge cannot penetrate the phospholipid bilayer and thus require other pathways of entry. While detailed studies of such routes are limited in plants, research on endocytic and non-endocytic pathways has given promising insight on the uptake of nanomaterials by the plant cell membrane [71].

## 3.5 Endocytic Pathways

Primarily the most widely accepted mechanism of plasma membrane absorption of nanoparticles in plants is Receptor-Mediated Endocytosis (RME). Based on the morphological properties of the nanoparticles, RME is classified into different types; nonetheless, the basic mechanism involves the binding of a ligand associated nanoparticle to a receptor present on the surface of the plasma membrane inducing a change in its configuration. Resultantly the cell membrane forms an infolding that generates an endosome, responsible for the transport of the enveloped nanoparticle to its destination [116].

### 3.5.1 Clathrin-Mediated Endocytosis (CME)

Specialized regions of the plant cell membrane recruit clathrin utilizing it to coat endocytic vesicles with an average diameter of 70–150 nm, that are thus confined to the transportation of nanoparticles falling within the stated range [73]. The formation of the vesicle and assembly of clathrin are simultaneously triggered by a ligand-receptor interaction on the membrane surface. The polygonal arrangement of clathrin, as demonstrated in Fig. 2, then envelopes the vesicle directing its internalization into the cell system and eventually dissociates once inside. The vesicle develops into an early endosome by fusing with other vesicles and eventually matures into a late endosome [95]. The receptors, enclosed within a vesicle, travel to the membrane and fuse with it in order to capture more ligands.

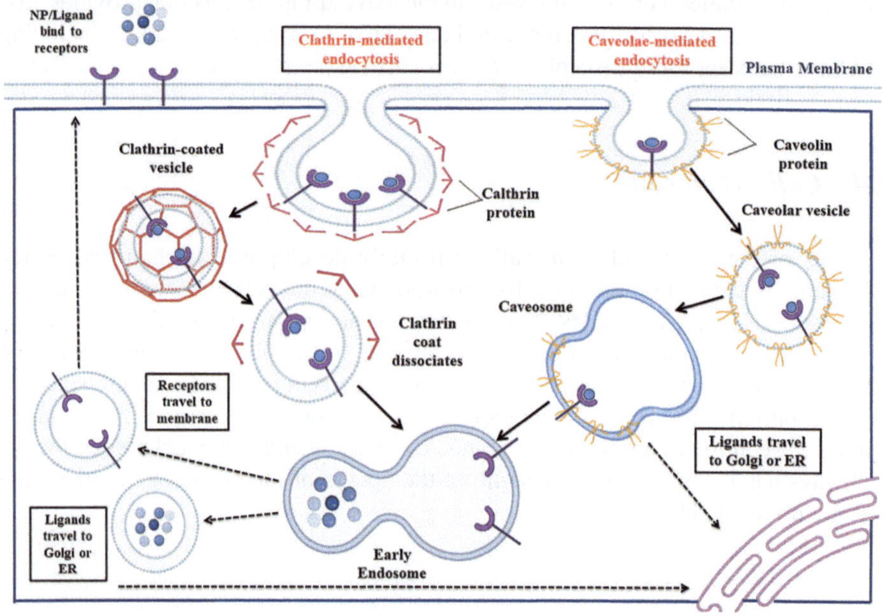


**Fig. 2** Two primary mechanisms involved in uptake of nanoparticles by Receptor Mediated Endocytosis (RME): Clathrin-Mediated Endocytosis and Claveolae-Mediated Endocytosis

### 3.5.2 Caveolin-Mediated Endocytosis (CVME)

Smaller nanoparticles ranging from 60 to 80 nm employ CVME to invade plant cells by causing the plasma membrane to invaginate, internalizing the nanoparticle as well as extracellular fluids. Unlike CME, the vesicle coating proteins of CVME such as caveolin-1 do not detach and remain bound via cholesterol molecules in the lipid of the vesicle. Furthermore, the caveolin vesicles formed, fuse with others of its kind to produce larger units known as caveosomes which eventually integrate with early endosomes and progress towards the Golgi-apparatus or the smooth endoplasmic reticulum [71].

## *3.6 Non-endocytic Pathways*

Aquaporins are channel proteins present within the cell membrane that are responsible for the maintenance of the turgor pressure of the cell by selectively transporting water molecules and other non-ionic solutes in and out of the cell [71]. The size restriction of aquaporins is up to 1 nm while structurally, they are only 0.2–0.25 nm wide at their mid-point, easily being prone to blockage by nanoparticles [55, 96]. Research reveals that genes encoding the activity of aquaporin proteins are significantly down regulated in response to water-stress and nanoparticle treatment, resulting in a decrease in uptake of water [37]. The outcome is hypothesized to be due to the blockage of the cell apoplast by the nanoparticles that disrupt the shape of the aquaporins, hindering water absorption [65]. Yet other mechanisms based on ligand-membrane interaction have only been studied on mammalian cells, they may potentially be true for plant cells too as their structures are comparable in thickness and the presence of a lipid bilayer. One such process is the snorkeling effect that involves the rearrangement of the bilayer core and is mostly observed in the uptake of amphiphilic nanoparticles [72]. Snorkeling and other similar mechanisms show that there is still much to learn about plant cell membrane absorption.

## *3.7 Plasmodesmata*

Nanoparticles that are unable to pass through the pores of the cell wall due to their incompatible size or charge are often moved by symplastic transportation through the plasmodesmata, a specialized cylindrical structure in plant systems that allows direct communication between adjacent cells through a cytoplasmic bridge [58]. The organelle responsible for this stream of cell-to-cell continuity is the endoplasmic reticulum that is connected in each neighboring cell allowing the movement of nanoparticles ranging in size from <15 to 40 nm [55]. However, limited availability of data and unclear observation techniques to analyze the function of symplastic transport causes perplexity in the contribution of the plasmodesmata in the transport of nanoparticles. Typically, nanoparticles are discovered adopting the apoplastic pathway rather than the symplast [110].

The proteins involved in forming the desmotubule in the plasmodesmata are assumed to be flexible, thus, nanoparticles <20 nm may also pass the space between the cell membrane and the desmotubule (other than the symplastic pathway) during transportation [44]. This was later validated by research as scientists used STEM-EDS to detect a significant concentration of aggregates conjugated with silver in various longitudinal channels and regions of the cell wall that were presumed to be the plasmodesmata [35]. Furthermore, certain molecules have been reported to momentarily enlarge the plasmodesmata channels by physical pressure induced via changes in the concentration gradient in order to transport larger particles [27, 80]. The external aperture of the plasmodesmata may widen to accommodate the passing of larger molecules similar to when plant viruses adjust the diameter of channel in order to make way [30]. Nonetheless, the larger the size of the nanoparticle, the slower will be its movement.

## 3.8 Stomata

Stomata are guarded openings present abundantly on the lower surface of leaves, and in fewer ratios on the remaining aerial parts of the plant. Their primary function is to transport gases and allow transpiration in most terrestrial phototrophic plants. Both these processes occur at high rates during the day as most plants open their apertures when sunlight is available. Structurally, stomata lack a layer of cuticle that aids in a more seamless diffusion of gases and has a rough texture due to the presence of salt precipitates that favors the attachment of nanoparticles [12]. Stomata generally range in diameter from 10 to 100 μm but their size and density may differ in distinctive plant species. For example, monocotyledons commonly possess a narrower extracellular aperture whereas dicotyledons, such as Citrus trees, not only have wider pores but higher stomatal density which is highly conducive to the uptake of nanoparticles [50, 97]. Owing to the peculiar geometric design of the stomata, the exact SEL of the pores of the stomata for the diffusion of nanoparticles still remains unclear [40].

It has been demonstrated that stomata are the largest pores among the various apertures in plants and are thus the least restrictive biological barriers (in comparison to the cell wall and cell membrane), consequently allowing more absorption of nanoparticles through leaves [136]. Nevertheless, a major drawback of their increased permeability is the clogging of the stomatal pores by particles measured in μm to nm that eventually pose a negative impact on the plants internal temperature, rate of transpiration and photosynthesis, and growth [29]. Furthermore, foliar application of nanoparticles increases the risk of accumulation of heavy metals in different regions of the plant that eventually enter the food chain. Researchers treated cucumber leaves with cerium dioxide ($CeO_2$) nanoparticles in order to study their leaf-shoot translocation and discovered that an estimated 3% of the total cerium absorbed was found in the roots, suggesting the active movement of cerium ions in the plant. Additionally, 73–81% of the $CeO_2$ nanoparticles that were applied were retained on the outer surface of the leaf [45].

Nanoparticle exposure through the roots can cause stomatal pores to close resulting in slower transpiration of the plant. The suggested correlation between the two phenomena is that the uptake of nanoparticles from the roots interferes with the flux of water, blocking the vasculature and eventually the stomata from within the plant system [4].

### 3.9 *Root Hair*

As mentioned earlier, roots secrete chemicals referred to as mucilage and exudates that allow nanoparticles to adsorb on their surface and deposit within the rhizosphere [130]. Moreover, the negatively charged surface of the tip of the root hairs displays increased affinity for nanoparticles carrying a positive charge thus, their concentration around the roots is often relatively high [67]. Plants such as Citrus trees tend to develop far reaching lateral roots that provide new adsorption surfaces and a higher probability of penetration within the root column [39, 91]. Furthermore, as the tips of root hairs contain a number of immature cells with an under developed epidermis, they are vulnerable to penetration by nanoparticles and often provide direct entry into the plant [97]. Mature roots that contain a fully developed epidermal layer have pores within their cell wall that prevent the invasion of foreign particles making the root system semi-permeable [93]. However, certain large sized nanoparticles can dismantle the root cell wall by inducing the formation of wider pores and forcefully crossing the secondary barrier, the cell membrane [2, 127]. Once absorbed, the nanoparticles further move into the plant tissue by damage, carrier protein binding, or endocytosis [67].

## 4 Translocation Pathways of Nanoparticles in Citrus Trees

Foliarly administered nanoparticles enter the plant through the stomata and cuticle and are further transported via the symplast (plastid pathway) or the apoplast (extracellular pathway) [75]. The plastid pathway refers to the movement of nanoparticles through an intercellular channel known as the plasmodesmata that is formed by the extension of the endoplasmic reticulum of each neighboring cell [19]. The nanoparticles that adopt this route must pass through the cytoplasm and often accumulate therein further being translocated to the endothelial layer and Casparian strip of the plant [75]. The apoplastic pathway on the other hand directs the nanoparticles through the extracellular spaces between the cell wall, the middle lamella and eventually the xylem [32]. The nanoparticles do not directly enter the cell through this route and are often blocked from further movement beyond the cortex due to the presence of the Casparian band [16]. The average size exclusion limit of nanoparticles that can be transported through the apoplastic pathway is 50–200 nm while all nanomaterials less than 50 nm are led through the symplastic channel [99]. Eventually, the final recipient of the nanoparticles from the leaves is the phloem, one of the chief conducting tubes of the vascular bundle. Since the distance between the sieve plates present within the phloem is quite wide, particles up to 0.45 μm in size can easily be transported along with water, nutrients and cell sap.

Nanoparticles taken up by the roots follow similar pathways by selectively penetrating the cell wall of the root hair (present abundantly in the rhizosphere), crossing the epidermis, cortex and entering the endothelial layer via the symplastic and apoplastic pathway [126]. Initially, nanoparticles transported through the exoplast are faced by a hindrance as they are unable to pass the Casparian strip after crossing the epidermis and endothelium. Often a large number of nanoparticles accumulate in the endothelium while some travel along the radius of the Casparian strip. The lateral root junction, however, displays an exception by allowing the nanoparticles to cross the immature, under-developed Casparian band and reaching the vascular bundle [110]. Lastly, unlike the final destination of nanoparticles absorbed by the leaves, uptake by the roots directs the nanoparticles into the xylem vessel that continues their upward translocation [126]. Figure 1 highlights the pathways stated.

## 5 Factors Influencing Nanoparticle Uptake and Translocation

Despite a common pathway, different nanoparticles administered through the same route demonstrate varying rates of absorption, translocation and accumulation in the plant. That is because a number of factors govern their uptake including the physiology and species of the plant, the nature and dimensions of the nanomaterial, and the interaction of the nanoparticles with the environment.

## 6 Plant Physiology and Morphology

With reference to physiology, plants that are tolerant to droughts and have a low rate of transpiration tend to translocate fewer nanomaterials as both the traits correlate to rare incidences of stomatal opening. Moreover, morphological differences such as a taller plant, tougher cell wall, the presence of a thick cuticle, a compact root system, and narrow, less dense stomatal pores can also hinder the uptake of nanoparticles in plants [110]. For instance, dicotyledons including the Citrus tree possess irregularly shaped, scattered stomata on their leaves as opposed to the neatly patterned pores of monocotyledons. Furthermore, the developmental phase of the plant can also impact its ability to absorb foreign particles as immature leaves and flowers often have an undeveloped, weak cuticle layer that is more prone to invasion. Similarly, leaves that are nearing the end of their life cycle due to senescence also have a thin cuticle that provides more opportunity of nanoparticle entrance [47, 57]. Additionally, certain diseases of the leaf such as chlorosis, necrosis, blight and leaf mold or abrasive wounds can further increase the vulnerability of the plant by damaging its protective barriers especially the cuticle, cell wall, and cell membrane [106]. Other than variations from specie to specie, different regions of the same plant can also possess contrasting traits such as unsteady sap composition and flow rate with which nanoparticles translocate, fluctuating sizes of apertures in porous membranes, and degree of association of the conducting vessels—the xylem and phloem [118].

### 6.1 Size of Nanomaterials

The size, chemical composition, surface and surface coating of nanomaterials govern their rate of uptake and movement within a plant [119]. Moving from the outside towards the inside, the permeability of each porous membrane in a plants structure tends to decrease as a result of which nanoparticles larger than the size exclusion limit are unable to cross the barriers completely. Certain metals have been reported to display a higher rate of uptake as compared to others and the core reason behind this affinity remains undiscovered. Generally, metal based nanoparticles exceeding the size of 100 nm cannot be absorbed by the plant roots [5]. However, an experiment revealed the successful absorption of Si nanoparticles as large as 200 nm by the roots of an *Arabidopsis* plant [114]. Yet another study utilized TEM and confocal microscopy to observe that sugar cane roots were also prosperously penetrated by Zein nanoparticles with an average diameter of 135 nm.

### 6.2 Surface Charge of Nanomaterials

Surface charge is a significant characteristic which decides the fate of nanomaterials in plants. It mediates the bonds that are formed with the plant system. As stated earlier, the negative charge in the rhizosphere creates an electrostatic force of attraction for positively charged nanoparticles causing them to accumulate within that vicinity and thus hindering their uptake through the leaves while negatively charged nanoparticles are easily absorbed [10]. Neutral or negatively charged NPs are more likely to internalize in plant tissues as compared to positively charged NPs [145]. This is due to the surface properties of the cell wall, which has free carboxyl groups on pectin moieties. It gives negative charge to cell wall which attracts positively charged NPs hindering their ability to cross membranes [101]. However, it varies according to the plant species and method of exposure of NPs [145]. Avellan et al. [3] described that negatively charged mucilage adsorbed AuNPs of size about 12 nm having positive charge and inhibit their translocation, while the translocation of Au NPs with negative charge was not inhibited.

### 6.3 *Membrane Potential*

Another factor that greatly influences the translocation of nanoparticles across membranes is the electrochemical gradient also known as membrane potential. This potential favors the translocation and can act as a driving force for the movement of charged nanoparticles. Membrane potential and its role in the efficient delivery of nanoparticles is rarely addressed and is worthy of investigation [134]. Studies have demonstrated that small nanoparticles with size less than 10 nm in diameter have high zeta potential (>40 mV) and can be delivered with great efficiency in protoplasts as compared to neutral nanoparticles [135]. Nanomaterials with high zeta potential can efficiently cross the cytosol and can penetrate the chloroplasts as well [63].

## 7 Plant Tissue Reactions to Nanomaterials: Physicochemical Insights

After successful entry into plants, NMs initiate a range of physiological and biochemical interactions, as evidenced by a wealth of research studies mostly in artificial and controlled environments. Although a large number of reports have unveiled positive interactions, their inhibitory effects cannot be ignored. NMs, when applied in optimal concentrations, have been reported to have significant impact on the seed germination, mitigating different types of stress, increasing the yield and improving the biomass of plants. Conversely, there are reports where the same NMs can cause inhibition of the aforementioned processes. The main reason for the occurrence of these inhibitory effects is the overdose of the NMs [55].

Seed germination is the first step in plant growth and development. NMs have been reported to not only break seed dormancy but also enhance the rate of seed germination [83, 138]. Additionally, recent studies have illuminated that nanomaterial-treated seeds exhibit the ability to activate multiple genes during the germination process. This phenomenon is attributed to several other mechanisms, including the formation of nanopores in seed coats, the introduction of reactive oxygen species (ROS), heightened enzyme activity at starch-degrading sites, and the infusion of ROS into the seed coat [112].

NMs have a pivotal role in fortifying membrane stability and facilitating nutrient and water uptake in plants. Additionally, they serve as a shield for the plant's photosynthetic machinery, safeguarding it from detrimental effects induced by the stress, ultimately resulting in enhanced plant growth even under stress conditions [140]. Furthermore, NMs promote the accumulation of stress-protective hormones,

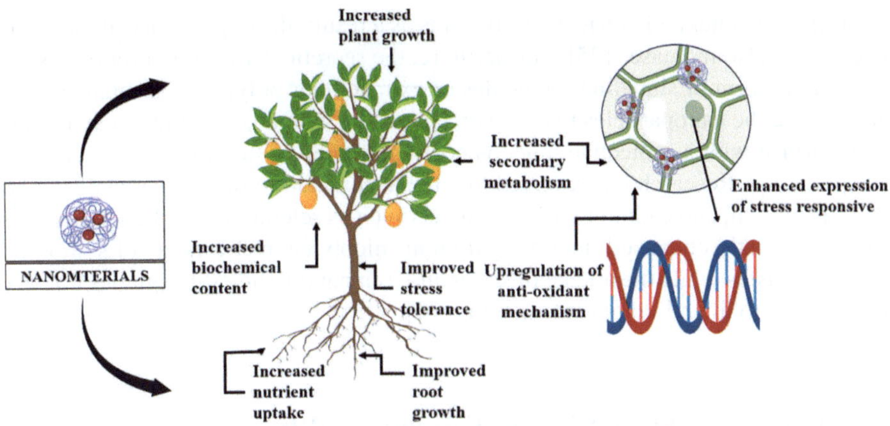


**Fig. 3** General responses of plants under the influence of nanomaterials

osmolytes, and phenolic compounds [48]. Moreover, they boost the expression of stress-responsive and antioxidant genes, significantly bolstering the plant's defense mechanisms against stress [102]. Various studies have shown that exposure to nanomaterials results in the increased photosynthetic efficiency, elongation of roots and shoots and improvement in the plant biomass along with the enhanced biochemical production [49, 92, 124, 129].

Secondary metabolites (SMs) are a diverse group of bioactive compounds produced by plants to adapt to their surroundings, protect them against stressors, and interact with their environment [43]. Their commercial value extends across multiple industries, making them important for both plant biology and various human applications, including pharmaceuticals, cosmetics, food production, and agriculture. The strategy called "nano-elicitation" is being widely applied to enhance the production of SMs in plants by the use of NMs [52] (see Fig. 3).

Citrus plants are not only rich in vitamin C as mentioned before but are a reservoir of numerous other metabolites such as flavonols, carotenoids, limonoids and terpenes which are all secondary metabolites [104]. Thus, not only are NMs playing a vital role in the growth and development of plants but they also make them economically and medicinally valuable by enhancing production of these SMs.

## 8 Nanoparticle Interaction with the Soil Environment

The phyllosphere contains a myriad of symbiotic bacteria and mycorrhizal fungi that not only form pertinent partnerships with plant roots but also release extracellular secretions into the environment that alter the chemistry of certain nanoparticles. Firstly, fungi symbionts penetrate root nodes increasing the surface area for absorption of water and nutrients by 10 folds as a result; the opportunity of nanoparticle uptake also increases [25]. Furthermore, the secretions by the microorganisms, often in the form of signaling molecules or extracellular polymeric substances, can either cause the nanoparticles to dissolve, enhancing their absorbability or shield the plant surface with a protective mucous coating, hindering the uptake of nanoparticles [64, 142]. Research has revealed that the accumulation of heavy metal such as zinc, chromium, and cadmium, of non-metals such as selenium and of quantum dots was significantly enhanced in non-leguminous dicotyledons by virtue of symbiotic microorganisms while the uptake of silver and iron nanoparticles in legumes notably reduced due to the microbial interactions [38].

## 9 Potential Risks of NMs on Human Health and the Environment

The potential risks associated with nanomaterials raise concerns regarding their impact on both environment and human health. There is relatively limited record of studies exploring the effects of nanomaterials exposure. Application of nanomaterials in soil not only benefits the plants but alternatively can have adverse effects on soil environment and its biodiversity as well [8]. Enzymatic activity and respiration in soil indicates the impact of NMs on soil community. A study revealed that NMs can deteriorate the reproductive cycle in earthworms resulting in demise [98]. You et al. [139] investigated the effect of ZnO, $Fe_3O_4$, $CeO_2$ and $TiO_2$ on bacterial diversity in soil and activity of invertase, urease, phosphatase and catalase enzymes. A decrease in activities was observed threatening nitrogen fixation in soil as well. Higher concentrations of NMs negatively affect the dehydrogenase activity of microbes in soil as well as influence the rate of self-cleaning and balance of nutrients, which forms the basis of nutrition regulation and soil fertility [70].

Toxicological investigations have revealed that NMs can impact both unicellular and larger aquatic organisms [34]. When carbon dots, characterized by their numerous surface functional groups, even dispersion, and photoluminescent properties, are introduced into the aquatic environment, they undergo rapid photocatalysis. Similarly, carbon nanotubes (CNTs) and their byproducts have shown toxic effects on marine organisms such as *Thalassiosira pseudonana* and *Tigriopus japonicus* [60]. Moreover, nano-ZnO has been found to affect the growth phase of algae and exhibit toxic effects on various aquatic microorganisms, including *Escherichia coli* and *Aeromonas hydrophila* [20]. Both nano-$TiO_2$ and nano-ZnO are reported to harm aquatic bacteria by damaging their cell membranes and display antibacterial activity, particularly against *E. coli* [125]. The exposure to CNTs also negatively impacted the larvae of marine organisms, potentially inducing physical and oxidative stress.

Investigations into the potential harm of NPs on human health commenced in the early 2000s with the advent of CNTs and their reported impact on aquatic life. Since then, researchers have conducted numerous studies to assess the possible negative effects of NPs exposure on various vital organs, including the lungs, liver, kidneys, and brain [115]. The studies have unveiled that NMs exposed to plants can infiltrate the human body through inhalation or ingestion of modified agri-foods, and skin contact, leading to damage to cells, tissues, and organs. Recent research endeavors have been primarily focused on elucidating the intricate mechanisms behind NPs' toxicity and pinpointing the contributing factors to their harmful effects.

Silver nanoparticles (AgNPs) are reported to toxicologically affect the immune system in the human body by inhibiting the cytokine expression in blood cells even at levels as low as 15 ppm [85]. Platelet aggregation and thrombosis have been observed in the cardiovascular system [22]. As NPs travel through the bloodstream, they eventually reach sensitive target locations, including lymph nodes, the spleen, kidneys, liver, pancreas, bone marrow, and the brain [123]. When NPs breach cell membranes and accumulate within various cellular compartments, such as mitochondria and nucleus, they can trigger harmful responses within these vital organelles [9]. These responses encompass inflammation, immunotoxicity, cytotoxicity, genotoxicity, and even the potential for malignancy, all stemming from the oxidative stress induced by nanoparticle exposure [117]. It is worth noting that exposure to quartz and carbon black NPs, in particular, have been associated with notable effects such as interstitial fibrosis and inflammation in the airways [62].

## 10 Strategies for Effective and Safe Administration of NMs

Despite various workshops, discussion, research reports and reviews, there remains a significant dearth regarding the safety regulations. Currently we lack effective applications of NMs in living systems and therefore face challenges in completely assessing the risks associated with NMs. To address these knowledge gaps and ensure the responsible utilization of NMs, it is imperative to outline key strategies for their safe and effective administration.

### *10.1 Optimizing Nanomaterial Design and Customization for Enhanced Applications*

The ability to modify surface coatings has been demonstrated to influence the ease of entry and/or translocation of NMs. A study reported by Avellan et al. [3] emphasized the effects of gold nanoparticles (AuNPs) size and coating chemistry on interactions with wheat leaves and internal plant transport. VP-coated AuNPs exhibited strong adhesion to wheat leaf surfaces and effective penetration of the cuticle layer. However, their transport through mesophyll cells was comparatively limited, affecting wheat photosynthesis. On the other hand, citrate-coated AuNPs showed incomplete leaf uptake but displayed efficient translocation to the plant vasculature.

Likewise magnetic coatings for the targeted delivery of nanoparticles in plants have garnered special attention in the past few years and proved to be highly effective. Iron-coated carbon nanoparticles were reported for their delivery by using the magnetic fields to immobilize and concentrate them in specific plant organs susceptible to pathogen attacks in *Cucurbita pepo* living plants [105].

In recent years, controlled release formulations have emerged as a promising frontier in the agricultural sector, mirroring the advancements in drug delivery systems within the biomedical field. By nano-encapsulating agrochemicals, controlled release systems ensure that nutrients or protective agents are released gradually and strategically, promoting crop health and environmental sustainability [28]. These formulations are designed to optimize the application of agrochemicals, such as fertilizers, pesticides, and herbicides [132].

Oliveira et al. [84] developed chitosan nanoparticles loaded with the NO donor S-nitroso-mercaptosuccinic acid (S-nitroso-MSA) to provide controlled and sustained release of nitric oxide (NO), showing superior efficacy in mitigating salt stress effects on maize plants compared to conventional NO delivery methods. The impact of azoxystrobin encapsulated in porous hollow $SiO_2$ nanocarriers on soil and plant health was assessed by Bueno et al. [11]. Encapsulated pesticide significantly improved plant growth and reduced phytotoxicity compared to non-encapsulated treatment. Similarly, Nanoparticles loaded with atrazine exhibit enhanced weed control effectiveness, even at lower application doses. Radiometric studies reveal faster and more substantial absorption of nanoatrazine in mustard leaves, leading to increased inhibition of photosystem II activity [121]. This nanoencapsulation approach not only potentiated the herbicidal activity of atrazine but also provided a two-fold improvement in weed control in field conditions, offering more efficient performance while minimizing environmental risks.

A novel approach is the use of biorecognition motifs, specifically a chloroplast guiding peptide, for the targeted delivery of NM to chloroplasts in plants as reported by Santana et al. [107]. By coating hydrophilic quantum dots with this, a conserved chloroplast targeting peptide, rationally designed from Rubisco small subunit 1 A, the researchers were able to achieve specific manipulation of chloroplast redox status and enhance colocalization with chloroplasts. This approach shows promise for applications in plant biology and agrochemical delivery, highlighting the importance of incorporating engineered biomolecule coatings and acquired coronas for accurate predictions of nanoparticle distribution in other parts of the plants.

## 10.2 Compliance with Nanomaterial Regulations to Mitigate Potential Risks

It is essential to note that the development and effective utilization of NMs in agriculture necessitate adherence to regulatory standards. Concerns about potential environmental and health risks have prompted regulatory bodies worldwide to establish guidelines for safe use [59]. Regulatory oversight varies by country, with the Environmental Protection Agency (EPA) and U.S. Department of Agriculture (USDA) overseeing agri-products in the United States, while the European Chemicals Agency (ECHA) and European Food Safety Authority (EFSA) managing them in the European Union. These agencies require rigorous risk assessments, including toxicity evaluations and environmental impact assessments. Labeling of agri-products containing nanomaterials is mandatory to inform consumers. International standards, like ISO/TS 80004-1, provide terminology and definitions for nanomaterials [100]. Collaboration between researchers, manufacturers, regulators, and consumers is vital for their continued safety and effectiveness. Regulatory agencies worldwide share the common goal of safeguarding nanotechnology's use in agriculture while adhering to applicable regulations [103].

## 11 Concluding Remarks and Future Prospects

This chapter comprehensively explores the schematic mechanisms underlying the processes of uptake, translocation and assimilation of nanoparticles in citrus plants. NMs are exposed to the plants via different methods such as foliar, trunk or root exposure. After crossing various barriers, these NMs are transported to different parts of the plants through symplastic and apoplastic pathways. Different endocytic and non-endocytic pathways allow nanomaterials to enter plant cells and tissues where they physiochemically influence the growth and development of the plants. As mentioned before, NMs materials can facilitate growth rate at low concentrations but prove detrimental for plants at high concentrations. In addition to it, NMs also facilitate the production of secondary metabolites in the plants, increasing their economic value in different sectors.

Nanotechnology has the potential to revolutionize agriculture by offering innovative and modernized solutions for crop management, pest control, nutrient delivery, and more. Over recent years, there has been a significant increase in research focused on understanding the interaction between nanomaterials and plants. While we have made significant strides in understanding these processes, many questions remain for both agricultural practice and environmental safety.

The need for cautious and thoughtful use of nanomaterials in citrus agriculture remains till date. As we harness the potential benefits of these novel materials to enhance crop productivity and resilience, we should also remain vigilant about potential risks to human health and the environment. The regulatory landscape in this domain is evolving, and it is incumbent upon researchers and stakeholders to contribute to the development of guidelines and best practices that ensure the safe and responsible application of nanomaterials in agriculture.

## References


1. Abdelmoaty S, Khandaker M, Badaluddin NA, Mohd K, Abdullahi U, Mat Shaari N, Khairil M (2022) The importance of lemon (Citrus limon) and the future of its cultivation by using bio-fertilizers. Biosci Res, 889–898
2. Ali S, Mehmood A, Khan N (2021) Uptake, translocation, and consequences of nanomaterials on plant growth and stress adaptation. J Nanomater 2021:6677616. https://doi.org/10.1155/2021/6677616
3. Avellan A, Yun J, Zhang Y, Spielman-Sun E, Unrine JM, Thieme J, Li J, Lombi E, Bland G, Lowry GV (2019) Nanoparticle size and coating chemistry control foliar uptake pathways, translocation, and leaf-to-rhizosphere transport in wheat. ACS Nano 13:5291–5305. https://doi.org/10.1021/acsnano.8b09781
4. Ballikaya P, Brunner I, Cocozza C, Grolimund D, Kaegi R, Murazzi ME, Schaub M, Schönbeck LC, Sinnet B, Cherubini P (2023) First evidence of nanoparticle uptake through leaves and roots in beech (Fagus sylvatica L.) and pine (Pinus sylvestris L.). Tree Physiol 43:262–276. https://doi.org/10.1093/treephys/tpac117
5. Banerjee K, Pramanik P, Maity A, Joshi D, Wani S, Krishnan P (2019) Methods of using nanomaterials to plant systems and their delivery to plants (Mode of entry, uptake, translocation, accumulation, biotransformation and barriers). In: Advances in phytonanotechnology. Elsevier, pp 123–152
6. Bauer P, Elbaum R, Weiss IM (2011) Calcium and silicon mineralization in land plants: transport, structure and function. Plant Sci 180:746–756. https://doi.org/10.1016/j.plantsci.2011.01.019
7. Behzadi S, Serpooshan V, Tao W, Hamaly MA, Alkawareek MY, Dreaden EC, Brown D, Alkilany AM, Farokhzad OC, Mahmoudi M (2017) Cellular uptake of nanoparticles: journey inside the cell. Chem Soc Rev 46:4218–4244. https://doi.org/10.1039/C6CS00636A
8. Bimová P, Barbieriková Z, Grenčíková A, Šípoš R, Škulcová AB, Krivjanská A, Mackuľak T (2021) Environmental risk of nanomaterials and nanoparticles and EPR technique as an effective tool to study them—a review. Environ Sci Pollut Res 28:22203–22220. https://doi.org/10.1007/s11356-021-13270-5
9. Borm PJ, Robbins D, Haubold S, Kuhlbusch T, Fissan H, Donaldson K, Schins R, Stone V, Kreyling W, Lademann J (2006) The potential risks of nanomaterials: a review carried out for ECETOC. Part Fibre Toxicol 3:1–35. https://doi.org/10.1186/1743-8977-3-11
10. Bosker T, Bouwman LJ, Brun NR, Behrens P, Vijver MG (2019) Microplastics accumulate on pores in seed capsule and delay germination and root growth of the terrestrial vascular plant Lepidium sativum. Chemosphere 226:774–781. https://doi.org/10.1016/j.chemosphere.2019.03.163
11. Bueno V, Wang P, Harrisson O, Bayen S, Ghoshal S (2022) Impacts of a porous hollow silica nanoparticle-encapsulated pesticide applied to soils on plant growth and soil microbial community. Environ Sci Nano 9:1476–1488. https://doi.org/10.1039/D1EN00975C
12. Burkhardt J, Basi S, Pariyar S, Hunsche M (2012) Stomatal penetration by aqueous solutions—an update involving leaf surface particles. New Phytol 196:774–787. https://doi.org/10.1111/j.1469-8137.2012.04307.x
13. Calderan-Rodrigues MJ, Guimarães Fonseca J, de Moraes FE, Vaz Setem L, Carmanhanis Begossi A, Labate CA (2019) Plant cell wall proteomics: a focus on monocot species, Brachypodium distachyon, Saccharum spp. and Oryza sativa. Int J Mol Sci 20. https://doi.org/10.3390/ijms20081975
14. Cao Y, Lim E, Xu M, Weng J-K, Marelli B (2020) Precision delivery of multiscale payloads to tissue-specific targets in plants. Adv Sci 7:1903551. https://doi.org/10.1002/advs.201903551
15. Castle W (1978) Citrus root systems: their structure, function, growth and relationship to tree performance. Proc Int Soc Citric 1:62
16. Chen R, Ratnikova TA, Stone MB, Lin S, Lard M, Huang G, Hudson JS, Ke PC (2010) Differential uptake of carbon nanoparticles by plant and mammalian cells. Small 6:612–617. https://doi.org/10.1002/smll.200901911

17. Coelho G (2017) Ecosystem services in Brazilian's southern agroforestry systems. Trop Subtrop Agroecosystems 20:475–492. https://doi.org/10.56369/tsaes.2421
18. Cornelis G, Hund-Rinke K, Kuhlbusch T, Van den Brink N, Nickel C (2014) Fate and bioavailability of engineered nanoparticles in soils: a review. Crit Rev Environ Sci Technol 44:2720–2764. https://doi.org/10.1080/10643389.2013.829767
19. Cornu JY, Bussière S, Coriou C, Robert T, Maucourt M, Deborde C, Moing A, Nguyen C (2020) Changes in plant growth, Cd partitioning and xylem sap composition in two sunflower cultivars exposed to low Cd concentrations in hydroponics. Ecotoxicol Environ Saf 205:111145. https://doi.org/10.1016/j.ecoenv.2020.111145
20. Das B, Dash SK, Mandal D, Ghosh T, Chattopadhyay S, Tripathy S, Das S, Dey SK, Das D, Roy S (2017) Green synthesized silver nanoparticles destroy multidrug resistant bacteria via reactive oxygen species mediated membrane damage. Arab J Chem 10:862–876. https://doi.org/10.1016/j.arabjc.2015.08.008
21. Dietz K-J, Herth S (2011) Plant nanotoxicology. Trends Plant Sci 16:582–589. https://doi.org/10.1016/j.tplants.2011.08.003
22. Djibril Sekou K, Patel H (2023) A review on the interaction between nanoparticles and toxic metals in soil: meta-analysis of their effects on soil, plants and human health. Soil Sediment Contam: Int J 32:417–447. https://doi.org/10.1016/j.tplants.2011.08.003
23. Driouich A, Follet-Gueye M-L, Vicré-Gibouin M, Hawes M (2013) Root border cells and secretions as critical elements in plant host defense. Curr Opin Plant Biol 16:489–495. https://doi.org/10.1016/j.pbi.2013.06.010
24. Driouich A, Follet-Gueye M-L, Vicré-Gibouin M, Hawes M (2013b) Root border cells and secretions as critical elements in plant host defense 16:489–495
25. Durán P, Acuña JJ, Jorquera M, Azcón R, Borie F, Cornejo P, Mora M (2013) Enhanced selenium content in wheat grain by co-inoculation of selenobacteria and arbuscular mycorrhizal fungi: a preliminary study as a potential Se biofortification strategy. J Cereal Sci 57:275–280. https://doi.org/10.1016/j.jcs.2012.11.012
26. Eichert T, Kurtz A, Steiner U, Goldbach HE (2008) Size exclusion limits and lateral heterogeneity of the stomatal foliar uptake pathway for aqueous solutes and water-suspended nanoparticles. Physiol Plant 134:151–160. https://doi.org/10.1016/j.jcs.2012.11.012
27. Erwee MG, Goodwin PB (1985) Symplast domains in extrastelar tissues of Egeria densa Planch. Planta 163:9–19. https://doi.org/10.1016/j.jcs.2012.11.012
28. Esfanjani AF, Assadpour E, Jafari SM (2018) Improving the bioavailability of phenolic compounds by loading them within lipid-based nanocarriers. Trends Food Sci Technol 76:56–66. https://doi.org/10.1016/j.jcs.2012.11.012
29. Eveling D (2008) Effects fo spraying plants with suspensions of inert dust. Ann Appl Biol 64:139–151. https://doi.org/10.1111/j.1744-7348.1969.tb02864.x
30. Faulkner CR, Blackman LM, Collings DA, Cordwell SJ, Overall RL (2009) Anti-tropomyosin antibodies co-localise with actin microfilaments and label plasmodesmata. Eur J Cell Biol 88:357–369. https://doi.org/10.1016/j.ejcb.2009.02.184
31. Galloway AF, Knox P, Krause K (2020) Sticky mucilages and exudates of plants: putative microenvironmental design elements with biotechnological value. New Phytol 225:1461–1469. https://doi.org/10.1111/nph.16144
32. Gangwar P, Johri P, Datta R, Singh S, Trivedi M (2023) Overview on 1 phytopharmaceuticals and biotechnology of herbal plants. In: Phytopharmaceuticals and biotechnology of herbal plants. CRC Press, pp 1–17
33. Gao M, Chang J, Wang Z, Zhang H, Wang T (2023) Advances in transport and toxicity of nanoparticles in plants. J Nanobiotechnol 21:75. https://doi.org/10.1186/s12951-023-01830-5
34. Gao M, Zhang Z, Lv M, Song W, Lv Y (2018) Toxic effects of nanomaterial-adsorbed cadmium on Daphnia magna. Ecotoxicol Environ Saf 148:261–268. https://doi.org/10.1016/j.ecoenv.2017.10.038
35. Geisler-Lee J, Wang Q, Yao Y, Zhang W, Geisler M, Li K, Huang Y, Chen Y, Kolmakov A, Ma X (2013) Phytotoxicity, accumulation and transport of silver nanoparticles by Arabidopsis thaliana. Nanotoxicology 7:323–337. https://doi.org/10.3109/17435390.2012.658094

36. Goldschmidt EE (1997) Basic and practical aspects of citrus trees' carbohydrate economy. Citrus Flowering Fruiting Short Course Proceedings, Citrus Research Education Center, IFAS, Univ. of Florida, Lake Alfred, FL
37. Gong C, Wang L, Li X, Wang H, Jiang Y, Wang W (2019) Effect of $Y_2O_3$ nanoparticles on growth of maize seedlings. In: IOP conference series: earth and environmental science. IOP Publishing. https://doi.org/10.1088/1755-1315/300/5/052049
38. Guo J, Chi J (2014) Effect of Cd-tolerant plant growth-promoting rhizobium on plant growth and Cd uptake by Lolium multiflorum Lam. and Glycine max (L.) Merr. in Cd-contaminated soil. Plant Soil Sediment Contam: Int J 375:205–214. https://doi.org/10.1007/s11104-013-1952-1
39. Gupta G, Paul S, Singh S, Pietramellara G, Pathan SI, Danish S, Jha PN (2022) Exploring functional diversity and community structure of diazotrophic endophytic bacteria associated with Pennisetum glaucum growing under field in a semi-arid region. Land 11(7):991
40. Ha N, Seo E, Kim S, Lee SJ (2021) Adsorption of nanoparticles suspended in a drop on a leaf surface of Perilla frutescens and their infiltration through stomatal pathway. Sci Rep 11:11556. https://doi.org/10.1038/s41598-021-91073-x
41. Hameed A, Fatma S, Wattoo JI, Yaseen M, Ahmad S (2018) Accumulative effects of humic acid and multinutrient foliar fertilizers on the vegetative and reproductive attributes of citrus (Citrus reticulata cv. kinnow mandarin). J Plant Nutr 41:2495–2506. https://doi.org/10.1080/01904167.2018.1510506
42. Hatami M, Kariman K, Ghorbanpour M (2016) Engineered nanomaterial-mediated changes in the metabolism of terrestrial plants. Sci Total Environ 571:275–291. https://doi.org/10.1016/j.scitotenv.2016.07.184
43. Hatami M, Naghdi Badi H, Ghorbanpour M (2019) Nano-elicitation of secondary pharmaceutical metabolites in plant cells: a review. فصلنامه علمی پژوهشی گیاهان دارویی 18:6–36. https://doi.org/10.29252/jmp.3.71.6
44. Haywood V, Kragler F, Lucas WJ (2002) Plasmodesmata: pathways for protein and ribonucleoprotein signaling. Plant Cell 14(Suppl):S303–325. https://doi.org/10.1105/tpc.000778
45. Hong J, peralta-videa J, Rico C, Sahi S, Viveros M, Bartonjo J, Zhao L, Gardea-Torresdey J (2014) Evidence of trans location and physiological impacts of foliar applied $CeO_2$ nanoparticles on cucumber (Cucumis sativus) plants. Environ Sci Technol 48. https://doi.org/10.1021/es404931g
46. Hong J, Wang C, Wagner DC, Gardea-Torresdey JL, He F, Rico CM (2021) Foliar application of nanoparticles: mechanisms of absorption, transfer, and multiple impacts. Environ Sci Nano 8:1196–1210. https://doi.org/10.1039/D0EN01129K
47. Honour SL, Bell JNB, Ashenden TW, Cape JN, Power SA (2009) Responses of herbaceous plants to urban air pollution: effects on growth, phenology and leaf surface characteristics. Environ Pollut 157:1279–1286. https://doi.org/10.1016/j.envpol.2008.11.049
48. Hu J, Guo H, Li J, Gan Q, Wang Y, Xing B (2017) Comparative impacts of iron oxide nanoparticles and ferric ions on the growth of Citrus maxima. Environ Pollut 221:199–208. https://doi.org/10.1016/j.envpol.2016.11.064
49. Hu J, Guo H, Li J, Wang Y, Xiao L, Xing B (2017) Interaction of $\gamma$-$Fe_2O_3$ nanoparticles with Citrus maxima leaves and the corresponding physiological effects via foliar application. J Nanobiotechnology 15:51. https://doi.org/10.1186/s12951-017-0286-1
50. Hu P, An J, Faulkner MM, Wu H, Li Z, Tian X, Giraldo JP (2020) Nanoparticle charge and size control foliar delivery efficiency to plant cells and organelles. ACS Nano 14:7970–7986. https://doi.org/10.1021/acsnano.9b09178
51. Hussain HI, Yi Z, Rookes JE, Kong LX, Cahill DM (2013) Mesoporous silica nanoparticles as a biomolecule delivery vehicle in plants. J Nanopart Res 15:1–15. https://doi.org/10.1007/s11051-013-1676-4
52. Inam M, Attique I, Zahra M, Khan AK, Hahim M, Hano C, Anjum S (2023) Metal oxide nanoparticles and plant secondary metabolism: unraveling the game-changer nano-elicitors. Plant Cell Tissue Organ Cult, 1–18. https://doi.org/10.1007/s11240-023-02587-3

53. Jain T, Srivastava K, Singh R, Ansari MJ, Singh S, Dutta PK (2022) Role of nanotechnology 18 in the field of phytopharmaceuticals for the delivery of herbal drugs
54. Kaiser H (2014) Stomatal uptake of mineral particles from a sprayed suspension containing an organosilicone surfactant. J Plant Nutr Soil Sci 177:869–874. https://doi.org/10.1002/jpln.201300607
55. Khan MR, Adam V, Rizvi TF, Zhang B, Ahamad F, Jośko I, Zhu Y, Yang M, Mao C (2019) Nanoparticle-plant interactions: two-way traffic. Small 15:e1901794. https://doi.org/10.1002/smll.201901794
56. Khare N, Bhardwaj M, Chawla S, Praveen R, Singh S (2023) Redox responsive smart nanomaterials to tackle hypoxia associated oxidative damage and inflammatory mediators using phytocompounds. in smart nanomaterials targeting pathological hypoxia.Springer Nature Singapore, Singapore, pp 313–325
57. Khare P, Kishore K, Sharma DK (2017) A study on the standardization parameters of Cassia angustifolia. Asian J Pharm Clin Res 10(7):329–332
58. Kim JY (2005) Regulation of short-distance transport of RNA and protein. Curr Opin Plant Biol 8:45–52. https://doi.org/10.1016/j.pbi.2004.11.005
59. Kumari R, Suman K, Karmakar S, Mishra V, Lakra SG, Saurav GK, Mahto BK (2023) Regulation and safety measures for nanotechnology-based agri-products 5. https://doi.org/10.3389/fgeed.2023.1200987
60. Kwok KW, Leung KM, Flahaut E, Cheng J, Cheng SH (2010) Chronic toxicity of double-walled carbon nanotubes to three marine organisms: influence of different dispersion methods 5:951–961. https://doi.org/10.2217/nnm.10.59
61. Larue C, Castillo-Michel H, Sobanska S, Trcera N, Sorieul S, Cécillon L, Ouerdane L, Legros S, Sarret G (2014) Fate of pristine $TiO_2$ nanoparticles and aged paint-containing $TiO_2$ nanoparticles in lettuce crop after foliar exposure. J Hazard Mater 273:17–26. https://doi.org/10.1016/j.jhazmat.2014.03.014
62. Lee S, Yun H-S, Kim S-H (2011) The comparative effects of mesoporous silica nanoparticles and colloidal silica on inflammation and apoptosis. Biomaterials 32:9434–9443. https://doi.org/10.1016/j.biomaterials.2011.08.042
63. Lew TTS, Wong MH, Kwak SY, Sinclair R, Koman VB, Strano MS (2018) Rational design principles for the transport and subcellular distribution of nanomaterials into plant protoplasts. Small 14:1802086. https://doi.org/10.1002/smll.201802086
64. Lindow SE, Brandl MT (2003) Microbiology of the phyllosphere. Appl Environ Microbiol 69:1875–1883. https://doi.org/10.1128/aem.69.4.1875-1883.2003
65. Lü P, Cao J, He S, Liu J, Li H, Cheng G, Ding Y, Joyce DC (2010) Nano-silver pulse treatments improve water relations of cut rose cv. Movie Star flowers. Postharvest Biol Technol 57:196–202. https://doi.org/10.1016/j.postharvbio.2010.04.003
66. Lv G, Du C, Ma F, Shen Y, Zhou J (2020) In situ detection of rice leaf cuticle responses to nitrogen supplies by depth-profiling Fourier transform photoacoustic spectroscopy. Spectrochim Acta Part A Mol Biomol Spectrosc 228:117759. https://doi.org/10.1016/j.saa.2019.117759
67. Lv J, Christie P, Zhang S (2019) Uptake, translocation, and transformation of metal-based nanoparticles in plants: recent advances and methodological challenges. Environ Sci Nano 6:41–59. https://doi.org/10.1039/C8EN00645H
68. Lv J, Zhang S, Luo L, Zhang J, Yang K, Christie P (2015) Accumulation, speciation and uptake pathway of ZnO nanoparticles in maize. Environ Sci Nano 2:68–77. https://doi.org/10.1039/C4EN00064A
69. Maddala VKS, Singh S, Bandi J (2024) Soil properties influencing nutrient signaling in plant soil systems. In: Essential minerals in plant-soil systems. Elsevier, pp 373–393
70. Maliszewska I (2016) Effects of the biogenic gold nanoparticles on microbial community structure and activities. Ann Microbiol 66:785–794. https://doi.org/10.1007/s13213-015-1158-2
71. Manzanares D, Ceña V (2020) Endocytosis: the nanoparticle and submicron nanocompounds gateway into the cell. Pharmaceutics 12. https://doi.org/10.3390/pharmaceutics12040371

72. Mazumdar S, Chitkara D, Mittal A (2021) Exploration and insights into the cellular internalization and intracellular fate of amphiphilic polymeric nanocarriers. Acta Pharmaceutica Sinica B 11:903–924. https://doi.org/10.1016/j.apsb.2021.02.019
73. McMahon HT, Boucrot E (2011) Molecular mechanism and physiological functions of clathrin-mediated endocytosis. Nat Rev Mol Cell Biol 12:517–533. https://doi.org/10.1038/nrm3151
74. Meddya S, Meshram S, Sarkar D, Datta R, Singh S, Avinash G, Thulasinathan T (2023) Plant stomata: an unrealized possibility in plant defense against invading pathogens and stress tolerance. Plants 12(19):3380
75. Miralles P, Church TL, Harris AT (2012) Toxicity, uptake, and translocation of engineered nanomaterials in vascular plants. Environ Sci Technol 46:9224–9239. https://doi.org/10.1021/es202995d
76. Mittal D, Kaur G, Singh P, Yadav K, Ali SA (2020) Nanoparticle-based sustainable agriculture and food science: recent advances and future outlook. Front Nanotechnol 2. https://doi.org/10.3389/fnano.2020.579954
77. Monica RC, Cremonini R (2009) Nanoparticles and higher plants. Caryologia 62:161–165. https://doi.org/10.1080/00087114.2004.10589681
78. Mourdikoudis S, Pallares RM, Thanh NT (2018) Characterization techniques for nanoparticles: comparison and complementarity upon studying nanoparticle properties. Nanoscale 10:12871–12934. https://doi.org/10.1039/C8NR02278J
79. Nadiminti PP, Dong YD, Sayer C, Hay P, Rookes JE, Boyd BJ, Cahill DM (2013) Nanostructured liquid crystalline particles as an alternative delivery vehicle for plant agrochemicals. ACS Appl Mater Interfaces 5:1818–1826
80. Nair R, Mohamed MS, Gao W, Maekawa T, Yoshida Y, Ajayan PM, Kumar DS (2012) Effect of carbon nanomaterials on the germination and growth of rice plants. J Nanosci Nanotechnol 12:2212–2220. https://doi.org/10.1166/jnn.2012.5775
81. Nair R, Varghese SH, Nair BG, Maekawa T, Yoshida Y, Kumar DS (2010) Nanoparticulate material delivery to plants. Plant Sci 179:154–163. https://doi.org/10.1016/j.plantsci.2010.04.012
82. Nazari M, Riebeling S, Banfield CC, Akale A, Crosta M, Mason-Jones K, Dippold MA, Ahmed MA (2020) Mucilage polysaccharide composition and exudation in maize from contrasting climatic regions. Front Plant Sci 11. https://doi.org/10.3389/fpls.2020.587610
83. Nile SH, Thiruvengadam M, Wang Y, Samynathan R, Shariati MA, Rebezov M, Nile A, Sun M, Venkidasamy B, Xiao J, Kai G (2022) Nano-priming as emerging seed priming technology for sustainable agriculture—recent developments and future perspectives. J Nanobiotechnology 20:254. https://doi.org/10.1186/s12951-022-01423-8
84. Oliveira HC, Gomes BCR, Pelegrino MT, Seabra AB (2016) Nitric oxide-releasing chitosan nanoparticles alleviate the effects of salt stress in maize plants. Nitric Oxide 61:10–19. https://doi.org/10.1016/j.niox.2016.09.010
85. Panyala NR, Peña-Méndez EM, Havel JJ (2008) Silver or silver nanoparticles: a hazardous threat to the environment and human health? J Appl Biomed 6
86. Parrotta L, Guerriero G, Sergeant K, Cai G, Hausman J-F (2015) Target or barrier? The cell wall of early- and later-diverging plants vs cadmium toxicity: differences in the response mechanisms. Front Plant Sci 6. https://doi.org/10.3389/fpls.2015.00133
87. Parveen R, Jain T, Parveen R, Singh S (2023) Genome-wide transcriptome profiling of crop plants. In: Genomics, transcriptomics, proteomics and metabolomics of crop plants. Academic Press, pp 145–171
88. Parveen R, Khare N, Singh S, Johri P (2023) An in silico outlook for the detection and surveillance of evolving and persistent plant pathogens. In: Detection, diagnosis and management of soil-borne phytopathogens. Springer Nature Singapore, Singapore, pp 17–40
89. Patani A, Patel A, Prajapati D, Khare N, Singh S (2023) Various agriculture crop plant-based bioactive compounds and their use in nanomaterial synthesis and applications. In: Nanomaterials from agricultural and horticultural products. Springer Nature Singapore, Singapore, pp 223–241

90. Patani A, Prajapati D, Shukla K, Patel M, Patani P, Patel A, Singh S (2024) Environmental stress–induced alterations in the micro-and macronutrients status of plant. In: Essential minerals in plant-soil systems. Elsevier, pp 181–195
91. Peng C, Duan D, Xu C, Chen Y, Sun L, Zhang H, Yuan X, Zheng L, Yang Y, Yang J, Zhen X, Chen Y, Shi J (2015) Translocation and biotransformation of CuO nanoparticles in rice (Oryza sativa L.) plants. Environ Pollut 197:99–107. https://doi.org/10.1016/j.envpol.2014.12.008
92. Pérez Velasco EA, Betancourt Galindo R, Valdez Aguilar LA, González Fuentes JA, Puente Urbina BA, Lozano Morales SA, Sánchez Valdés S (2020) Effects of the morphology, surface modification and application methods of ZnO-NPs on the growth and biomass of tomato plants. Molecules 25:1282. https://doi.org/10.3390/molecules25061282
93. Pérez-de-Luque A (2017) Interaction of nanomaterials with plants: what do we need for real applications in agriculture? Front Environ Sci 5. https://doi.org/10.3389/fenvs.2017.00012
94. Poole CP and Owens FJ (2003) Introduction to nanotechnology
95. Popova N, Deyev I, Petrenko A (2013) Clathrin-mediated endocytosis and adaptor proteins. Acta Naturae 5:62–73. https://doi.org/10.32607/20758251-2013-5-3-62-73
96. Porter GA (1985) Assimilate transfer and accumulation within the maize pedicel (phloem unloading, assimilate partitioning, translocation). The Pennsylvania State University.
97. Rajput V, Minkina T, Mazarji M, Shende S, Sushkova S, Mandzhieva S, Burachevskaya M, Chaplygin V, Singh A, Jatav H (2020) Accumulation of nanoparticles in the soil-plant systems and their effects on human health. Ann Agric Sci 65:137–143. https://doi.org/10.1016/j.aoas.2020.08.001
98. Rajput V, Minkina T, Sushkova S, Behal A, Maksimov A, Blicharska E, Ghazaryan K, Movsesyan H, Barsova N (2020) ZnO and CuO nanoparticles: a threat to soil organisms, plants, and human health. Environ Geochem Health 42:147–158. https://doi.org/10.1007/s10653-019-00317-3
99. Raliya R, Saharan V, Dimkpa C, Biswas P (2018) Nanofertilizer for precision and sustainable agriculture: current state and future perspectives. J Agric Food Chem 66:6487–6503. https://doi.org/10.1021/acs.jafc.7b02178
100. Ramos D and Almeida L (2022) Overview of standards related to the occupational risk and safety of nanotechnologies 2:83–89. https://doi.org/10.3390/standards2010007
101. Rani S, Kumari N, Sharma V (2023) Uptake, translocation, transformation and physiological effects of nanoparticles in plants. Arch Agron Soil Sci 69:1579–1599. https://doi.org/10.1080/03650340.2022.2103549
102. Rasheed A, Li H, Tahir MM, Mahmood A, Nawaz M, Shah AN, Aslam MT, Negm S, Moustafa M, Hassan MU, Wu Z (2022) The role of nanoparticles in plant biochemical, physiological, and molecular responses under drought stress: a review 13. https://doi.org/10.3389/fpls.2022.976179
103. Sagar SA, Neha T, Sangram KL (2021) Prospects of nano-and peptide-carriers to deliver CRISPR cargos in plants to edit across and beyond central dogma. Nanotechnol Environ Eng 6:22. https://doi.org/10.1007/s41204-021-00118-z
104. Saini RK, Ranjit A, Sharma K, Prasad P, Shang X, Gowda KGM, Keum YS (2022) Bioactive compounds of citrus fruits: a review of composition and health benefits of carotenoids, flavonoids, limonoids, and terpenes. Antioxidants (Basel) 11. https://doi.org/10.3390/antiox11020239
105. Samrot AV, Sahithya CS, Selvarani AJ, Purayil SK, Ponnaiah P (2021) A review on synthesis, characterization and potential biological applications of superparamagnetic iron oxide nanoparticles. Curr Res Green Sustain Chem 4:100042. https://doi.org/10.1016/j.crgsc.2020.100042
106. Sankaran S, Mishra A, Ehsani R, Davis C (2010) A review of advanced techniques for detecting plant diseases. Comput Electron Agric 72:1–13. https://doi.org/10.1016/j.compag.2010.02.007
107. Santana I, Wu H, Hu P, Giraldo JP (2020) Targeted delivery of nanomaterials with chemical cargoes in plants enabled by a biorecognition motif. Nat Commun 11:2045. https://doi.org/10.1038/s41467-020-15731-w

108. Schreiber L (2005) Polar paths of diffusion across plant cuticles: new evidence for an old hypothesis. Ann Bot 95:1069–1073. https://doi.org/10.1093/aob/mci122
109. Schwab F, Bucheli TD, Lukhele LP, Magrez A, Nowack B, Sigg L, Knauer KJ (2011) Are carbon nanotube effects on green algae caused by shading and agglomeration? Environ Sci Technol 45:6136–6144. https://doi.org/10.1021/es200506b
110. Schwab F, Zhai G, Kern M, Turner A, Schnoor JL, Wiesner MR (2016) Barriers, pathways and processes for uptake, translocation and accumulation of nanomaterials in plants—critical review. Nanotoxicology 10:257–278. https://doi.org/10.3109/17435390.2015.1048326
111. Schwabe F, Tanner S, Schulin R, Rotzetter A, Stark W, von Quadt A, Nowack B (2015) Dissolved cerium contributes to uptake of Ce in the presence of differently sized $CeO_2$-nanoparticles by three crop plants. Metallomics 7:466–477. https://doi.org/10.1039/C4MT00343H
112. Shelar A, Nile SH, Singh AV, Rothenstein D, Bill J, Xiao J, Chaskar M, Kai G, Patil R (2023) Recent advances in nano-enabled seed treatment strategies for sustainable agriculture: challenges, risk assessment, and future perspectives. Nano-Micro Lett 15:54. https://doi.org/10.1007/s40820-023-01025-5
113. Singh A, Sengar RS, Singh AK, Singh S, Kumar A, Ahmad K (2019) Impact of genetic engineering on agriculture food crops. Biotech Today: Int J Biol Sci 9(1):17–24
114. Slomberg DL, Schoenfisch MH (2012) Silica nanoparticle phytotoxicity to Arabidopsis thaliana. Environ Sci Technol 46:10247–10254. https://doi.org/10.1021/es300949f
115. Smita S, Gupta SK, Bartonova A, Dusinska M, Gutleb AC, Rahman Q (2012) Nanoparticles in the environment: assessment using the causal diagram approach. Environ Health 11:S13. https://doi.org/10.1186/1476-069X-11-S1-S13
116. Stewart MP, Langer R, Jensen KF (2018) Intracellular delivery by membrane disruption: mechanisms, strategies, and concepts. Chem Rev 118:7409–7531. https://doi.org/10.1021/acs.chemrev.7b00678
117. Stone V, Nowack B, Baun A, van den Brink N, von der Kammer F, Dusinska M, Handy R, Hankin S, Hassellöv M, Joner E (2010) Nanomaterials for environmental studies: classification, reference material issues, and strategies for physico-chemical characterisation. Sci Total Environ 408:1745–1754. https://doi.org/10.1016/j.scitotenv.2009.10.035
118. Su Y, Ashworth V, Kim C, Adeleye AS, Rolshausen P, Roper C, White J, Jassby D (2019) Delivery, uptake, fate, and transport of engineered nanoparticles in plants: a critical review and data analysis. Environ Sci Nano 6:2311–2331. https://doi.org/10.1039/C9EN00461K
119. Sun X-D, Yuan X-Z, Jia Y, Feng L-J, Zhu F-P, Dong S-S, Liu J, Kong X, Tian H, Duan J-L (2020) Differentially charged nanoplastics demonstrate distinct accumulation in Arabidopsis thaliana. Nat Nanotechnol 15:755–760. https://doi.org/10.1038/s41565-020-0707-4
120. Suri S, Singh A, Nema PK (2022) Current applications of citrus fruit processing waste: a scientific outlook. Appl Food Res 2:100050. https://doi.org/10.1016/j.afres.2022.100050
121. Takeshita V, de Sousa BT, Preisler AC, Carvalho LB, Pereira AdES, Tornisielo VL, Dalazen G, Oliveira HC, Fraceto LF (2021) Foliar absorption and field herbicidal studies of atrazine-loaded polymeric nanoparticles. J Hazard Mater 418:126350. https://doi.org/10.1016/j.jhazmat.2021.126350
122. Taylor AF, Rylott EL, Anderson CW, Bruce NC (2014) Investigating the toxicity, uptake, nanoparticle formation and genetic response of plants to gold. PLoS One 9:e93793. https://doi.org/10.1371/journal.pone.0093793
123. Thomas T, Bahadori T, Savage N, Thomas K (2009) Moving toward exposure and risk evaluation of nanomaterials: challenges and future directions. Wiley Interdiscip Rev: Nanomed Nanobiotechnol 1:426–433. https://doi.org/10.1002/wnan.34
124. Tombuloglu H, Slimani Y, Tombuloglu G, Almessiere M, Baykal A, Ercan I, Sozeri H (2019) Tracking of $NiFe_2O_4$ nanoparticles in barley (Hordeum vulgare L.) and their impact on plant growth, biomass, pigmentation, catalase activity, and mineral uptake. Environ Nanotechnol Monit Manag 11:100223. https://doi.org/10.1016/j.enmm.2019.100223
125. Tong T, Wilke CM, Wu J, Binh CTT, Kelly JJ, Gaillard J-F, Gray KA (2015) Combined toxicity of nano-ZnO and nano-$TiO_2$: from single- to multinanomaterial systems. Environ Sci Technol 49:8113–8123. https://doi.org/10.1021/acs.est.5b02148

126. Tripathi DK, Shweta SS, Singh S, Pandey R, Singh VP, Sharma NC, Prasad SM, Dubey NK, Chauhan DK (2017) An overview on manufactured nanoparticles in plants: uptake, translocation, accumulation and phytotoxicity. Plant Physiol Biochem 110:2–12. https://doi.org/10.1016/j.plaphy.2016.07.030
127. Tungare K, Shahu R, Zambare V, Agarwal P, Jobby R, Nisar N, Jha P (2022) Toxicity mitigation of textile dye reactive blue 4 by hairy roots of Helianthus annuus and testing its effect in in vivo model systems. Biomed Res Int 2022
128. Uzu G, Sobanska S, Sarret G, Munoz M, Dumat C (2010) Foliar lead uptake by lettuce exposed to atmospheric fallouts. Environ Sci Technol 44:1036–1042. https://doi.org/10.1021/es902190u
129. Van Nguyen D, Nguyen HM, Le NT, Nguyen KH, Nguyen HT, Le HM, Nguyen AT, Dinh NTT, Hoang SA, Van Ha C (2022) Copper nanoparticle application enhances plant growth and grain yield in maize under drought stress conditions. J Plant Growth Regul 41:364–375. https://doi.org/10.1007/s00344-021-10301-w
130. Verma N, Sao P, Srivastava A, Singh S (2021) Physiological and molecular responses to drought, submergence and excessive watering in plants. Harsh environment and plant resilience: molecular and functional aspects, 305–321
131. Vora Z, Pandya J, Vaikuntapu PR, Singh S, Asha S, Purama RK (2023) Genome-wide association of defense hormone crosstalk in plants. In: Hormonal cross-talk, plant defense and development. Academic Press, pp 353–371
132. Wani TA, Masoodi FA, Baba WN, Ahmad M, Rahmanian N, Jafari SM (2019) Chapter 11—nanoencapsulation of agrochemicals, fertilizers, and pesticides for improved plant production. In: Ghorbanpour M, Wani SH (eds.) Advances in phytonanotechnology. Academic Press, pp 279–298
133. Werrie P-Y, Burgeon C, Le Goff GJ, Hance T, Fauconnier M-L (2021) Biopesticide trunk injection into apple trees: a proof of concept for the systemic movement of mint and cinnamon essential oils 12. https://doi.org/10.3389/fpls.2021.650132
134. Wu H, Li Z (2022) Nano-enabled agriculture: how do nanoparticles cross barriers in plants? Plant Commun 3:100346. https://doi.org/10.1016/j.xplc.2022.100346
135. Wu H, Shabala L, Barry K, Zhou M, Shabala S (2013) Ability of leaf mesophyll to retain potassium correlates with salinity tolerance in wheat and barley. Physiol Plant 149:515–527. https://doi.org/10.1111/ppl.12056
136. Xu T, Zheng F, Zhao Y (2023) Chapter 6—biophysicochemical transformations of ENMs in air. In: La Rosa GD, Peralta-Videa JR (eds) Physicochemical interactions of engineered nanoparticles and plants, vol 4. Academic Press, pp 143–173
137. Yang C, Powell CA, Duan Y, Shatters R, Zhang M (2015) Antimicrobial nanoemulsion formulation with improved penetration of foliar spray through citrus leaf cuticles to control citrus huanglongbing. PLoS ONE 10:e0133826
138. Yang Y, Li R, Wang L, Bi H, Peng Z, Li J, Guo C, Bi Y, Lai Y, Guo D (2023) Enhanced germination and growth of alfalfa with seed presoaking and hydroponic culture in $Fe_2O_3$ magnetic nanoparticles. J Nanomater 2023:9783977. https://doi.org/10.1155/2023/9783977
139. You T, Liu D, Chen J, Yang Z, Dou R, Gao X, Wang L (2018) Effects of metal oxide nanoparticles on soil enzyme activities and bacterial communities in two different soil types. J Soils Sediments 18:211–221. https://doi.org/10.1007/s11368-017-1716-2
140. Zhang Y, Liu N, Wang W, Sun J, Zhu LJ (2020) Photosynthesis and related metabolic mechanism of promoted rice (Oryza sativa L.) growth by $TiO_2$ nanoparticles. Front Environ Sci Eng 14:1–12. https://doi.org/10.1007/s11783-020-1282-5
141. Zhang Z, He X, Zhang H, Ma Y, Zhang P, Ding Y, Zhao Y (2011) Uptake and distribution of ceria nanoparticles in cucumber plants. Metallomics 3:816–822. https://doi.org/10.1039/c1mt00049g
142. Zhao L, Ortiz C, Adeleye AS, Hu Q, Zhou H, Huang Y, Keller AA (2016) Metabolomics to detect response of lettuce (Lactuca sativa) to $Cu(OH)_2$ nanopesticides: oxidative stress response and detoxification mechanisms. Environ Sci Technol 50:9697–9707. https://doi.org/10.1021/acs.est.6b02763

143. Zhao L, Peralta-Videa JR, Varela-Ramirez A, Castillo-Michel H, Li C, Zhang J, Aguilera RJ, Keller AA, Gardea-Torresdey JL (2012) Effect of surface coating and organic matter on the uptake of $CeO_2$ NPs by corn plants grown in soil: insight into the uptake mechanism. J Hazard Mater 225:131–138. https://doi.org/10.1016/j.jhazmat.2012.05.008
144. Zhu J, Li J, Shen Y, Liu S, Zeng N, Zhan X, White JC, Gardea-Torresdey J, Xing B (2020) Mechanism of zinc oxide nanoparticle entry into wheat seedling leaves. Environ Sci Nano 7:3901–3913. https://doi.org/10.1039/D0EN00658K
145. Zhu Z-J, Wang H, Yan B, Zheng H, Jiang Y, Miranda OR, Rotello VM, Xing B, Vachet RW (2012) Effect of surface charge on the uptake and distribution of gold nanoparticles in four plant species. Environ Sci Technol 46(12391):12398. https://doi.org/10.1021/es301977w

# Potential Effects of Nanopesticides on Honeybees

A. V. Moorthy, Renu Pandey, Pramod Mall, and K. Aravinthraju

**Abstract** Nanotechnology has found diverse applications across agriculture, industry, and medicine. In agriculture, the prominent focus has been on developing nanomaterials to combat plant diseases and pests. The imperative to satisfy the expanding global food demand, along with rapid nanotechnology progress, has driven the emergence of nanopesticides as potential alternatives to conventional pesticides. These nanopesticides utilize active ingredients formulated at the nanoscale, offering improved stability, heightened efficacy, even dispersion, and controlled release to target organisms, thereby reducing overall pesticide usage. However, the improved chemical stability that enhances nanopesticide performance also raises concerns about their persistence, and the optimized dispersion of these active ingredients raises the possibility of unintended interactions with non-target organisms. Consequently, evaluating the potential toxicity of nanopesticides on non-target organisms, such as honeybees that play a vital role in crop pollination, becomes crucial. The impact of nanopesticides on honeybees has gained significant attention, as their unintended consequences could contribute to the ongoing decline in honeybee populations. Despite the fact that nanopesticides are specifically designed to target pests while minimizing harm to non-target species, traces of these nanoparticles have been identified in pollen grains collected and transported by bees to their hives. This accumulation of nanopesticides in beeswax poses a persistent threat to bee health over time. This chapter addresses the benefits offered by nanopesticides, including enhanced stability, but also sheds light on their potential negative impact on honeybees. The complex interactions between nanoparticles and pollen particles during collection are examined, along with recommended practices aimed at safeguarding honeybee populations from the adverse effects of nanopesticides.

A. V. Moorthy (✉) · R. Pandey · P. Mall
Department of Entomology, College of Agriculture, G B Pant University of Agriculture and Technology, Pantnagar, Uttarakhand, India
e-mail: moorthyagri96@gmail.com

K. Aravinthraju
Department of Agricultural Entomology, Tamil Nadu Agricultural University, Coimbatore, Tamil Nadu, India

 
D. Jabborova et al. (eds.), *Nanomaterials in Agroforestry Systems*, Smart Nanomaterials Technology, https://doi.org/10.1007/978-981-96-1337-3_18

**Keywords** Nanotechnology · Nanopesticide · Honey bee · Electrostatic conduction · Toxic effects · Symptoms · Management

## 1 Introduction

In the past few decades, nanotechnology has surfaced as a prominent field of study with numerous applications, and agriculture has not been an exception to its influence. Nanotechnology has revolutionized the agricultural field by introducing high-tech practices and innovative nanoproducts [118]. This advancement has become essential in developing efficient pest control strategies and combating resistance to conventional formulations, which has become a pressing need due to increasing pest-related economic losses and production challenges [129]. Products enhanced by nanotechnology, such as nanofertilizers and nanopesticides, have garnered attention for their desirable properties, including stress tolerance, reduced transportation costs, and eco-friendliness [11]. However, addressing the environmental impact of pesticides becomes crucial, considering the escalating growing global need for food and increasing pest resistance. The widespread utilization and manufacture of pesticides over the years have raised concerns about their environmental footprint [124]. Additionally, soil degradation and the impacts of climate change are impacting crop yields, and a substantial increase in production is anticipated to meet future demands [81]. Addressing these challenges is further complicated by inefficiencies in food usage, with a significant portion of harvested food going to waste [113]. To overcome these issues, nanotechnology-based pesticides have gained prominence and are being adopted worldwide [11, 58]. These pesticides offer advantages such as reduced active ingredient amounts, enhanced solubility, and decreased use of surfactants and adjuvants found in conventional formulations [18]. Nanotechnology also allows for the regulated release of agricultural chemicals, leading to longer-lasting effects and potentially minimizing application, leaching, and runoff [129]. This renders nanotechnology-driven pesticides a more effective and eco-friendly method for safeguarding crops and enhancing yields. Metal-infused nanopesticides, utilizing nanoparticles have gained popularity owing to their straightforward customization, resulting in strong bonding interactions with pesticide compounds [18, 96, 110]. Various nanoformulations, including nanoemulsions, nano-encapsulates, nanogels, and electrospun nano-fibres, have also been explored [2, 106]. Nevertheless, the potential adverse effects of nanomaterials and their genuine eco-safety have prompted concerns, particularly regarding their implications for health and the environment, particularly in water bodies and non-target organisms. Despite the promise of nanotechnology-based pesticides, there is still limited research on their ecotoxicity, leading to inconclusive results [11]. Concerning the toxicity mechanisms of nanotechnology-based pesticides, they can infiltrate surface water bodies and detrimentally affect ecosystems.

Nanoparticles (NPs), frequently employed in nanopesticide formulations, can induce toxicological effects owing to their inherent nanoscale characteristics, broad dispersion, and accumulation in water and soil environments [30, 71, 131]. Nanoparticles (NPs) can function as a "Trojan horse," amplifying the toxic effects of nanopesticides. Various factors, including particle size, surface area, charge, and materials, influence their biocidal effects. For example, smaller nanopesticides exhibit higher efficacy as they can better distribute on crop leaves [18, 96, 110]. The environmental destiny of pesticides based on nanotechnology is an important concern as their widespread use increases. While these pesticides can be designed to decrease application rates in comparison to conventional alternatives, they also possess properties that can lead to different contamination problems in soils and aquatic bodies due to improved transportation, persistence, and toxicity [128]. Understanding the fate of nanopesticides is crucial for assessing their environmental risk and benefits. Nanopesticides may interact with microorganisms in the environment, affecting their decomposition and nutrient-recycling capabilities [114]. Additionally, aggregation of nanoparticles can further impact their fate in aquatic environments, influencing sediment accumulation and potential toxicity to aquatic life [41, 44, 75]. Lastly, the safety of nanotechnology-based pesticides is an ongoing debate. While some research suggests that nanopesticides are environmentally safe due to their optimized application and prolonged release of active ingredients [8, 27, 37], there is still limited information and inconclusive results regarding their ultimate eco-safety. The potential impacts of nanomaterials on non-target species, coupled with their ability to enter organisms through various routes, raise concerns about their persistence and mobility in soil and water [6]. Nanotechnology-based pesticides hold promise for more efficient and sustainable pest control and increased crop production. However, their potential adverse effects on the environment and non-target organisms necessitate further research and robust studies to precisely assess their benefits and risks [82]. Understanding the environmental fate and potential eco(un)safety of nanopesticides is crucial in developing regulatory guidelines to minimize environmental risks and ensure a sustainable agricultural future [94]. Hence, the objective of this chapter is to furnish a contemporary comprehension of these nanopesticides from an ecotoxicological perspective.

## 2 Nanopesticides: A Revolution in Agriculture's Future

Nanotechnology-based pesticides (NBPs), known as nanopesticides, are being addressed as a potentially revolutionary advancement in agriculture, tackling the formidable challenge of fulfilling the continually growing global demand for food, fibre, and fuel [81]. These innovative formulations offer numerous advantages over traditional pesticides, including enhanced solubility, stability, and efficacy. Conventional pesticide formulations frequently feature descriptors such as "controlled release," "improved rainfastness," "UV light protection," or "extended residual control." These indicators illustrate how nano-based pesticides safeguard active ingredients from physical and microbial degradation processes, ensuring their effectiveness over a longer period [48, 105].

One of the key benefits of NBPs lies in their engineered properties, enabling the controlled release of the crop protection agent under specific conditions. These conditions can include dehydration, changes in pH or temperature, interactions with enzymes or antigens, or other triggers [120]. This controlled release mechanism allows for more precise and targeted application, reducing the amount of active ingredient required while increasing the deposition of the pesticide on the intended target [101]. As a result, NBPs contribute to more efficient and sustainable pest management practices. Moreover, NBP formulations offer environmental advantages, as they reduce the reliance on volatile petroleum solvents commonly used in traditional pesticide formulations to deliver poorly soluble active ingredients [83]. The reduced use of these solvents decreases the risk to both the environment and pesticide applicators. By minimizing the release of volatile compounds, nanotechnology-based pesticides promote safer and more environmentally friendly agricultural practices [62]. Nanotechnology-based pesticides, or nanopesticides, have the potential to revolutionize modern agriculture by providing increased solubility, stability, and efficacy over traditional formulations. Their ability to release crop protection agents in a controlled manner, along with reduced reliance on volatile solvents, makes them an attractive option for achieving sustainable and efficient pest management while meeting the growing global demand for agricultural products [92, 95].

## 2.1 *Nanotechnology in Crop Protection*

In agriculture, nanotechnology is harnessed to augment food production, striving to attain comparable or even superior nutritional value, quality, and safety in crops. One of the key ways to improve crop production is by efficiently using fertilizers, pesticides, herbicides, and plant growth regulators. Nanocarriers play a crucial role in achieving controlled release of these agricultural chemicals [93]. As an illustration, poly (epsilon-caprolactone) nanocapsules have been engineered as carriers for herbicides such as atrazine. When mustard plants were treated with nanocapsules, it led to heightened herbicidal efficacy in contrast to commercial atrazine, leading to reduced net photosynthetic rates, stomatal conductance, and overall growth of the plants [21]. Similar nanocarriers like silica nanoparticles and polymeric nanoparticles [42] have also been developed for the controlled release of pesticides. These precision farming strategies can improve crop yields while minimizing soil and water damage [104]. Furthermore, nanotechnology has been used for gene or DNA transfer in plants to develop insect-resistant varieties [121]. Certain nanomaterials themselves can act as pesticides due to their enhanced toxicity and sensitivity. For instance, metal oxide nanomaterials like ZnO, TiO2, and CuO have been studied for their ability to protect plants from pathogen infections. ZnO nanoparticles, for instance, exhibit strong antifungal and antibacterial activity against various harmful microbes [67]. Nanofertilizers have emerged as a solution to address the inefficiencies and high losses associated with conventional mineral fertilizers. These nanofertilizers, particularly micro-nutrients at the nanoscale, such as Magnesium, Copper, Iron, Zinc,

Molybdenum, and Boran, can reduce nutrient losses and enhance nutrient assimilation by crops and soil microorganisms. Other nanomaterials, like carbon nano-onions and chitosan nanoparticles [7], have also shown promise in increasing crop growth and quality. The adoption of novel nanofertilizers is expected to revolutionize the fertilizer production industry in the near future. Nanosensors, especially, wireless nanosensors have been created to monitor crop and environmental conditions in the field. These specially designed nanosensors can detect chemicals at trace levels in agricultural systems. Real-time monitoring using nanosensors can help prevent can mitigate potential crop losses and enhance crop production when paired with the appropriate application of nanofertilizers, nanopesticides, and nanoherbicides. For example, copper-doped montmorillonite [1] has been used as a nanosensor to monitor the fungicide propineb in aquatic environments, demonstrating the potential for in situ and real-time monitoring to support agricultural practices. Nanotechnology in agriculture offers various beneficial aspects, including the use of nanocarriers for controlled release of agricultural chemicals, nanofertilizers to improve nutrient uptake and reduce losses, and nanosensors for real-time monitoring of crop health and environmental conditions. These advancements have the potential to significantly enhance food production and sustainability in the agricultural sector.

## 2.2 *Precision in Action of Nanopesticides*

Numerous pesticide active ingredients display hydrophobic characteristics or possess other characteristics that create challenges in formulating aqueous solutions for their effective application. Nanopesticides address this issue by packaging crop protection mediators in elements of optimized size to enhance solubility or dispersion. In some cases, active ingredients can be subjected to a process of crystallization and milling, resulting in the creation of nanoscale particles. This size reduction increases the solubility of the pesticide because of the increased surface area, thereby enhancing dissolution rates [99]. Another approach to achieve increased solubility involves incorporating the pesticide active ingredients into or onto the surfaces of unstructured particles [51].

To facilitate communication and categorization of different pesticide formulations, particulate pesticide formulations are assigned specific formulation codes. However, the precise details and compositions of pesticide formulations are often treated as proprietary business data and are not publicly disclosed [17, 32]. In the formulation of nanopesticides, NBP particles can be enveloped or suspended within inert ingredients and other substances. These additional materials endow the NBP particles with properties that may not be present in the raw active ingredient. For example, the inclusion of UV protectants can enhance the stability of the pesticide under sunlight, while other components may contribute to extending the shelf life of the formulation [49]. Nanotechnology-based pesticides address the solubility and dispersion challenges associated with certain pesticideactive ingredients. By engineering pesticide agents into nanoscale particles or incorporating them into particulate formulations, nanopesticides improve the effectiveness and application precision of crop protection measures. Additionally, the inclusion of specific inert ingredients further enhances the overall performance and longevity of the nanopesticide formulation.

## 3 Understanding Nanoscale Risks

Nanoscale materials and substances possess distinct properties compared to the similar compound with larger structures, making them highly sought-after for diverse communal and marketable applications. However, these special properties may also lead to different behaviours than conventional chemicals, requiring special regulatory scrutiny. Particles at the lower end of this nanoscale entities are of specific regulatory concern due to the potential for innovative functional or toxicological attributes within this size series. Nanoscale materials are unique due to their size-dependent properties, resulting from quantum effects and increased surface-to-volume ratios. When materials are at the nanoscale, their physicochemical characteristics, such as solubility, reactivity, and toxicity, may differ significantly from their larger counterparts. These properties have sparked interest in developing various nanotechnology-based products for diverse applications, including agrotechnology. The regulatory landscape for nanoscale materials is still evolving, as their special properties may warrant specific safety assessments beyond conventional chemicals. Recognizing this, the International Organization for Standardization (ISO) has defined nanoscale as ranging from roughly ranging from 1 to 100 nm. Nanoparticles falling within this range, especially those at the lower end of the nanoscale spectrum, have attracted regulatory interest because they can display unique properties and interactions that are not evident in larger-scale materials. To address the potential risks associated with nanomaterials, especially in agrotechnology, regulatory agencies like the United States Environmental Protection Agency (EPA) have taken steps to regulate nanomaterial pesticides. They have set a working definition of nanoscale as spanning from 1 to 100 nm, enabling them to focus on nano-sized particles in their assessments. Nanosilver is one such example of a nanopesticide, known for its antimicrobial activity, and its particle sizes typically fall between 1.5 and 5 nm. The intention behind such regulation is to ensure that nanoscale materials, including nanopesticides, undergo proper safety evaluations, taking into account their unique characteristics and potential risks. By setting a defined range for nanoscale, regulatory authorities aim to foster safe and responsible use of nanotechnology-based products in agriculture and other sectors.

## 3.1 Behaviour and Fate of NBP Formulations

The literature review conducted on pesticide formulations suggests that these particles may possess nanoscale structures such as layers, pores, coatings, or other characteristics that significantly increase their surface area available for interactions with the pesticide's active ingredients. Several types of NBP formulations have been identified, including those derived from nanoparticles or microparticles, as well as emulsions containing conventional pesticide active ingredients. These formulations may involve coatings or encapsulation by a nanolayer of another substance, or adsorption or entrapment within, a polymer. For instance, This acts as a water-dispersible carrier, enclosing a core or reservoir containing the active ingredient. The capsule design allows the controlled release of the pesticide contents after application. The shell may consist of single or many layers of synthetic, or biodegradable polymers, potentially modifying environmental properties and toxicity [49]. Monolithic Polymers involve the homogeneous accumulation of active ingredients, which are then processed into spherical structures to facilitate the gradual release of the pesticide over time. Similarly, hard lipid nanoparticles represent another approach with similarities to Monolithic Polymeric Spheres. Additionally, polymers and hydrogels, are cross-linked to form a gel, are used to attach the pesticide active ingredient, further diversifying NBP formulations. Each of these formulations presents unique characteristics that influence their behaviour, fate, and potential risks in the environment. Suspension NBPs involve the milling of crystallized active ingredients to achieve submicron size particles, which are then coated with specific compounds. This coating enables the suspension of the crystals in aqueous solutions, allowing for convenient application as pesticides [23] (see Fig. 1).

## 3.2 Impact of Nanomaterial Carriers on Pesticide

Porous silica and zeolites are examples of nanomaterials that can act as carriers for pesticides. Porous silica consists of silicates and aluminosilicates with attached organic moieties. Conversely, zeolites are a varied group of porous, crystalline aluminosilicates, derived from either regular or artificial sources. Both materials function as inorganic polymers that facilitate slow release of pesticides, offering extended effectiveness [122]. Natural clays have a layered silicate sheets and provide an area for the adsorption of pesticides. In the context of pesticide formulations, organoclays and clay composites are particularly noteworthy. They contain cations, between the coatings, enhancing their adsorption and delivery capabilities [97]. Layered double hydroxides are characterized by a diverse, positively charged layer structure balanced with anions in the interlayer. This unique structure also serves as a potential carrier for pesticides, allowing for controlled release over time [24]. The use of clay particles for protecting, stabilizing, and slowly releasing crop protection agents has been a practice employed in agriculture for decades [73]. Metal nanoparticles, particles

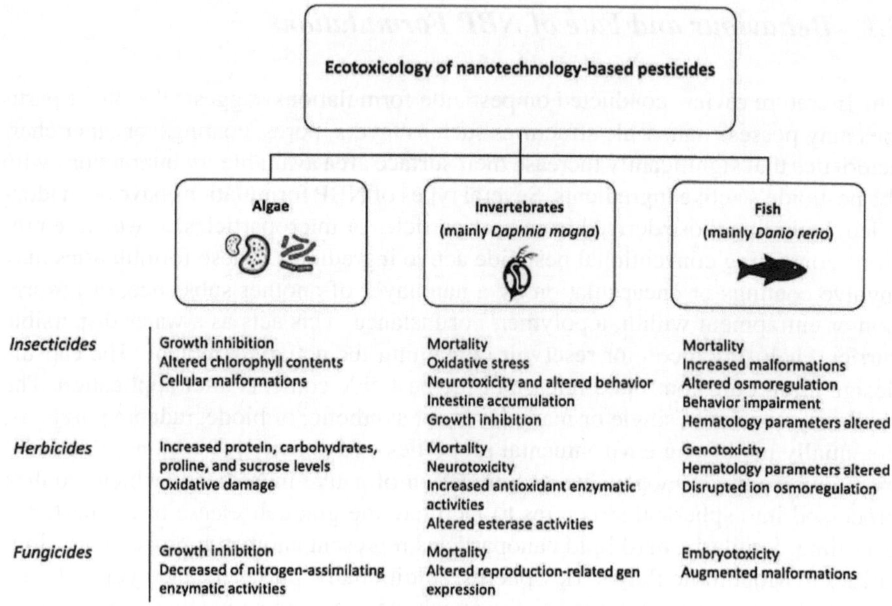


**Fig. 1** Summary of the primary ecotoxicological impacts of pesticides derived from nanotechnology on organisms not intended as targets [6]

with a diameter below 100 nm, exhibit functional activity without necessitating the addition of conventional pesticide active ingredients. While there is significant interest in employing metal nanoparticles regulatory concerns persist. Similar to those encountered with nanosilver [67, 77]. Nanoemulsions are water-based comprising nano-sized hydrophobic droplets. These nanoemulsions serve as colloidal carriers for pesticides, facilitating their dispersion and application [123]. Apart from the examples, numerous additional ingredients and fusion particles are currently being proposed or used as carriage systems for plant defence agents.

Studies conducted by Kah et al. [61] have projected a definition for nanopesticides, which includes preparations that purposely incorporate entities up to 1000 nm. Additionally, the designation of a "nano" prefix or the claim of new stuffs allied with minor size also falls under the scope of nanopesticides. By incorporating these criteria, many currently used pesticides, even those above 100 nm, fit Kah's definition of nanopesticides [61]. Regardless of the mass or structure of the particles in pesticide formulations, they have the potential to impact the fate of active ingredients in the environment. This uncertainty underscores the importance of considering formulation risks.

### 3.3 *Pollution Puzzle: PM's Impact on Ecological Systems*

The properties of nanosilver are primarily attributed to its huge surface area relative to silver elements. This increased surface area facilitates a higher discharge of silver ions outside, which contributes to its enhanced antimicrobial activity. The EPA has approved conditional registration for nanosilver as an antimicrobial pesticide [65, 66]. However, this registration process has faced delays and legal disagreements due to data breaches and uncertainties surrounding environmental impacts associated with nanosilver. In contrast to nanosilver, nanotechnology-based pesticide (NBP) particles are typically larger and more heterogeneous. As a result, NBPs have not undergone the same level of regulatory scrutiny as nanosilver. One possible reason for this distinction is that nanosilver functions as an active ingredient itself, whereas NBP particles serve as carriers for active ingredients, and typically, their dimensions exceed 100 nm. EFSA acknowledges that larger particles may still exhibit size-related properties warranting regulation. However, there is currently no universally agreed definition for "nanopesticide." Unlike nanosilver, NBPs are presently introduced into the environment through farming [59].

Additionally, manmade activities accidentally release particles into the environment. Many industrial processes contribute to the emission of particulate matter (PM). PM is categorized into coarse and fine particulate matter based on their aerodynamic diameter, with PM 2.5 referring to particles lesser than 2.5 μm. The impact of PM, especially ultrafine particles (PM 0.1), on ecological systems and non-target species, including arthropods critical for pollinating croplands, has been a subject of concern and limited research.

An investigation into various farming and housing pesticides using SEM revealed particles ranging from 50 nm to several microns. This suggests that many of these particles exceed the ISO size criterion for nanoscale. If airborne, the particles would predominantly fall within the size range between PM 0.1 and PM 2.5, indicating potential overlap between NBP dimensions and particulate matter in the environment. Some of the examined particles displayed varying degrees of homogeneity and complexity, with different types of particles coexisting.

### 3.4 *Nanopesticide—Risk to Biodiversity*

According to the most current dose–response science, nanomaterials have positive impacts on environment. However, these effects on biodiversity may have unidentified negative values. To ensure a comprehensive approach, a broader perspective should be taken into account, especially in the context of ecological risk assessment. Neglecting to include the entire dose–response continuum in this process may result in improper estimates and the establishment of hazardous governing criteria [56].

Hormesis is an essential concept to understand when assessing the ecological effects of nanomaterials and nanopesticides. It refers to the stimulation by low concentrations. In other words, at low levels of exposure, nanomaterials and nanopesticides may have a beneficial effect on organisms, while adverse effects are more likely to occur at high levels of exposure [3]. Research has revealed that hormesis is an extensive phenomenon experiential in various organisms when exposed to stress-inducing agents, including pesticides and nanomaterials. For instance, numerous pesticides, including widely used herbicides and insecticides, have been found to induce hormesis in various organisms [33]. Similarly, nanomaterials, have been revealed to encourage hormesis in crops, soil microbes, insects, and nematodes. At low doses, nanomaterials can act as a conditioning medium, reducing toxicities caused by other stressors present at higher concentrations. It is important to note that hormesis occurs at concentrations or doses significantly lower than those that lead to adverse effects. Therefore, even though concerns have been high about the toxicity of nanomaterials and additives in nanopesticides, hundreds of dose–response studies have demonstrated optimistic effects of low concentrations nanomaterials on various organisms [19]. While the ecological risk assessment of nanopesticides and nanofertilizers should consider the combined effects of nanomaterials and pesticides, the interactions between these components are not yet fully understood [38]. However, given that both individually induce hormesis, it is reasonable to expect that hormesis will also occur at low concentrations of nanopesticides. Understanding the mechanisms of action and chemical interactions between these compounds is crucial to assessing the potential risks and benefits of nanopesticides accurately. In conclusion, considering hormesis in the risk assessment of nanopesticides and incorporating the full dose–response continuum will provide a more comprehensive understanding of their potential ecological impacts. Taking into account the positive and negative effects at various concentrations will help ensure the safe and sustainable use of nanotechnology in agriculture while safeguarding biodiversity and the natural environment [130] (see Table 1).

## 4 Honey Bee Decline—Current Situation

Honey bees are the most important and commercially dominant pollinators for food crop production worldwide. Research indicates that honeybees play a vital role in pollinating 87.5% of all blooming and edible plants. Bee variety is vital for long-term pollination services. However, bee populations have been dropping, putting a strain on key commodities such as fruits, vegetables, and fodder crops. In the United States, colony collapse disorder, characterized by an abrupt and rapid loss of honeybee populations, accounts for 30–40% of colony disappearances [76]. Furthermore, several native bee species in North America and Mexico are vulnerable, and 26% of bumble bee species are threatened [60]. Other regions, such as the United Kingdom and China, have also experienced significant losses in honeybee populations [68, 98]. India has seen a decline of more than 40% in honeybees over the past 25 years [47]. The decline of honeybees, considered the most important pollinators of agricultural crops, poses a severe threat to global agriculture, as one-third

**Table 1** The main categories of nanopesticides presently in use, their applications, and their behaviour in the environment are subjects of current interest and research

| Nanopesticide | Applications | Environmental fate | References |
|---|---|---|---|
| Al-based | This functions by adhering to cuticle of the insect, thereby disrupting the protective wax layer. This disruption leads to dehydration in insects | No studies concerning the environmental fate were discovered. Regarding organisms' exposure, their toxicity was indicated to be low | Rani et al. [100] |
| Nanocarriers polysaccharides | This acts as insecticides, herbicides, or fungicides | It was presumed that they exhibit low persistence upon reaching environments, although their characteristics have been inadequately researched | Ding et al. [40] |
| Metallic-based | Acting primarily as a biocide, particularly for antibacterial purposes, by causing damage to cellular membranes and releasing ions | In certain environments, there is a possibility of nanoparticle dissolution, leading to ion release. Agglomeration and/or sedimentation may also occur. Additionally, particles could be soothed by organic substances. The presence of algae can further enhance ion release due to interactions with their exudates | Andrade et al. [9] |
| Silica-based | The insecticide induces dehydration by adhering to the lipid | They exhibit considerable stability, with no occurrence of photochemical degradation or speciation in aquatic environments, although changes in particle size may result from accumulation or cluster. Suspension might happen based on pH and the presence of organic acid salts. Limited poisonousness has been indicated for non-target organisms, and their perseverance in muscles is negligible. They can adhere to the surfaces of the cell and potentially modify structure and integrity of membrane | Ale et al. [5] |

(continued)

**Table 1** (continued)

| Nanopesticide | Applications | Environmental fate | References |
|---|---|---|---|
| Solid lipid-based | The extent of pesticide loading, for instance with herbicide or oil-loaded antiparasitic, determines the outcome | Insufficiently researched and greatly reliant on the level of pesticide charging | Nemati et al. [89] |
| Nanoemulsions | Typically infused with traditional pesticides | The deadly effects on both target and non-target organisms were elevated compared to their conventional counterparts due to increased absorption | Nemati et al. [89] |

of all food consumed globally relies on pollinators, especially bees. Without bees, the diet of various organisms, including humans, would become less nutritious, and food prices would increase. Nutritional crops like fruits, nuts, and vegetables that depend on pollination would be replaced with basic crops family include leguminosae, leading to an imbalanced diet. Crops such as coffee, almonds, tomatoes, and cocoa, which rely on pollination, would face extinction without bees and other pollinators. To counter this threat, countries should implement more pollinator-friendly food policies and systems. The global decline in bee populations poses a significant risk to essential plants that contribute to human well-being and livelihoods. Hence, it is essential for countries to take more measures to help safeguard these essential friends in the fight against hunger and malnutrition.

### *4.1 Role of Electric Fields in Pollen Capture by Bees*

Bees, along with other pollinators, possess remarkable adaptations that enable them to efficiently collect and transport pollen. In the case of honey bees, they employ specialized hair-like structures called setae that cover almost their whole body, including their eyes. These setae act as effective pollen traps, allowing bees to actively collect pollen from flowers or gather it passively through electrostatic forces [26]. An intriguing aspect of bee behaviour is their ability to accumulate a positive charge while flying. As they approach blossoms, the presence of the bee induces an image charge, creating an electric field that plays a crucial role in the final capture of pollen [116]. The process of pollen capture through electrostatic forces is fascinating. As bees fly through the air, the friction generated during flight results in a positive charge on their body. In contrast, flowers carry a negative charge, which is more pronounced at their tips and edges. When bees come near a flower, they can sense the electric field emanating from the flower. As they move even closer, the electrostatic forces come into play, facilitating the transfer of pollen from the flower to the bee's body [116].

Recent research has shed light on the bee's ability to use electric charge as a cue to assess the pollination status of flowers [25, 50]. The exploration of this electroreceptive ability in bees is an area of emerging study [111]. It highlights the incredible adaptations that bees have evolved over time to be highly efficient pollinators, contributing significantly to plant reproduction and ecosystem health. As environmental sentinels, bees' behaviours and responses to changes in their habitats can provide valuable insights into the overall health of ecosystems and the potential impact of environmental stressors. Monitoring and studying bees as environmental indicators can aid in understanding ecological changes and inform conservation efforts to safeguard pollinator populations and the critical ecosystem services they provide.

## *4.2 Electrostatics and Non-pollen Particle Accumulation*

While in flight, honey bees engage in a fascinating process of pollen collection and transportation back to their colony. They meticulously clean the pollen from their head and mouthparts and transfer it to their hind legs. Using their corbicula, commonly known as the pollen basket, bees push the pollen into this specialized structure for easy transport back to their hive [28]. However, during their foraging activities, pollinators may unintentionally collect various types of particles, including non-pollen particles or pollen contaminated with particulates. Although pollen grains are significantly larger than the nanotechnology-based pesticides (NBPs) discussed in this context, electrostatic effects likely play a role in the accumulation of non-pollen particles or particulate-contaminated pollen on bees' bodies. Honey bees gather these pollen grains, along with any pollutants present, and combine them with nectar to ferment into "bee bread," a protein-rich food source for their emerging larvae [28]. Upon close examination of bees collected from the field using SEM, researchers observed numerous unidentified non-pollen particles adhering to diverse setae distributed across various body segments of honey bees.

Owing to their wide-ranging foraging activities that span large areas and their unique physical characteristics, honey bees have the remarkable ability to prefer small concentrations of chemicals present in the flowers. These contaminants, which might be present in widely dispersed forms typically undetectable by laboratory analysis, become strenuous in hive materials and even the bees themselves, making their amount feasible. Researchers have utilized honey bees to detect a range of organic materials, including PCB and heavy metals. They have also studied the degeneracy of Cesium-137 years after the Chernobyl accident [64, 126]. As a result, numerous recent publications have reported the presence of multiple pesticides in various honey bee hive components worldwide, including beeswax, pollen, honey, and bees themselves. Additionally, colony matrices may contain chemicals like antibiotics and miticides used by beekeepers to maintain the health of the bees [29]. Hence, honey bees are considered vital bioindicators of environmental pollution, playing a crucial role in monitoring the presence and effects of various contaminants in the ecosystem [107].

## 4.3 Impact of Nanopesticides on Honeybees

Nanopesticides show a crucial role in the decline of pollinators. Researchers continue to study the impact of various insecticides and application strategies on bee health, with a particular focus on a group of pesticides called "neonicotinoids." These systemic compounds enter and spread to all tissues of plants, effectively protecting it from pests. They are operative after a single application and target insects, making them less harmful to other animals. In theory, these nanopesticides should not harm bees because they feed on pollen and honey, not plant tissues. However, trace amounts of nanopesticides have been found in pollen grains, which bees transport back to their colonies. While a single pollen grain with trace chemicals may not be harmful, scientists have discovered that these pollutants accumulate to dangerous levels within beeswax.

For example, some pesticide formulations, such as Optimate CS and Warrior II with Zeon Technology, exhibited a capsule suspension structure, while Natria and Rovral 4F were flowable formulations containing specific active ingredients. Tourismo, Protocol, and Bravo Weather Stik were fungicides with different chemical compositions and formulations. The investigation provided valuable insights into the potential environmental fate and exposure risks associated with NBP particles, highlighting the need for further research and regulatory considerations concerning these novel pesticide carriers. Intrepid 2F is an insect growth regulator manufactured by Dow AgroSciences (Indianapolis, IN, USA) with a formulation code "2F," which indicates that it contains 2 pounds of active ingredient per gallon in a flowable formulation. This pesticide includes 22.6% methoxyfenozide, the active ingredient responsible for its insecticidal properties. Bayer Advanced All-In-One Lawn Weed & Crabgrass Killer is a ready-to-use (RTU) herbicide designed for lawn weed and crabgrass control. It contains three active ingredients: 2,4-D, quinclorac, and dicamba. Upon observation, small particles were noted, some of which appeared separate while others were mixed with larger particles. Tempo SC Ultra is an insecticide produced by Bayer (Leverkusen, Germany) that contains 11.8% beta-cyfluthrin. SC stands for soluble concentrate. The pesticide formulation comprises sets of particles that exhibit distinct differences from one another. Safari 2SG is an insecticide sold by Valent (Walnut Creek, CA, USA) containing 20% Dinotefuran. 2SG stands for soluble granules, referring to the type of pesticide formulation used. The composition and type of pesticide formulations are classified as private business information. As a result, the particles' precise composition is unknown save for the presence of the pesticide active component. Nonetheless, the picture gives useful information on the many types of nanotechnology-based pesticide (NBP) formulations now available on the market.

### 4.4 Electrostatic Adhesion of Nanoparticles in Honey Bees

In the 1970s, (microencapsulated methyl parathion product) Penncap-M (microencapsulated methyl parathion product) was introduced for insect pest management. Methyl parathion is extremely poisonous to bees, and the capsules, which were roughly the size of pollen grains, stuck electrostatically to bees and remained longer in the field and in pollen stored in the hive than expected from the active ingredient alone [15]. Beekeepers experienced significant colony losses due to their colonies' exposure to this organophosphate insecticide, leading to the cancellation of its use in the US in 2011. This incident emphasized the importance of avoiding bee exposure to encapsulate and dust pesticide formulations [57]. However, contemporary encapsulated NBP pesticide formulations have much smaller particle sizes. More recently, beekeepers have reported new honey bee colony losses due to fugitive dust from planting insecticide-coated seeds. The seeds were pre-coated with neonicotinoids. As the seedlings grew, they absorbed the systemic insecticide, protecting themselves from insect pests. Initially, this method seemed like an efficient way to apply pesticides with minimal contact with bees. However, the coated seeds tended to cling together in the vacuum seed planter, necessitating lubrication with talcum or graphite powder. During the planting operation, the seed coating was abraded and bound to the lubricant powder, which was released as dust from the planter exhaust. This fugitive dust was transmitted over the terrain to trees, woody plants, and adjacent fields where bees graze. It was linked to increased mortality in honey bee colonies, even in colonies located many miles away from the planting site [70]. Low quantities of neonicotinoids may also persist in surface soils, migrating after wind erosion [79]. Similar circumstances have been reported in Europe, the United States, and Canada, emphasizing the need for more research into the environmental fate of purposely produced NBP particles. Unintentional dust incidences, such as those involving neonicotinoid-coated seeds, have inspired efforts to find alternate lubricants and best practices to mitigate the problem [90], it is unknown if purposely produced NBP particles subsidize atmospheric particulate matter (PM) (see Fig. 2).

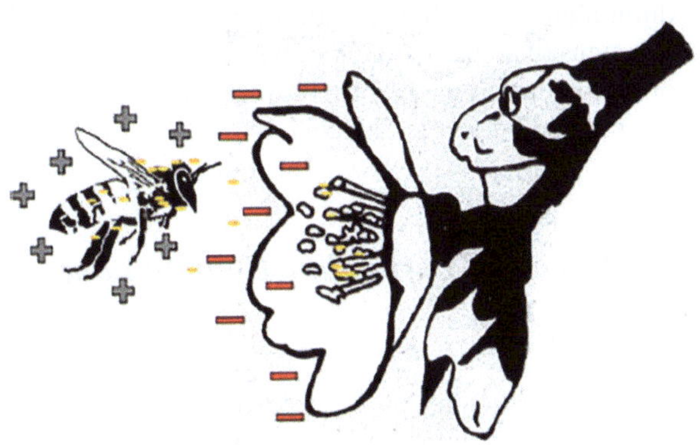

**Fig. 2** Electrostatic phenomena play a role in transferring pollen. Bees possess specialized structures like setae that aid in pollen accumulation. Additionally, bees collect pollen actively using their forelegs and mandibles [57]

### 4.5 Routes of Exposure to Nanopesticides

Nanopesticides are applied to crops using different methods, such as direct spray, soil treatments, and seed applications, to protect them from various threats like weeds, pathogens, and insects. These application methods expose bees and other pollinators that visit crops to nanopesticides in various ways. Bees can be directly exposed to insecticides and die on contact, which does not harm the queen, brood, or nurse bees, allowing the colony to survive. They can also be exposed to nanopesticides by bringing them back to the colony through pollen or nectar they collect from treated plants. Additionally, bees can encounter active residues of nanopesticides on foliage and flowers, or they can pick up nanopesticide particles from dust formulations via wind drift.

### 4.6 Modes of Intake of Nanopesticide

Toxicants can enter bees through various modes of intake. Foraging worker bees help with the oral intake of nanoinsecticides when they collect nectar and pollen from treated fields. Some nanopesticides are absorbed through the respiratory organs, and others are absorbed through direct contact with the bee's body surface. Bees can also ingest nanopesticides by consuming or touching contaminated water or honeydew [72].

### 4.7 Symptoms of Bee Poisoning

Bee poisoning due to nanopesticides can result in various visible symptoms. Bees may die or show signs of poisoning near the hive entrance if they come into direct contact with nanoinsecticides. Nanopesticide-exposed bees regurgitate honey and exhibit abnormal behaviour, becoming more aggressive or agitated. They may also show signs of stupefaction, paralysis, or jerky, whirling motions. Colonies can suffer from a disruption in the brood cycle, and the hive may contain a moist and sticky mass of dead bees (see Table 2).

### 4.8 Effects of Particulate Contaminants on Bees Olfactory System

Apart from pesticides, other types of PM, such as soot particles from diesel exhaust, may also pose hazards for bees. Recent research reveals that air pollution and diesel exhaust impair with bees capacity to accept olfactory cues from flowers and it disrupts

**Table 2** Classification of toxicants to honey bees

| Toxicity symbol | Classification | Acute $LD_{50}$ to adult bees (μg/bee) |
|---|---|---|
| 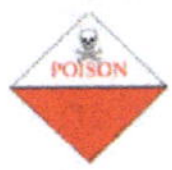  | Highly toxic | <2 |
| 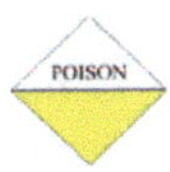  | Moderately toxic | 2–10.99 |
|   | Slightly toxic | $LD_{50}$ 11–100 |
| 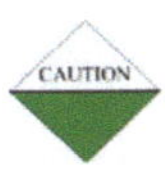  | Nontoxic | $LD_{50} > 100$ |

AV et al. [12]

floral scents, leading to increased foraging times [46]. Volcanic ash, a usual source of nanoparticles, may similarly affect plant–pollinator interactions [84]. Bees can unintentionally gather a variety of biological particles, including airborne bacteria, viruses, and fungal spores, and they can transfer plant infections. Additionally, bees have been studied as potential carriers of biocontrol agents [78]. This underscores the fact that bees, along with other pollinators who collect and ingest pollen are inadvertently exposed to particles in the air and terrestrial environment, potentially increasing their exposure to harmful compounds [88]. Therefore, the potential risks posed by particulate contaminants on pollinators should be considered a significant research priority, taking into account their impacts on ecological systems and pollination networks.

## 5 Uncertainties Surrounding NBP Impact on Honey Bees

The size of Novel Binding Particles (NBPs) may have implications for toxicity in various organisms, including aquatic systems. Initial laboratory investigations have hinted at possible harmful effects of nanosilver on honey. However, in order to fully understand how NBPs may harm bees, it is necessary to address the practical administration of pesticide particles in the field and how this interacts with pollinators' particle-collecting abilities. Pesticides are often administered via electrostatic spray nozzles, which produce a cloud of charged droplets. The high charge-to-mass ratio of these droplets leads to their deposition on the intended target. Many variables, such as the spray device and interaction with the surrounding air, can impact the final deposition on the target surface [86]. Coatings that increase the electrostatic properties of particles have been shown to enhance pesticide availability to mosquitoes, and similar electrostatic techniques are used for other problem species [10, 74]. Charged droplets and particles are more likely to be attracted to honey bee pollen.

Label precautions normally ban the use of bee-hazardous insecticides during pollination. However, sprays can drift considerable distances from the application site [36], potentially exposing non-target plants and organisms, including bees, to pesticides [80]. Newer electrostatic spray technologies minimize drift but do not completely eliminate it. There is a dearth of quantified exposure data for non-target sites and organisms [34], efforts are being made to improve drift modelling, with a focus on droplet size [112]. The particles contained in formulations are not expected to significantly effect droplet formation or drift potential [55]. However, the drift of particles after the water has evaporated from droplets in the air, as well as the aeolian effects on particulate residues settled on foliage or in soil, are largely unknown and could be better modelled using approaches used to describe atmospheric dispersion of particulate matter. Interestingly, investigations of pesticides in the atmosphere have linked current-use insecticides to mineral-based particles [31, 39]. Given that NBPs are made up of clay and other minerals, and pesticides can bind to soil particles, there may be a link. Some pesticides have even been discovered in areas remote from their point of application, which contradicts the known qualities of the active ingredient [85]. If NBP drift contributes to the atmospheric pool of particulate matter, and bees collect such particles as they travel through the air, it may help explain the complex pesticide combinations reported in hive materials.

Mechanical pollination devices use the electrostatic forces involved in pollen transport from flower anthers to bees and from bees to stigma [13]. It is not surprising that pollen attracts particulate matter particles [88], and there have been observations of particles clinging to almond pollen collected from the field that resembled NBPs. Plant leaves and petals have complex morphology, surface topology, and chemistry, all of which may influence particle deposition and behaviour, as well as particle transport to pollinators. The tips and edges of leaves and flowers are supposed to have the largest negative charge, however, the electric fields surrounding plants can change polarity under variable weather circumstances [88].

## 6 NBPs and Bee-Pollinator Interactions

NBPs have the ability to reach target locations at larger dosages than traditional formulations [69]. Bees interact with plants at the projecting reproductive organs of flowers, which may alter the amount and type of NBPs they are exposed. Additionally, bees can passively accumulate particles and actively gather pollen [88]. These two activities, passive particle buildup and active pollen collecting, may enhance their exposure to environmental pollutants, such as NBPs. However, the current EPA's Bee Rex model, which calculates contact and ingestion exposures to individual bees based on application rate, fails to account for potential variability in the behaviour of NBP particles, which could affect their exposure [115].

After pesticide droplets evaporate, there is little public information available about how tightly or efficiently NBP particles or residues stick to foliage and flowers. This uncertainty begs the question of whether NBP particles may easily migrate from foliage to pollinators, and how this varies over time and under different situations. The use of controlled release NBP formulations extends the time of efficacy for pest management but also results in longer residual toxicity for non-target organisms. This is especially significant in agricultural settings, where the timing of regulated pollinator arrival and departure must be synchronized with pesticide applications [88].

While direct contact with certain insecticides can kill bees in the field, controlled release NBP formulations protect bees from immediate exposure while allowing them to transfer particles, posing a delayed risk to the colony. Complex pesticide mixes are frequently discovered in numerous bee-related products such as nectar, honey, pollen, bee bread, and beeswax [14]. The transmission of pesticide residues with pollen is a rising concern because pollen is the primary protein source for larval development [16]. Honey bee larvae, especially during their final instars, are directly fed modest amounts of pollen, while nursing bees ingest considerable amounts of pollen to make brood food for developing larvae [125]. Because bees forage over great distances, even hives near organically maintained farms or isolated places are frequently contaminated with pesticides. Historical comparisons of pesticide active components, sample preparation, and analysis methodologies might be tricky [20]. Consequently, laboratory and field investigations are required to examine whether NBP formulations promote the deposition of certain pesticides in hive matrices.

## 6.1 *Trophic Transfer of NBP Particles: Implications for Pollinators*

When analysing pesticide dangers for bees, residues in hive components are a substantial source of uncertainty [88]. Environmental fate models for pesticide active ingredients rely on hydrolysis, photolysis in soil, water solubility, vapour pressure, n-octanol–water partition coefficient (KOW), Henry's Law Constant, and dissociation constant in water (pKa or pKb) are all used to estimate dissipation processes [91]. Many pesticide active components are hydrophobic, which is taken into account when modelling their accumulation and persistence inside hive matrices [108]. This leads to the accumulation of numerous pesticides in beeswax, which can potentially affect bees adversely [127], even though risk assessors generally consider the risk of pesticide exposure from wax to bees to be low [45].

NBPs, on the other hand, are often to be water-soluble, which may complicate the toxicokinetics modelling of hydrophobic compounds [109]. If hydrophobic active ingredients when transferred within the colony, they may collect in high-risk compartments such as nectar, honey, pollen, bee bread, or even within the bees themselves. This accumulation may alter pesticide exposure to developing larvae and could disrupt the critical bacteria responsible for digesting pollen into nourishing bee bread [22, 119]. Furthermore, the preservation of active chemicals within NBP particles may impair their digestion by bees and the colony's microbiome, confounding pesticide destiny predictions in hive materials. This situation may result in delayed and persistent pesticide exposures to developing bees, which can have far-reaching effects on the colony's health [108].

Furthermore, our current understanding of pesticide drift is mostly concerned with the impacts of wind and weather on droplets during application and the evaporation of volatile pesticides. The forces that may influence the destiny, mobility, physical, and trophic transmission of NBP particles in terrestrial habitats remain largely unknown [109]. This knowledge gap is especially important in understanding how bees and other pollinators are exposed to different environmental pollutants. To completely assess the impact of NBPs on bees and other pollinators, a better understanding of the behaviour and destiny of NBP particles in various habitats is required.

## 7 Nanopesticide Application: Safeguarding Honey Bees

To safeguard pollinators, including honeybees, from potential exposure to nanopesticides, several important factors should be carefully considered during the application process:

1. Time of Application: It is crucial to apply nanopesticides only when necessary and preferably in the evening when bees are less active. Avoid spraying when bees are actively foraging during the day to minimize direct contact.
2. Nanopesticides on Blossoms: To protect bees, refrain from using insecticides on blooming crops and remove attractive blooms from weeds before treatment. This prevents bees from coming into contact with nanopesticides while foraging for nectar and pollen.
3. Toxicity of Nanopesticides: When choosing nanopesticides, opt for products with the least harm to bees and those with shorter residual activity. This reduces the chances of prolonged exposure to pollinators.
4. Consideration in Application: Employ integrated pest management (IPM) strategies, which involve a combination of techniques to minimize pesticide use while maintaining crop health. By using alternative pest control methods, the reliance on nanopesticides can be reduced.
5. Distance from Treated Areas: It has been observed that honeybee mortality due to nanopesticides decreases as bee colonies move further away from treated regions. Thus, it is essential to consider the proximity of beehives to treated fields.

6. Residual Action: Be mindful of the residual activity of nanopesticides and avoid using formulations with extended residual toxicity to bees. Opt for products that break down more quickly and have a lower impact on pollinators.
7. Recovery from Nanopesticide Exposure: In cases where colonies are exposed to nanopesticides, there is a possibility of recovery if proper precautions are taken. This may involve removing contaminated combs and providing the affected colonies with adequate nourishment.
8. Nanopesticide Formulation: Choose nanopesticide formulations that are less hazardous to bees. Some formulations, such as solutions, emulsifiable concentrates, and granular formulations, may present lower risks to pollinators.

By adhering to these protective measures and following label guidelines, it is possible to minimize the harmful effects of nanopesticides on honeybees and other vital pollinators. By preserving the health of pollinators, we ensure their crucial role in maintaining global food security and preserving biodiversity.

## 8 Potential of NBPs in Pollinator Conservation

The impact of pesticide use on colony losses among bees is often enigmatic, as evidenced by the substantial decline of honey bee colonies during California almond pollination in 2014, with only recent tentative attributions to a cause [53]. The connection between certain pesticides in colonies and Colony Collapse Disorder has been suggested but not conclusively proven [117]. Moreover, concerns persist about the role of neonicotinoids in the decline of pollinators [35]. Wild pollinators, including bumble bee species, monarchs, and butterflies, are facing challenges, and insecticides may aggravate the effects of other stressors on them [103]. These uncertainties emphasize the importance of comprehending pesticide exposure to bees and other pollinators, particularly concerning Novel Binding Particle (NBP) formulations.

NBPs have the ability to change the route, quantity, and residual toxicity of non-target organisms, therefore these factors must be considered while addressing these issues. On the one hand, NBPs may reduce pollinator risks by lowering drift, solvent usage, and the total amount of pesticides required for effective application. They could lengthen the half-life of less stable molecules, allowing the delivery of less harmful and more focused techniques such as RNAi [63]. Additionally, NBPs could be designed with pollinator conservation in mind, releasing active ingredients only upon interaction with specific pests and pathogens [87]. These attributes of NBPs could be particularly beneficial in combatting the Varroa destructor, an ectoparasitic mite that poses a severe threat to honey bees [102].

# 9 Conclusion

The absence of specific information about NBP formulations raises questions about their exposure and potential benefits to pollinators. Therefore, it is critical for the agricultural and scientific communities to thoroughly evaluate not only the possible benefits but also the hazards connected with new pesticide formulation methods, as NBPs have already entered the market [52]. Current pesticide usage, including NBPs, in agricultural environments worldwide amounts to a staggering 5.6 billion pounds [4]. These agrochemical pollutants are identified as significant contributors to the global decline in insect populations, including bee pollinators [103]. The threats and extinctions faced by insects and pollinators, as well as disruptions in ecological interaction networks, are becoming increasingly alarming [43]. Researchers and regulators must obtain a better knowledge of the intricate mechanisms involved in pesticide exposure to individual bees, as well as how these compounds accumulate within beehives. This understanding also includes the environmental behaviour of NBP particles in agricultural and residential contexts, where urban pollinators may be equally affected [54]. Pollinators' unique structural adaptations to accumulate minute particles, such as electrostatic pollen collection, make them susceptible to higher exposure risks. As a result, honey bees are an excellent model organism for studying how various chemical compounds migrate through the troposphere by attaching to both manmade and naturally occurring particles.

# References


1. Abbaci A, Azzouz N, Bouznit Y (2014) A new copper doped montmorillonite modified carbon paste electrode for propineb detection. Appl Clay Sci 90:130–134. https://doi.org/10.1016/j.clay.2013.12.036
2. Abdollahdokht D, Gao Y, Faramarz S, Poustforoosh A, Abbasi M, Asadikaram G (2022) Conventional agrochemicals towards nano-biopesticides: an overview on recent advances. Chem Biol Technol Agric 9:1–19. https://doi.org/10.1186/s40538-021-00281-0
3. Agathokleous E, Calabrese EJ (2019) Hormesis: the dose response for the 21st century: the future has arrived. Toxicology 425:152249. https://doi.org/10.1016/j.tox.2019.152249
4. Alavanja MC (2009) Introduction: pesticides use and exposure extensive worldwide. Rev Environ Health 24(4):303–309. https://doi.org/10.1515/reveh.2009.24.4.303
5. Ale A, Gutierrez MF, Rossi AS, Bacchetta C, Desimone MF, Cazenave J (2021) Ecotoxicity of silica nanoparticles in aquatic organisms: an updated review. Environ Toxicol Pharmacol 87:103689
6. Ale A, Andrade VS, Gutierrez MF, Bacchetta, C, Rossi AS, Santo Orihuela P, Desimone MF, Cazenave J (2023) Nanotechnology-based pesticides: environmental fate and ecotoxicity. Toxicol Appl Pharmacol 116560
7. Ale A (2023) Nanomaterials and safety concerns to end users. Mater Res Found, 135
8. Amjad S, Sharma AK, Serajuddin M (2018) Toxicity assessment of cypermethrin nanoparticles in Channa punctatus: behavioural response, micronuclei induction and enzyme alteration. Regul Toxicol Pharmacol 100:127–133. https://doi.org/10.1016/j.yrtph.2018.10.004
9. Andrade VS, Ale A, Antezana PE, Desimone MF, Cazenave J, Gutierrez MF (2023) Ecotoxicity of nanosilver on cladocerans and the role of algae provision. Environ Sci Pollut Res 30(10):27137–27149

10. Andriessen R, Snetselaar J, Suer RA, Osinga AJ, Deschietere J, Lyimo IN, Mnyone LL, Brooke BD, Ranson H, Knols BGJ, Farenhorst M (2015) Electrostatic coating enhances bioavailability of insecticides and breaks pyrethroid resistance in mosquitoes. Proc Natl Acad Sci USA 112(39):12081–12086. https://doi.org/10.1073/pnas.1510801112
11. Arora S, Murmu G, Mukherjee K, Saha S, Maity D (2022) A comprehensive overview of nanotechnology in sustainable agriculture. J Biotechnol 355:21–41. https://doi.org/10.1016/j.jbiotec.2022.06.007
12. Av M, Pandey R, Mall P (2023) Protecting honeybees from pesticides: a call to action. Biodiversity 24(3):117–123
13. Banerjee S, Law SE (6–10 Oct 1996) Electrostatic induction charging of pollen suspensions. In: Proceedings of the 1996 IEEE industry applications conference thirty-first IAS annual meeting, San Diego, CA, United States, pp 1775–1781
14. Berenbaum MR (2016) Does the honey bee "Risk Cup" runneth over? Estimating aggregate exposures for assessing pesticide risks to honey bees in agroecosystems. J Agric Food Chem 64(1):13–20. https://doi.org/10.1021/acs.jafc.5b01067
15. Burgett M, Fisher GC (1980) Recovery of Penncap-M from foraging honey bees and pollen Storage-Cells. Environ Entomol 9(4):430–431. https://doi.org/10.1093/ee/9.4.430
16. Burlew DA (2010) The Effects of pesticide-contaminated pollen on larval development of the honey bee, Apis mellifera [PhD Thesis]. Evergreen State College
17. CIPAC. Formulation codes. https://www.cipac.org/index.php/methods-publications/further-information/formulation-codes. Accessed 20 Oct 2019
18. Cáceres M, Vassena CV, Garcerá MD, Santo-Orihuela PL (2019) Silica nanoparticles for insect pest control. Curr Pharm Des 25(37):4030–4038. https://doi.org/10.2174/1381612825666191015152855
19. Calabrese EJ, Blain RB (2011) The hormesis database: the occurrence of hormetic dose responses in the toxicological literature. Regul Toxicol Pharmacol 61(1):73–81. https://doi.org/10.1016/j.yrtph.2011.06.003
20. Calatayud-Vernich P, Calatayud F, Simó E, Picó YE (2016) Efficiency of QuEChERS approach for determining 52 pesticide residues in honey and honey bees. MethodsX 3:452–458. https://doi.org/10.1016/j.mex.2016.05.005
21. Cao L, Zhou Z, Niu S, Cao C, Li X, Shan Y, Huang Q (2018) Positive-charge functionalized mesoporous silica nanoparticles as nanocarriers for controlled 2, 4-dichlorophenoxy acetic acid sodium salt release. J Agric Food Chem 66(26):6594–6603. https://doi.org/10.1021/acs.jafc.7b01957
22. Chen WY (2016) Toxicokinetic modeling challenges for aquatic nanotoxicology. Front Mar Sci 2:114. https://doi.org/10.3389/fmars.2015.00114
23. Chin CP, Wu HS, Wang SS (2011) New approach to pesticide delivery using nanosuspensions: research and applications. Ind Eng Chem Res 50(12):7637–7643. https://doi.org/10.1021/ie2001007
24. Choy JH, Choi SJ, Oh JM, Park T (2007) Clay minerals and layered double hydroxides for novel biological applications. Appl Clay Sci 36(1–3):122–132. https://doi.org/10.1016/j.clay.2006.07.007
25. Clarke D, Whitney H, Sutton G, Robert D (2013) Detection and learning of floral electric fields by bumblebees. Science 340(6128):66–69. https://doi.org/10.1126/science.1230883
26. Clarke D, Morley E, Robert D (2017) The bee, the flower, and the electric field: electric ecology and aerial electroreception. J Comp Physiol A, Neuroethol Sens Neural Behav Physiol 203(9):737–748. https://doi.org/10.1007/s00359-017-1176-6
27. Clemente Z, Grillo R, Jonsson M, Santos NZ, Feitosa LO, Lima R, Fraceto LF (2014) Ecotoxicological evaluation of poly (ε-caprolactone) nanocapsules containing triazine herbicides. J Nanosci Nanotechnol 14(7):4911–4917. https://doi.org/10.1166/jnn.2014.8681
28. Connor LJ, Muir RG (2013) Pollen and bee bread. Am Bee J 153:727–729
29. Conti ME, Botrè F (2001) Honeybees and their products as potential bioindicators of heavy metals contamination. Environ Monit Assess 69(3):267–282. https://doi.org/10.1023/a:1010719107006

30. Corsi I, Desimone MF, Cazenave J (2022) Building the bridge from aquatic nanotoxicology to safety by design silver nanoparticles. Front Bioeng Biotechnol 10:836742. https://doi.org/10.3389/fbioe.2022.836742
31. Coscollà C, Muñoz A, Borrás E, Vera T, Ródenas M, Yusà V (2014) Particle size distributions of currently used pesticides in ambient air of an agricultural Mediterranean area. Atmos Environ 95:29–35. https://doi.org/10.1016/j.atmosenv.2014.06.022
32. Cox C, Surgan M (2006) Unidentified inert ingredients in pesticides: implications for human and environmental health. Environ Health Perspect 114(12):1803–1806. https://doi.org/10.1289/ehp.9374
33. Cutler GC, Rix RR (2015) Can poisons stimulate bees? Appreciating the potential of hormesis in bee–pesticide research. Pest Manag Sci 71(10):1368–1370. https://doi.org/10.1002/ps.4042
34. Damalas CA (2015) Pesticide drift: seeking reliable environmental indicators of exposure assessment. In: Armon HR, Hänninen O (eds) Environmental indicators, pp 251–26
35. David A, Botías C, Abdul-Sada A, Nicholls E, Rotheray EL, Hill EM, Goulson D (2016) Widespread contamination of wildflower and bee-collected pollen with complex mixtures of neonicotinoids and fungicides commonly applied to crops. Environ Int 88:169–178. https://doi.org/10.1016/j.envint.2015.12.011
36. Davis BNK, Williams CT (1990) Buffer zone widths for honeybees from ground and aerial spraying of insecticides. Environ Pollut 63(3):247–259. https://doi.org/10.1016/0269-7491(90)90158-9
37. de Albuquerque FP, de Oliveira JL, dos Santos ML, Richardi VS, da Silva MAN, Pompêo MLM, Fraceto LF, Carlos VM (2021) Use of nontarget organism Chironomus sancticaroli to study the toxic effects of nanoatrazine. Ecotoxicology 30(4):733–750. https://doi.org/10.1007/s10646-021-02400-x
38. De Sousa A, Saleh AM, Habeeb TH, Hassan YM, Zrieq R, Wadaan MAM, Hozzein WN, Selim S, Matos M, Abd Elgawad H (2019) Silicon dioxide nanoparticles ameliorate the phytotoxic hazards of aluminum in maize grown on acidic soil. Sci Total Environ 693:133636. https://doi.org/10.1016/j.scitotenv.2019.133636
39. Degrendele C, Okonski K, Melymuk L, Landlová L, Kukučka P, Audy O, Kohoutek J, Čupr P, Klánová J (2016) Pesticides in the atmosphere: a comparison of gas-particle partitioning and particle size distribution of legacy and current-use pesticides. Atmos Chem Phys 16(3):1531–1544. https://doi.org/10.5194/acp-16-1531-2016
40. Ding Y, Xiao Z, Chen F, Yue L, Wang C, Fan N, Ji H, Wang Z (2023) A mesoporous silica nanocarrier pesticide delivery system for loading acetamiprid: effectively manage aphids and reduce plant pesticide residue. Sci Total Environ 863:160900
41. Doucet FJ, Lead JR, Santschi PH (2007) Colloid-trace element interactions in aquatic systems. IUPAC Ser Anal Phys Chem Environ Syst 10:95
42. Duhan JS, Kumar R, Kumar N, Kaur P, Nehra K, Duhan S (2017) Nanotechnology: the new perspective in precision agriculture. Biotechnol Rep 15:11–23. https://doi.org/10.1016/j.btre.2017.03.002
43. Dunn RR (2005) Modern insect extinctions, the neglected majority. [Extinciones Modernas de Insectos, la Mayoría Desatendida]. Conserv Biol 19(4):1030–1036. https://doi.org/10.1111/j.1523-1739.2005.00078.x
44. Filella M (2007) Colloidal properties of submicron particles in natural waters. IUPAC Ser Anal Phys Chem Environ Syst 10:17
45. Fischer D, Moriarty T (2011) Pesticide risk assessment for pollinators: summary of a SETAC Pellston workshop. https://c.ymcdn.com/sites/www.setac.org/resource/resmgr/publications_and_resources/executivesummarypollinators_.pdf?hhSearchTerms=S. Accessed 3 Dec 2019. Society of Environmental Toxicology and Chemistry (SETAC), p 29
46. Fuentes JD, Chamecki M, Roulston TA, Chen B, Pratt KR (2016) Air pollutants degrade floral scents and increase insect foraging times. Atmos Environ 141:361–374. https://doi.org/10.1016/j.atmosenv.2016.07.002
47. Gallai N, Salles JM, Settele J, Vaissière BE (2009) Economic valuation of the vulnerability of world agriculture confronted with pollinator decline. Ecol Econ 68(3):810–821. https://doi.org/10.1016/j.ecolecon.2008.06.014

48. Gangwar P, Johri P, Datta R, Singh S, Trivedi M (2023) Overview on 1 phytopharmaceuticals and biotechnology of herbal plants. In: Phytopharmaceuticals and biotechnology of herbal plants. CRC Press, pp 1–17
49. Green JM, Beestman GB (2007) Recently patented and commercialized formulation and adjuvant technology. Crop Prot 26:320–327
50. Greggers U, Koch G, Schmidt V, Dürr A, Floriou-Servou A, Piepenbrock D, Göpfert MC, Menzel R (2013) Reception and learning of electric fields in bees. Proc Biol Sci 280(1759):20130528. https://doi.org/10.1098/rspb.2013.0528
51. Hancock BC, Parks M (2000) What is the true solubility advantage for amorphous pharmaceuticals? Pharm Res 17(4):397–404. https://doi.org/10.1023/a:1007516718048
52. Harper S, Usenko C, Hutchison JE, Maddux BLS, Tanguay RL (2008) In vivo biodistribution and toxicity depends on nanomaterial composition, size, surface functionalisation and route of exposure. J Exp Nanosci 3(3):195–206. https://doi.org/10.1080/17458080802378953
53. Henein M, California H (2019) Almonds are killing bees. http://www.honeycolony.com/article/california-almonds-killing-bees/. Accessed 10 Jul 2019
54. Hennig EI, Ghazoul J (2012) Pollinating animals in the urban environment. Urban Ecosyst 15(1):149–166. https://doi.org/10.1007/s11252-011-0202-7
55. Hilz E, Vermeer AWP (2013) Spray drift review: the extent to which a formulation can contribute to spray drift reduction. Crop Prot 44:75–83. https://doi.org/10.1016/j.cropro.2012.10.020
56. Holden PA, Gardea-Torresdey JL, Klaessig F, Turco RF, Mortimer M, Hund-Rinke K, Cohen Hubal EA, Avery D, Barceló D, Behra R, Cohen Y, Deydier-Stephan L, Ferguson PL, Fernandes TF, Herr Harthorn B, Henderson WM, Hoke RA, Hristozov D, Johnston JM, Nel AE (2016) Considerations of environmentally relevant test conditions for improved evaluation of ecological hazards of engineered nanomaterials. Environ Sci Technol 50(12):6124–6145. https://doi.org/10.1021/acs.est.6b00608
57. Hooven L, Sagili R, Johansen E (2013) How to reduce bee poisoning from pesticides. Oregon State University Extension Service, Corvallis, OR
58. Jabborova D, Davranov K, Jabbarov Z, Bhowmik SN, Ercisli S, Danish S, Datta R (2022) Dual inoculation of plant growth-promoting Bacillus endophyticus and Funneliformis mosseae improves plant growth and soil properties in ginger. ACS Omega 7(39):34779–34788
59. Jain T, Srivastava K, Singh R, Ansari MJ, Singh S, Dutta PK (2022) Role of nanotechnology 18 in the field of phytopharmaceuticals for the delivery of herbal drugs
60. Janousek WM, Douglas MR, Cannings S, Clément MA, Delphia CM, Everett JG, Hatfield RG, Keinath DA, Koch JBU, McCabe LM, Mola JM, Ogilvie JE, Rangwala I, Richardson LL, Rohde AT, Strange JP, Tronstad LM, Graves TA (2023) Recent and future declines of a historically widespread pollinator linked to climate, land cover, and pesticides. Proc Natl Acad Sci USA 120(5):e2211223120. https://doi.org/10.1073/pnas.2211223120
61. Kah M, Beulke S, Tiede K, Hofmann T (2013) Nanopesticides: state of knowledge, environmental fate, and exposure modeling. Crit Rev Environ Sci Technol 43(16):1823–1867. https://doi.org/10.1080/10643389.2012.671750
62. Kah M, Kookana RS, Gogos A, Bucheli TD (2018) A critical evaluation of nanopesticides and nanofertilizers against their conventional analogues. Nat Nanotechnol 13(8):677–684. https://doi.org/10.1038/s41565-018-0131-1
63. Katoch R, Sethi A, Thakur N, Murdock LL (2013) RNAi for insect control: current perspective and future challenges. Appl Biochem Biotechnol 171(4):847–873. https://doi.org/10.1007/s12010-013-0399-4
64. Kevan PG (1999) Pollinators as bioindicators of the state of the environment: species, activity and diversity. Agr Ecosyst Environ 74:373–393
65. Khare P, Kishore K, Sharma DK (2017) A study on the standardization parameters of Cassia angustifolia. Asian J Pharm Clin Res 10(7):329–332
66. Khare P, Kishore K, Sharma DK, Khare N (2024) Investigation of memory enhancing activity of combination extracts of bauhinia variegata and madhuca longifolia leaves against colchicine: an experimental study and biochemical alterations in mice. Ind J Pharm Edu Res 58(1s):s282–s288

67. Khot LR, Sankaran S, Maja JM, Ehsani R, Schuster EW (2012) Applications of nanomaterials in agricultural production and crop protection: a review. Crop Prot 35:64–70. https://doi.org/10.1016/j.cropro.2012.01.007
68. Kluser S, Peter N, Chauzat MP, Pascal P, Ron W, Mwangi T (2010) Global honey bee colony disorders and other threats to insect pollinators 16:1–16
69. Koch K, Bhushan B, Barthlott W (2009) Multifunctional surface structures of plants: an inspiration for biomimetics. Prog Mater Sci 54(2):137–178. https://doi.org/10.1016/j.pmatsci.2008.07.003
70. Krupke CH, Holland JD, Long EY, Eitzer BD (2017) Planting of neonicotinoid-treated maize poses risks for honey bees and other non-target organisms over a wide area without consistent crop yield benefit. J Appl Ecol 54(5):1449–1458. https://doi.org/10.1111/1365-2664.12924
71. Kuhlbusch TAJ, Wijnhoven SWP, Haase A (2018) Nanomaterial exposures for worker, consumer and the general public. NanoImpact 10:11–25. https://doi.org/10.1016/j.impact.2017.11.003
72. Kumar G, Singh S, Nagarajaiah RPK (2020) Detailed review on pesticidal toxicity to honey bees and its management Modern beekeeping-bases for sustainable production
73. Lagaly G (2001) Pesticide–clay interactions and formulations. Appl Clay Sci 18(5–6):205–209. https://doi.org/10.1016/S0169-1317(01)00043-6
74. Latheef MA, Carlton JB, Kirk IW, Hoffmann WC (2009) Aerial electrostatic-charged sprays for deposition and efficacy against sweet potato whitefly (Bemisia tabaci) on cotton. Pest Manag Sci 65(7):744–752. https://doi.org/10.1002/ps.1748
75. Lead JR, Wilkinson KJ (2007) Environmental colloids and particles: current knowledge and future developments. IUPAC Ser Anal Phys Chem Environ Syst 10:1
76. Lebuhn G, Droege S, Connor EF, Gemmill-Herren B, Potts SG, Minckley RL, Ollerton J, Winfree R, Tarrant S (2011) How many flowering plants are pollinated by animals? Oikos 120(3):321–326. https://doi.org/10.1111/j.1600-0706.2010.18644.x
77. Li N, Georas S, Alexis N, Fritz P, Xia T, Williams MA, Horner E, Nel A (2016) A work group report on ultrafine particles (American Academy of Allergy, Asthma & Immunology): why ambient ultrafine and engineered nanoparticles should receive special attention for possible adverse health outcomes in human subjects. J Allergy Clin Immunol. Am Acad Allergy Asthma Immunol 138(2):386–396. https://doi.org/10.1016/j.jaci.2016.02.023
78. Lighthart B, Prier K, Loper GM, Bromenshenk J (2000) Bees scavenge airborne bacteria. Microb Ecol 39(4):314–321
79. Limay-Rios V, Forero LG, Xue Y, Smith J, Baute T, Schaafsma A (2016) Neonicotinoid insecticide residues in soil dust and associated parent soil in fields with a history of seed treatment use on crops in southwestern Ontario. Environ Toxicol Chem 35(2):303–310. https://doi.org/10.1002/etc.3257
80. Long EY, Krupke CH (2016) Non-cultivated plants present a season-long route of pesticide exposure for honey bees. Nat Commun 7:11629. https://doi.org/10.1038/ncomms11629
81. Lowry GV, Avellan A, Gilbertson LM (2019) Opportunities and challenges for nanotechnology in the agri-tech revolution. Nat Nanotechnol 14(6):517–522. https://doi.org/10.1038/s41565-019-0461-7
82. Maddala VKS, Singh S (2023) Essential oils from plants and their role in nanomaterial synthesis characterization and applications. In: Secondary metabolites based green synthesis of nanomaterials and their applications. Springer Nature Singapore, Singapore, pp 191–207
83. Maddala VKS, Singh S, Bandi J (2024) Soil properties influencing nutrient signaling in plant soil systems. In: Essential minerals in plant-soil systems. Elsevier, pp 373–393
84. Martínez AS, Masciocchi M, Villacide JM, Huerta G, Daneri L, Bruchhausen A, Rozas G, Corley JC (2013) Ashes in the air: the effects of volcanic ash emissions on plant-pollinator relationships and possible consequences for apiculture. Apidologie 44(3):268–277. https://doi.org/10.1007/s13592-012-0177-2
85. Mast MA, Foreman WT, Skaates SV (2007) Current-use pesticides and organochlorine compounds in precipitation and lake sediment from two high-elevation national parks in the Western United States. Arch Environ Contam Toxicol 52(3):294–305. https://doi.org/10.1007/s00244-006-0096-1

86. Meredith AN, Harper B, Harper SL (2016) The influence of size on the toxicity of an encapsulated pesticide: a comparison of micron- and nano-sized capsules. Environ Int 86:68–74. https://doi.org/10.1016/j.envint.2015.10.012
87. Meyer WL, Gurman P, Stelinski LL, Elman NM (2015) Functional nano-dispensers (FNDs) for delivery of insecticides against phytopathogen vectors. Green Chem 17(8):4173–4177. https://doi.org/10.1039/C5GC00717H
88. Negri I, Mavris C, Di Prisco G, Caprio E, Pellecchia M, Bees H (2015) Honey bees (Apis mellifera, L.) as active samplers of airborne particulate matter. PLOS One 10(7):e0132491. https://doi.org/10.1371/journal.pone.0132491
89. Nemati S, Mohammad Rahimi H, Hesari Z, Sharifdini M, Jalilzadeh Aghdam N, Mirjalali H, Zali MR (2022) Formulation of Neem oil-loaded solid lipid nanoparticles and evaluation of its anti-Toxoplasma activity. BMC Complement Med Ther 22(1):122
90. Nuyttens D, Devarrewaere W, Verboven P, Foqué D (2013) Pesticide-laden dust emission and drift from treated seeds during seed drilling: a review. Pest Manag Sci 69(5):564–575. https://doi.org/10.1002/ps.3485
91. Orrick G, Rothman G, Bohaty R, White K, Koper C. Miller R, Liu L (2012) Guidance for reviewing environmental fate studies; environmental fate and E_ects division. USEPA
92. Parveen R, Jain T, Parveen R, Singh S (2023) Genome-wide transcriptome profiling of crop plants. In: Genomics, transcriptomics, proteomics and metabolomics of crop plants. Academic Press, pp 145–171
93. Parveen R, Khare N, Singh S, Johri P (2023) An in silico outlook for the detection and surveillance of evolving and persistent plant pathogens. In: Detection, diagnosis and management of soil-borne phytopathogens. Springer Nature Singapore, Singapore, pp 17–40
94. Patani A, Patel A, Prajapati D, Khare N, Singh S (2023) Various agriculture crop plant-based bioactive compounds and their use in nanomaterial synthesis and applications. In: Nanomaterials from agricultural and horticultural products. Springer Nature Singapore, Singapore, pp 223–241
95. Patani A, Prajapati D, Shukla K, Patel M, Patani P, Patel A, Singh S (2024) Environmental stress–induced alterations in the micro-and macronutrients status of plant. In: Essential minerals in plant-soil systems. Elsevier, pp 181–195
96. Peixoto S, Henriques I, Loureiro S (2021) Long-term effects of Cu $(OH)_2$ nanopesticide exposure on soil microbial communities. Environ Pollut 269:116113. https://doi.org/10.1016/j.envpol.2020.116113
97. Pérez-de-Luque A, Hermosín MC (2013) Nanotechnology and its use in agriculture. In: Bagchi D (ed) Bio-nanotechnology. Blackwell Publishing Ltd., pp 383–398
98. Potts SG, Biesmeijer JC, Kremen C, Neumann P, Schweiger O, Kunin WE (2010) Global pollinator declines: trends, impacts and drivers. Trends Ecol Evol 25(6):345–353. https://doi.org/10.1016/j.tree.2010.01.007
99. Qian WY, Sun DM, Zhu RR, Du XL, Liu H, Wang SL (2012) pH-sensitive strontium carbonate nanoparticles as new anticancer vehicles for controlled etoposide
100. Rani N, Duhan A, Pal A, Kumari P, Beniwal RK, Verma D, Goyat A, Singh R (2023) Are nano-pesticides really meant for cleaner production? An overview on recent developments, benefits, environmental hazards and future prospectives. J Clean Prod, 137232. Release Int J Nanomedicine 7: 5781–5792. https://doi.org/10.2147/IJN.S34773
101. Rizwan M, Ali S, Qayyum MF, Ok YS, Adrees M, Ibrahim M, Zia-Ur-Rehman M, Farid M, Abbas F (2017) Effect of metal and metal oxide nanoparticles on growth and physiology of globally important food crops: a critical review. J Hazard Mater 322(A):2–16. https://doi.org/10.1016/j.jhazmat.2016.05.061
102. Rosenkranz P, Aumeier P, Ziegelmann B (2010) Biology and control of Varroa destructor. J Invertebr Pathol 103:96-S119. https://doi.org/10.1016/j.jip.2009.07.016
103. Sánchez-Bayo F, Wyckhuys KAG (2019) Worldwide decline of the entomofauna: a review of its drivers. Biol Cons 232:8–27. https://doi.org/10.1016/j.biocon.2019.01.020
104. Sekhon BS (2014) Nanotechnology in agri-food production: an overview. Nanotechnol Sci Appl 7:31–53. https://doi.org/10.2147/NSA.S39406

105. Shang YF, Hasan MK, Ahammed GJ, Li MQ, Yin HQ, Zhou J (2019) Applications of nanotechnology in plant growth and crop protection: a review. Molecules 24(14):2558. https://doi.org/10.3390/molecules24142558
106. Singh A, Sengar RS, Singh AK, Singh S, Kumar A, Ahmad K (2019) Impact of genetic engineering on agriculture food crops. Biotech Today: Int J Biol Sci 9(1):17–24
107. Smith KE, Weis D, Amini M, Shiel AE, Lai VWM, Gordon K (2019) Honey as a biomonitor for a changing world. Nat Sustain 2(3):223–232. https://doi.org/10.1038/s41893-019-0243-0
108. Smodis Skerl MI, Kmecl V, Gregorc A (2010) Exposure to pesticides at sublethal level and their distribution within a honey bee (Apis mellifera) colony. Bull Environ Contam Toxicol 85(2):125–128. https://doi.org/10.1007/s00128-010-0069-y
109. Stone D, Harper BJ, Lynch I, Dawson K, Harper SL (2010) Exposure assessment: recommendations for nanotechnology-based pesticides. Int J Occup Environ Health 16(4):467–474. https://doi.org/10.1179/107735210799160066
110. Sun Y, Liang J, Tang L, Li H, Zhu Y, Jiang D, Song B, Chen M, Zeng G (2019) Nano-pesticides: a great challenge for biodiversity? Nano Today 28:100757. https://doi.org/10.1016/j.nantod.2019.06.003
111. Sutton GP, Clarke D, Morley EL, Robert D (2016) Mechanosensory hairs in bumblebees (Bombus terrestris) detect weak electric fields. Proc Natl Acad Sci USA 113(26):7261–7265. https://doi.org/10.1073/pnas.1601624113
112. Teske ME, Thistle HW, Schou WC, Miller PCH, Strager JM, Richardson B, Ellis MCB, Barry JW, Twardus DB, Thompson DG (2011) A review of computer models for pesticide deposition prediction. Trans ASABE 54(3):789–801. https://doi.org/10.13031/2013.37094
113. Tscharntke T, Clough Y, Wanger TC, Jackson L, Motzke I, Perfecto I, Vandermeer J, Whitbread A (2012) Global food security, biodiversity conservation and the future of agricultural intensification. Biol Conserv 151(1):53–59. https://doi.org/10.1016/j.biocon.2012.01.068
114. Tungare K, Shahu R, Zambare V, Agarwal P, Jobby R, Nisar N, Jha P (2022) Toxicity mitigation of textile dye reactive blue 4 by hairy roots of Helianthus annuus and testing its effect in in vivo model systems. Biomed Res Int 2022
115. United States Environmental Protection Agency (2014) Guidance for assessing pesticide—Risks to bees. United States Environmental Protection Agency
116. Vaknin Y, Gan-Mor S, Bechar A, Ronen B, Eisikowitch D (2000) The role of electrostatic forces in pollination. Plant Syst Evol 222:133–142
117. Vanengelsdorp D, Evans JD, Donovall L, Mullin C, Frazier M, Frazier J, Tarpy DR, Hayes J, Pettis JS (2009) Entombed Pollen: a new condition in honey bee colonies associated with increased risk of colony mortality. J Invertebr Pathol 101(2):147–149. https://doi.org/10.1016/j.jip.2009.03.008
118. Verma N, Sao P, Srivastava A, Singh S (2021) Physiological and molecular responses to drought, submergence and excessive watering in plants. Harsh environment and plant resilience: molecular and functional aspects, 305–321
119. Villa S, Vighi M, Finizio A, Serini GB (2000) Risk assessment for honeybees from pesticide-exposed pollen. Ecotoxicology 9:287–297
120. Vishwakarma SK, Ilyas T, Shahid M, Malviya D, Kumar S, Singh S, Singh HV (2024) Bacillus spp.: nature's gift to agriculture and humankind. In: Applications of bacillus and bacillus derived genera in agriculture, biotechnology and beyond. Springer Nature Singapore, Singapore, pp 1–36
121. Vora Z, Pandya J, Vaikuntapu PR, Singh S, Asha S, Purama RK (2023) Genome-wide association of defense hormone crosstalk in plants. In: Hormonal cross-talk, plant defense and development. Academic Press, pp 353–371
122. Wang Y, Cui H, Sun C, Zhao X, Cui B (2014) Construction and evaluation of controlled-release delivery system of abamectin using porous silica nanoparticles as carriers. Nanoscale Res Lett 9(1):2490. https://doi.org/10.1186/1556-276X-9-655
123. Wang L, Li X, Zhang G, Dong J, Eastoe J (2007) Oil-in-water nanoemulsions for pesticide formulations. J Colloid Interface Sci 314(1):230–235. https://doi.org/10.1016/j.jcis.2007.04.079

124. Wang Y, Tian J, Wang Z, Li C, Li X (2022) Crop-safe pyraclostrobin-loaded multiwalled carbon nanotube delivery systems: higher fungicidal activity and lower acute toxicity. ACS Agric Sci Technol 2(3):534–545. https://doi.org/10.1021/acsagscitech.1c00293
125. Winston ML (1987) The biology of the honey bee. Harvard University Press
126. Woodcock BA, Ridding L, Freeman SN, Pereira MG, Sleep D, Redhead J, Aston D, Carreck NL, Shore RF, Bullock JM, Heard MS, Pywell RF (2018) Neonicotinoid residues in UK honey despite European Union moratorium. PLoS ONE 13(1):e0189681. https://doi.org/10.1371/journal.pone.0189681
127. Wu JY, Anelli CM, Sheppard WS (2011) Sub-lethal effects of pesticide residues in brood comb on worker honey bee (Apis mellifera) development and longevity. PLoS ONE 6(2):e14720. https://doi.org/10.1371/journal.pone.0014720
128. Yadav J, Jasrotia P, Kashyap PL, Bhardwaj AK, Kumar S, Singh M, Singh GP (2021) Nanopesticides: current status and scope for their application in agriculture. Plant Prot Sci 58(1):1–17. https://doi.org/10.17221/102/2020-PPS
129. Zhang Y, Goss GG (2022) Nanotechnology in agriculture: comparison of the toxicity between conventional and nano-based agrochemicals on non-target aquatic species. J Hazard Mater 439:29559. https://doi.org/10.1016/j.jhazmat.2022.129559
130. Zhang R, Zhang Y, Xu Q, Li J, Zhu F (2019) Hormetic effects of mixtures of dimethachlone and prochloraz on Sclerotinia sclerotiorum. Plant Dis 103(3):546–554. https://doi.org/10.1094/PDIS-06-18-1071-RE
131. Zielińska A, Costa B, Ferreira MV, Miguéis D, Louros JMS, Durazzo A, Lucarini M, Eder P, Chaud MV, Morsink M, Willemen N, Severino P, Santini A, Souto EB (2020) Nanotoxicology and nanosafety: safety-by-design and testing at a glance. Int J Environ Res Public Health 17(13):4657. https://doi.org/10.3390/ijerph17134657

# Statistical Approach

# Optimization of Green Synthesis of Nanoparticles Using Response Surface Methodology

**Ajith S., Karthik R., Manoj Kanti Debnath, Laxmanarayanan M., Deepranjan Sarkar, Rakesh S., Rahul Datta, and Sachidanand Singh**

**Abstract** The properties of nanoparticles synthesized from green synthesis are determined by the combined effect of many factors involved in the process of green synthesis. Despite the significant growth in the plant-extract-mediated synthesis of nanoparticles, the issue of optimization of process parameters in biosynthesis still needs to be addressed. The optimization of various controlling factors which are profound determinants of green synthesis is an important aspect in standardizing the most effective and quality nanomaterial. Response Surface Methodology (RSM) is a robust statistical method to design an experiment to evaluate the combined effect of several factors for obtaining the optimum conditions that yield desirable

Ajith S.
International Maize and Wheat Improvement Centre (CIMMYT), Delhi, India

Ajith S. (✉) · M. K. Debnath
Department of Agricultural Statistics, Uttar Banga Krishi Viswavidyalaya, Cooch Behar, West Bengal, India
e-mail: ajithagristat@gmail.com

Karthik R.
Department of Entomology, Assam Agricultural University, Jorhat, Assam, India

Laxmanarayanan M.
ICAR-National Bureau of Soil Survey and Land Use Planning, Nagpur, Maharashtra, India

D. Sarkar
Agricultural Systems and Engineering, Department of Food, Agriculture and Natural Resources, School of Environment, Resources and Development, Asian Institute of Technology, Klong Luang, Pathum Thani, Thailand

Rakesh S.
International Crops Research Institute for the Semi-Arid Tropics, Patancheru, Hyderabad, Telangana, India

R. Datta
Faculty of Forestry and Wood Technology, Department of Geology and Pedology, Mendel University in Brno, Brno, Czech Republic

S. Singh
Department of Biotechnology, School of Energy Technology, Pandit Deendayal Energy University, Gandhinagar, Gujarat, India



D. Jabborova et al. (eds.), *Nanomaterials in Agroforestry Systems*, Smart Nanomaterials Technology, https://doi.org/10.1007/978-981-96-1337-3_19

output. The RSM is a systematic fusion of the design of the experiment, statistical modeling, and optimization method. This chapter discusses the practical considerations in designing and analyzing RSM methodology to optimize the response. The stepwise procedure of RSM which includes a selection of controlling factors, determination of factor levels, coding the factor, running the experiment, fitting second-order response model, assessment of the significance of factor effects, validation of the fitted model, and finally optimization concept has been discussed. Further, the concept of RSM has been illustrated using an arbitrarily chosen dataset to optimize the temperature, reaction time, and pH that maximize the size of Silver Nanoparticles (AgNPs).

**Keywords** Optimization · Green synthesis · Nanoparticles · Design of experiments · Response surface methodology · Central composite design

## 1 Green Synthesis of Nanoparticles

The particles at the smaller dimension with a size range from 1 to 100 nm are called nanoparticles (NPs) and they exhibit various unique biological and physical properties. The synthesis of nanomaterials has gained interest among researchers as these can be used in different scientific fields such as agriculture, aerospace, medicine, electronics, physics, chemistry, and biology [50]. In general, NPs are synthesized via physical, chemical, and biological methods [42]. The physical and chemical methods are top-down approaches while the biological methods are bottom-up approaches [29]. The biological route of synthesis, i.e., green synthesis of NPs is generally preferred over physical and chemical methods [58] owing to its distinct advantages in terms of less energy consumption, non-toxic to the environment and human beings, less expensive, and sustainability [34].

In green synthesis, the NPs are synthesized using various biological organisms (plants and microorganisms), enzymes, and biomolecules [49]. In the case of microorganisms, fungi, bacteria, and algae are commonly used, and plant-based synthesis uses various plant parts such as leaves, seeds, roots, and flowers [63]. The biological organism contains capping and stabilizing agents which are needed for effective nanoparticle synthesis [34]. In this way, the NPs having a homogenous chemical composition can be synthesized [28]. In an in vitro condition, a single-step bioreduction process is involved where the reduction of metal precursors into the size and shape of NPs of our desired level takes place using the extracts of biological organisms [33].

**Table 1** Nanoparticles synthesized via greener route using forest trees as a source

| Sl. no. | Nanoparticle | Tree species and their parts used for the nanoparticle synthesis | References |
|---|---|---|---|
| 1 | AuNPs | Leaf extract of *Cassia auriculata* | Priyatharishini et al. [51] |
| 2 | AuNPs | Leaf extract of *Thuja orientalis* | Noruzi et al. [46] |
| 3 | AgNPs | Leaf extract of *Thuja occidentalis* | Kanawaria et al. [32] |
| 4 | AgNps | Pod extract of *Acacia nilotica* | Edison and Sethuraman [25] |
| 5 | AgNps | Leaf and fruit extract of *Quercus infectoria* | Chahardooli et al. [22] |
| 6 | CuNPs | Cone and flower extract of *Pinus merkusii* | Masruri et al. [41] |
| 7 | FeNPs | Leaf extract of Eucalyptus | Wang et al. [62] |
| 8 | Iron oxide NPs | Extract from leaves and needles of *Pinus eldarica* | Kheshtzar et al. [35] |
| 9 | PdNPs | Leaf extract of *Filicium decipiens* | Sharmila et al. [57] |
| 10 | Zinc oxide NPs | Extract from leaves and needles of *Texus baccata* | Sarli and Ghasemi [56] |

## 2 Green Synthesis of NPs Using Forest Trees

Among all the biological organisms, plants are the major source for the green synthesis of NPs due to their easy availability [39]. Recently, the interest in the synthesis of NPs using forest trees as a source has been increased [62]. Research studies with green synthesis of NPs using different forest trees are presented in Table 1.

## 3 Factors Influencing the Green Synthesis of NPs

The dimension and size of NPs are greatly determined by the nature of biological organisms [6]. For instance, silver NPs (AgNPs) of the size 25–50 nm could be synthesized using *Terminalia cuneata* [24], however, the desirable size could not be achieved with the extract of *Papaver somniferum* [60]. It has also been reported that the amount of NPs is based on the type of extract from the biological organism as in the case of AgNPs synthesized from *Sesuvium portulacastrum* where callus extract produced more silver nanoparticles than leaf extract [45]. The process of green synthesis of NPs not only depends on the biotic factor, i.e., the living organism used in synthesis, but also on abiotic factors such as reaction temperature, pH of the reaction medium, reaction time, and salt concentration [26]. For example, the gold nanoparticles (AuNPs) synthesized from *Ziziphus ziziphus* where the researchers found that 3 min reaction time was proved to be better for the stability of AuNPs when compared to other reaction times tested [3]. In the case of temperature, under 37 °C, the AgNPs could not be synthesized from *Courouptia guianemsis* [61]. The size of NPs is also controlled by the pH of the medium [25].

The optimization of various controlling factors which are profound determinants of nanoparticle synthesis and properties of synthesized nanoparticles is an important aspect of standardization of the most effective and quality nanomaterial [1, 9, 30]. Despite the great attention on plant-extract-mediated biosynthesis of nanoparticles, an issue on optimization of process parameters still needs to be addressed [8].

## 4 Response Surface Methodology

Response Surface Methodology (RSM) is a robust statistical technique used to design an experiment that evaluates the combined effect of several factors for obtaining the optimum conditions that yield desirable output [2]. The optimization process in RSM is implemented by formulating a mathematical relationship between the response and factor variables of a system [21]. The notion of RSM is to identify the best combination of various input variables or treatment factor levels that maximize or minimize the response variable with fewer experimental runs [48].

For example, the RSM can be used for the optimization of levels of nitrogen (N), phosphorous (P), and potassium (K) that maximize crop yield [12, 31]. An entomologist can use RSM to optimize the combination of pesticide concentration, droplet size, and rotational speed of the nozzle to minimize pest infestation on the crop. An economist may have an interest in identifying the optimum combination of investment in various aspects of business that maximize profit.

The RSM is the systematic fusion of design of experiment, statistical modeling, and optimization method. In the first step, the observations are obtained through statistically designed experiments. Then, a polynomial interaction effect model is to be fitted by taking the treatment factors as independent variables and observed values of the response variable aroused due to the combined effect of treatment factors as the dependent variable. Subsequently, an optimization problem is to be formulated to optimize the combination of levels of treatment factors that maximize or minimize the response.

There are many advantages of using RSM compared to regular experimental designs as it needs fewer experimental runs; it examines individual as well as interaction effects of factors on response and it also identifies the best combination of factor levels that maximize or minimize the targeted response [7]. The concept of RSM is applied in various fields such as material science [53], bioscience [52], chemical engineering [65], microbiology [5], food science [55], and so on for product as well as process optimization.

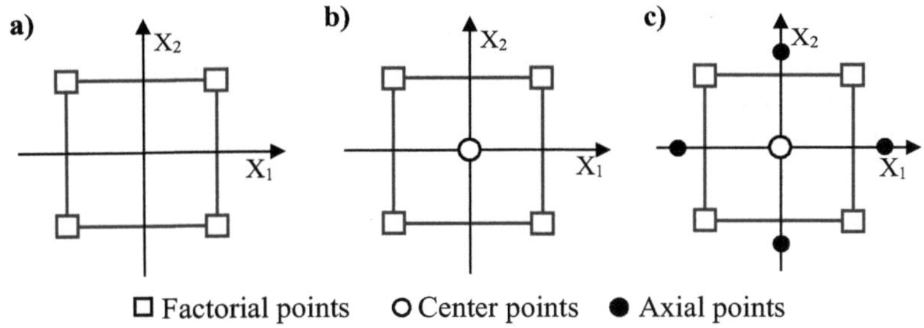


**Fig. 1** Central composite design for two-factor variables. **a** Factorial points; **b** Center points with factorial points; **c** Axial points with factorial and center points

## *4.1 Central Composite Design (CCD)*

The RSM can be implemented by employing specialized experimental designs viz. central composite design (CCD) and box behnken design (BBD) [38]. The central composite design (CCD) which was developed by Box and Wilson [19] is the most popular and efficient second-order response surface design [4, 54]. The usual factorial experiment uses a first-order model that estimates only the main and interaction effects of factors, but it is inadequate when there is a curvature in the true response surface [44]. The CCD is implemented by employing a second-order model that assesses the quadratic effect of factors on the response and the same cannot be estimated in the usual factorial designs [11].

For a better understanding of the concept assume there are two treatment factors ($X_1$ and $X_2$) with two levels of each (high and low). This experimental setup is similar to a $2^2$ full factorial experiment. The CCD is characterized by three experimental points viz. factorial, center, and axial points.

### 4.1.1 Factorial Points

The treatment combinations of a full factorial design are represented as factorial points ($n_f$). These factorial points are located at the corners of a square (Fig. 1a). It is placed at the vertices of a cube when there are three treatment factors. These factorial points characterize the first-order model and they are designed to test the hypothesis test. In general, $2^k$ factorial points are required for $2^k$ experimental design [36].

### 4.1.2 Center Points

The factorial points are further augmented with center points ($n_0$) which are the average of all the levels of each factor variable (Fig. 1b). These points are located at the center of the design. These center points enable the estimation of experimental error, and assessment of curvature at the region of interest on the response surface, and also provide adequate power to test the lack of fit of the fitted model. The number of center points is to be decided by the experimenter and it is generally recommended to have four or five center points [16].

### 4.1.3 Axial Points

Axial points ($n_\alpha$) are placed in all directions of the square at a fixed distance ($\alpha$) from the design center (Fig. 1c). The axial points allow us to estimate the pure quadradic effect in the region of interest [37]. In general, $2^k$ number of axial points are required for $2^k$ experimental design. The distance of axial points from center points can be calculated as [47]

$$\alpha = 2^{\frac{k}{4}} \tag{1}$$

where $k$ is the number of factors. The total number of experimental runs ($N$) required for $2^k$ experimental setup is [15]

$$N = n_f + n_\alpha + n_O = 2^k + 2k + n_O \tag{2}$$

where $n_f$, $n_O$, and $n_\alpha$ are the number of factorial, center, and axial points, respectively.

### 4.1.4 Coding of Factors

As the factors are measured in different units and their magnitudes are not similar, the factor levels are to be coded to obtain dimensional values [17].

$$x_{ij} = \frac{X_{ij} - X_i{}^*}{\Delta X_i} \tag{3}$$

where $x_{ij}$ is code for $j$th level of $i$th factor, $X_{ij}$ is $j$th original level of $i$th factor, $X_i{}^*$ is original level at center point of $i$th factor, and $\Delta X_i$ is the step change value which is equal to the difference of two consecutive levels of a factor.

### 4.1.5 Illustration of CCD of $2^2$ Experimental Designs Augmented with Four Central Points

The CCD of $2^2$ experimental designs augmented with four central points has 12 experimental runs (Table 2). The lowest and highest levels of factors are assigned with the code −1 and +1, respectively. The average of two levels of the factors (center points) are coded with 0. The axial points are positioned at a distance of 1.41 ($\alpha$) from center points in all directions (Fig. 2).

**Table 2** Central composite design (CCD) for $2^2$ experimental designs with four central points

| Run | Factor $X_1$ | Factor $X_2$ | Experiment points |
|---|---|---|---|
| 1 | −1 | −1 | Factorial points |
| 2 | −1 | +1 | |
| 3 | +1 | −1 | |
| 4 | +1 | +1 | |
| 5 | 0 | 0 | Center points |
| 6 | 0 | 0 | |
| 7 | 0 | 0 | |
| 8 | 0 | 0 | |
| 9 | 0 | +1.41 | Axial points |
| 10 | 0 | −1.41 | |
| 11 | +1.41 | 0 | |
| 12 | −1.41 | 0 | |

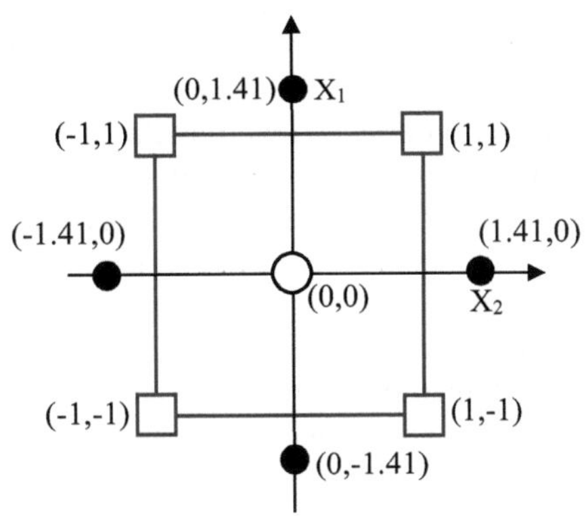


**Fig. 2** Central composite design (CCD) for $2^2$ experimental design

## 4.2 Second-Order Polynomial Model

After framing the experimental setup as given in Sect. 4.1, the experiment has to be carried out in the field or lab. The responses aroused due to the effect of each treatment combination have to be recorded. Then, a second-order polynomial model has to be fitted by taking observations of response variables as dependent variable and factor variables as independent variables. The notion of model fitting is to verify the statistical significance of included factors on the response. The second-order polynomial equation for an experiment with $k$ factors is given by Box and [18].

$$y = \beta_0 + \sum_{i=1}^{k} \beta_i x_i + \sum_{i=1}^{k} \beta_{ii} x_i^2 + \sum_{i=1, j=1 \,\&\, i \neq j}^{k} \beta_{ij} x_i x_j + \varepsilon \tag{4}$$

where $y$ is the response variable, $x_i$ and $x_j$ are $i$th and $j$th factors (coded), respectively, $x_i^2$ is the square of $i$th factor which is assumed as a quadratic term of $i$th factor, $x_ix_j$ is the interaction term of $i$th and $j$th factors, $\beta_0$ is a constant term, $\beta_i$ is coefficient of the linear term of $i$th factor, $\beta_{ii}$ is coefficient of the quadratic term of $i$th factor, $\beta_{ij}$ is coefficient of interaction term of $i$th and $j$th factors, and $\varepsilon$ is the error which is assumed to follow normal distribution $N(0, \sigma^2)$.

For a better understanding of the above equation, the second-order polynomial regression equation for an experiment with two factors $x_1$ and $x_2$ with two levels of each $\pm 1$ is given by

$$y = \beta_0 + \beta_1 x_1 + \beta_2 x_2 + \beta_{11} x_1^2 + \beta_{22} x_2^2 + \beta_{12} x_1 x_2 + \varepsilon \tag{5}$$

where $y$ is the response variable, $\beta_0$ is the constant term, $\beta_1$ is the coefficient of the linear term of factor variable $x_1$ which measures the mean effect of the factor $x_1$, $\beta_{11}$ is the coefficient of the quadratic term of factor variable $x_1$, $\beta_{12}$ is coefficient of the two-factor interaction, and $\varepsilon$ is the random error.

The regression coefficients $\beta$'s can be estimated using the ordinary least square (OLS) estimation procedure [10]. Further, an Analysis of Variance (ANOVA) has to be carried out to investigate the statistical significance of each linear, quadratic, and interaction effect as well as the lack of fit of the model [13]. A significant lack of fit indicates that the fitted model is inadequate to represent average response as the function of factor variables. If there is no lack of fit and significance of any or all of the included effects namely linear, quadratic, and interaction effects implies that the fitted model is sufficient to explain the average response by the respective significant factor effects [23]. The effects that correspond to significant regression coefficients are retained in the model. In case the quadratic term is not significant, the quadratic term is to be removed from the model and the equation remains linear.

## 4.3 Optimization

The vital aspect of RSM is the optimization. The second-order model fitted as given in Sect. 4.2 can be used to examine the response surface as long as there is no significant lack of fit. Then either path of steepest ascent or path of steepest descent is to be followed to climb on the response surface toward the maximum and minimum of the response, respectively [43]. The path of the steepest ascent or path of steepest descent on the response surface is determined based on the sign and magnitude of the estimated regression coefficient of the fitted model.

For a unique treatment combination, the response neither increases nor decreases, and the tangent surface at that point will be a plane which is termed as stationary point. At the stationary point, the average response is either maximum or minimum. The status of the response at the stationary point can be identified by rewriting Eq. (4) in canonical form. This computation involves a complex derivation and interested readers can refer to [14] for a detailed derivation of the gradient search algorithm for optimization. However, statistical software can handle these complex calculations.

The optimization model equation can be visually represented by a response surface plot and contour plot [64]. These plots describe the changes in the response variable for changes in the levels of factor variables. There is an either increase or decrease in the response variables on the response surface plot for every increase in the combinations of levels of factor variables and the maximum or minimum is obtained for a particular combination of levels of factor variables. The targeted point which indicates either the maximum or minimum in the contour plot is represented by a circular or elliptical pattern [20].

## 5 Steps Involved in Designing and Analysis of RSM

**Step 1: Identification of controlling factors**

The first step in the implementation of RSM is to identify the governing factors or controlling variables of the targeted response variable. The response, as well as factor variables, should be quantitative in the sense that it should be a measurable numerical variable such as yield (kg), concentration (ppm), time (hours), and temperature (°C) and it should not be a qualitative variable such as variety, color, shape, etc. In our present context of green synthesis of NPs, the response variable may be the quantity of NPs produced or the size of the NPs. The factor variables may be temperature, pH, reaction time, salt concentration, etc.

**Step 2: Determination of levels of controlling factors**

The levels of controlling factors that significantly influence the response can be determined by the experience of the researcher or by performing screening experiments with few runs using fractional factorial or Taguchi experiments [59]. The uppermost level and lowest possible level of each factor have to be identified.

**Step 3: Selection of design**

Experiments can be carried out by using any of the response surface designs viz. CCD and BBD. The main differences between these designs are the number of runs required and the choices of experimental points.

**Step 4: Determination of treatment combinations to be experimented**

The treatment combinations of the full factorial experiment are the factorial points. The center points are determined by averaging the levels of each factor. Each factor levels have to be coded as given in Sect. 4.1.4. The axial points are to be determined by locating points at a fixed distance ($\alpha$) from the coded design center (0,0) in all the directions of the square or cube. This level of the axial points is coded values as given in Sect. 4.1.4. The actual levels of axial points of a factor can be computed by multiplying its center points in the original level (average of high and low levels) with α. Once the factor levels corresponding to factorial points, center points, and axial points are fixed, the corresponding treatment combinations are determined.

**Step 5: Running the experiment**

After determining the treatment combinations to be experimented with, an experiment is to be undertaken in the field or lab condition. Each treatment combination has to be applied to a distinct and independent plot or run in the sense that a particular treatment combination should not influence its preceding or succeeding plot or run. The observation of our targeted response variable from each plot or run corresponding to a specific treatment combination has to be recorded.

**Step 6: Model fitting and evaluation of factor effects**

A second-order model as given in Eq. (4) is to be fitted using the data obtained from the experiment. The significance of various linear, quadratic, and interaction effects as well as the lack of fit of the fitted model can be verified using ANOVA analysis. The non-significance of lack of fit and significance of any or all of the linear, quadratic, and interaction effects are desired.

**Step 7: Validation of the model**

The fitted model is to be validated to ensure the model's adequacy in terms of proper approximation of experimental data. The chi-square test or Welch's *t*-test can be used to check the agreement between the observed and predicted values of the response variable [27]. The goodness of fit of the model can be verified using $R^2$. The adequacy of the model can also be verified graphically using observed versus predicted plot.

**Step 8: Optimization**

After assessing the model fitness and validation, the maximum or minimum of the response can be achieved by maximization or minimization of the fitted equation, respectively. The steps involved in the implementation of RSM are summarized in Fig. 3.

## 6 Statistical Software Available to Analyze RSM Data

The advent of advanced statistical software is a boon for researchers to carry out any complex statistical analysis in an easier way. Accordingly, almost every statistical software has an option to carry out RSM analysis. The most commonly used software to analyze RSM are Design-Expert, R, SAS, STATA, Minitab, etc.

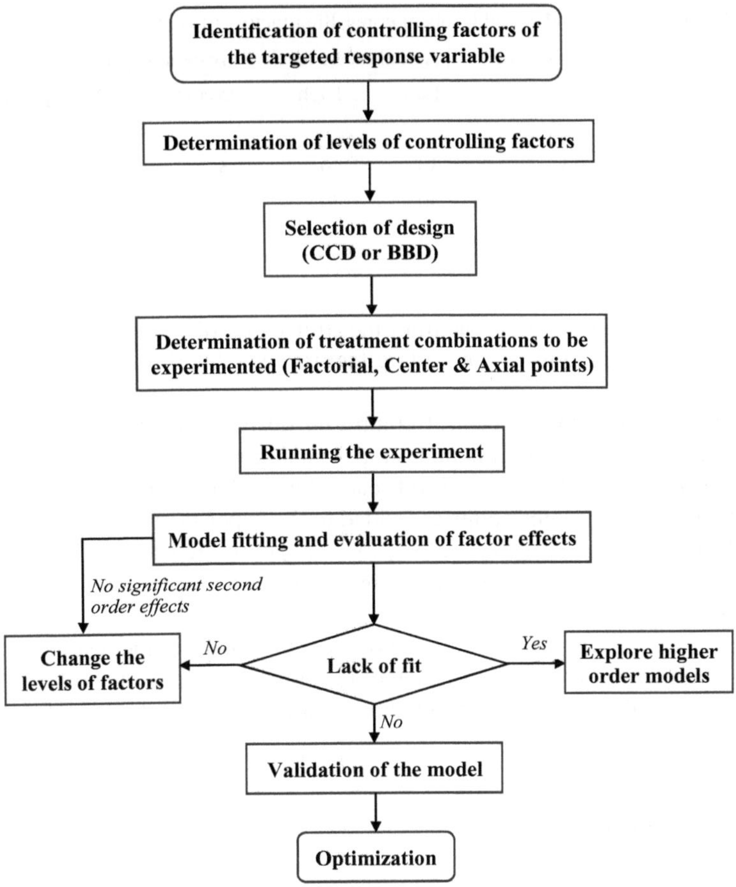


**Fig. 3** Roadmap in the implementation of RSM

## 7 Example

The concept of RSM has been illustrated using an arbitrarily chosen dataset for the sake of understanding the concept. The designing and analysis of RSM are carried out in R software using the "rsm" package [40]. The stepwise R codes used in the analysis are provided in the appendix.

### *7.1 Designing the Experiment*

Let us assume that an experiment is conducted to synthesize silver nanoparticles (AgNPs) using leaf extract of *Cassia auriculata*. The key determinants of the size of

**Table 3** Levels of actual and coded levels of controlling factors of AgNPs

| Controlling factors | Symbol | Actual factor levels corresponding to coded levels | | | | |
|---|---|---|---|---|---|---|
| | | Low | High | Average | Axial points | |
| | | −1 | +1 | 0 | −1.7 | +1.7 |
| Temperature (°C) | $x_1$ | 30 | 40 | 35 | 26.3 | 43.7 |
| Reaction time (min) | $x_2$ | 30 | 70 | 50 | 15.4 | 84.6 |
| pH | $x_3$ | 3 | 9 | 6 | 0.8 | 11.2 |

AgNPs are temperature (°C), reaction time (min), and pH of the reaction mixture. The levels of the above three controlling factors considered for the experiment are given in Table 3.

The experiment setup of central composite design (CCD) is derived using R software (Table 4). This experimental setup is analogous to a $2^3$ factorial experiment since there are three factors at two levels each (low and high). Hence, there are eight factorial points. Four center points are added to the experiment as the average levels of each factor. As there are three factors, six axial points are added to the experiment at a distance of 1.68 ($2^{3/4}$) from the design center. Therefore, the total number of experimental runs is 18.

Then, the experiment is carried out to observe the values of the response variable, i.e., size of the synthesized NPs for each of the eighteen treatment combinations and the same is recorded against corresponding treatment combinations (Table 4).

### 7.2 Model Fitting

Next, the second-order polynomial model is fitted to the observed data. The summary of the fitted model is given in Table 5. It can be observed that both reaction time and pH of the reaction medium play significant roles in the determination of the size of AgNPs in linear as well as pure quadratic form ($p \leq 0.05$). The interaction of reaction time and pH and the interaction of temperature and pH are found to have significant effect on the size of AgNPs. The linear as well as pure quadratic effects of temperature and the interaction of temperature and reaction time are not significant ($p > 0.05$). It is also found that three-factor interaction is non-significant.

From the ANOVA, it can be witnessed that linear, pure quadratic, and two-way interaction effects are significant ($p \leq 0.05$) (Table 6). The three-way interaction effect is not significant ($p > 0.05$) which is in line with the results of Table 5. There is no sufficient evidence of a lack of fit in the fitted model since the lack of fit of the model is not significant ($p > 0.05$). The overall model is fitted very well to the data with $p < 0.001$. Further, the multiple $R^2$ and Adjusted $R^2$ are close to one confirming the goodness of fit of the model. Hence, the model adequately fits the observed data.

**Table 4** Experiment design and observed size of synthesized AgNPs

| Exp. run | Coded levels | | | Actual levels | | | Response variable |
|---|---|---|---|---|---|---|---|
| | $x_1$ | $x_2$ | $x_3$ | Temperature (°C) | Reaction time (min) | pH | Size of nanoparticle (nm) |
| 1 | 1 | 1 | 1 | 40 | 70 | 9 | 90 |
| 2 | 0 | 0 | 0 | 35 | 50 | 6 | 95 |
| 3 | −1 | 1 | −1 | 30 | 70 | 3 | 86 |
| 4 | −1 | −1 | −1 | 30 | 30 | 3 | 48 |
| 5 | 0 | 0 | 0 | 35 | 50 | 6 | 95 |
| 6 | −1 | 1 | 1 | 30 | 70 | 9 | 97 |
| 7 | 0 | 0 | 0 | 35 | 50 | 6 | 95 |
| 8 | 1 | −1 | −1 | 40 | 30 | 3 | 70 |
| 9 | −1 | −1 | 1 | 30 | 30 | 9 | 32 |
| 10 | 0 | 0 | 0 | 35 | 50 | 6 | 95 |
| 11 | 1 | −1 | 1 | 40 | 30 | 9 | 23 |
| 12 | 1 | 1 | −1 | 40 | 70 | 3 | 96 |
| 13 | −1.7 | 0 | 0 | 26.3 | 50 | 6 | 96 |
| 14 | 0 | 1.7 | 0 | 35 | 84.6 | 6 | 98 |
| 15 | 0 | 0 | 1.7 | 35 | 50 | 11.2 | 24 |
| 16 | 0 | 0 | −1.7 | 35 | 50 | 0.8 | 65 |
| 17 | 1.7 | 0 | 0 | 43.7 | 50 | 6 | 89 |
| 18 | 0 | −1.7 | 0 | 35 | 15.4 | 6 | 25 |
| 10 | 1 | 1 | 1 | 40 | 70 | 9 | 90 |

**Table 5** Summary of the fitted second-order polynomial regression model

| Factors | Coefficient | Std. error | *t*-value | *p*-value |
|---|---|---|---|---|
| Intercept | 94.92 | 2.58 | 36.73 | <0.001 |
| *Linear effect* | | | | |
| $x_1$ | 0.30 | 1.39 | 0.21 | 0.835 |
| $x_2$ | 23.23 | 1.39 | 16.76 | <0.001 |
| $x_3$ | −9.27 | 1.39 | −6.69 | <0.001 |
| *Pure quadratic effect* | | | | |
| $x_1^2$ | 0.30 | 1.39 | 0.21 | 0.837 |
| $x_2^2$ | 23.23 | 1.39 | 16.67 | <0.001 |
| $x_3^2$ | −9.27 | 1.39 | −6.65 | <0.001 |
| *Interaction effect* | | | | |
| $x_1x_2$ | −0.31 | 1.43 | −0.22 | 0.835 |
| $x_1x_3$ | −11.04 | 1.43 | −7.70 | 0.011 |
| $x_2x_3$ | −16.92 | 1.43 | −11.81 | 0.002 |
| $x_1x_2x_3$ | 1.75 | 1.83 | 0.96 | 0.370 |

**Table 6** Analysis of variance (ANOVA) of the effects of fitted model

| Sources | Degrees of freedom | Sum of square | Mean square | *F*-value | *p*-value |
|---|---|---|---|---|---|
| Linear effects | 3 | 8620 | 2873 | 107 | <0.001 |
| Two-way interaction effects | 3 | 879 | 293 | 11 | 0.005 |
| Pure quadratic effects | 3 | 4781 | 1594 | 60 | 0.000 |
| Three-way interaction effect | 1 | 25 | 25 | 1 | 0.370 |
| Lack of fit | 4 | 187 | 47 | 258,370 | 0.220 |
| Residuals | 7 | 187 | 27 | | |
| Overall $p$-value < 0.001 | | | | | |
| Multiple $R^2 = 0.987$ | | | | | |
| Adjusted $R^2 = 0.969$ | | | | | |

## 7.3 Updating the Model

As some of the effects do not significantly influence the response variable, the fitted model is updated by retaining only the significant factors in the model. Now, all the retained linear, pure quadratic, and two-way interaction effects are significantly influencing the size of AgNPs (Table 7). The ANOVA table also supports the above results (Table 8).

**Table 7** Summary of the updated model

| Factors | Coefficient | Std. error | *t*-value | *p*-value |
|---|---|---|---|---|
| Intercept | 94.57 | 1.80 | 52.65 | <0.001 |
| *Linear effect* | | | | |
| $x_2$ | 23.23 | 1.22 | 18.99 | <0.001 |
| $x_3$ | −9.27 | 1.22 | −7.58 | <0.001 |
| *Pure quadratic effect* | | | | |
| $x_2^2$ | −10.97 | 1.23 | −8.94 | <0.001 |
| $x_3^2$ | −16.85 | 1.23 | −13.74 | <0.001 |
| *Interaction effect* | | | | |
| $x_1x_3$ | −6.00 | 1.61 | −3.74 | <0.001 |
| $x_2x_3$ | 8.50 | 1.61 | 5.30 | <0.001 |

**Table 8** Analysis of variance (ANOVA) of the effects of the updated model

| Sources | Degrees of freedom | Sum of square | Mean square | $F$-value | $p$-value |
|---|---|---|---|---|---|
| **Linear effects** | 2 | 8619 | 4310 | 209 | <0.001 |
| Pure quadratic effects | 2 | 4780 | 2390 | 116 | <0.001 |
| $x_1x_3$ | 1 | 288 | 288 | 14 | 0.003 |
| $x_2x_3$ | 1 | 578 | 578 | 28 | <0.001 |
| Lack of fit | 3 | 125 | 42 | 3 | 0.080 |
| Residuals | 11 | 227 | 21 | | |
| Overall $p$-value < 0.001 | | | | | |
| Multiple $R^2 = 0.985$ | | | | | |
| Adjusted $R^2 = 0.976$ | | | | | |

## 7.4 Model Validation

The multiple $R^2$ and Adjusted $R^2$ are not decreased substantially even after dropping some of the non-significant factors and lack of fit is not significant. Further, Welch's $t$-test is employed to test whether there exists a significant difference between observed and predicted values of the size of AgNPs. The results revealed that there is no significant difference between observed and predicted values and $p$-value of one indicates high association between observed and predicted values of AgNPs. The goodness of fit is also examined graphically using a scatterplot of observed versus predicted values (Fig. 4). The data points are not scattered in the plot and no pattern of distribution is observed.

From the above results, it is evident that the updated model adequately fits the observed data. The updated model can be written in terms of coded value as

$$\textbf{Size of nanoparticles (nm)} = \mathbf{94.57 + 23.23x_2 - 9.27x_3 - 10.97x_2^2 - 16.85x_3^2 - 6.00x_1x_3 + 8.50x_2x_3} \quad (6)$$

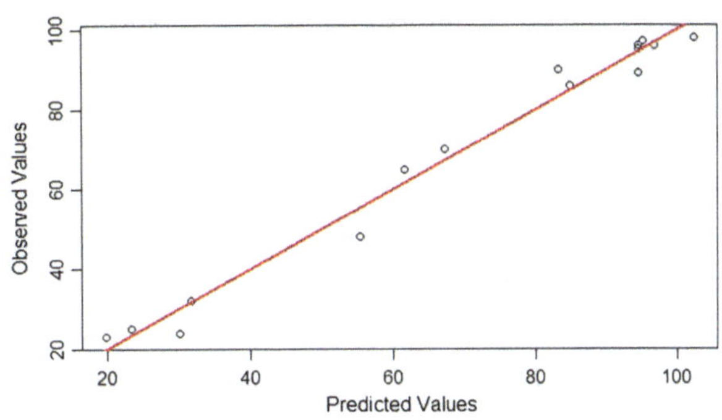


**Fig. 4** Scatterplot of observed versus predicted size of AgNPs

It can be observed that the magnitude of coefficients corresponding to pH is negative in both linear and quadratic effects. Therefore, an increase in pH alone negatively influences the AgNP's size. But pH is positively influencing the response when it is in interaction with reaction time. There is a positive and negative impact of reaction time on AgNP size in linear and quadratic effects, respectively. The interaction of temperature and pH harms the AgNP size.

## 7.5 Optimization

As the updated model adequately fits the data, it can be used for optimization. The response surface plot is plotted for reaction time versus pH at the center point of temperature (35°C) since the interaction of pH and reaction time significantly influences size of AgNPs (Fig. 5a). By examining the surface plot, it is evident that the size of the AgNPs is increasing as both reaction time and pH are increasing between 20 min and 2 min, respectively. The maximum level is attained at a certain point and plummets after that. The levels of reaction time and pH at which the size of AgNPs attains the maximum are stationary points and the corresponding size of the AgNPs is the maximum possible size.

The peak of the response surface is depicted by a contour plot (Fig. 5b). The center point of the ellipse or circle is the maximum point. The maximum size of the AgNPs is attained when the reaction time ranges from 70 to 80 min and pH ranges from 5 to 7. The exact stationary points and the corresponding maximum of the response variable can be predicted using the "predict" function in R software. The maximum attainable size of AgNPs is 105.67 nm which can be obtained when the reaction time, pH, and temperature are 71 min, 5.17, and 35°C, respectively.

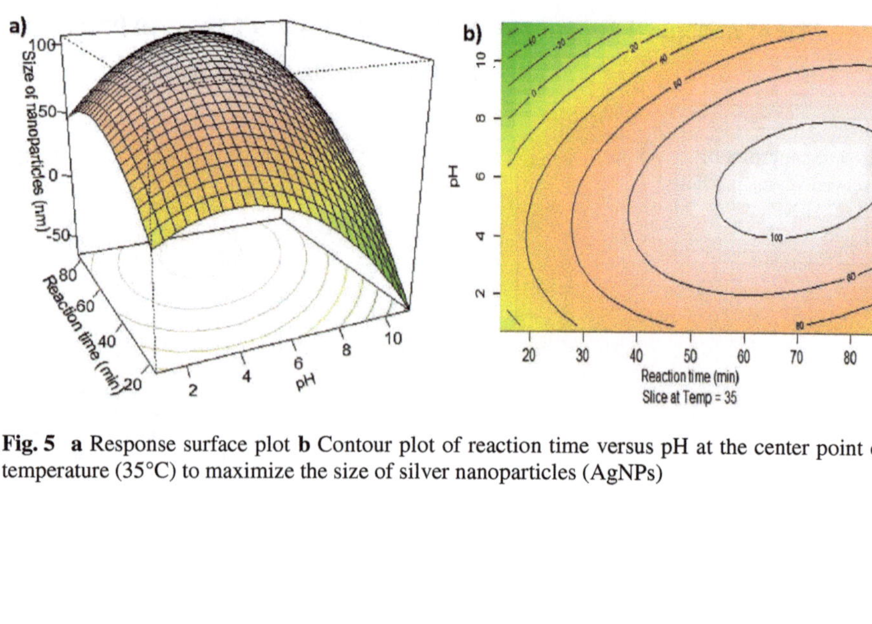


**Fig. 5** **a** Response surface plot **b** Contour plot of reaction time versus pH at the center point of temperature (35°C) to maximize the size of silver nanoparticles (AgNPs)

## 8 Conclusion

The present study attempted to discuss various practical considerations in designing and analysis of RSM for effective optimization of silver nanoparticles (AgNPs). This optimization of levels of factors involved in the green synthesis process yields the nanoparticles of desired properties which makes them effective for various applications. The success in the implementation of RSM for optimization of the quality end product depends on the selection of the most influencing factors on response and identification of their levels as well as proper designing of the experiment. The RSM has wider application in almost all science fields where there exists a problem of either product or process optimization. The readers are highly encouraged to refer core mathematical concept of RSM which is available in theoretical research papers listed in the reference section. Further, machine learning algorithms such as Artificial Neural Network (ANN) or Genetic Algorithm (GA) can also be coupled with RSM for effective optimization.

## Appendix

### Designing and Analysis of Response Surface Design Using R Software

```
### Installing "rsm" package
install.packages(rsm)
### Loading "rsm" package
library(rsm)
### Creating 2*3 design with four center points
des <- cube (3, n0 = 4)
### Adding axial points to the above design
des <- djoin(des, star(alpha = "spherical", n0 = 0))
### Decoding the levels to original levels (Decoded by reverse action of the Eq. 3)
des$Temp <-des$ × 1*5 + 35
des$Reac.time <-des$ × 2*20 + 50
des$pH <-des$ × 3*3 + 6
print(des)
### Importing data (Data of coded levels of all treatment combinations and corresponding
observations of response variable)
ccd.data <-read.delim("clipboard")
### Establishing relationship between coded and original levels of factor variables
ccd1 <-as.coded.data(ccd.data,
   x1 ~ (Temp - 35)/5,
   x2 ~ (Reac.time - 50)/20,
   x3 ~ (pH - 6)/3)
str(ccd1)
### Fitting second-order polynomial model
model <-rsm(Nanoparticle_size ~ FO(x1, x2, x3) + TWI(formula = ~x 1*x2*x3) + PQ(x1,
x2, x3) + x1:x2:x3, data = ccd1)
summary(model)
####Note: FO, TWI, and PQ stand for First-Order, Two-way Interaction, and Pure Quadratic
effects, respectively
### Updating the model by removing non-significant effects
model1 <-rsm(Nanoparticle_size ~ FO(x2, x3) + (x1:x3) + (x2:x3) + PQ(x2, x3), data = ccd1)
summary(model1)
### t-test for goodness of fit of model
predicted <-predict(model1)
t.test(ccd.data$Nanoparticle_size, predicted)
### Validation of fitted model using scatter plot of actual vs. predicted values
plot(predict(model1),
ccd.data$Nanoparticle_size,
xlab = "Predicted Values",
ylab = "Observed Values")
abline(a = 0,
b = 1,
col = "red",
lwd = 2)
### Plotting surface plot
persp(model1, x1 ~ x3,
col = terrain.colors(50),
contours = "colors",
zlab = "Size of nanoparticles (nm)",
xlabs = c("Reaction time (min)", "pH"))
### Plotting contour plot
contour(model1, ~x1 + x3,
image = TRUE,
xlabs = c("Reaction time (min)", "pH"))
### Prediction
maxi <-data.frame(x1 = 0, x2 = 1.058917, x3 = −0.274974)
predict(model1,maxi)
### Note: The values of x1, x2, and x2 are the stationary points (coded) which are
availed from summary (model1)
```

## References


1. Acharya NN, Lin DK (2008) Understanding a ZnO nanorods fabrication process: a supersaturated design approach. Int J Nanomanuf 2(4):319–330. https://doi.org/10.1504/IJNM.2008.022559
2. Ahmad AL, Wong SS, Teng TT, Zuhairi A (2007) Optimization of coagulation–flocculation process for pulp and paper mill effluent by response surface methodological analysis. J Hazard Mater 145(1–2):162–168. https://doi.org/10.1016/j.jhazmat.2006.11.008
3. Aljabali AA, Yazan A, Mazhar SA, Khalid MA, Bahaa A, Osama AA, Alaaldin MA, Mourad B, David JE (2018) Synthesis of gold nanoparticles using leaf extract of Ziziphus zizyphus and their antimicrobial activity. Nanomaterials 8(3):174
4. Alkhatib MF, Mamun AA, Akbar I (2015) Application of response surface methodology (RSM) for optimization of color removal from POME by granular activated carbon. Int J Environ Sci Technol 12:1295–1302. https://doi.org/10.1007/s13762-014-0504-4
5. Almeida DG, Soares S, Luna JM, Rufino RD, Santos VA, Sarubbo LA (2017) Response surface methodology for optimizing the production of biosurfactant by Candida tropicalis on industrial waste substrates. Front Microbiol 8:157. https://doi.org/10.3389/fmicb.2017.00157
6. Aromal SA, Vidhu VK, Philip D (2012) Green synthesis of well-dispersed gold nanoparticles using Macrotyloma uniflorum. Spectrochim Acta Part A Mol Biomol Spectrosc 85(1):99–104
7. Aydar AY (2018) Utilization of response surface methodology in optimization of extraction of plant materials. Statistical approaches with emphasis on design of experiments applied to chemical processes, 157–169
8. Bao Y, He J, Song K, Guo J, Zhou X, Liu S (2021) Plant-extract-mediated synthesis of metal nanoparticles. J Chem 2021:1–14. https://doi.org/10.1155/2021/6562687
9. Barglik-Chory C, Remenyi C, Strohm H, Müller G (2004) Adjustment of the band gap energies of biostabilized CdS nanoparticles by application of statistical design of experiments. J Phys Chem B 108(23):7637–7640. https://doi.org/10.1021/jp036476x
10. Baş D, Boyacı İH (2007) Modeling and optimization I: usability of response surface methodology. J Food Eng 78(3):836–845. https://doi.org/10.1016/j.jfoodeng.2005.11.024
11. Behera SK, Meena H, Chakraborty S, Meikap BC (2018) Application of response surface methodology (RSM) for optimization of leaching parameters for ash reduction from low-grade coal. Int J Min Sci Technol 28(4):621–629
12. Bevan L, Jones M, Zheng Y (2021) Optimisation of nitrogen, phosphorus, and potassium for soilless production of Cannabis sativa in the flowering stage using response surface analysis. Front Plant Sci 2587. https://doi.org/10.3389/fpls.2021.764103
13. Bezerra MA, Santelli RE, Oliveira EP, Villar LS, Escaleira LA (2008) Response surface methodology (RSM) as a tool for optimization in analytical chemistry. Talanta 76(5):965–977. https://doi.org/10.1016/j.talanta.2008.05.019
14. Biles WE (1975) A response surface method for experimental optimization of multi-response processes. Ind Eng Chem Process Des Dev 14(2):152–158
15. Biswas G, Kumari M, Adhikari K, Dutta S (2017) Application of response surface methodology for optimization of biosorption of fluoride from groundwater using Shorea robusta flower petal. Appl Water Sci 7:4673–4690. https://doi.org/10.1007/s13201-017-0630-5
16. Borkowski JJ (1995) Spherical prediction-variance properties of central composite and Box-Behnken designs. Technometrics 37(4):399–410. https://doi.org/10.1080/00401706.1995.10484373
17. Box GE, Draper NR (2007) Response surfaces, mixtures, and ridge analyses. Wiley
18. Box GE, Wilson KB (1992) On the experimental attainment of optimum conditions. In: Breakthroughs in statistics: methodology and distribution. Springer New York, New York, NY, pp 270–310
19. Box GEP, Wilson KB (1951) On the experimental attainment of optimum conditions. J Roy Stat Soc B 13:1–45

20. Breig SJM, Luti KJK (2021) Response surface methodology: a review on its applications and challenges in microbial cultures. Mater Today: Proc 42:2277–2284. https://doi.org/10.1016/j.matpr.2020.12.316
21. Brightman HJ (1978) Optimization through experimentation: applying response surface methodology. Decis Sci 9(3):481–495
22. Chahardooli M, Khodadadi E, Khodadadi E (2014) Green synthesis of silver nanoparticles using oak leaf and fruit extracts (Quercus) and its antibacterial activity against plant pathogenic bacteria. Int J Biosci 4(7):97–103
23. Dean A, Voss D, Draguljić D, Dean A, Voss D, Draguljić D (2017) Response surface methodology. Design and analysis of experiments, 565–614
24. Edison TNJI, Lee YR, Sethuraman MG (2016) Green synthesis of silver nanoparticles using Terminalia cuneata and its catalytic action in reduction of direct yellow-12 dye. Spectrochim Acta Part A Mol Biomol Spectrosc 161:122–129
25. Edison TNJI, Sethuraman MG (2013) Electrocatalytic reduction of benzyl chloride by green synthesized silver nanoparticles using pod extract of Acacia nilotica. ACS Sustain Chem Eng 1(10):1326–1332
26. Gericke M, Pinches A (2006) Biological synthesis of metal nanoparticles. Hydrometallurgy 83(1–4):132–140
27. Goemaere I, Punj D, Harizaj A, Woolston J, Thys S, Sterck K, Braeckmans K (2023) Response surface methodology to efficiently optimize intracellular delivery by photoporation. Int J Mol Sci 24(4):3147. https://doi.org/10.3390/ijms24043147
28. Gopinath K, Shanmugam VK, Gowri S, Senthilkumar V, Kumaresan S, Arumugam A (2014) Antibacterial activity of ruthenium nanoparticles synthesized using Gloriosa superba L. leaf extract. J Nanostruct Chem 4:83
29. Horwat D, Zakharov DI, Endrino JL, Soldera F, Anders A, Migot S, Pierson JF (2011) Chemistry, phase formation, and catalytic activity of thin palladium-containing oxide films synthesized by plasma-assisted physical vapor deposition. Surf Coat Technol 205:S171–S177
30. Hou TH, Su CH, Liu WL (2007) Parameters optimization of a nano-particle wet milling process using the Taguchi method, response surface method and genetic algorithm. Powder Technol 173(3):153–162. https://doi.org/10.1016/j.powtec.2006.11.019
31. Jahan M, Amiri MB (2018) Optimizing application rate of nitrogen, phosphorus and cattle manure in wheat production: an approach to determine optimum scenario using response-surface methodology. J Soil Sci Plant Nutr 18(1):13–26
32. Kanawaria SK, Sankhla A, Jatav PK, Yadav RS, Verma KS, Velraj P, Kachhwaha S, Kothari SL (2018) Rapid biosynthesis and characterization of silver nanoparticles: an assessment of antibacterial and antimycotic activity. Appl Phys A 124:1–10
33. Kaushik N, Thakkar KN, Mhatre SS, Parikh RY (2010) Biological synthesis of metallic nanoparticles. Nanomed Nanotechnol Biol Med 6(2):257–262
34. Kharissova OV, Dias HR, Kharisov BI, Pérez BO, Pérez VMJ (2013) The greener synthesis of nanoparticles. Trends Biotechnol 31(4):240–248
35. Kheshtzar R, Berenjian A, Taghizadeh SM, Ghasemi Y, Asad AG, Ebrahiminezhad A (2019) Optimization of reaction parameters for the green synthesis of zero valent iron nanoparticles using pine tree needles. Green Process Synth 8(1):846–855
36. Khuri AI, Mukhopadhyay S (2010) Response surface methodology. Wiley Interdiscip Rev: Comput Stat 2(2):128–149. https://doi.org/10.1002/wics.73
37. Krajnik P, Kopac J, Sluga A (2005) Design of grinding factors based on response surface methodology. J Mater Process Technol 162:629–636. https://doi.org/10.1016/j.jmatprotec.2005.02.187
38. Kumari M, Gupta SK (2019) Response surface methodological (RSM) approach for optimizing the removal of trihalomethanes (THMs) and its precursor's by surfactant modified magnetic nanoadsorbents (sMNP)-an endeavor to diminish probable cancer risk. Sci Rep 9(1):18339. https://doi.org/10.1038/s41598-019-54902-8
39. Lee HJ, Lee G, Jang NR, Yun JH, Song JY, Kim BS (2011) Biological synthesis of copper nanoparticles using plant extract. Nanotechnology 1(1):371–374

40. Lenth RV (2010) Response-surface methods in R, using RSM. J Stat Softw 32:1–17
41. Masruri M, Pangestin DN, Ulfa SM, Riyanto S, Srihardyastutie A, Rahman MF (2018) A potent Staphylococcus aureus growth inhibitor of a dried flower extract of Pinus merkusii Jungh & De Vriese and copper nanoparticle. In: IOP conference series: materials science and engineering, vol 299(1). IOP Publishing, p 012072
42. Mohanpuria P, Rana NK, Yadav SK (2008) Biosynthesis of nanoparticles: technological concepts and future applications. J Nanopart Res 10:507–517
43. Myers RH, Khuri AI, Carter WH (1989) Response surface methodology: 1966–l988. Technometrics 31(2):137–157
44. Myers RH, Montgomery DC, Anderson-Cook CM (2016) Response surface methodology: process and product optimization using designed experiments. Wiley
45. Nabikhan A, Kandasamy K, Raj A, Alikunhi NM (2010) Synthesis of antimicrobial silver nanoparticles by callus and leaf extracts from saltmarsh plant, Sesuvium portulacastrum L. Colloids Surf, B 79(2):488–493
46. Noruzi M, Zare D, Davoodi D (2012) A rapid biosynthesis route for the preparation of gold nanoparticles by aqueous extract of cypress leaves at room temperature. Spectrochim Acta Part A Mol Biomol Spectrosc 94:84–88
47. De Oliveira LG, de Paiva AP, Balestrassi PP, Ferreira JR, da Costa SC, da Silva Campos PH (2019) Response surface methodology for advanced manufacturing technology optimization: theoretical fundamentals, practical guidelines, and survey literature review. Int J Adv Manuf Technol 104:1785–1837. https://doi.org/10.1007/s00170-019-03809-9
48. Panwar V, Sharma DK, Kumar KP, Jain A, Thakar C (2021) Experimental investigations and optimization of surface roughness in turning of en 36 alloy steel using response surface methodology and genetic algorithm. Mater Today: Proc 46:6474–6481. https://doi.org/10.1016/j.matpr.2021.03.642
49. Parveen K, Banse V, Ledwani L (2016) Green synthesis of nanoparticles: their advantages and disadvantages. In: AIP conference proceedings, vol 1724(1). AIP Publishing
50. Pearce JM (2012) Make nanotechnology research open-source. Nature 491(7425):519–521
51. Priyatharishini PSNC, Saraswathy NC, Smila KH, Yuvaraj D, Chandran M, Vivek P (2014) Green synthesis of gold nano particles from Cassia auriculata leaf aqueous extract and its cytotoxicity effect on in vitro cell line. Int J ChemTech Res 6(9):4241–4250
52. Raza A, Li F, Xu X, Tang J (2017) Optimization of ultrasonic-assisted extraction of antioxidant polysaccharides from the stem of Trapa quadrispinosa using response surface methodology. Int J Biol Macromol 94:335–344. https://doi.org/10.1016/j.ijbiomac.2016.10.033
53. Reddy M, Rao VR, Chaitanya KN, Khed VC (2021) Optimization of bentocrete parameters using response surface methodology (RSM). AIMS Mater Sci 8(2). https://doi.org/10.3934/matersci.2021015
54. Roy R, Mostofa MG, Wang J, Sikdar A, Sarker T (2020) Improvement of growth performance of Amorpha fruticosa under contrasting regime of water and fertilizer in coal-contaminated spoils using response surface methodology. BMC Plant Biol 20:1–15. https://doi.org/10.1186/s12870-020-02397-1
55. Samaram S, Mirhosseini H, Tan CP, Ghazali HM, Bordbar S, Serjouie A (2015) Optimisation of ultrasound-assisted extraction of oil from papaya seed by response surface methodology: oil recovery, radical scavenging antioxidant activity, and oxidation stability. Food Chem 172:7–17. https://doi.org/10.1016/j.foodchem.2014.08.068
56. Sarli S, Ghasemi N (2020) Optimization of biosynthesized Zn nanoparticles by poisonous Taxus baccata leaves extract and evaluation of their effect on the bacterias and MCF-7 cancer cells. Eurasian Chem Commun 2:302–318
57. Sharmila G, Fathima MF, Haries S, Geetha S, Kumar NM, Muthukumaran C (2017) Green synthesis, characterization and antibacterial efficacy of palladium nanoparticles synthesized using Filicium decipiens leaf extract. J Mol Struct 1138:35–40
58. Singh A, Singh NB, Hussain I, Singh H, Singh SC (2015) Plant nanoparticle interaction: an approach to improve agricultural practices and plant productivity. Int J Pharm Sci Inven 4:25–40

59. Taguchi G (1986) Introduction to quality engineering: designing quality into products and processes. The Asian Productivity Organization, Tokyo. http://worldcat.org/isbn/9283310845
60. Vijayaraghavan K, Nalini SK, Prakash NU, Madhankumar D (2012) One step green synthesis of silver nano/microparticles using extracts of Trachyspermum ammi and Papaver somniferum. Colloids Surf B: Biointerfaces 94:114–117
61. Vimala RTV, Sathishkumar G, Sivaramakrishnan S (2015) Optimization of reaction conditions to fabricate nano-silver using Couroupita guianensis Aubl.(leaf & fruit) and its enhanced larvicidal effect. Spectrochim Acta Part A Mol Biomol Spectrosc 135:110–115
62. Wang T, Jin X, Chen Z, Megharaj M, Naidu R (2014) Green synthesis of Fe nanoparticles using eucalyptus leaf extracts for treatment of eutrophic wastewater. Sci Total Environ 466:210–213
63. Ying S, Guan Z, Ofoegbu PC, Clubb P, Rico C, He F, Hong J (2022) Green synthesis of nanoparticles: current developments and limitations. Environ Technol Innov 26:102336
64. Yolmeh M, Jafari SM (2017) Applications of response surface methodology in the food industry processes. Food Bioprocess Technol 10(3):413–433. https://doi.org/10.1007/s11947-016-1855-2
65. Yıldız N, Kapucu H, Çalımlı A (2000) Response surface optimization of the phenol adsorption onto HDTMA-bentonite. Rev Chem Eng 16(1):55–70. https://doi.org/10.1515/REVCE.2000.16.1.55

MIX
Papier aus verantwortungsvollen Quellen
Paper from responsible sources
FSC® C105338

If you have any concerns about our products,
you can contact us on
**ProductSafety@springernature.com**

In case Publisher is established outside the EU,
the EU authorized representative is:
**Springer Nature Customer Service Center GmbH**
**Europaplatz 3, 69115 Heidelberg, Germany**

Printed by Libri Plureos GmbH
in Hamburg, Germany